Atlas of EEG in Critical Care

Atlas of EEG in Critical Care

Lawrence J. Hirsch, MD

Comprehensive Epilepsy Center, Neurological Institute, Columbia University, New York, New York, U.S.A.

Richard P. Brenner, MD

Department of Neurology, University of Pittsburgh School of Medicine, Pittsburgh, Pennsylvania, U.S.A.

WILEY-BLACKWELL

A John Wiley & Sons, Ltd, Publication

Wiley-Blackwell is an imprint of John Wiley & Sons, formed by the merger of Wiley's global Scientific, Technical and Medical business with Blackwell Publishing.

Registered office: John Wiley & Sons Ltd, The Atrium, Southern Gate, Chichester, West Sussex, PO19 8SQ, UK

Other Editorial Offices:
9600 Garsington Road, Oxford, OX4 2DQ, UK
111 River Street, Hoboken, NJ 07030-5774, USA

For details of our global editorial offices, for customer services and for information about how to apply for permission to reuse the copyright material in this book please see our website at www.wiley.com/wiley-blackwell

Library of Congress Cataloging-in-Publication Data

Atlas of EEG in critical care / edited by Lawrence J. Hirsch, Richard P. Brenner.
p. ; cm.
Includes bibliographical references.
ISBN 978-0-4709-8786-5 (cloth : alk. paper) 1. Electroencephalography—Atlases. 2. Critical care medicine—Atlases. I. Hirsch, Lawrence J. II. Brenner, Richard P.
[DNLM: 1. Electroencephalography—methods—Atlases. 2. Critical Care—Atlases. 3. Intensive Care—Atlases. WL 17 A8825 2009]
RC386.6.E43A85 2009
616.8′047547—dc22

2009021619

ISBN 978-0-4709-8786-5

British Library Cataloguing in Publication Data

A catalogue record for this book is available from the British Library

Typeset in 11.25/14 pt Times by Aptara, New Delhi, India
Printed and bound in Malaysia by Vivar Printing Sdn Bhd
First impression 2010

Dr Brenner dedicates this atlas to his wife Elizabeth and his children, Jennifer Brenner Moel, Alex Brenner and Dr Daniel Brenner.

Dr Hirsch dedicates this atlas to his wife Gaetane and his two boys, Calvin and Toby.

Both authors thank their families for putting up with the many hours of work, including at odd hours, required to complete this.

Contents

Preface ix

List of contributors xi

1 EEG basics **1**
- 1.1 Electrode nomenclature, polarity and referential vs. bipolar montages 1
- 1.2 Normal EEG: awake and asleep 4
- Suggested reading 6
- Figures 1.0–1.12 7

2 EEG in encephalopathy **39**
- 2.1 Nonspecific patterns of encephalopathy 39
- 2.2 Patterns suggesting specific diagnoses 39
- 2.3 Findings in specific clinical scenarios 40
- 2.4 Medication effects 40
- Suggested reading 41
- Figures 2.1–2.35 43

3 Seizures and status epilepticus **89**
- Suggested reading 89
- Figures 3.1–3.10 91

4 Periodic discharges and other controversial EEG patterns **129**
- 4.1 PLEDs, BIPLEDs, GPEDs and triphasic waves 129
- 4.2 SIRPIDs 130
- 4.3 Standardized nomenclature 130
- Suggested reading 130
- Figures 4.1–4.18 132

5 EEG in cerebrovascular disease **161**
- 5.1 Ischemia 161
- 5.2 Hemorrhage 161
- Suggested reading 162
- Figures 5.1–5.18 163

6 Artifacts that can mimic seizures or other physiologic patterns **187**
- Suggested reading 190
- Figures 6.1–6.20 191

7 Prolonged EEG monitoring and quantitative EEG techniques for detecting seizures and ischemia **217**
- Suggested reading 219
- Figures 7.1–7.10 Quantitative EEG (QEEG) basics 222
- Figures 7.11–7.17 Basics of seizure detection 240
- Figures 7.18–7.21 Cyclic seizures and PLEDs 250
- Figures 7.22–7.25 Other QEEG techniques and uses in patients with seizures 256
- Figures 7.26–7.31 Detecting other (non-seizure) events 262
- Figures 7.32–7.35 Long-term trends 272
- Figures 7.36–7.46 ICU artifacts 276
- Figures 7.47–7.48 Spreading depression/peri-injury depolarizations 288
- Figures 7.49–7.54 Multimodality monitoring and intracranial EEG in the ICU 290

8 Evoked and event-related potentials in the ICU **299**
8.1 Median nerve somatosensory evoked potentials 301
8.2 Brainstem auditory evoked potentials 303
8.3 Flash visual evoked potentials 308
8.4 Event-related potentials 308
Suggested reading 312

Appendix ACNS Standardized EEG Research Terminology and Categorization for the investigation of rhythmic and periodic patterns encountered in critically ill patients: July 2009 version **315**

Index **329**

Preface

Synopsis

As the population ages, technology improves, intensive care medicine expands and neurocritical care advances, the use of EEG monitoring in the critically ill is gaining an increasingly important role. Neurologists and intensivists need to become familiar with the use of routine brain monitoring with EEG, or 'neurotelemetry', as they have with routine cardiovascular monitoring. This atlas begins with a section on the basics of EEG interpretation geared towards someone with minimal, if any, EEG experience. It then demonstrates EEG patterns seen in encephalopathy – both nonspecific and specific, nonconvulsive seizures, status epilepticus, periodic EEG patterns and controversial patterns on the ictal-interictal continuum in a variety of clinical settings. Confusing artifacts, including ones that are often misinterpreted or that mimic seizures, are also shown and explained. EEG findings are highlighted and labeled in detail within the tracings themselves. The new proposed American Clinical Neurophysiology Society standardized nomenclature for these patterns is included.

After the major section on EEG patterns from both a basic and advanced viewpoint, there is an extensive color section on prolonged continuous digital EEG monitoring, including quantitative EEG techniques to aid in the interpretation of prolonged EEGs, such as compressed spectral array. These techniques can facilitate the efficient recognition of seizures, ischemia and other neurological events, and can help visualize long-term trends. Examples of multimodality brain monitoring in neurocritical care patients are also included. Finally, there is a section on evoked potentials and their applications in critical care, including using these for prognostication in coma.

Who should use this atlas?

This atlas is geared towards all healthcare professionals involved in critical care medicine, including practitioners, fellows, residents, technologists, physician assistants, nurse practitioners and researchers. Although it may be of particular interest to those in neurology, epilepsy and clinical neurophysiology, it is also appropriate for intensivists with an interest in maintaining brain health during critical illness of any etiology. It covers the basics as well as advanced material.

Acknowledgments

Dr Hirsch would like to thank those who have helped develop and maintain the continuous EEG monitoring program, both clinical and research aspects, at Columbia University Medical Center for the past 8 years, with special thanks to Ronald G. Emerson, Lewis L. Kull, Stephan Mayer, Jan Claassen and the Columbia Epilepsy/EEG fellows. Thanks to Bin Tu, the EEG technologists, and to the neurological ICU nurses, nurse practitioners, residents, fellows and attendings for caring for these patients so diligently and for helping to use this technology to its fullest potential, both in the past and in the future.

Dr Brenner would like to thank those neurologists, EEG technologists, neurophysiology fellows and neurology residents at the University of Pittsburgh Medical Center who have helped over many years in this endeavor. Special thanks to Drs Mark L. Scheuer and Anne C. Van Cott, and EEG technologists Susan Burkett and Cheryl Plummer. The authors would also like to thank those at Persyst Development Corporation (Prescott, AZ) for their digital and quantitative EEG software development used to prepare most of the images in this atlas, for addressing our never-ending requests for improvements, and for expert technical assistance for the past several years.

Lawrence J. Hirsch, MD and **Richard P. Brenner, MD**

List of contributors

Authors

Lawrence J. Hirsch, MD
Comprehensive Epilepsy Center, Neurological Institute, Columbia University, Box NI-135, 710 W. 168th St. New York 10032, NY, USA

Richard P. Brenner, MD
Department of Neurology, University of Pittsburgh School of Medicine, Kaufmann Medical Building, 3471 Fifth Avenue, Suite 810 Pittsburgh, PA 15213, USA

Contributors

G. Bryan Young, MD
Department of Clinical Neurological Sciences, London Health Sciences Centre, 339 Windermere Road, London, Ontario, Canada N6A 5A5

David Houlden, MD
Sunnybrook Health Sciences Centre and Department of Surgery, University of Toronto, Toronto, Ontario, Canada

1 EEG basics

1.1 Electrode nomenclature, polarity and referential vs. bipolar montages

Electroencephalography (EEG) is a technique that measures the spatial distribution of voltage fields on the scalp and their variation over time. The origin of this activity is thought to be due to the fluctuating sum of excitatory and inhibitory postsynaptic potentials. These potentials arise primarily from apical dendrites of pyramidal cells in the outer (superficial) layer of the cerebral cortex and are modified by input from subcortical structures, particularly the thalamus and ascending projections of the ascending reticular activating system. Structures in the thalamus serve as a 'pacemaker'. This produces widespread synchronization and rhythmicity of cortical activity over cerebral hemispheres.

The dendritic generators are vertically oriented and have two poles, one relatively negative and the other relatively positive. This is termed a dipole. Dipoles are sources of electrical current consisting of two charges of opposite polarity separated by relatively small distances. Since cerebral potentials are produced by dendritic generators radially oriented to the surface, a scalp electrode usually detects only one end of the generator at one point in time. In general, approximately $10\,\text{cm}^2$ of cortex needs to be discharging synchronously for the signal to be appreciated on scalp EEG.

The hardware necessary to record the EEG employs differential amplifiers. Each amplifier records the potential difference between two scalp electrodes (the electrode pair is referred to as a derivation or channel). Each amplifier has two inputs connected to scalp electrodes. By convention, when input 1 (historically referred to as grid 1 or G1) is relatively negative compared to input 2 (grid 2 or G2), there is an upward deflection; when input 1 is relatively more positive than input 2, there is a downward deflection. It is the relationship between the two inputs that determines the direction and amplitude, and not the absolute values. Simply put, the tracing at each channel (derivation) displays G1 minus G2, with negative values causing upward deflections. Table 1.1 shows some examples to help further demonstrate these principles.

In the following four examples the inputs are switched (Table 1.2).

As can be seen from both tables, there are no 'positive' or 'negative' deflections, there are only upward or downward deflections. When there is no deflection, inputs are equipotential and are either equally active or inactive.

When looking at only a single derivation (a one-channel recording of the potential difference between an electrode pair), one can only state the relationship of input 1 to input 2, i.e. it is either more or less negative or positive. However, it is not possible to localize cerebral activity or determine its polarity without further derivations/channels. Understanding polarity, as well as accurately assessing other factors such as the frequency of the activity being evaluated (cycles/second), its morphology, location, voltage, reactivity and symmetry in conjunction with the age and state of the patient are necessary for proper interpretation

Atlas of EEG in Critical Care Lawrence J. Hirsch and Richard P. Brenner

TABLE 1.1 Polarity

Input 1	Input 2	Difference	Deflection direction
+50	+20	+30	Down
+50	+50	0	—
+50	+70	−20	Up
+50	−50	+100	Down

of the EEG. In order to adequately represent the topography of the voltage, additional amplifiers and channels are needed for the sequential display of the EEG data, and this display of multiple channels is termed a montage. A montage refers to a collection of derivations for multiple channels recorded simultaneously and arranged in a specific order. Montages enable the technologist and electroencephalographer to systematically visualize the field of electrical activity of the brain.

Electrodes are applied to the scalp in accordance with the International 10-20 System (Figure 1.0). Different regions of the brain are identified as Fp (frontopolar), F (frontal), C (central), P (parietal), O (occipital) and T (temporal). Odd numbers refer to the left side, even to the right, and Z to midline placements. 'A' signifies an ear channel (A1 for left ear, A2 for right). Electrode placement has been standardized with this system, with electrode sites determined by anatomical skull landmarks. Technologists measure the distance from the nasion to the inion and the head circumference, marking precise electrode locations based on 10% or 20% intervals of those distances, hence the name '10-20'.

Montages may be viewed as software that enhances the use of the EEG machine (hardware) to function as a form of brain imaging. There are two basic types of montages: bipolar and referential. These two recording methods can be compared to techniques used to determine altitude at different points on a mountain. The referential type of recording (formerly incorrectly termed 'monopolar') is comparable to measuring the elevation with reference to a particular point, either on land or at sea level. Bipolar sequential recording is similar to measuring the difference of elevation between nearby points, going serially in a particular direction. Another analogy that has been used to describe the electrical potential field on the scalp is that of the surface of the sea. In this example, a number of buoys (the electrodes) float on the sea's surface with varying vertical displacements representing fluctuations of electrical potential.

TABLE 1.2 Polarity with inputs switched

Input 1	Input 2	Difference	Deflection direction
+20	+50	−30	Up
+50	+50	0	—
+70	+50	+20	Down
−50	+50	−100	Up

With a bipolar sequential recording, scalp electrodes are linked in straight lines (either anterior–posterior or transverse) and each channel records the difference in potential between electrode pairs. In a referential montage, any electrode may be used as the reference point with respect to which the potentials of the other electrodes can be measured. In this type of recording, scalp electrodes are combined to one or two common reference sites, often ear(s), the vertex (Cz) or an average of all electrodes (termed a 'common average reference'). Again, an amplifier records the difference between electrode pairs in separate channels; in a referential recording, the second input (G2) is always the reference.

Some advantages and disadvantages of each type of recording are described below.

Short distance bipolar recording

Advantages

(1) Value of phase reversal in localization, particularly when this occurs at the same electrode in two montages run at right angles to each other. Phase reversal in a sequential bipolar montage refers to the opposite simultaneous deflection of pens in channels that contain a common electrode. It is important to realize that a phase reversal does not imply normality or abnormality. This instrumental phase reversal usually, but not always, indicates that the potential field is maximal at or near the common electrode. To be certain that one has accurately defined the site of maximal involvement,

it is necessary to use an additional bipolar montage at right angles to the first, or a referential recording.

(2) Bipolar montages usually display local abnormalities well, since a phase reversal is often present. The exception occurs when the discharge is maximal at either the beginning or the end of the sequential chain.

(3) Can help resolve ambiguous findings on referential montages due to an active reference.

Disadvantages

(1) Amplitudes can be misleading; in any given channel higher amplitude indicates a greater potential difference, not necessarily the most active site, while low amplitude could be due to two electrodes being equally active and canceling or both electrodes being inactive.

(2) Diffuse potentials with relatively flat gradients are not detected well.

(3) Waveforms might be distorted and sham frequencies can be introduced.

Referential recording

Advantages

(1) Amplitude can be used to localize the site of maximal involvement if the reference is inactive. In referential recordings, when the reference is inactive (or is the least active electrode), the site of maximal involvement is identified as the one having the greatest voltage (i.e. the greatest amplitude of deflection).

(2) Little distortion of frequency or waveforms.

(3) Diffuse patterns with flat gradients can be detected. In contrast to focal abnormalities, diffuse discharges are frequently better appreciated on referential montages, particularly when there is a flat gradient.

(4) Can help resolve difficulties in bipolar recordings due to equipotential areas, horizontal dipoles or unevenly sloping gradients.

Disadvantages

(1) The reference electrode may not be inactive or be the least active electrode – it may be very active. When the reference electrode is active, because it is located near the peak of the potential being studied, interpretation can be more difficult. A major problem with the use of referential montages is that it is often difficult to use an inactive reference or to realize that the reference is active.

A reference may be active because of artifact or it may be within the cerebral field under study. With an active reference there often appears to be a 'phase reversal' on a referential montage, i.e. some electrodes are more negative than the reference, while others are more positive. One has to look at relative polarity, as well as amplitude, to decide which is the most active site. For those electrodes that are more active than the reference, the greatest amplitude indicates the site of maximal involvement. In contrast, for sites less active than the reference, the largest amplitude indicates the least active area. The deflection of the maximal and minimal sites will be in opposite directions. When the reference is the most active site, deflections in all channels are in the same direction, i.e. there is no phase reversal. Furthermore, the largest amplitudes occur at those sites that are the least active. This type of situation can be confusing, since one cannot be sure if the reference is uninvolved or is the most active of all scalp electrodes.

(2) Greater problem with artifact – depends on the reference employed. No single reference electrode is ideal for all situations. The ear electrodes frequently are contaminated by temporal lobe spikes as well as electrocardiogram (EKG) and/or muscle artifact. The Cz electrode, which is often a very good choice in helping to display focal temporal abnormalities, is very active during sleep.

Other midline reference electrodes, such as Fz or Pz, also have limitations: during wakefulness Fz is in the field of vertical eye movements, while Pz is usually in the field of the posterior dominant 'alpha' rhythm field (see section below on alpha rhythm); thus these references are often active.

It should be realized that if the same electrodes are used on a bipolar and referential montage then the montages will contain equivalent information, i.e. although the arrangement may differ, the pieces are the same. The two types of montages, bipolar and referential, should be employed in recording the EEG, as each has its own advantages and disadvantages. *Often, utilizing a different reference or a bipolar montage helps clarify localization problems.*

The American EEG Society has published suggestions for standard montages to be used in clinical EEG. The montages listed below are not intended for some purposes, such as neonatal EEG, all-night sleep recordings or for verification of electrocerebral inactivity. Three types of montages were suggested:

(1) longitudinal bipolar (LB) montage

(2) referential (R) montage (such as ipsilateral ear)

(3) transverse bipolar (TB) montage.

1.2 Normal EEG: awake and asleep

EEGs can be performed on patients of all ages, including neonates. There are marked maturational changes that occur in infancy and early childhood, while in adults between the ages of 20 and 60 years, the EEG is relatively stable. Further fairly subtle changes occur in the elderly. Thus in different age groups different patterns characterize wakefulness, drowsiness and sleep.

The normal adult EEG contains a number of different background rhythms and frequencies. These include alpha, beta, delta, mu, theta and normal sleep activity (such as V-waves, spindles, K complexes and positive occipital sharp transients of sleep (POSTS)). EEG activity is conventionally divided into the following frequencies (number of waveforms/s or hertz (Hz)):

Delta – refers to frequencies below 4 Hz. Delta activity, which is the slowest waveform, is normal when present in adults during sleep. In normal elderly subjects, delta activity is sometimes seen in the temporal regions during wakefulness, and in a generalized distribution, maximal anteriorly, during drowsiness. It is usually abnormal under other circumstances.

Theta – ranges from 4 Hz to less than 8 Hz. It is often present diffusely in children and young adults during wakefulness, whereas in adults it occurs predominantly during drowsiness. Like delta activity, theta activity may occur in the temporal regions in normal elderly adults during wakefulness.

Alpha – ranges from 8 to 13 Hz.

Beta – above 13 Hz. This activity is usually most prominent anteriorly and is often increased during drowsiness and in patients receiving sedating medication, particularly barbiturates or benzodiazepines.

In the analysis of the EEG the following need to be evaluated:

(1) frequency

(2) voltage

(3) location

(4) morphology

(5) polarity

(6) state

(7) reactivity

(8) symmetry

(9) artifact.

An important feature of the EEG is the frequency of the *alpha rhythm*, also known as the posterior dominant rhythm. During wakefulness, the alpha rhythm is present over posterior regions of the head, maximal with the subject relaxed and eyes closed. It attenuates with eye opening. Its frequency ranges from 8 to 13 Hz in adults and is typically sinusoidal. Some normal individuals do not have an alpha rhythm during wakefulness. By itself, this is not abnormal. There is often an asymmetry of the alpha rhythm with the right side being of higher voltage. A consistent asymmetry of the alpha rhythm of 50% or more (expressed as a percentage of the higher side) is considered abnormal. Since the right is often slightly higher in voltage, an asymmetry of 35–50% may be significant and considered abnormal when the right is the lower amplitude side. Focal slowing of the alpha rhythm unilaterally is rare and a difference of 1 Hz or greater is significant. An asymmetry of reactivity or frequency is a better indicator of a focal abnormality than is a voltage asymmetry.

The *mu rhythm* (7–11 Hz) is present in some normal individuals in wakefulness and drowsiness; it arises from the Rolandic cortex (primary sensorimotor cortex) at rest. It is often asynchronous and asymmetric, and can be unilateral. The mu rhythm attenuates with voluntary movement of the opposite side, such as clenching a fist, or even thinking about moving the opposite side.

A *breach rhythm* is a sharply contoured central or midtemporal pattern, often resembling a mu rhythm, that is seen with a skull defect, including a craniotomy or a burr hole. It can persist following bone replacement. It is composed of normal patterns that appear accentuated in sharpness and often in amplitude; faster frequencies are more 'enhanced' (higher amplitude and sharper appearing) than slower frequencies. It is sometimes misinterpreted as epileptiform.

Low-voltage beta activity is usually present in the normal EEG. Beta activity can show a mild (35%) asymmetry; however, a consistent asymmetry, particularly when associated with other findings, is a sensitive indicator of a cortical abnormality on the lower amplitude side, assuming that there is not an extra-axial collection on that side or a skull defect on the opposite side.

Theta and delta activity are classified as rhythmic (also known as monomorphic) or arrhythmic (polymorphic), intermittent or continuous, and regional (or focal) or generalized. Focal slowing (theta or delta), particularly when persistent and of delta frequency, is often associated with a structural lesion. Arrhythmic slowing is classically seen with lesions affecting white matter, whereas rhythmic slowing is more suggestive of subcortical (gray) dysfunction. Attenuation or loss of faster frequencies suggests cortical dysfunction or a collection between the cortex and the recording electrodes (including extracranial fluid).

Drowsiness: During drowsiness there is a decrease in frequency or persistence of the alpha rhythm, appearance of slow lateral eye movements, decrease in myogenic artifact and increase in beta frequencies.

Sleep is divided into non-REM and REM sleep. Non-REM sleep includes stages I and II and slow wave sleep (delta sleep, formerly stages III and IV).

Activities present during non-REM sleep include:

POSTS: Positive occipital sharp transients of sleep. These occur in light stages (I and II) of non-REM sleep.

Vertex (V) waves: Sharp potential, maximal at the vertex but with a field extending to bilateral fronto-central regions, surface negative, appears at the end of stage I non-REM sleep and persists in deeper sleep.

Sleep spindles: Usually paroxysmal, sinusoidal, low-medium amplitude 12–14 Hz activity lasting about a second and maximal in the vertex and fronto-central regions. Spindles (and K-complexes) mark the beginning of stage II non-REM sleep.

K complexes: High voltage, diphasic slow wave (duration at least 0.5 s) frequently associated with a sleep spindle. They are related to the arousal process, usually maximal at the vertex and can occur spontaneously or in response to sudden sensory stimuli.

Slow wave sleep: This is characterized by delta activity $\leq$2 Hz and >75 uV occupying at least 20% of the recording.

REM (rapid eye movement) sleep: The EEG is low voltage and there are rapid eye movements. Saw-toothed waves also occur in central regions.

Sleep spindles and V-waves can be affected by cerebral lesions. A persistent asymmetry in sleep usually indicates an abnormality on the side of the lower voltage. Focal delta activity during sleep may also be present.

Figure list

Figure 1.1 Alpha rhythm and blinks.

Figure 1.2 Alpha rhythm reactivity.

Figure 1.3 Mu rhythm and eye movements.

Figure 1.4 Mu rhythm.

Figure 1.5 Excess beta and active reference.

Figure 1.6 Lambda waves.

Figure 1.7 Slow lateral eye movements of drowsiness.

Figure 1.8 Positive occipital sharp transients of sleep (POSTS).

Figure 1.9 Vertex waves and sleep spindles.

Figure 1.10 K-complexes and POSTS.

Figure 1.11 Rapid eye movement (REM) sleep.

Figure 1.12 Focal slowing.

Suggested reading

American Electroencephalographic Society (1994) Guidelines in EEG, Number 7. *Journal of Clinical Neurophysiology* **11**, 30–36.

Burgess, R.C., Iwasaki, M. and Nair, D. (2006) Localization and field determination in electroencephalography and magnetoencehalography. In: Wyllie, E., Gupta, A. and Lachhwani, D.K. (eds), *The Treatment of Epilepsy. Principles and Practice*, pp. 141–168. Lippincott, Williams and Wilkins, Philadelphia.

Connolly, M.B., Sharbrough, F.W. and Wong, P.K.H. (2003) Electrical fields and recording techniques. In: Ebersole, J.S. and Pedley, T.A. (eds), *Current Practice of Clinical Electroencephalography*, pp. 72–99. Lippincott, Williams and Wilkins, Philadelphia.

Erwin, C.W., Sommerville, E.R. and Radtke, R.A. (1984) A review of electroencephalographic features of normal sleep. *Journal of Clinical Neurophysiology* **1**, 253–274.

Gloor, P. (1971) Recording principles. Volume conductor theory. *Spike and Wave*. **2**, 1–48.

Klem, G.H. (2003) *Artifacts*. In: Ebersole, J.S. and Pedley, T.A. (eds), *Current Practice of Clinical Electroencephalography*, pp. 271–287. Lippincott, Williams and Wilkins, Philadelphia.

Knott, J.R. (1969) Electrode montages revisited: How to tell up from down. *American Journal of EEG Technology* **9**, 33–45.

Kozelka, J.W. and Pedley, T.A. (1990) Beta and mu rhythms. *Journal of Clinical Neurophysiology* **7**, 191–208.

Lesser, R.P., Luders, H., Dinner, D.S. *et al.* (1985) An introduction to the basic concepts of polarity and localization. *Journal of Clinical Neurophysiology* **2**, 45–61.

Markand, O.N. (1990) Alpha rhythms. *Journal of Clinical Neurophysiology* **7**, 163–189.

Niedemeyer, E. (2005) *The normal EEG of the waking adult*. In: Niedermeyer, E. and Lopes de Silva, F. (eds), *Electroencephalography: Basic principles, clinical applications and related fields*, pp. 161–166. Lippincott, Williams and Wilkins, Philadelphia.

Niedemeyer, E. (2005) *Sleep and EEG*. In: Niedermeyer, E. and Lopes de Silva, F. (eds), *Electroencephalography: Basic principles, clinical applications and related fields*, pp. 193–207. Lippincott, Williams and Wilkins, Philadelphia.

Tao, J.X., Baldwin, M., Hawes-Ebersole, S. *et al.* (2007) Cortical substrates of scalp EEG epileptiform discharges. *Journal of Clinical Neurophysiology* **24**, 96–100.

Tatum, W.O. 4th, Husain, A.M., Benbadis, S.R. *et al.* (2006) Normal adult EEG and patterns of uncertain significance. *Journal of Clinical Neurophysiology* **23**, 194–207.

Tyner, F.S., Knott, J.R. and Mayer, W.B. Jr. (1983) *Artifacts*. In: *Fundamentals of EEG Technology*, Volume **1**, pp. 280–311. Raven Press, New York.

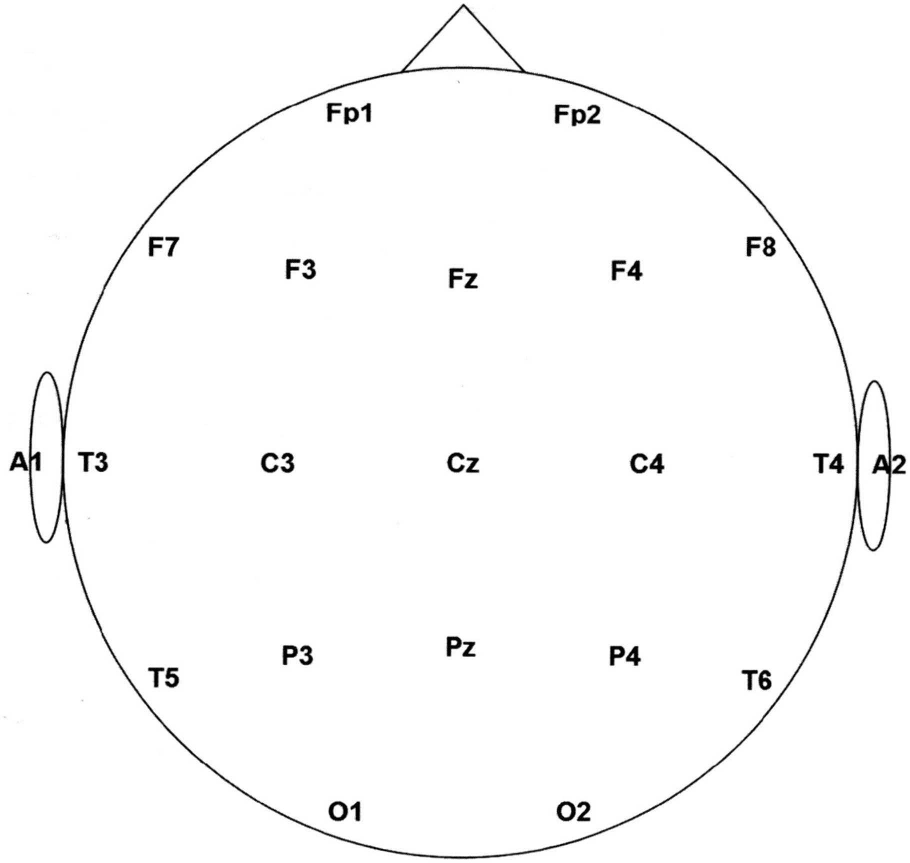

Figure 1.0 International 10–20 system.

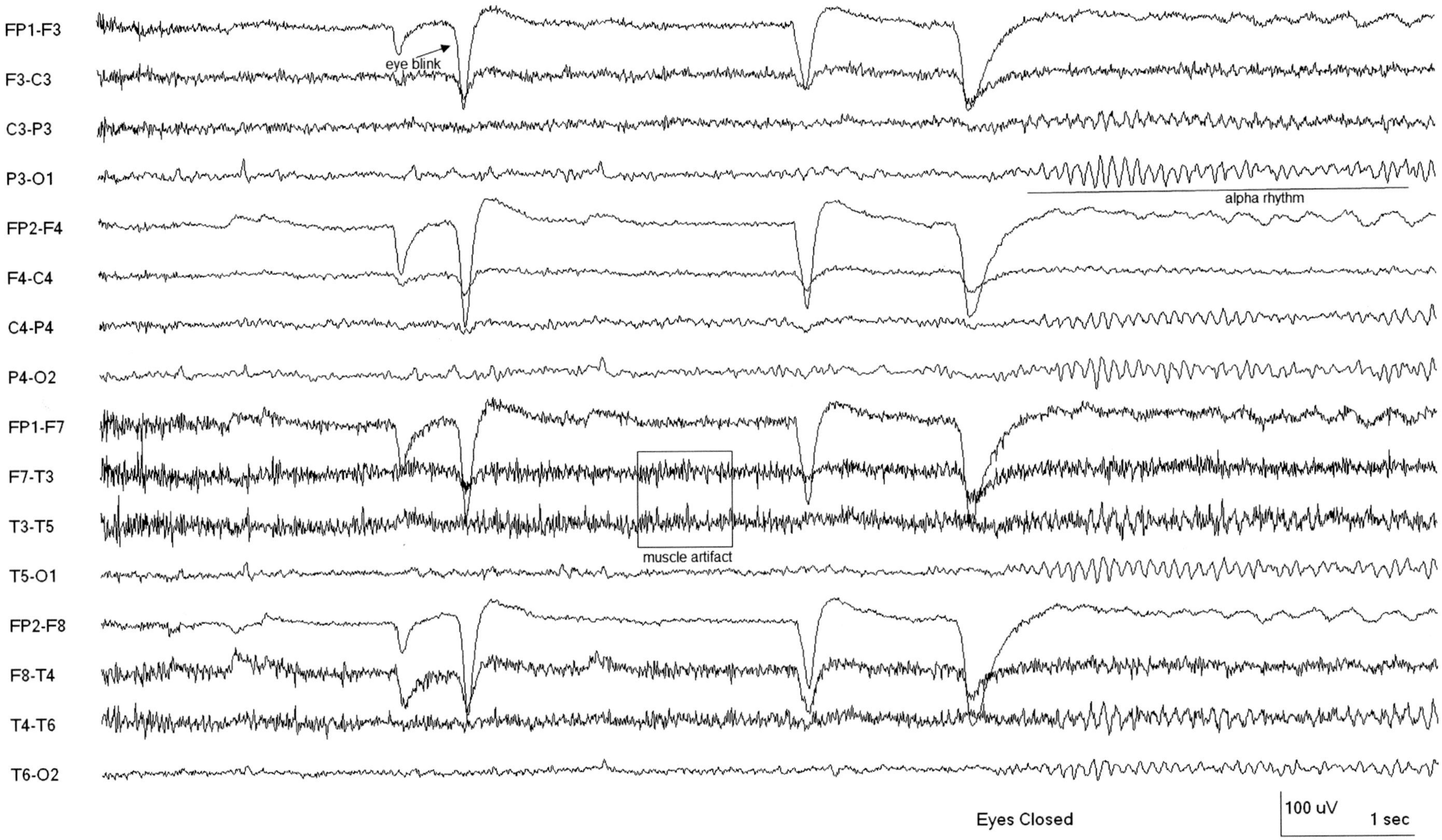

Figure 1.1 Alpha rhythm and blinks. (a) Following eye closure, rhythmic activity of 10 Hz is present posteriorly. This represents a normal alpha rhythm (sometimes referred to as the posterior dominant rhythm). The activity is maximal in O1 and O2 electrodes and seen to a lesser extent in parietal (P3/P4) and posterior temporal (T5/T6) regions.

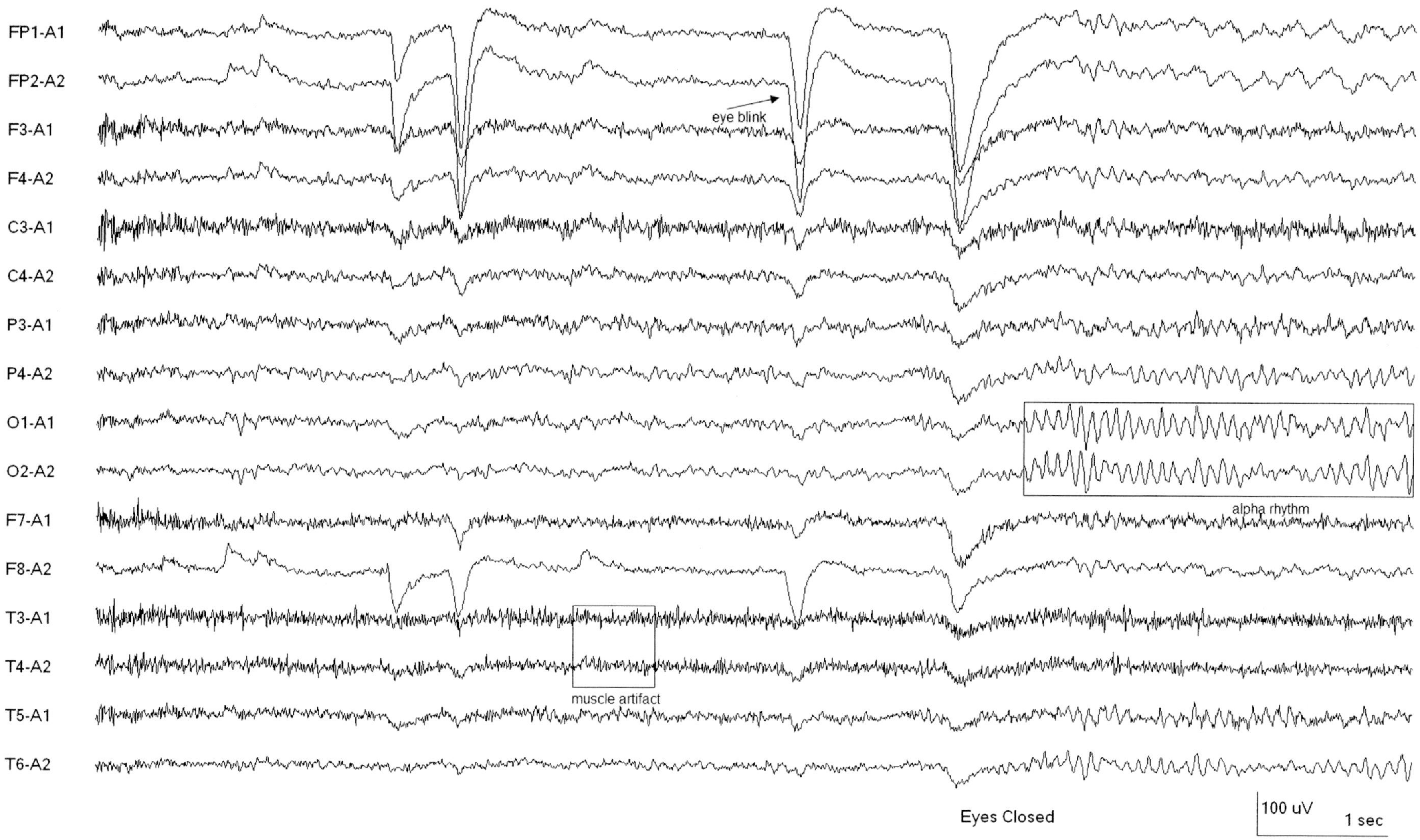

Figure 1.1 (*Continued*) (b) The same epoch in a referential montage, with ipsilateral ear reference. Blinks appear as prominent deflections on the EEG because the eye is a dipole, with the cornea being surface positive and the retina surface negative. During blinks the eyes go upward (Bell's phenomenon). This causes Fp1 and Fp2 electrodes to become relatively positive and there is a downgoing deflection in Fp1 and Fp2 channels. The opposite occurs if there is a downward movement of the eyes. Further monitoring of eye movements, utilizing electrodes inferior to orbits, is demonstrated in Figure 2.5c.

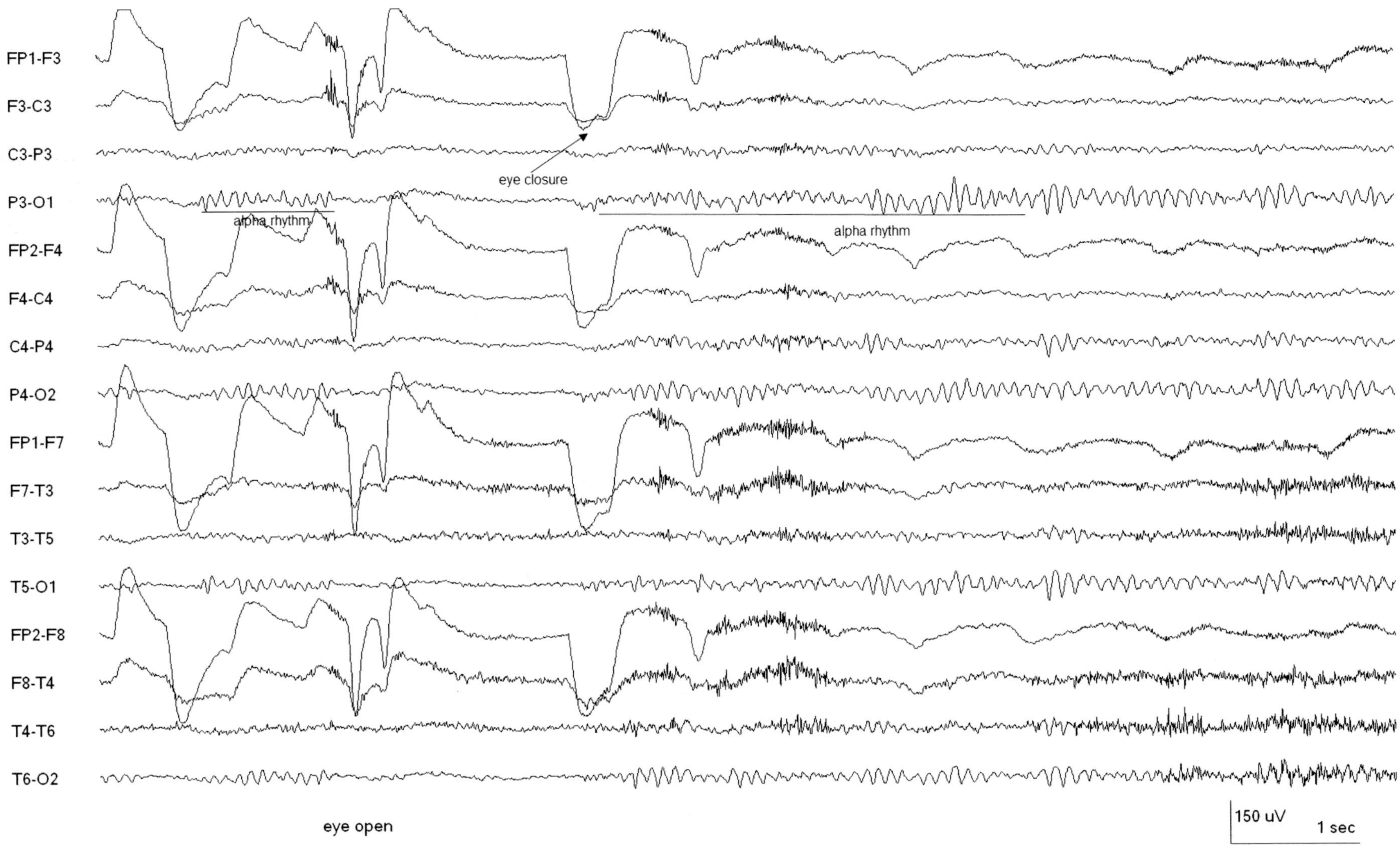

Figure 1.2 Alpha rhythm reactivity. Attenuation of the alpha rhythm following eye opening in a 72-year-old man. The alpha rhythm returns following eye closure, best seen in channels containing O1 and O2.

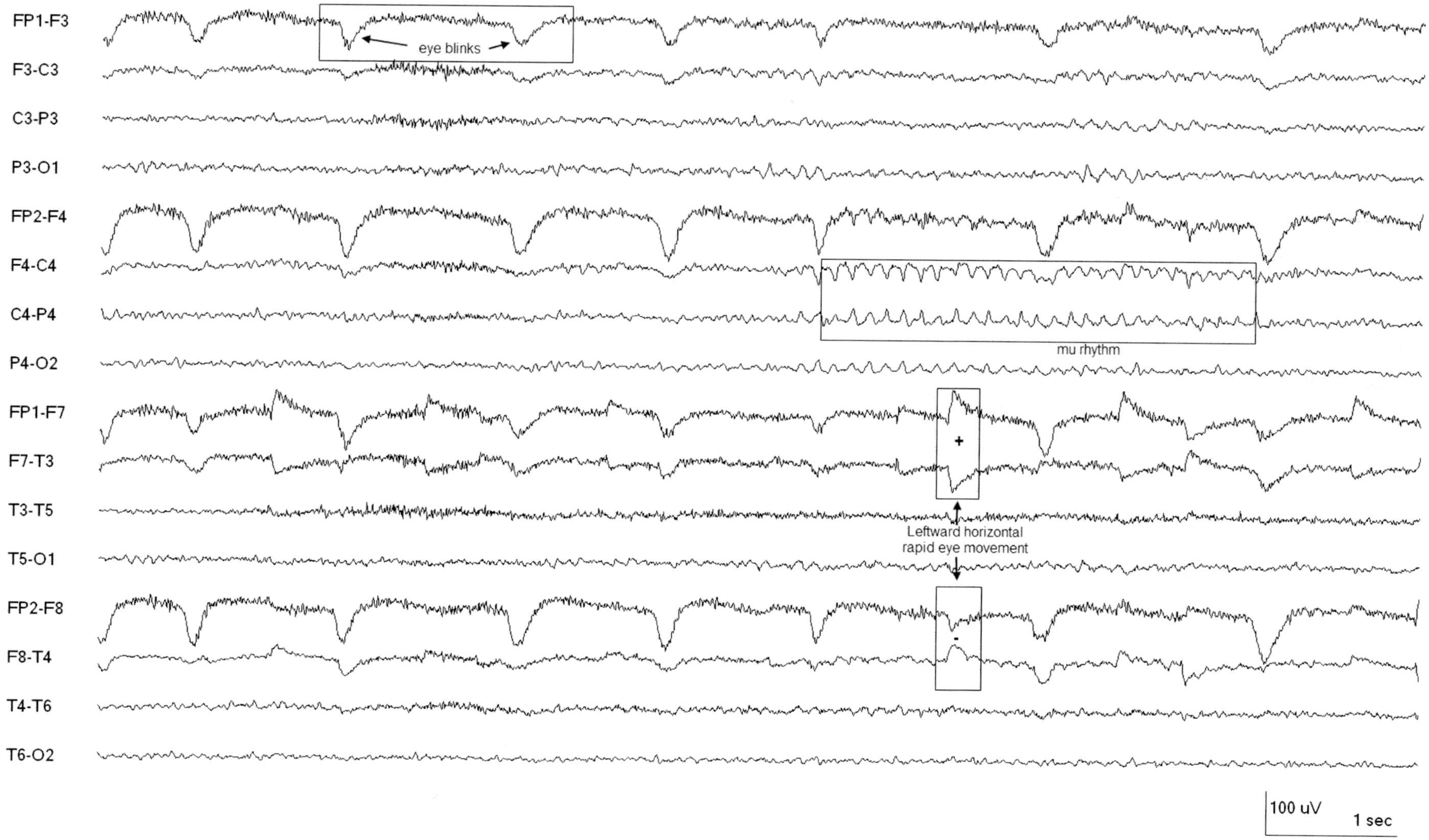

Figure 1.3 Mu rhythm and eye movements. (a) A mu rhythm prominent in the right parasagittal region in a 45-year-old man. The spike-like component is surface negative and maximal at electrode C4, as demonstrated by the phase reversal on this bipolar montage. This morphology, containing a sharp negative component alternating with a blunt positive component, as seen in F4-C4 and C4-P4, resembles the Greek letter mu giving this rhythm its name. There is also a typical leftward horizontal eye movement shown with a positivity at F7 (due to the cornea moving towards F7; deflections moving away from each other on bipolar) and negativity at F8 (deflections moving towards each other on bipolar).

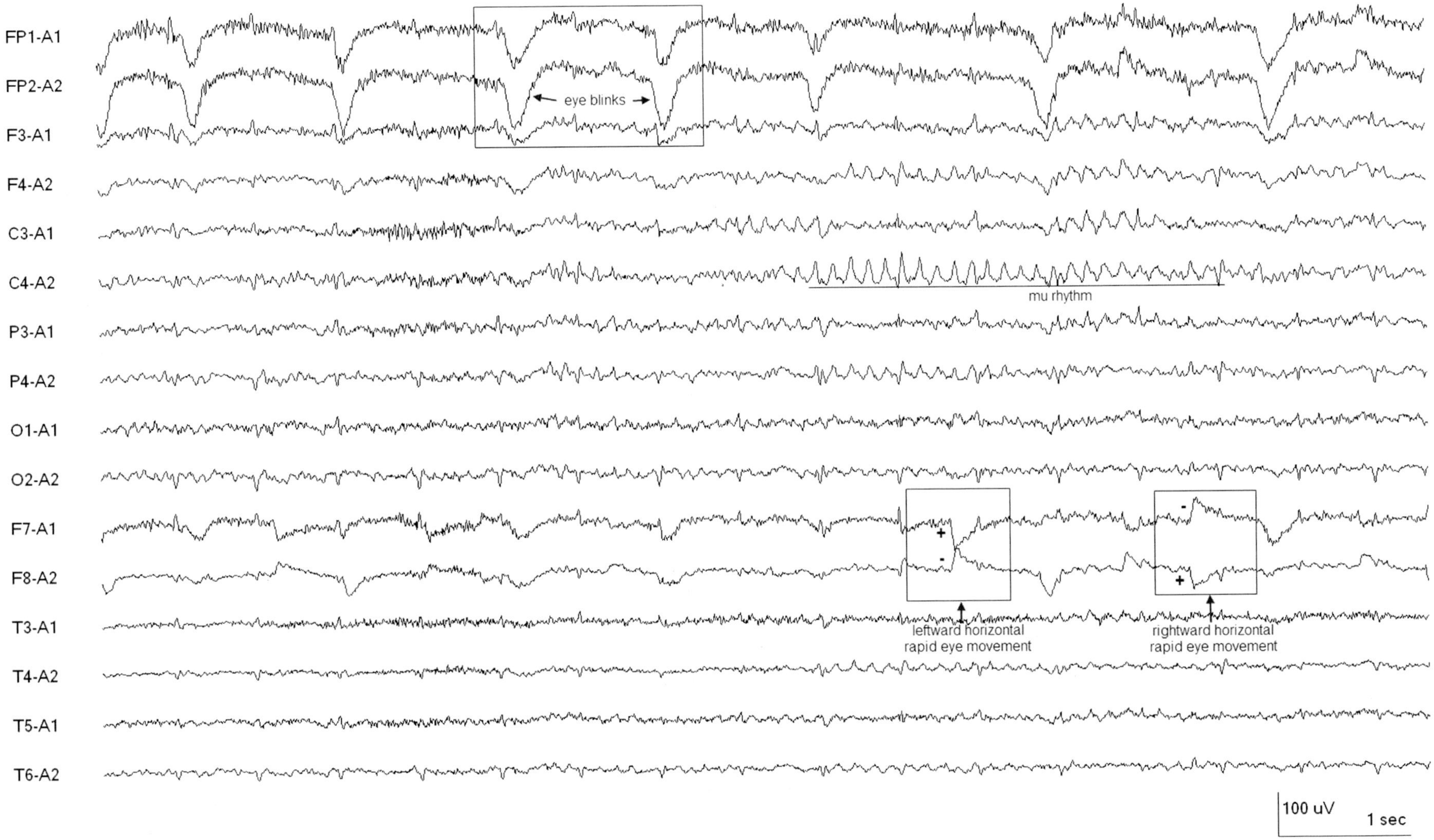

Figure 1.3 (*Continued*) (b) In this reformatted referential montage to ipsilateral ears, the same mu rhythm as seen in Figure 1.4 is best seen in the C4-A2 derivation, confirming that the maximum discharge is at C4 (electrode with the greatest amplitude on a referential recording, assuming an inactive reference). The spike-like component is upgoing indicating that C4 (input 1) is more negative than A2. Leftward (positivity at F7) and rightward (positivity at F8) rapid eye movements are shown as well.

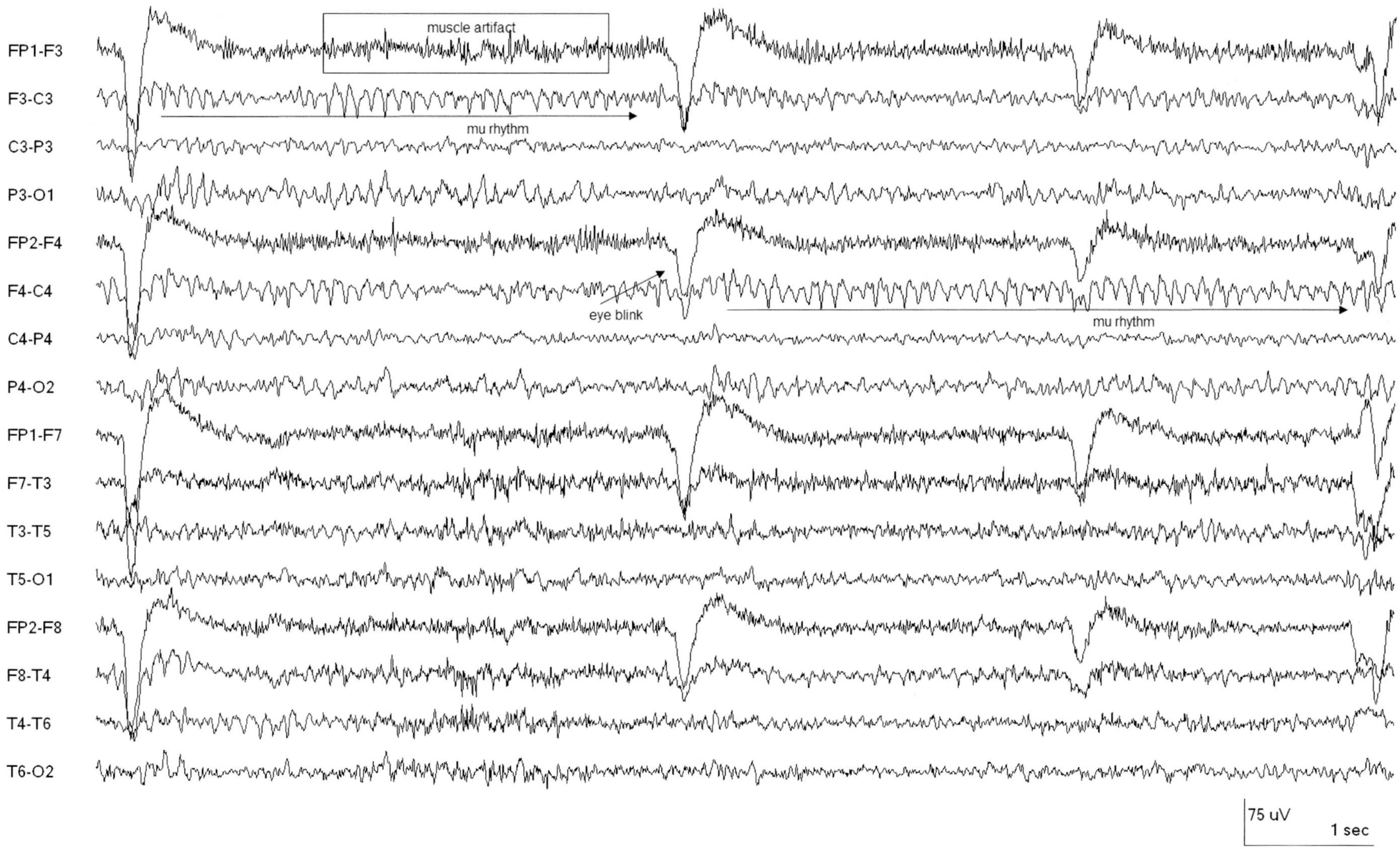

Figure 1.4 Mu rhythm. Rhythmic activity of 9 Hz is present, particularly in the F3-C3 followed by F4-C4 derivations. This is a normal mu rhythm. Unlike the alpha rhythm, mu can often occur asynchronously, as in this example.

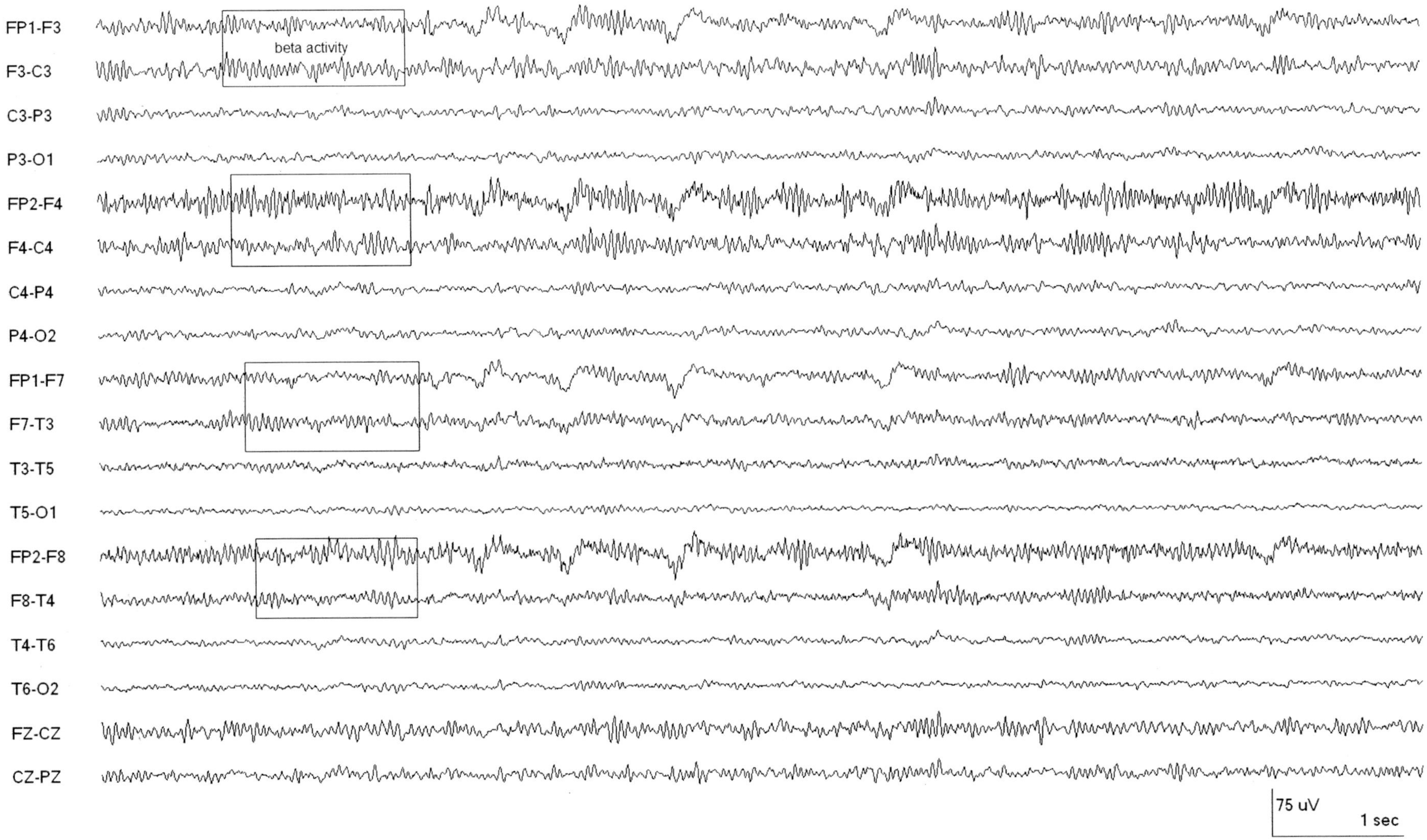

Figure 1.5 Excess beta and active reference. (a) The EEG in this 18-year-old man shows an excessive amount of beta activity anteriorly. The patient was receiving benzodiazepines.

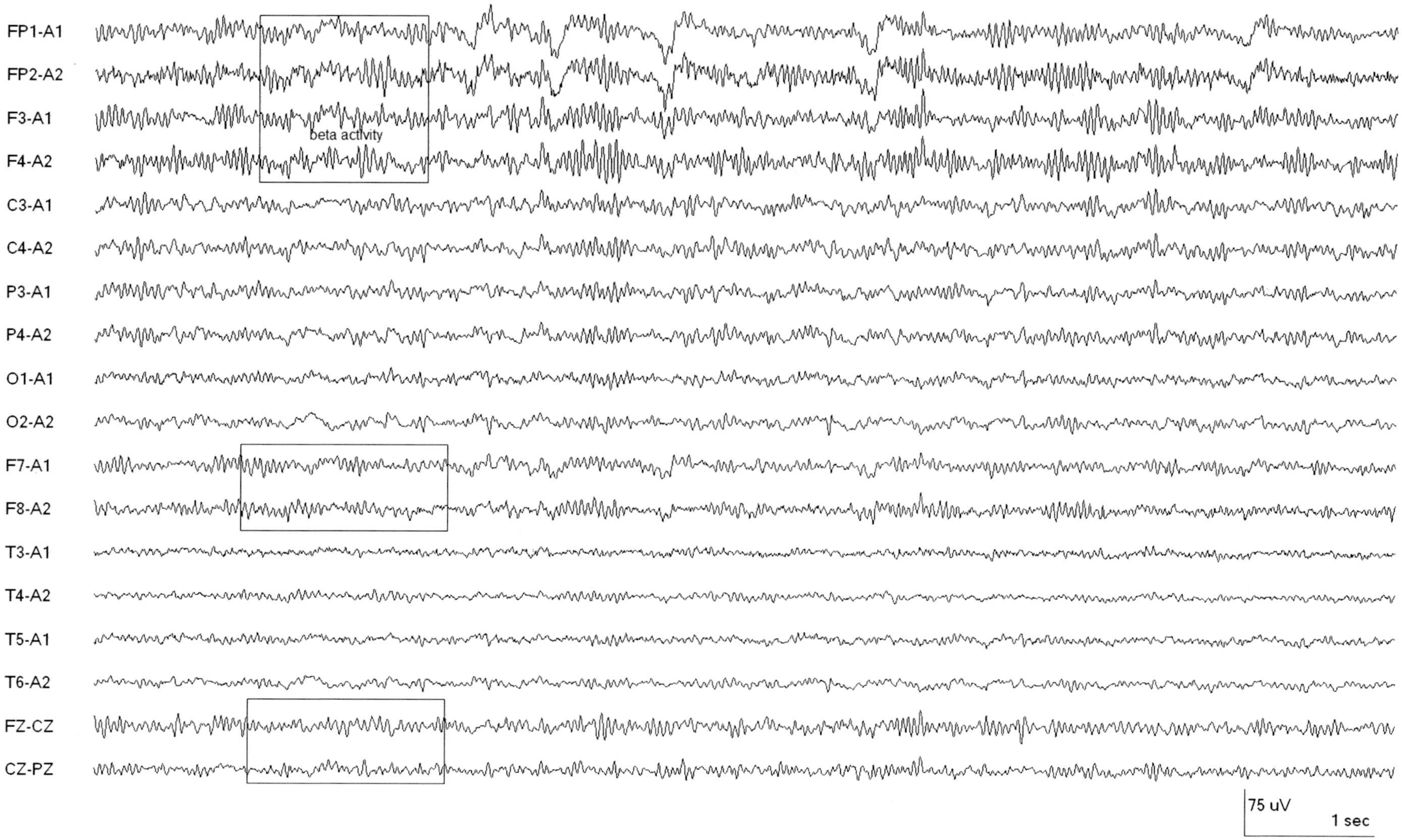

Figure 1.5 (*Continued*) (b) The same epoch reformatted to a referential montage to ipsilateral ears. Beta activity is most prominent in Fp1-A1, Fp2-A2, F3-A1 and F4-A2.

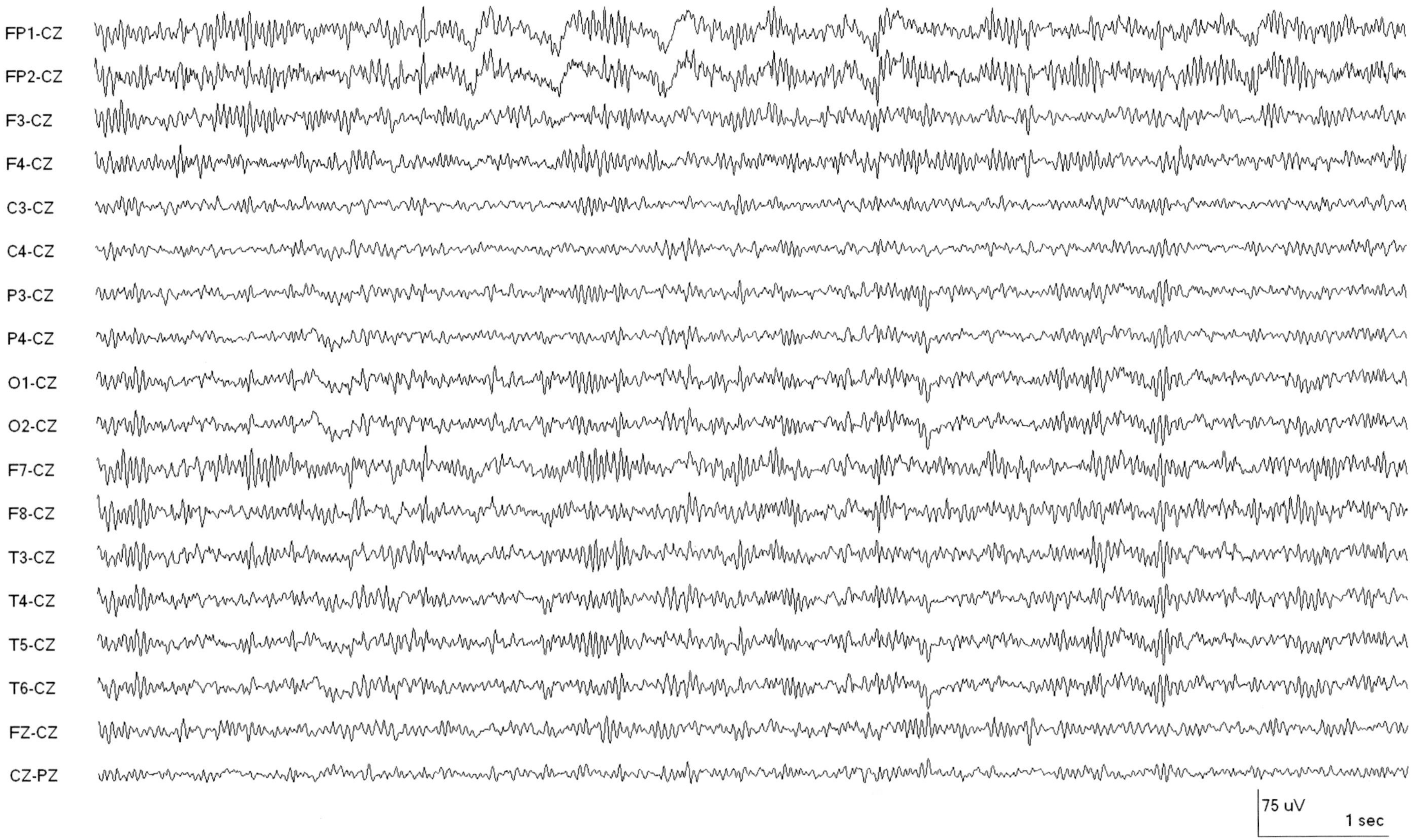

Figure 1.5 (*Continued*) (c) A referential montage to the midline vertex electrode (Cz). Note that the beta activity is well seen in mid and posterior temporal electrodes (T3, T4, T5 and T6), while this was not the case in the montage to ipsilateral ears (Figure 1.5b). This is because Cz is an active reference in this example, that is it is in a field of the beta activity. The beta activity present in T3-Cz, T4-Cz, T5-Cz and T6-Cz is due to difference between the temporal electrodes, which are relatively inactive, and the Cz electrode that is active. Beta activity is not prominent in the derivations C3-Cz and C4-C4 because of cancellation, i.e. both electrodes are equally active.

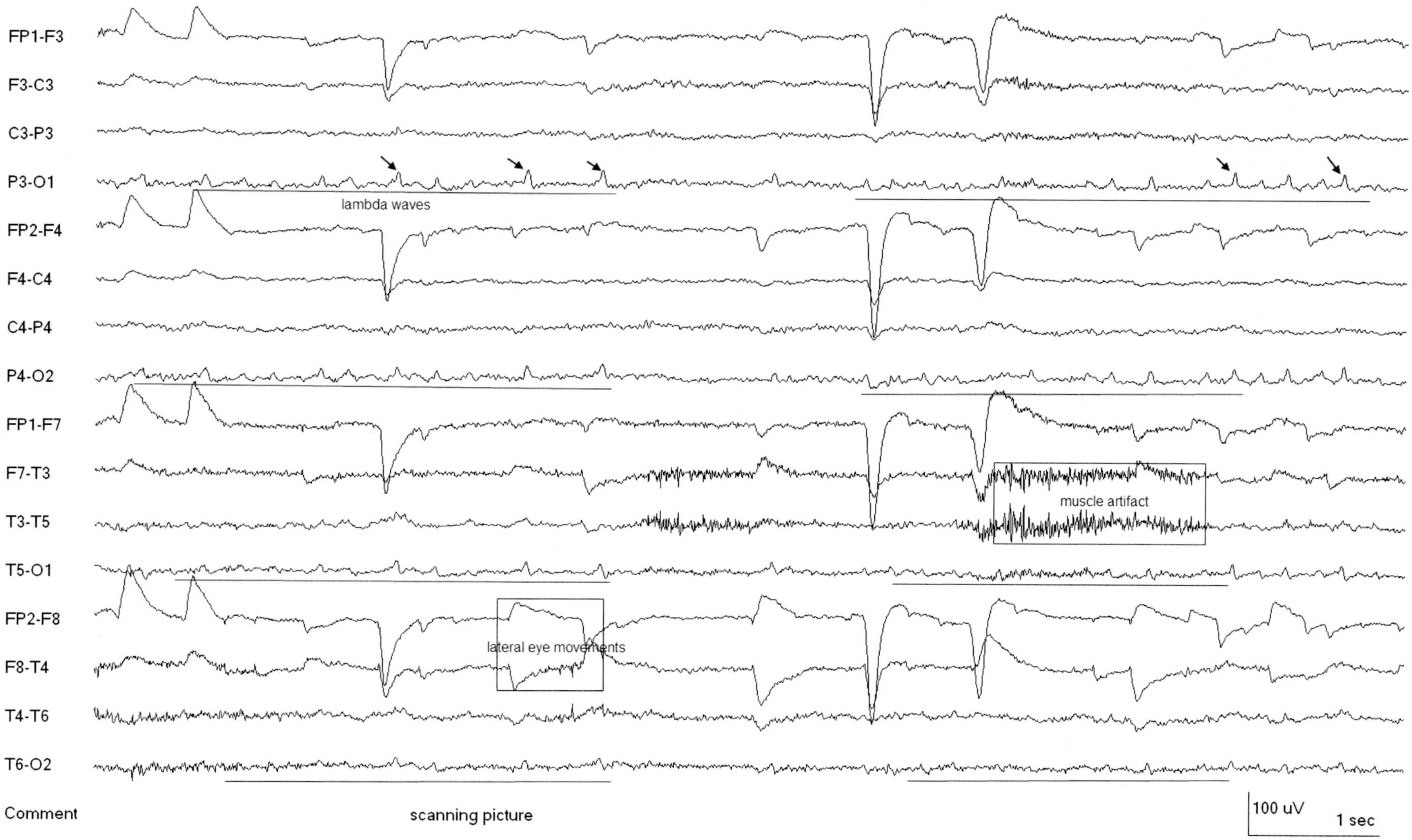

Figure 1.6 Lambda waves. (a) Low-voltage sharp waves are present bilaterally in posterior head regions (derivations P3-01, P4-02, T5-01 and T6-02) in this longitudinal bipolar montage. The sharp component is upgoing. This is because input 1 (electrodes P3, P4, T5 and T6) is relatively negative with respect to input 2 (electrodes 01 and 02); in this case this is because neutral minus positive = negative = upgoing. These represent lambda waves; surface positive potentials arising in the occipital area, with the polarity confirmed in the next figure. Lambda waves are normal and best seen during visual scanning; they are *not* evidence of epileptogenic potential. A few are labeled with arrows.

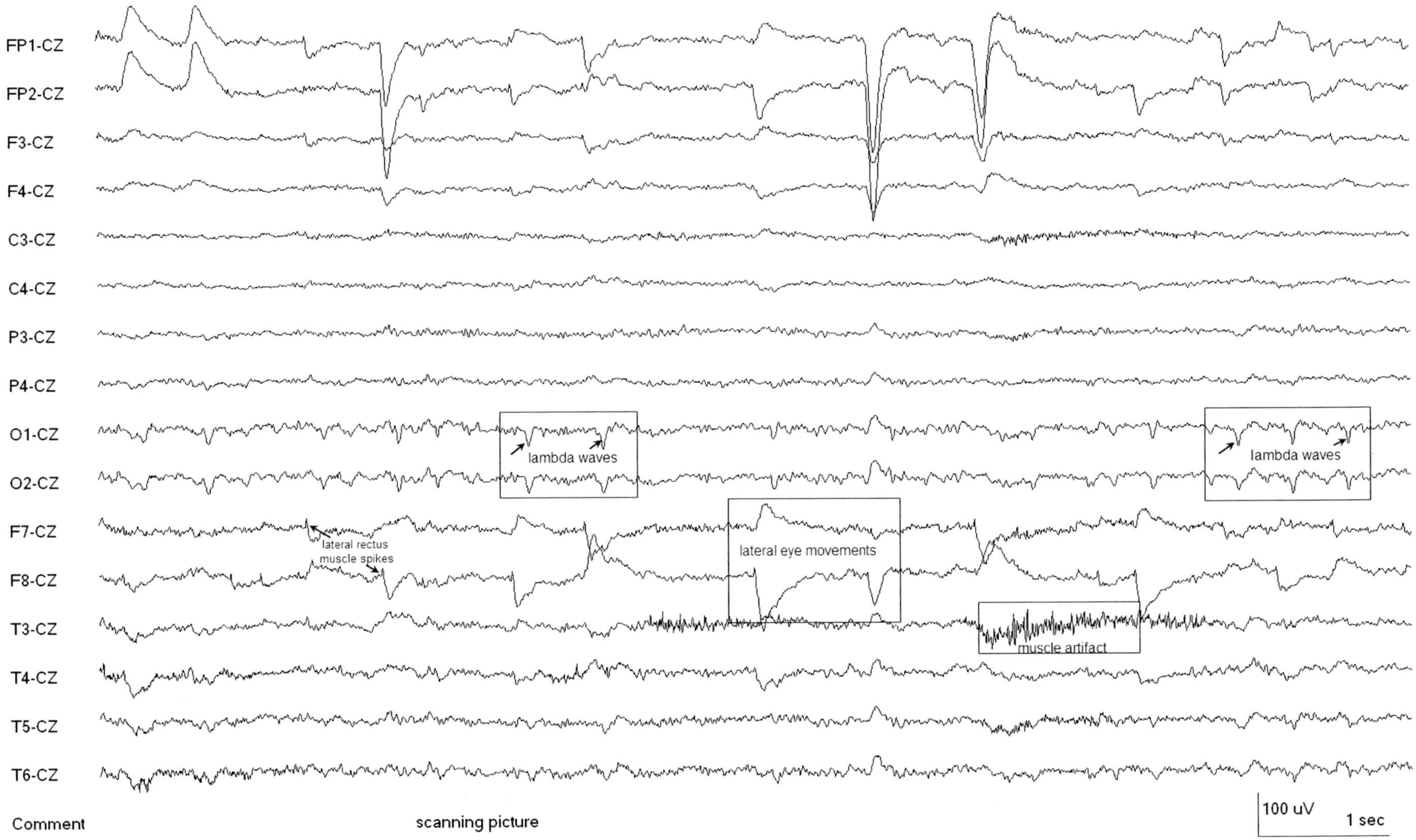

Figure 1.6 (*Continued*) (b). In a reformatted referential montage to the midline vertex electrode (Cz), the same lambda waves as seen in Figure 1.6a are well displayed in derivations O1-Cz and O2-Cz. The sharp component is downgoing because input 1 (O1 and O2) is positive with respect to input 2 (Cz), i.e. positive minus neutral = positive = downgoing. Lateral rectus muscle spikes can be seen at F7 and F8 in association with some of the horizontal eye movements as labeled.

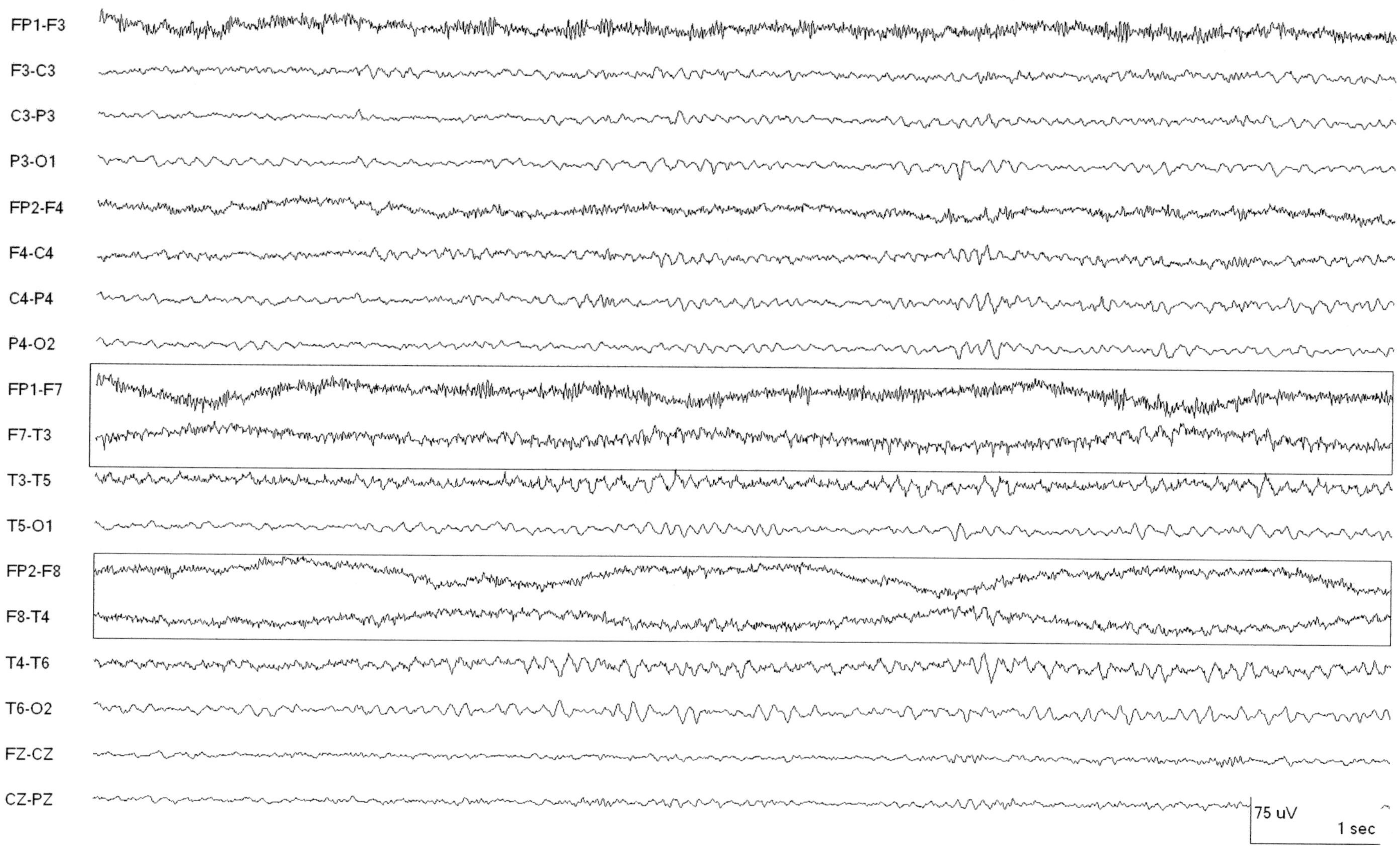

Figure 1.7 Slow lateral eye movements of drowsiness. (a) Slow lateral eye movements are prominent in this 32-year-old man during drowsiness, continuing smoothly in one direction, then the other. This is a normal feature of drowsiness. Note that F7 and F8 electrodes are out-of-phase; when one is surface positive (the cornea is moving towards this side), the other is negative (cornea moving away). This is consistent with lateral eye movements.

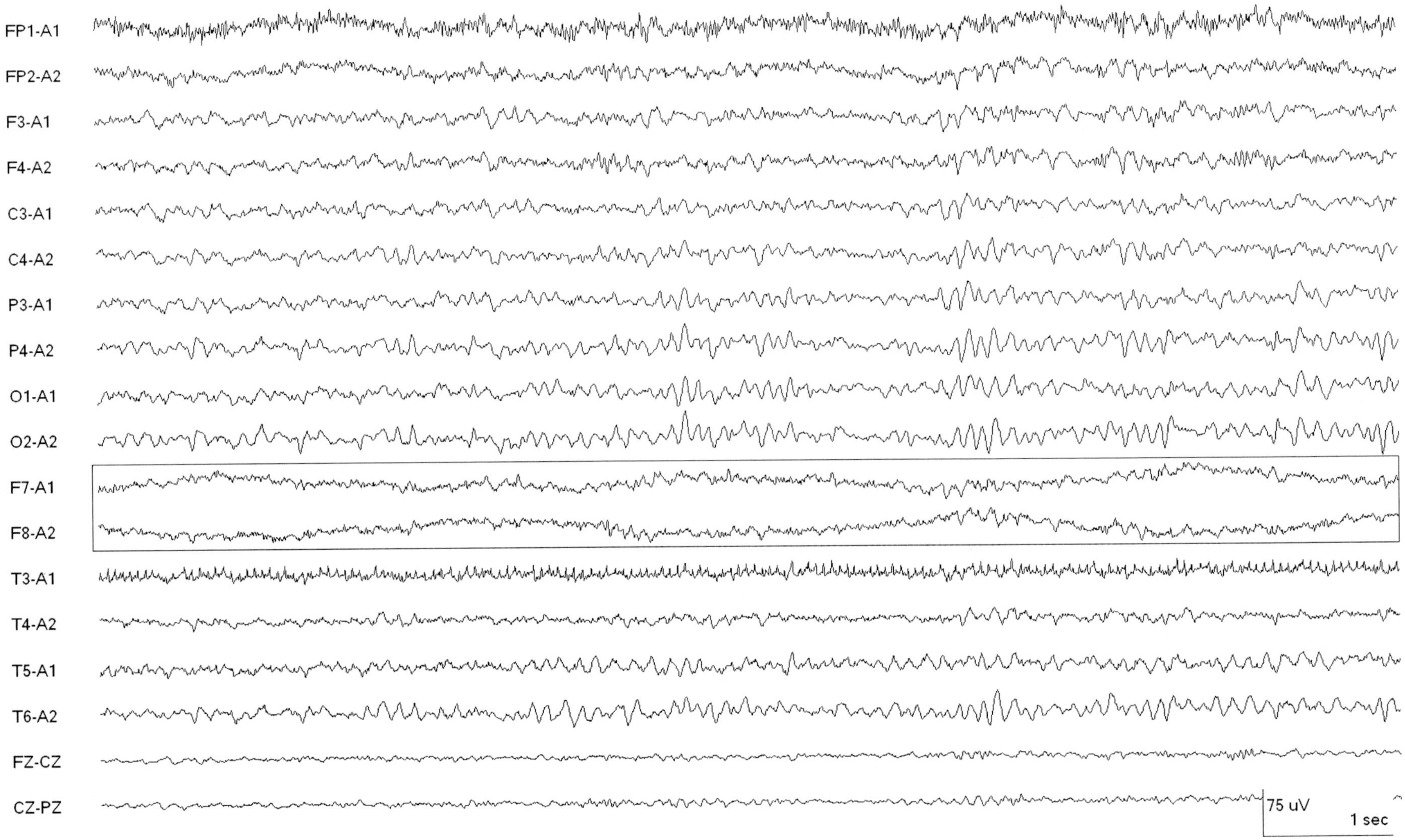

Figure 1.7 (*Continued*) (b) A reformatted referential montage to the ipsilateral ear showing the same roving, conjugate horizontal eye movements of drowsiness.

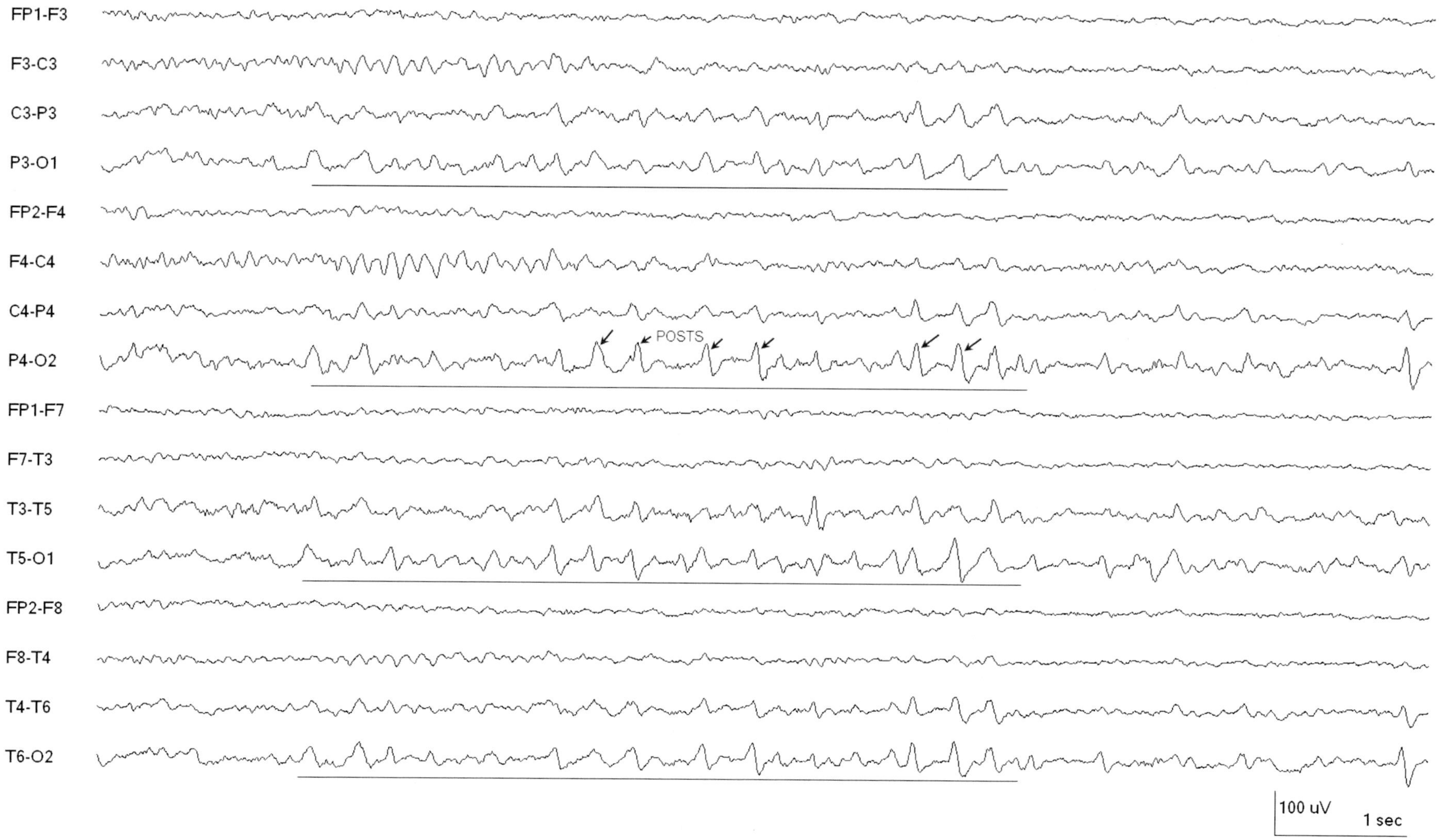

Figure 1.8 Positive occipital sharp transients of sleep (POSTS). (a) POSTS, longitudinal bipolar. Repetitive sharp activity is present bilaterally in the posterior head regions in this 31-year-old woman who is in non-REM sleep. This activity represents positive occipital sharp transients of sleep (POSTS). Polarity is confirmed with a referential montage in the Fig. 1.8b.

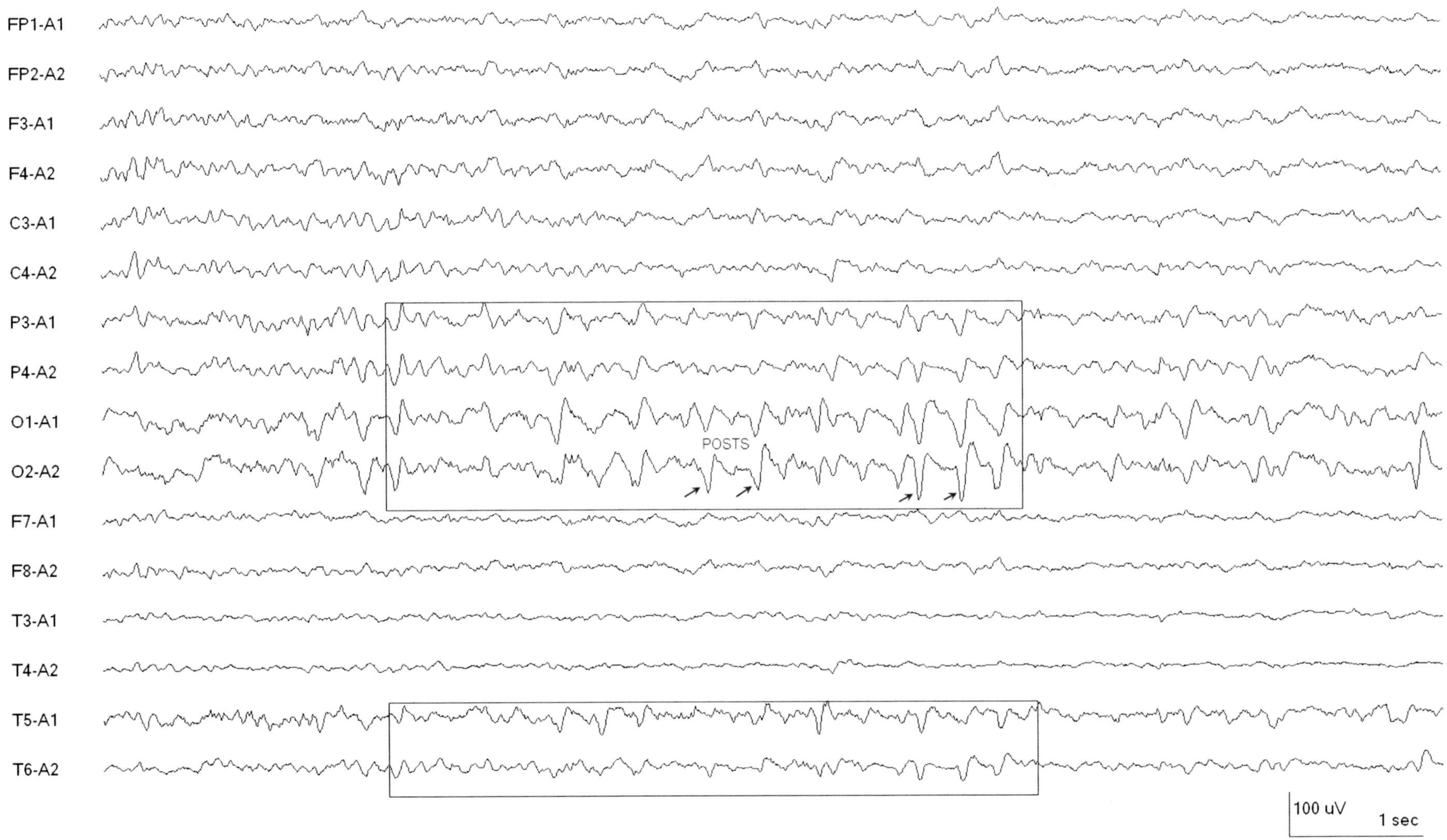

Figure 1.8 (*Continued*) (b) POSTS, referential. In a reformatted montage to ipsilateral ears the sharp activity is maximal in O1-A1 and O2-A2 derivations. The sharp activity is downgoing since O1 and O2 are relatively positive. The waveforms are also present to a lesser extent in parietal and posterior temporal areas.

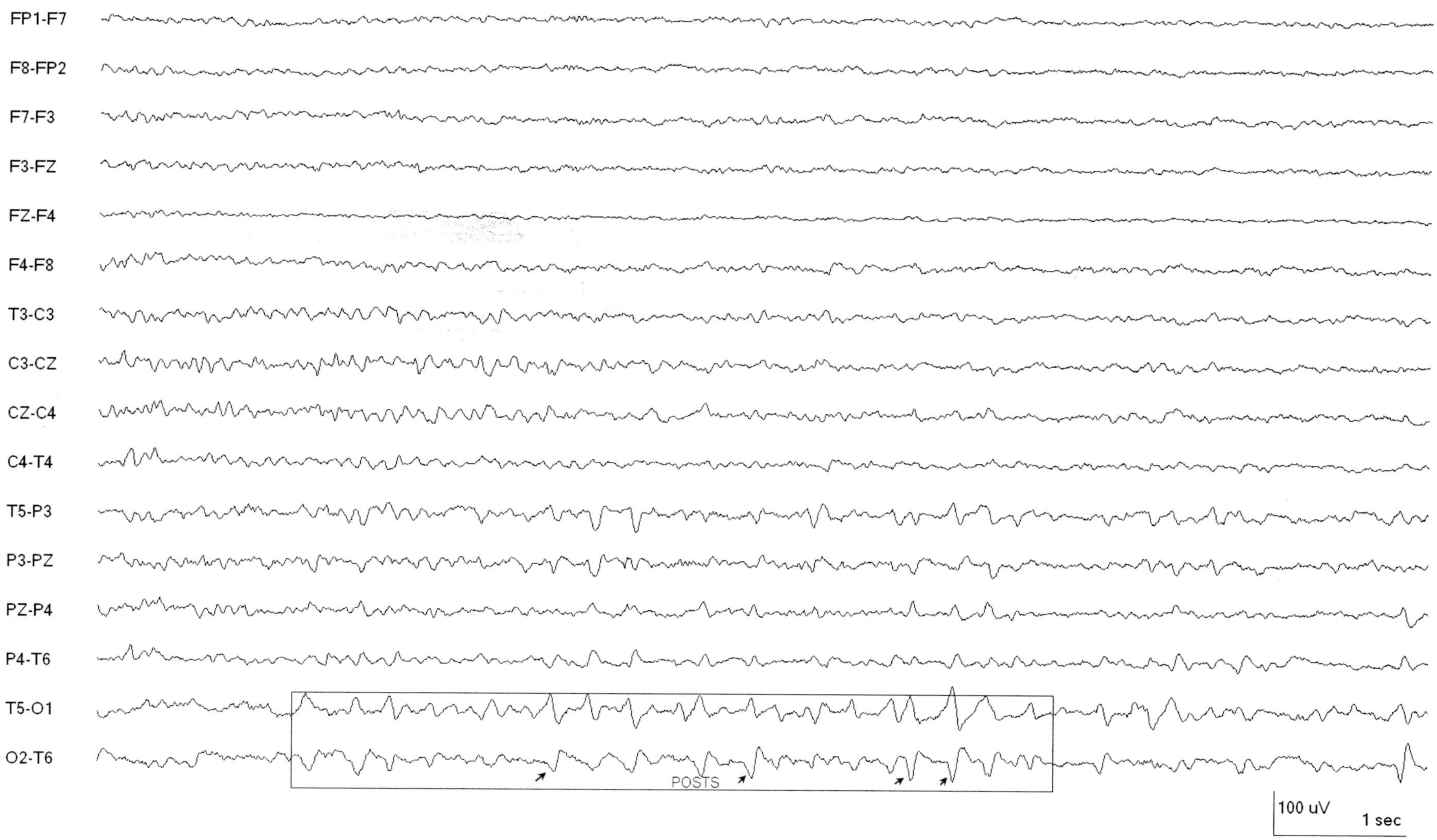

Figure 1.8 (*Continued*) (c) POSTS, transverse bipolar. In this transverse bipolar montage, complexes are seen best in the bottom two derivations (T5-01 and 02-T6). The sharp component is upgoing in T5-01 since T5 is relatively negative when compared to 01. In the 02-T6 derivations, since 02 is more positive than T6, there is a downgoing deflection.

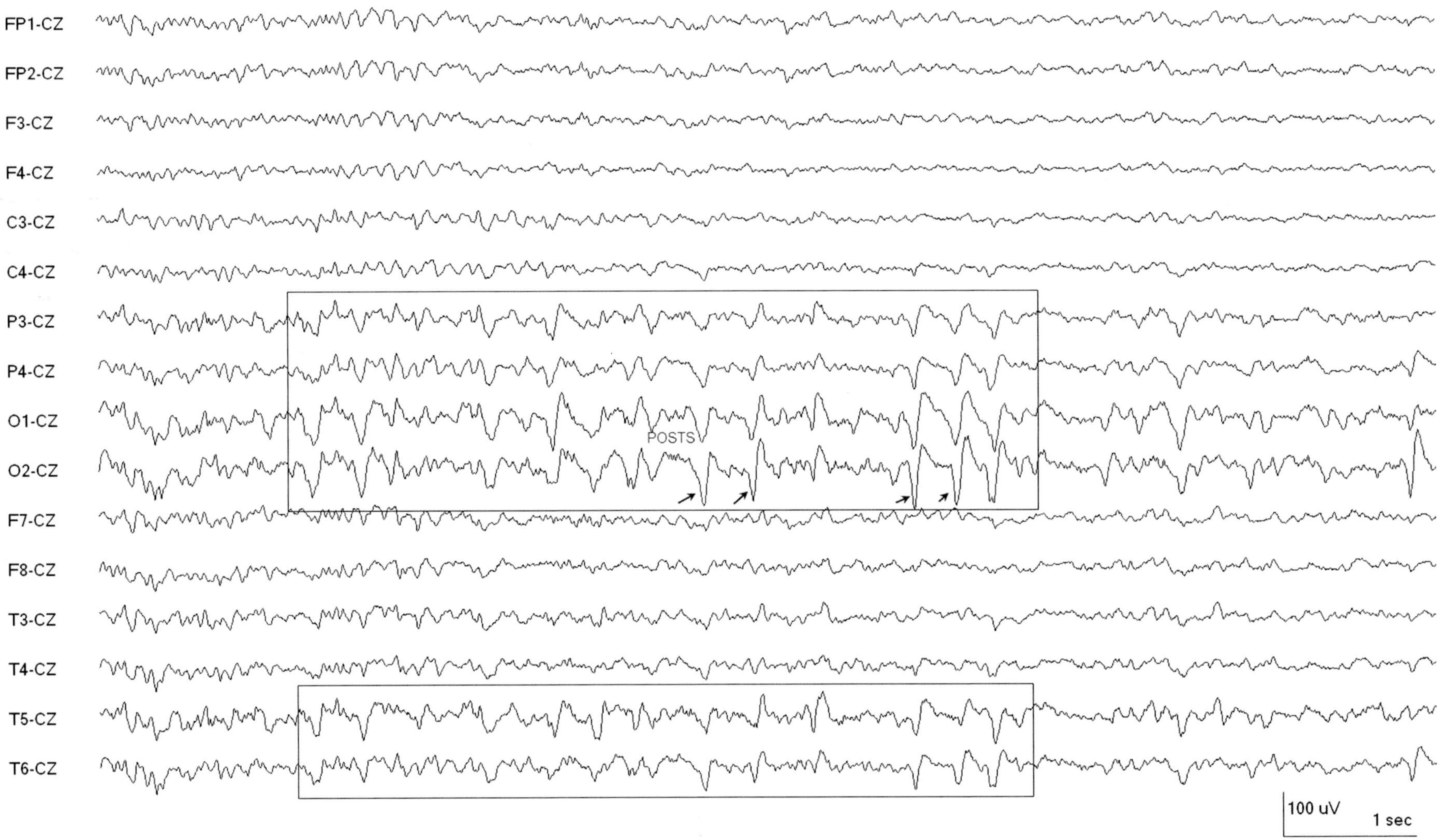

Figure 1.8 (*Continued*) (d) POSTS, Cz-reference. In this referential montage to Cz, sharp activity is seen again in the posterior head region, surface positive and maximal at O1 and O2. The Cz electrode is relatively uninvolved in this field, as was true of the A1 and A2 electrodes shown in Figure 1.8b. Thus, changing the reference in this case has little effect, since both references are relatively inactive.

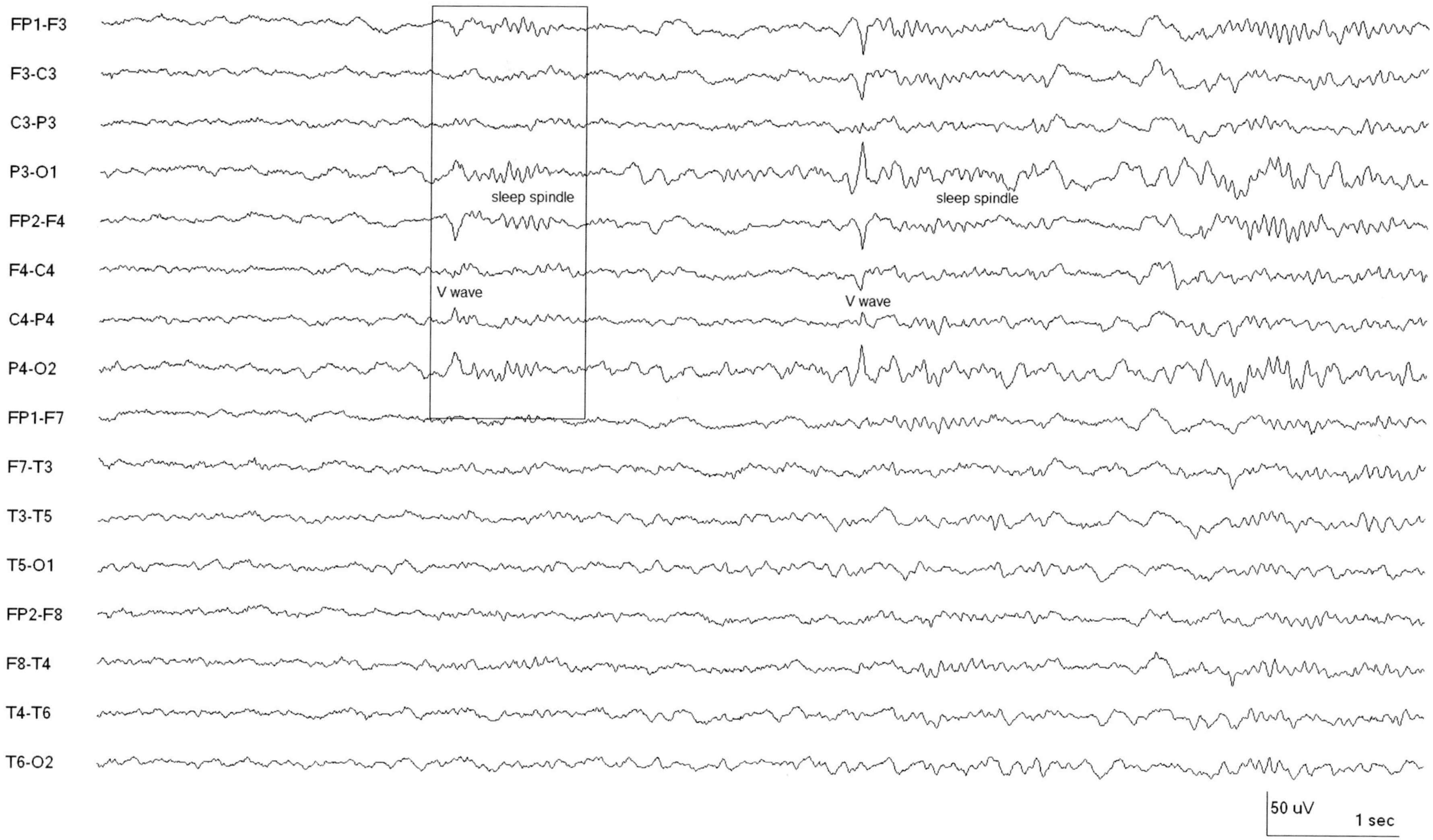

Figure 1.9 Vertex waves and sleep spindles (sleep transients). (a) Longitudinal bipolar. The vertex sharp waves (V-waves), sleep spindles and the defining features of normal stage-II sleep are prominent in this 30-year-old woman in non-REM sleep. On the right, there is a phase reversal at electrode C4, indicating maximal negativity at this site. On the left, the phase reversal is at C3-P3; the C3-P3 derivation does not show this activity since these areas are equipotential and canceling (confirmed in subsequent referential montages). The first labeled V-wave is more prominent on the right; this type of asymmetry is not unusual in early sleep and is not abnormal unless persistent.

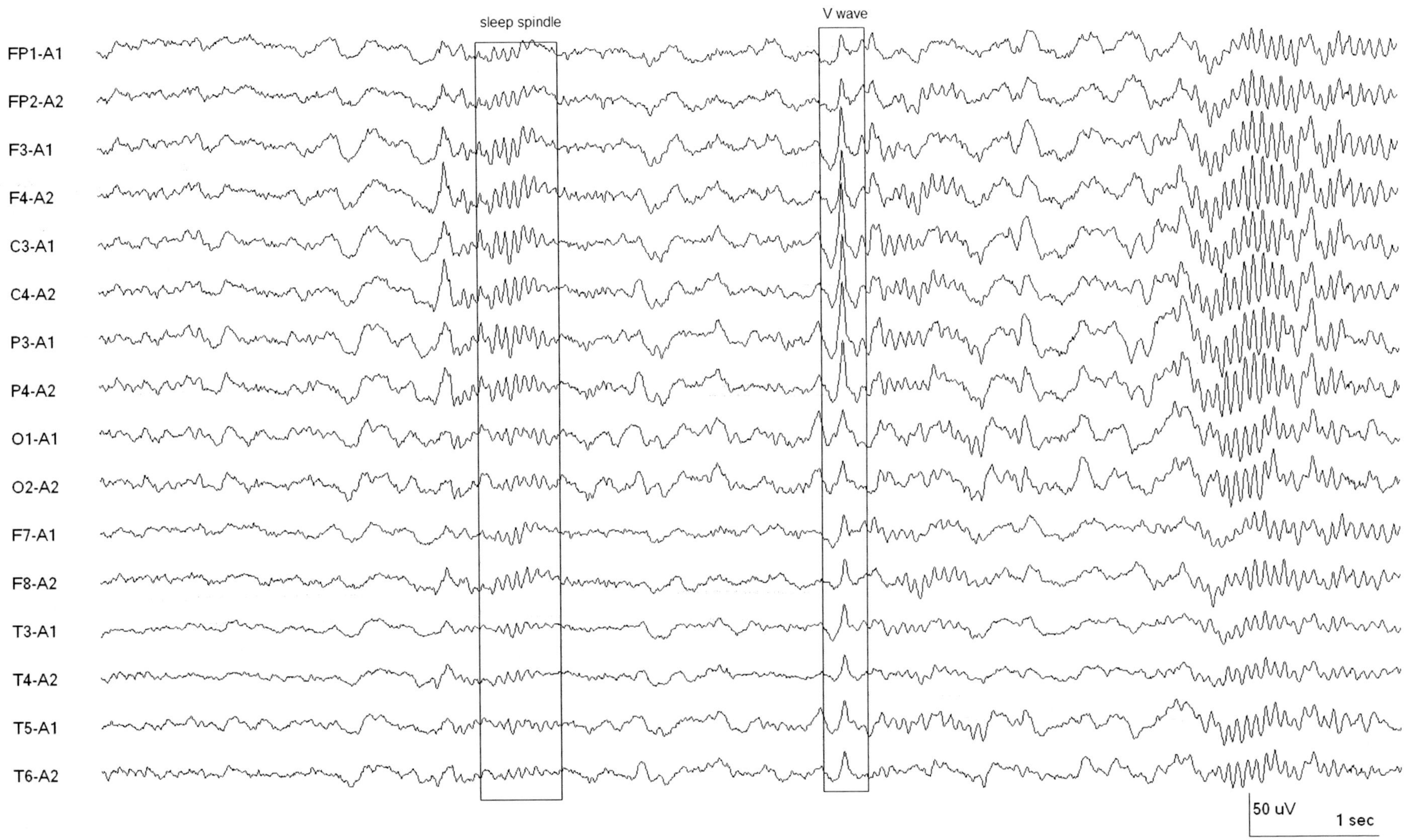

Figure 1.9 (*Continued*) (b) A referential montage to ipsilateral ears shows that V-waves and spindles are widespread in distribution in parasagittal regions and maximal in fronto-central regions, typical of normal sleep transients.

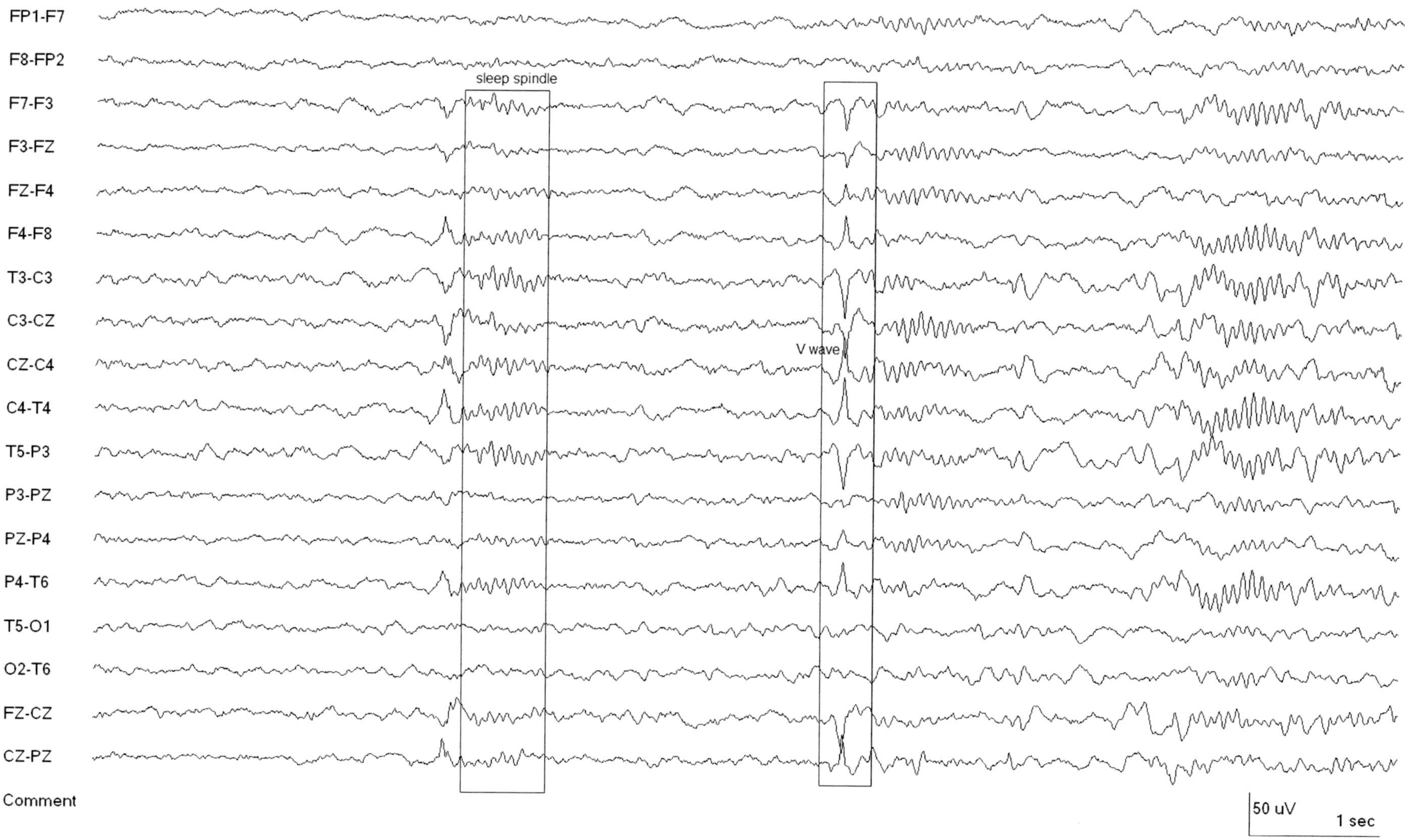

Figure 1.9 (*Continued*) (c) A transverse bipolar montage shows a phase reversal at several electrodes (Fz, Cz and Pz) simultaneously. In order to determine where this activity is maximal, one cannot use the amplitude from a bipolar montage, which indicates the difference in potential between two electrodes, to indicate the site of maximal involvement. Fz is being compared to frontal electrodes, Cz to central electrodes and Pz is to parietal electrodes. They need to be compared to each other or to the same reference. The midline derivations (Fz-Cz and Cz-Pz) are shown in the bottom two channels in a longitudinal direction (anterior to posterior). As demonstrated, the Fz-Cz and Cz-Pz derivations display a phase reversal at electrode Cz, with Cz being relatively surface negative compared to Fz or Pz. Thus Cz is the site of maximal negativity.

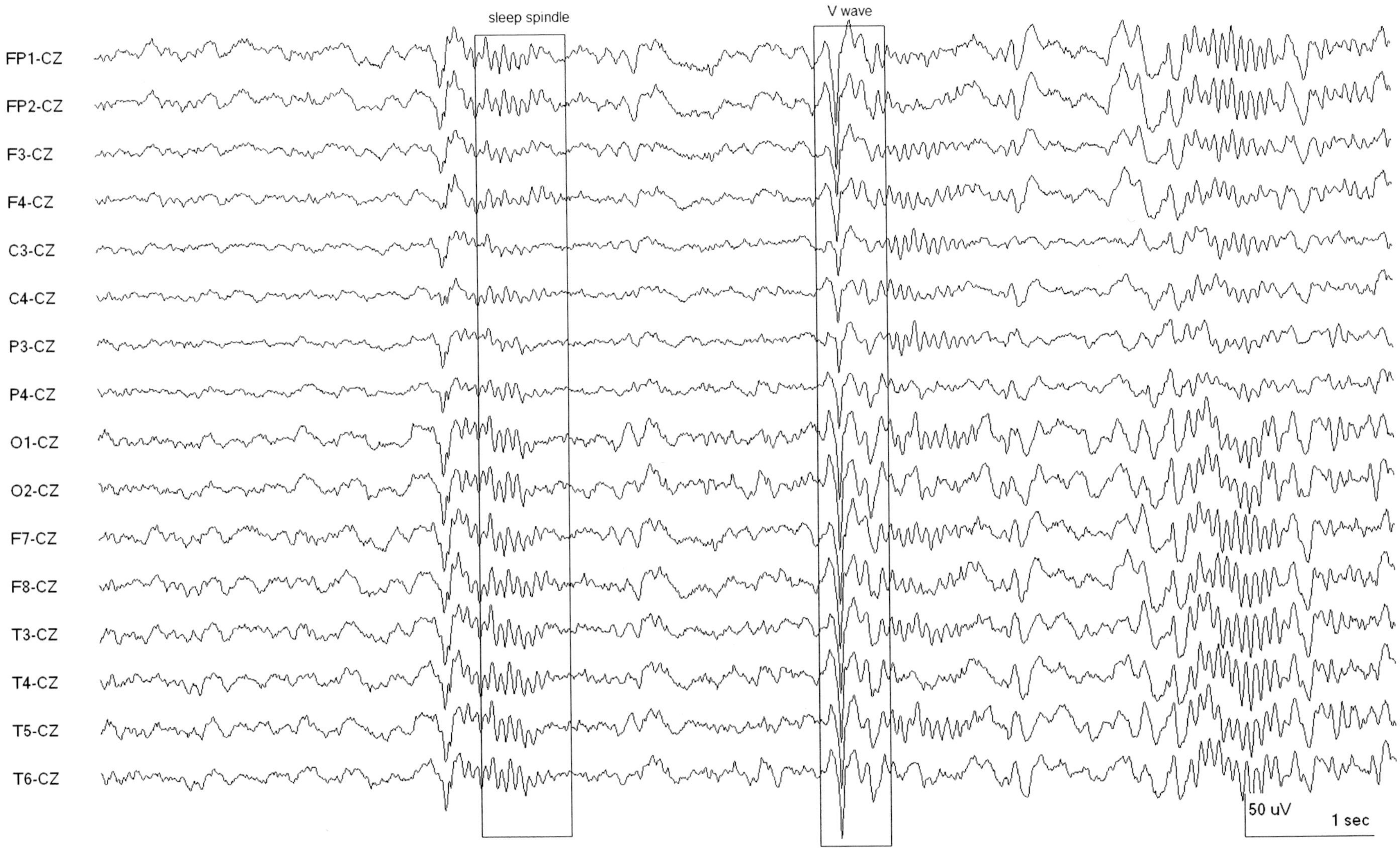

Figure 1.9 (*Continued*) (d) In this reformatted referential montage to the Cz, the sharp component of discharges are downgoing in all derivations. This is because electrode Cz is relatively more negative than all other electrodes, which are in input 1. This is another example of an active reference (Cz in this case).

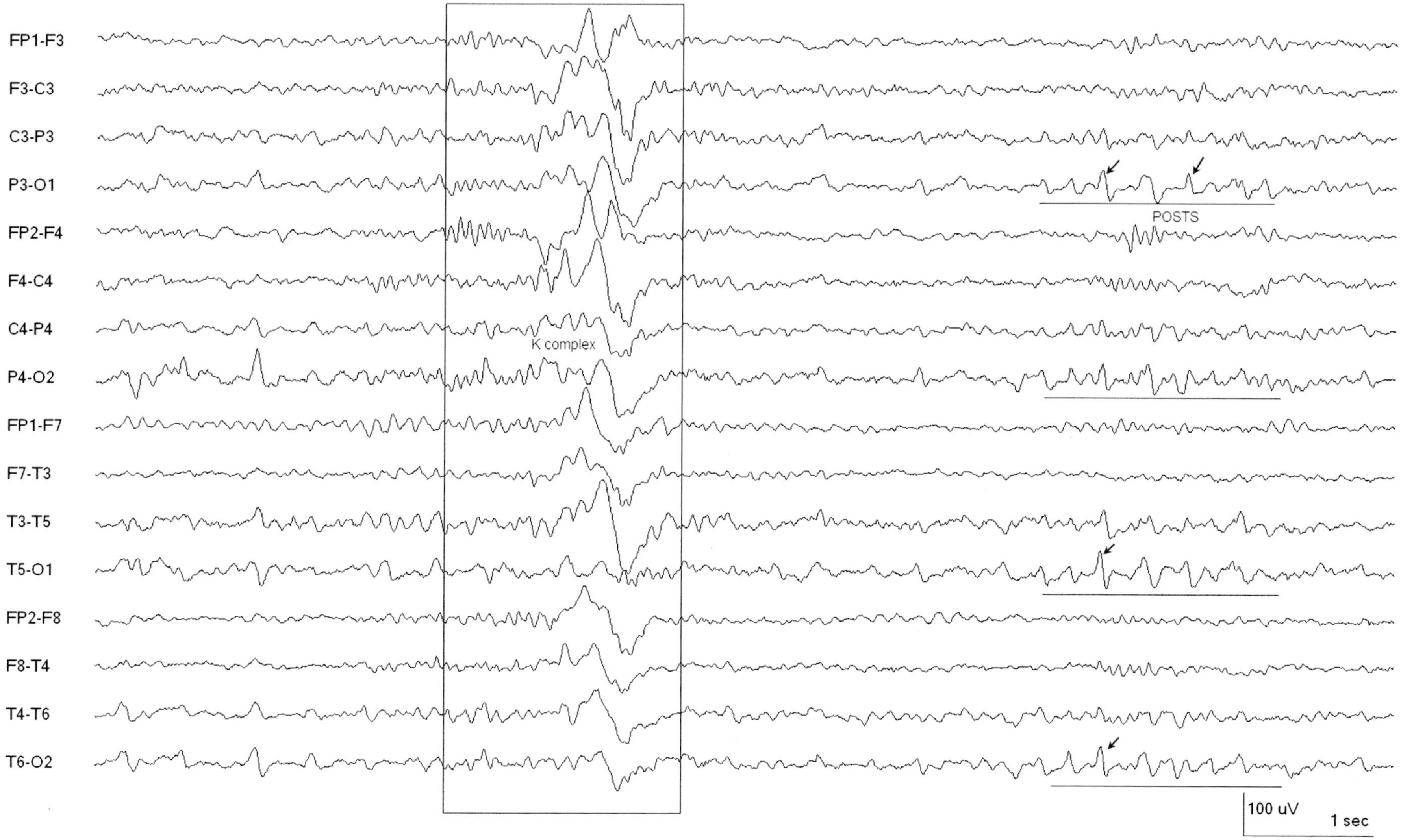

Figure 1.10 K-complex and POSTS. (a) Longitudinal bipolar. A slow wave preceded by faster activity is prominent in this longitudinal bipolar montage in a 31-year-old woman, who is in non-REM sleep. POSTS (positive occipital sharp transients of sleep) are also present, most evident in the last several seconds as labeled.

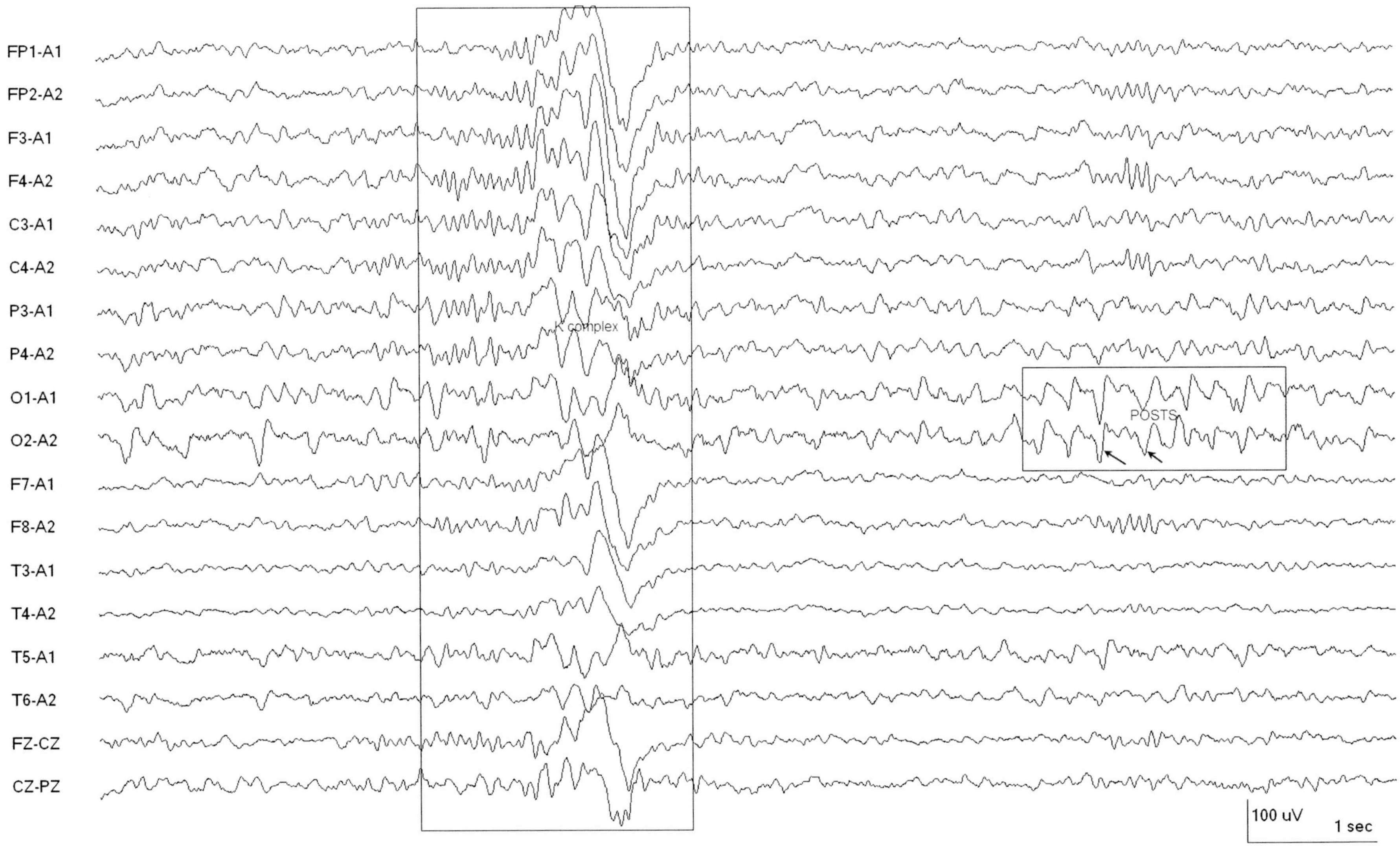

Figure 1.10 (*Continued*) (b) Referential. The referential montage to ipsilateral ears displays this activity, as well as better displays the preceding sleep spindle. The entire complex is referred to as a K-complex.

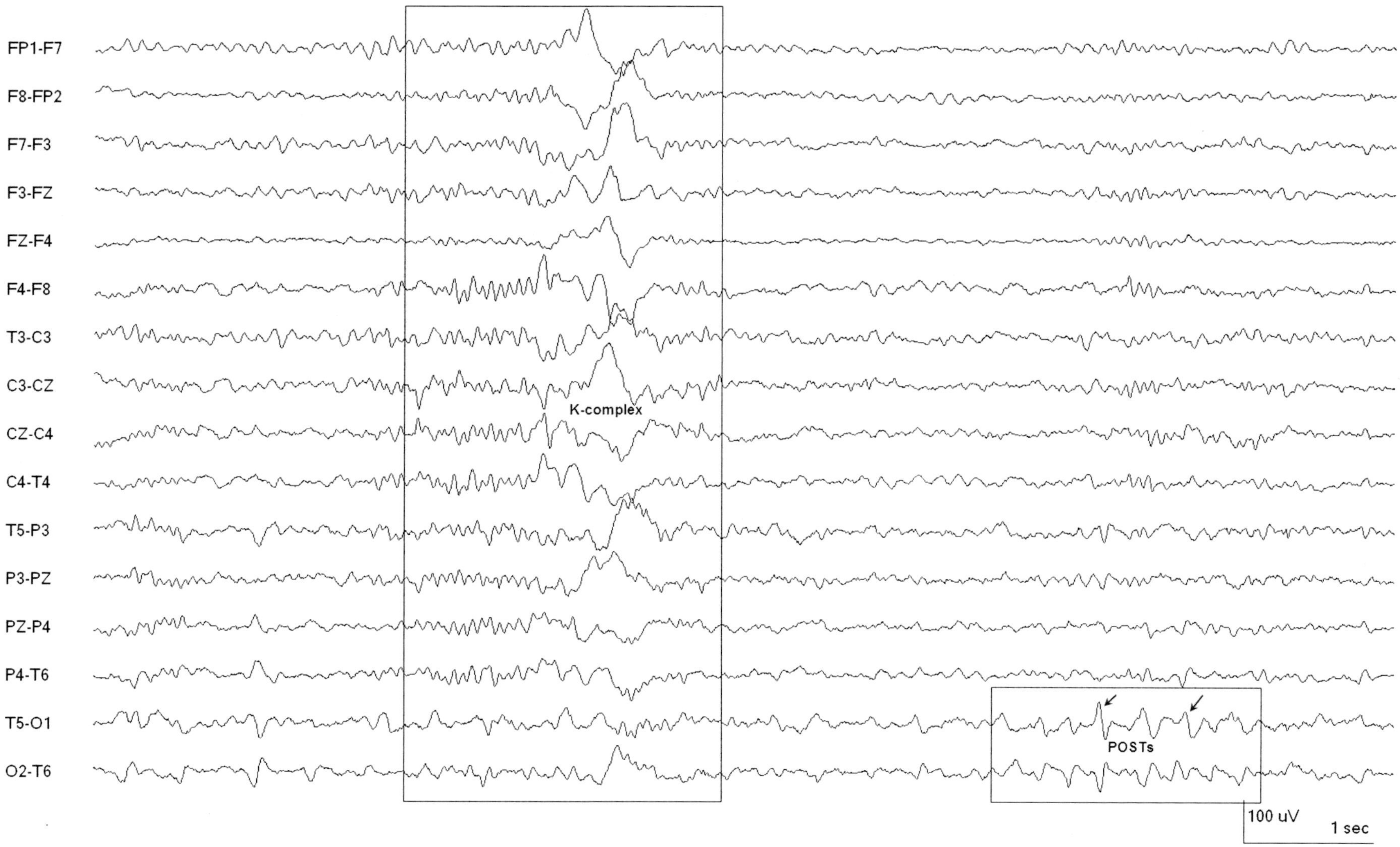

Figure 1.10 (*Continued*) (c) Transverse bipolar. Here the epoch has been reformatted to a transverse bipolar montage.

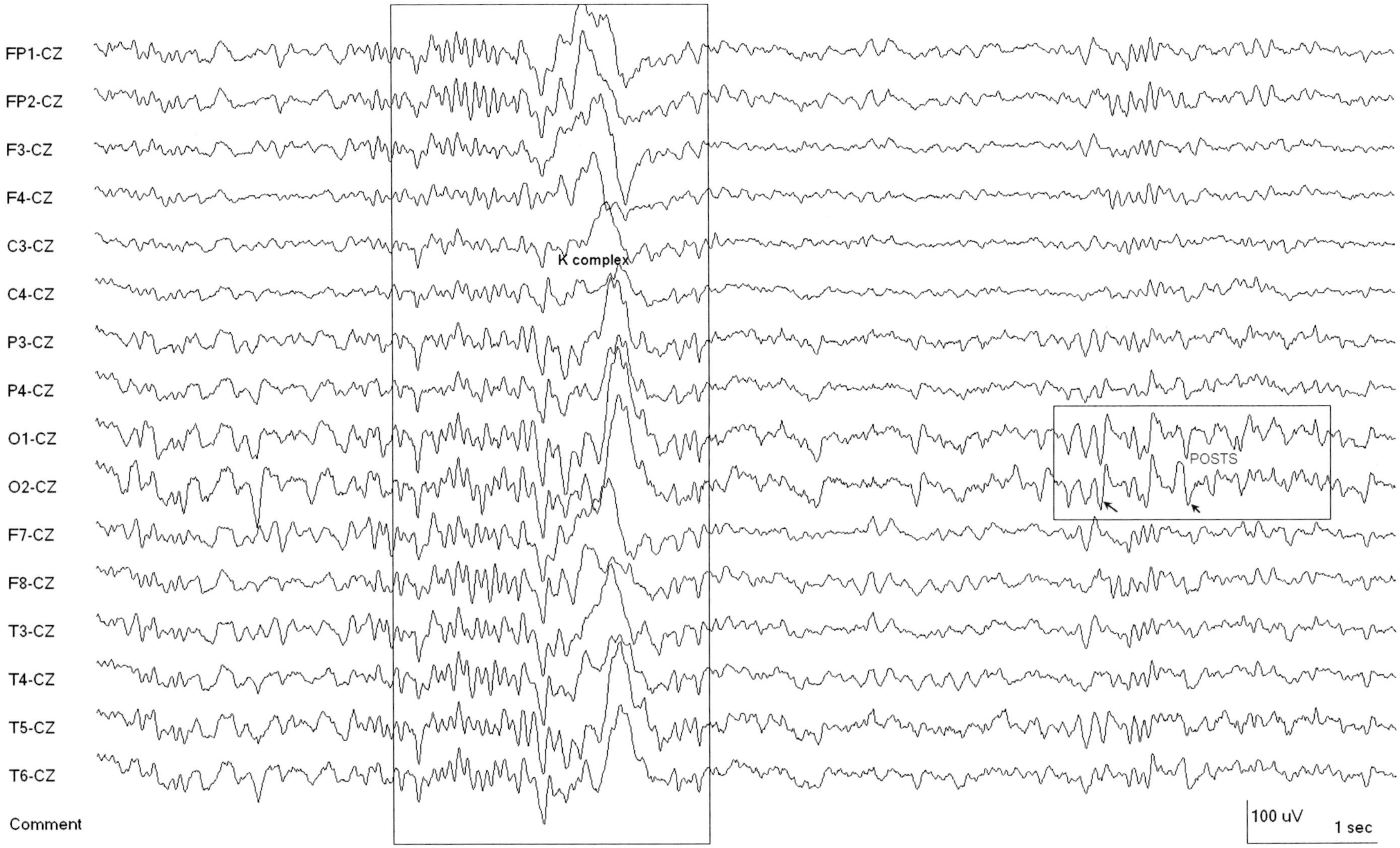

Figure 1.10 (*Continued*) (d) Cz-reference. Here the reference is electrode Cz, which is not often used as a reference during sleep because it is typically very active. Because of this, there is a considerable degree of cancelation, particularly in C3-Cz and C4-Cz derivations. Since this activity is maximal at the midline with relatively little spread to temporal regions, the temporal derivations show the K-complex, which is due to the active Cz-reference.

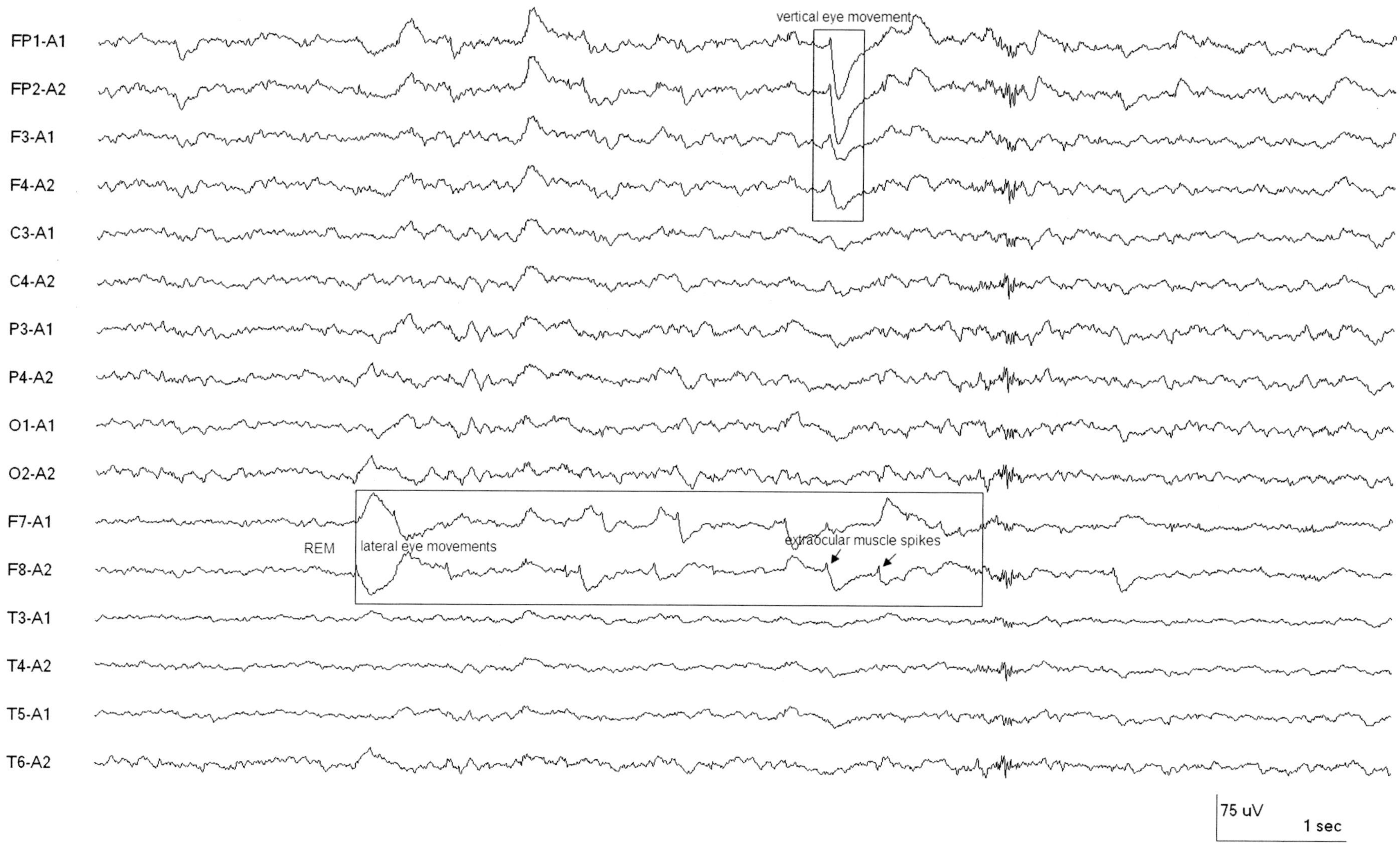

Figure 1.11 REM sleep. (a). Rapid eye movements are prominent in this 25-year-old man in REM (rapid eye movement) sleep. The majority of movements are lateral, at which time electrodes F7 and F8 are simultaneously out-of-phase. Leftward and rightward lateral eye movements are labeled (see also Figure 1.3), as well as one vertical eye movement. Small and sharp discharges can be seen with some of the rapid eye movements – these represent extraocular muscle spikes (mainly lateral rectus when seen at F7 and F8).

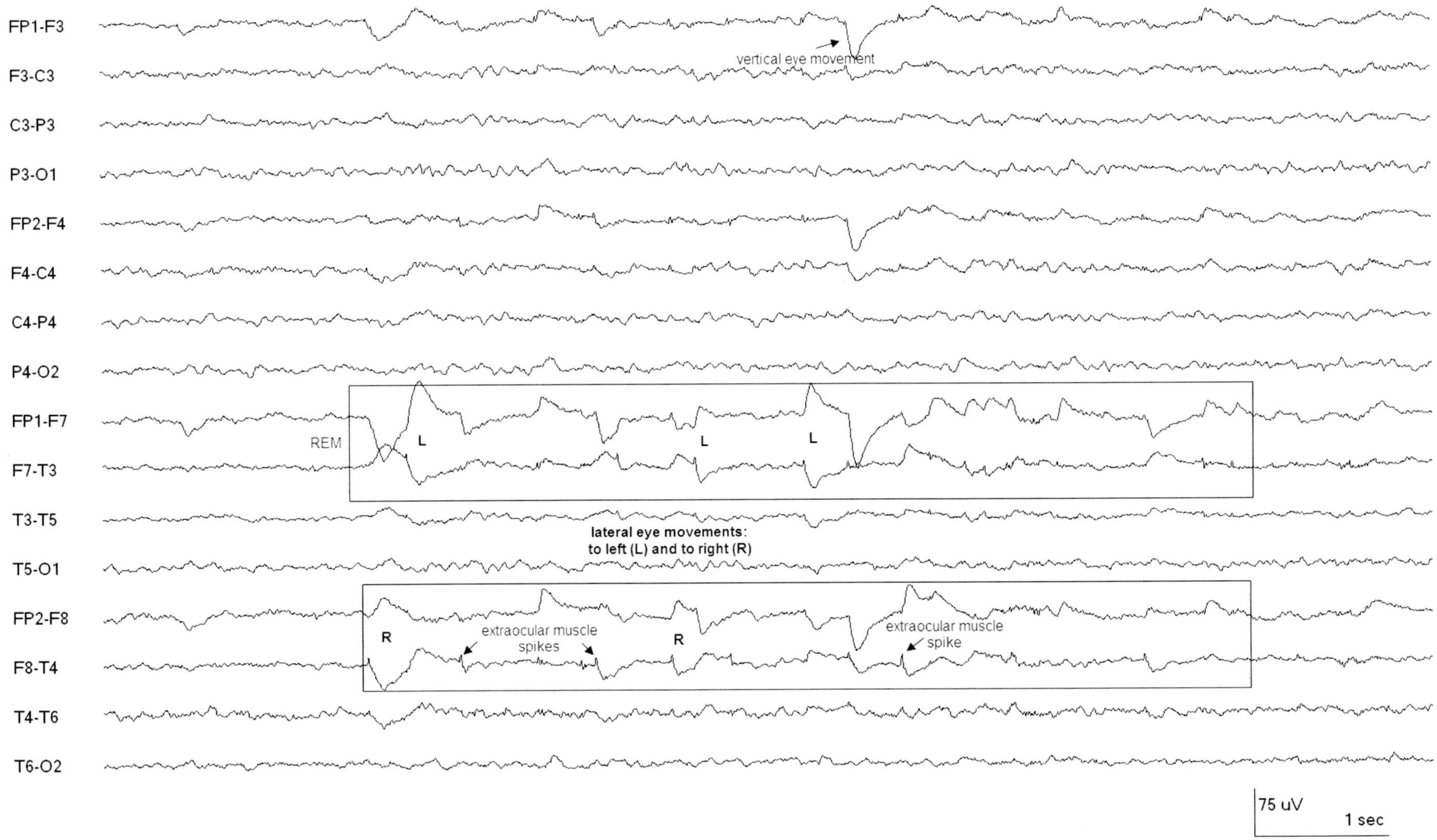

Figure 1.11 (*Continued*) (b) A reformatted referential montage to ipsilateral ears.

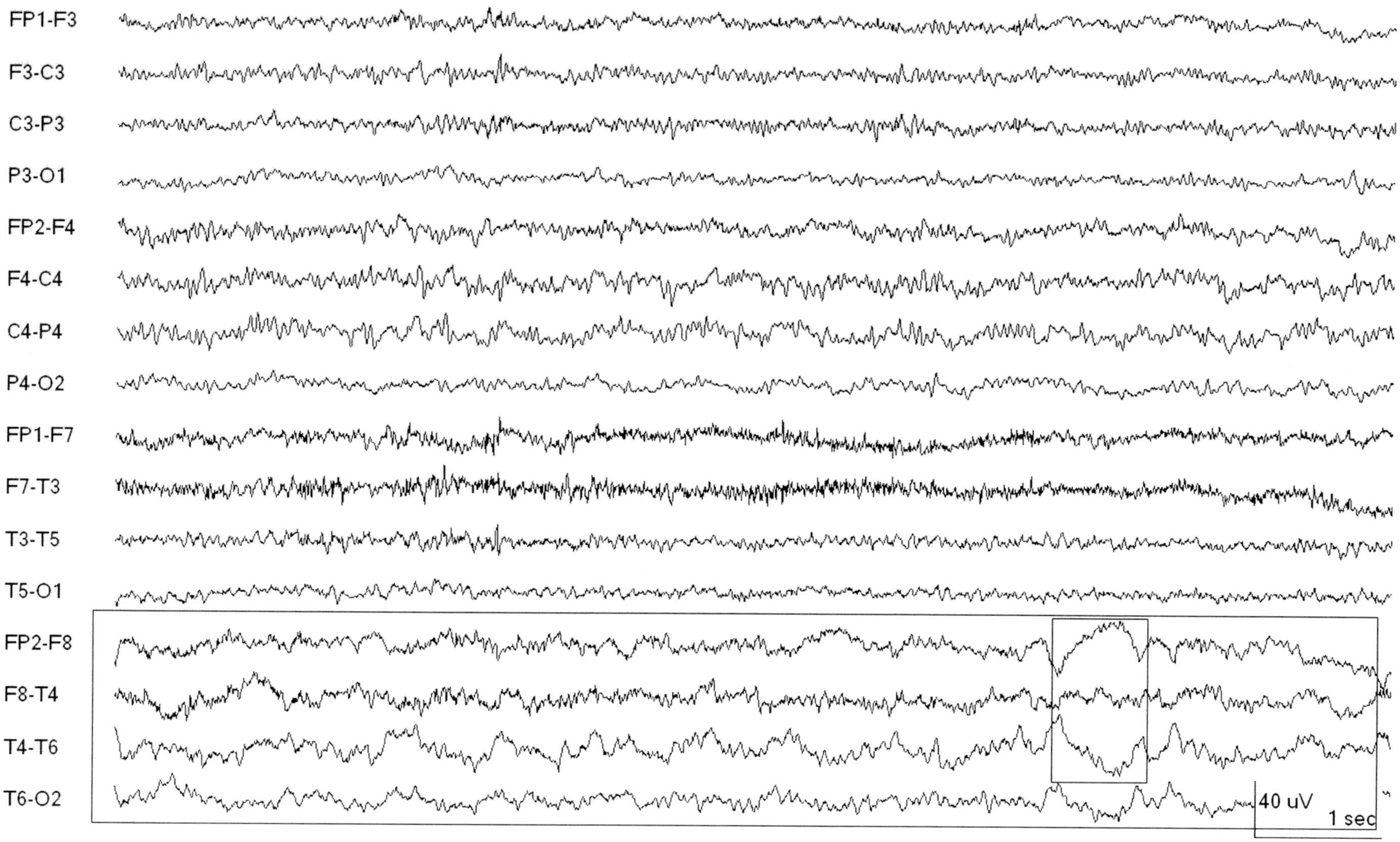

Figure 1.12 Focal slowing. (a) Longitudinal bipolar. Right temporal slowing consisting of arrhythmic (also known as polymorphic) delta activity is seen in the bottom four channels (large box); the small box highlights one particularly prominent slow wave. Most likely the activity is maximal at electrodes F8 and T4, as the F8-T4 channel demonstrates cancelation; this can be confirmed in a referential montage.

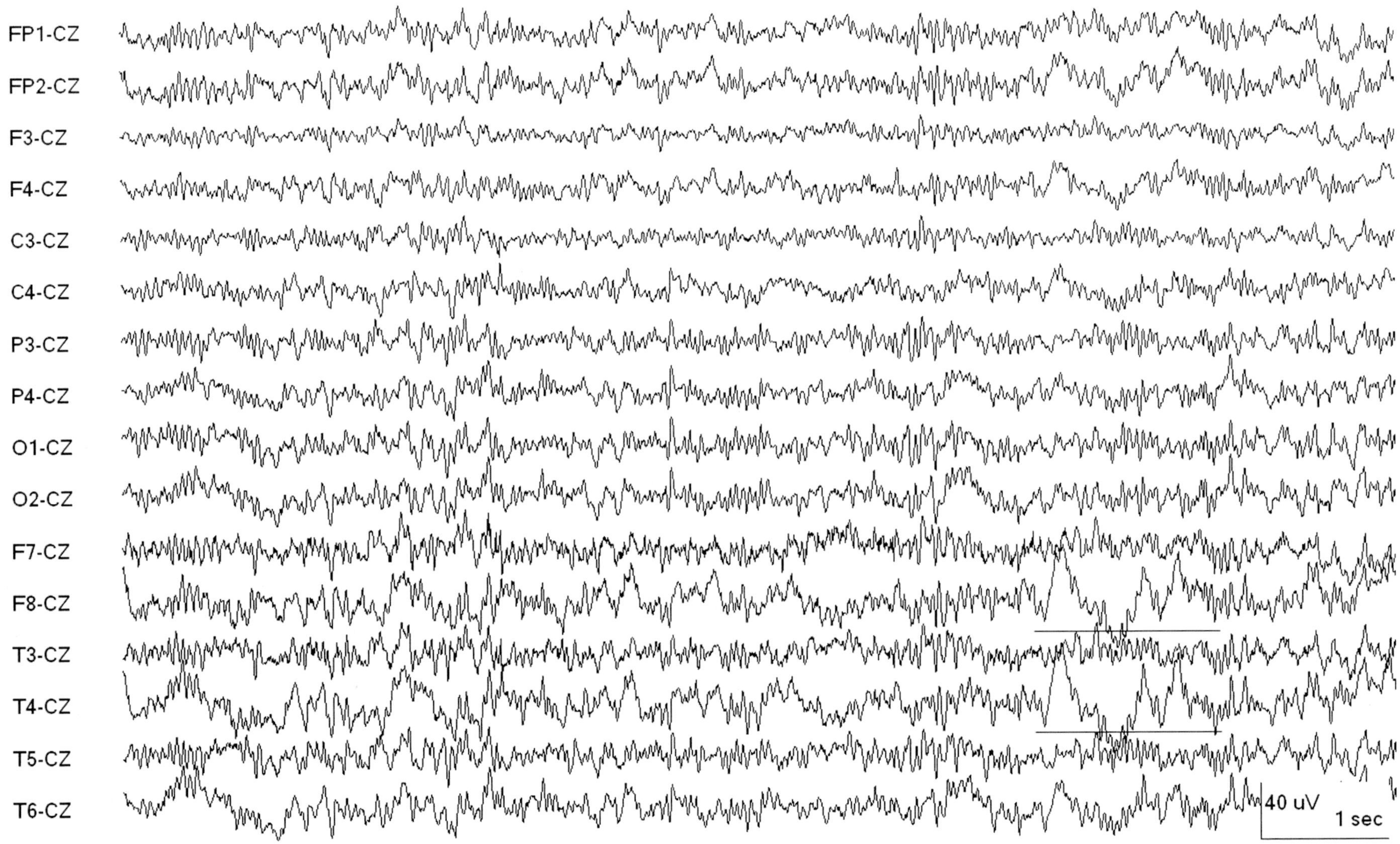

Figure 1.12 (*Continued*) (b) Cz-reference. The midline vertex electrode (Cz) is an excellent choice to display focal slow activity in the temporal region. In this case the intermittent slowing is most marked in F8 and T4 electrodes (underlined) and they are relatively equally active.

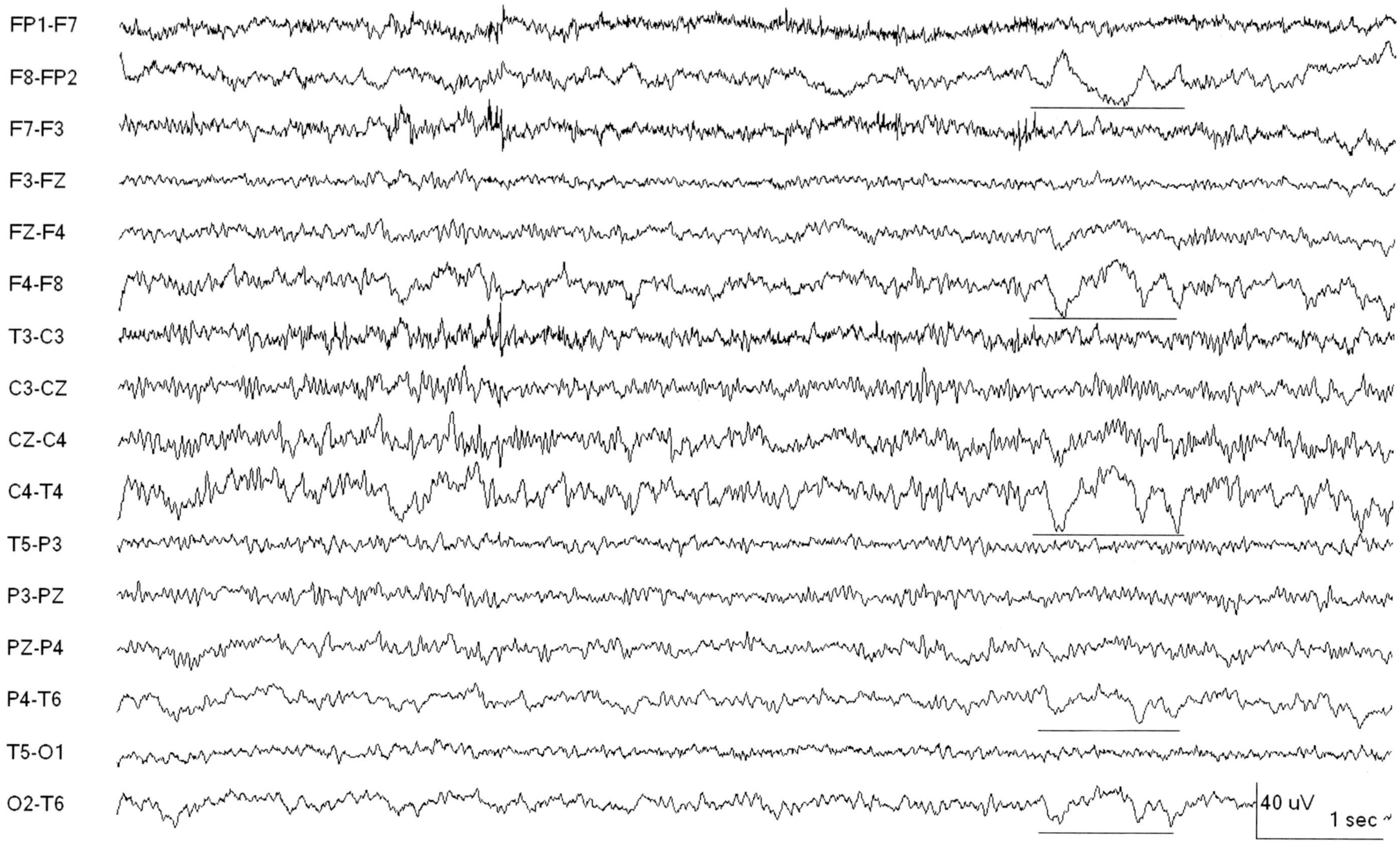

Figure 1.12 (*Continued*) (c) Transverse bipolar. Intermittent delta activity can again be appreciated in channels including the right temporal electrodes (F8/T4 > T6; underlined).

2 EEG in encephalopathy

2.1 Nonspecific patterns of encephalopathy

There are many nonspecific changes in EEG that occur during diffuse encephalopathies. Early changes include slowing of the alpha rhythm and excess slowing during wakefulness, first theta and then delta. This is followed by loss of alpha rhythm, more prominent slowing, loss of normal faster activity, loss or attenuation of normal sleep transients such as K-complexes and spindles, and sometimes periods of diffuse attenuation for a second or two. Abnormal arousal patterns and frontal intermittent rhythmic delta (FIRDA) may also be seen. Frontal intermittent rhythmic delta is most commonly seen in diffuse encephalopathy and is nonspecific, although it can sometimes be seen with raised intracranial pressure or with deep midline lesions.

As encephalopathy worsens, changes include loss of normal variability and state changes, loss of reactivity to external stimuli including pain, burst-suppression and ultimately electrocerebral inactivity (a 'flat' tracing). It is important to recognize that most or all of these patterns can be produced in a normal brain via the use of high-dose sedatives such as barbiturates, propofol and benzodiazepines.

2.2 Patterns suggesting specific diagnoses

Certain findings have diagnostic utility in the evaluation of encephalopathy, although they are rarely if ever pathognomonic. Generalized periodic discharges at approximately 1 per second in a patient with rapidly progressive dementia and myoclonus are highly suggestive of Creutzfeldt-Jacob disease. *Triphasic waves*, a subset of generalized periodic discharges, are suggestive of toxic/metabolic encephalopathy, although they can also be seen in patients with seizures, including nonconvulsive status epilepticus.

Periodic lateralized epileptiform discharges (PLEDs) are often seen with acute or subacute unilateral lesions. Although commonly associated with herpes simplex encephalitis, PLEDs can be seen in any acute or subacute process with a high association with seizures. Stroke is the most common cause.

Generalized periodic epileptiform discharges (GPEDs) can be seen in many circumstances, including postanoxic coma, after status epilepticus, medication toxicity (such as lithium, baclofen, ifosfamide and cefepime), Creutzfeldt-Jacob disease and metabolic encephalopathy.

Other useful EEG patterns in patients with encephalopathy include the following. A normal or near-normal EEG suggests a psychogenic process or brainstem disease, such as locked-in syndrome, in which the patient's mental status is actually normal or near-normal. Finding seizure activity will obviously affect management; the faster the diagnosis is made and the shorter the duration of nonconvulsive seizures, the more amenable to treatment they are and the better the outcome.

Atlas of EEG in Critical Care Lawrence J. Hirsch and Richard P. Brenner

2.3 Findings in specific clinical scenarios

In postanoxic coma, GPEDs, burst suppression, alpha coma and a low-amplitude nonreactive record are associated with poor prognosis, although all of the studies demonstrating this predated the era of therapeutic hypothermia for cardiac arrest. Thus, much of this needs to be reassessed.

All metabolic encephalopathies can cause diffuse slowing and generalized periodic discharges, including triphasic waves. Seizures and epileptiform discharges can also be seen in most of these conditions, especially renal failure, hyponatremia and Hashimoto's encephalopathy. Neuroleptic malignant syndrome, serotonin syndrome and some medication toxicities (as mentioned under GPEDs above) cause similar EEG patterns with diffuse slowing, GPEDs and seizures.

Neurosurgical procedures will produce breach rhythms due to skull defects. The skull defect causes a low-impedance pathway for electrical activity, resulting in accentuation of the underlying EEG, particularly higher frequencies. Normal underlying cerebral activity appears higher voltage and sharper, and can be misinterpreted as epileptiform.

The EEG is not usually helpful in patients in a vegetative or minimally conscious state as it can show a wide variety of degrees of diffuse dysfunction. EEG records cortical activity, not brainstem activity. Thus, in patients with primary brainstem injury, the EEG can appear remarkably 'healthy'. A completely flat EEG (electrocerebral inactivity) is seen with severe diffuse injury, with or without loss of brainstem function, which must be determined by other means (primarily examination, including apnea testing). There are detailed and formal guidelines for performing an EEG in order to document electrocerebral inactivity, although presently these are only used on rare occasions as part of the determination of brain death due to the limitations just mentioned.

2.4 Medication effects

Sedatives, particularly benzodiazepines and barbiturates, cause diffuse slowing as well as excess fast activity, primarily beta range. At higher levels, these can cause suppression-burst followed by electrocerebral inactivity at high enough doses. The suppression-burst pattern with barbiturates tends to have bursts of higher amplitude than with benzodiazepines; propofol is probably in between these two in that regard.

High doses of almost any centrally acting medication can cause diffuse slowing. Some tend to cause GPEDs as well (as mentioned above), most notoriously baclofen and lithium.

Figure list

Figure 2.1–2.4 Reactivity in coma.

Figure 2.5 Frontal intermittent rhythmic delta activity (FIRDA) vs. artifact; glossokinetic artifact; eye movement artifact.

Figure 2.6 FIRDA.

Figure 2.7–2.9 Diffuse slowing.

Figure 2.10 Intermittent suppression.

Figure 2.11 Unilateral attenuation.

Figure 2.12 Unilateral slowing.

Figure 2.13 Temporal slowing and sharp waves.

Figure 2.14 Periodic lateralized epileptiform discharges (PLEDs).

Figure 2.15–2.16 Breach rhythm.

Figure 2.17 Diffuse slowing and breach.

Figure 2.18 Triphasic waves.

Figure 2.19 14 Hz. Positive spikes.

Figure 2.20–21 Diffuse attenuation.

Figure 2.22 Electrocerebral inactivity.

Figure 2.23 Triphasic waves vs. generalized periodic epileptiform discharges (GPEDs).

Figure 2.24 Myoclonic status epilepticus.

Figure 2.25 Suppression-burst.

Figure 2.26 Suppression-burst plus muscle artifact.

Figure 2.27 Alpha coma.

Figure 2.28 Diffuse slowing.

Figure 2.29 Spindle coma.

Figure 2.30 Nonconvulsive status epilepticus vs. triphasic waves.

Figure 2.31 Nonconvulsive status epilepticus and propofol effect.

Figure 2.32 Barbiturate-induced suppression-burst.

Figure 2.33 Phenytoin toxicity.

Figure 2.34 Barbiturate-induced electrocerebral inactivity.

Figure 2.35 Baclofen toxicity.

Suggested reading

American Electroencephalographic Society (1994) Guideline three: Minimum technical standards for EEG recording in suspected cerebral death. *Journal of Clinical Neurophysiology* **11**, 10–13.

Bahamon-Dussan, J.E., Celesia, G.G. and Grigg-Damberger, M.M. (1989) Prognostic significance of EEG triphasic waves in patients with altered state of consciousness. *Journal of Clinical Neurophysiology* **6**, 313–319.

Banoczi, W.R. (2005) How some drugs affect the electroencephalogram. *American Journal of Endocrine Technology* **45**, 118–129.

Bickford, R.G. and Butt, H.R. (1955) Hepatic coma: The electroencephalographic pattern. *Journal of Clinical Investigation* **34**, 790–799.

Blume, W.T. (2006) Drug effects on EEG. *Journal of Clinical Neurophysiology* **23**, 306–311.

Brenner, R.P. (2005) The interpretation of the EEG in stupor and coma. *Neurologist* **11**, 271–284.

Brenner, R.P., Schwartzman, R.J. and Richey, E.T. (1975) Prognostic significance of episodic low amplitude or relatively isoelectric EEG patterns. *Disease of the Nervous System* **36**, 582–587.

Capparelli, F.J., Diaz, M.F., Hlavnika, A. *et al.* (2005) Cefepime- and cefixime-induced encephalopathy in a patient with normal renal function. *Neurology* **65**, 1840.

Chase, T.N., Moretti, L. and Prensky, A.L. (1968) Clinical and electroencephalographic manifestations of vascular lesions of the pons. *Neurology* **18**, 357–368.

Chatrian, G.E., White, L.W. and Daly, D. (1963) Electroencephalographic patterns resembling those of sleep in certain comatose states after injuries to the head. *Electroencephalography and Clinical Neurophysiology* **15**, 272–280.

Chatrian, G.E., Shaw, C.M. and Leffman, H. (1964) The significance of periodic lateralized epileptiform discharges in EEG: An electrographic, clinical, and pathological study. *Electroencephalography and Clinical Neurophysiology* **17**, 177–193.

Drury, I. (1988) The EEG in hypoxic–ischemic encephalopathy. *American Journal of EEG Technology* **70**, 1–8.

Fisch, B.J. and Klass, D.W. (1988) The diagnostic specificity of triphasic wave patterns. *Electroencephalography and Clinical Neurophysiology* **70**, 1–8.

Hansotia, P., Gottschalk, P., Green, P. *et al.* (1981) Spindle coma: Incidence, clinicopathologic correlates, and prognostic value. *Neurology* **31**, 83–87.

Herkes, G.K., Wszolek, Z.K., Westmoreland, B.F. *et al.* (1992) Effects of midazolam on electroencephalograms of seriously ill patients. *Mayo Clinic Procedure* **67**, 334–338.

Hockaday, J.M., Potts, F., Epstein, E. *et al.* (1965) Electroencephalographic changes in acute cerebral anoxia from cardiac or respiratory arrest. *Electroencephalography and Clinical Neurophysiology* **18**, 575–586.

Hormes, J.T., Benarroch, E.E., Rodriguez, M. *et al.* (1988) Periodic sharp waves in baclofen-induced encephalopathy. *Archives of Neurology* **45**, 814–815.

Hughes, J.R. (1980) Correlations between EEG and chemical changes in uremia. *Electroencephalography and Clinical Neurophysiology* **48**, 583–594.

Husain, A. (2006) Electroencephalographic assessment of coma. *Journal of Clinical Neurophysiology* **23**, 208–220.

Kaplan, P.W., Genoud, D., Ho, T.W. *et al.* (1999) Etiology, neurologic correlations, and prognosis in alpha coma. *Clinical Neurophysiology* **110**, 205–213.

Kaplan, P.W., Genoud, D., Ho, T.W. *et al.* (2000) Clinical correlates and prognosis in early spindle coma. *Journal of Clinical Neurophysiology* **111**, 584–590.

Karnaze, D.S. and Bickford, R.G. (1984) Triphasic waves: A reassessment of their significance. *Electroencephalography and Clinical Neurophysiology* **57**, 193–198.

Kuroiwa, Y. and Celesia, G.C. (1980) Clinical significance of periodic EEG patterns. *Archives of Neurology* **37**, 15–20.

Markand, O.N. (1976) Electroencephalogram in "locked-in" syndrome. *Electroencephalography and Clinical Neurophysiology* **40**, 529–534.

Rae-Grant, A.D., Strapple, C. and Barbour, P.J. (1991) Episodic low-amplitude events: an under-recognized phenomenon in clinical electroencephalography. *Journal of Clinical Neurophysiology* **8**, 203–11.

Reeves, A.L., Westmoreland, B.F. and Klass, D.W. (1997) Clinical accompaniments of the burst-suppression EEG pattern. *Journal of Clinical Neurophysiology* **14**, 150–153.

Schauble, B., Castillo, P.R., Boeve, B.F. *et al.* (2003) EEG findings in steroid-responsive encephalopathy associated with autoimmune thyroiditis. *Clinical Neurophysiology* **114**, 32–37.

Simonian, N.A., Gilliam, F.G. and Chiappa, K.H. (1993) Ifosfamide causes a diazepam-sensitive encephalopathy. *Neurology* **43**, 2700–2702.

Smith, S.J. and Kocen, R.S. (1988) A Creutzfeldt-Jakob like syndrome due to lithium toxicity. *Journal of Neurology, Neurosurgery & Psychiatry* **51**, 120–123.

Sundaram, M.B.M. and Blume, W.T. (1987) Triphasic waves: clinical correlates and morphology. *Canadian Journal of Neurological Sciences* **14**, 136–140.

Synek, V.M. (1988) Prognostically important EEG coma patterns in diffuse anoxic and traumatic encephalopathies in adults. *Journal of Clinical Neurophysiology* **5**, 161–174.

Van Cott, A.C. and Brenner, R.P. (2003) *Drug effects and toxic encephalopathies*. In: Ebersole, J.S. and Pedley, T.A. (eds), *Current Practice of Clinical Electroencephalography*, pp. 463–482. Lippincott, Williams and Wilkins, Philadelphia.

Westmoreland, B.F., Klass, D.W., Sharbrough, F.W. *et al.* (1975) Alpha-coma: electroencephalographic, clinical, pathologic and etiologic correlations. *Archives of Neurology* **32**, 713–718.

Wieser, H.G., Schindler, K. and Zumsteg, D. (2006) EEG in Creutzfeldt-Jakob disease. *Clinical Neurophysiology* **117**, 935–951

Wijdicks, E.F.M., Parisi, J.E. and Sharbrough, F.W. (1994) Prognostic value of myoclonus status in comatose survivors of cardiac arrest. *Annals of Neurology* **35**, 239–243.

Yamashita, S., Morinaga, T., Ohgo, S. *et al.* (1995) Prognostic value of electroencephalogram (EEG) in anoxic encephalopathy after cardiopulmonary resuscitation: relationship among anoxic period, EEG grading and outcome. *Internal Medicine* **34**, 71–76.

Yemisci, M., Gurer, G., Saygi, S. *et al.* (2003) Generalised periodic epileptiform discharges: Clinical features, neuroradiological evaluation and prognosis in 37 adult patients. *Seizure* **12**, 465–472.

Young, G.B., Blume, W.T., Campbell, V.M. *et al.* (1994) Alpha, theta and alpha-theta coma: a clinical outcome study utilizing serial recordings. *Electroencephalography and Clinical Neurophysiology* **91**, 93–99.

Young, G.B., McLachlan, R.S., Kreeft, J.H. *et al.* (1997) An electroencephalographic classification for coma. *Canadian Journal of Neurological Sciences* **24**, 320–325.

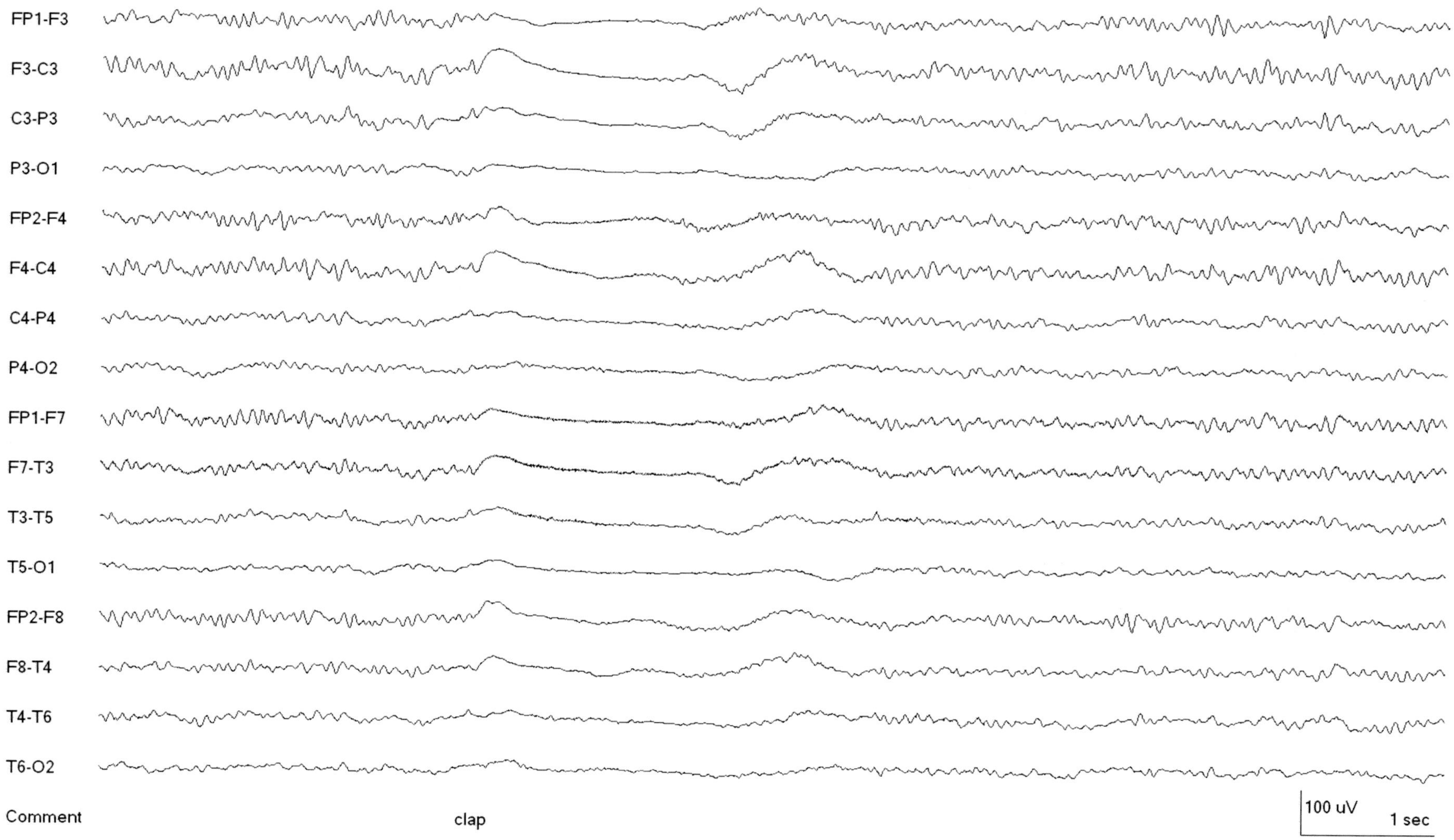

Figure 2.1 Reactivity in coma. A 32-year-old woman with decreased mental status and an elevated ammonia level. Alerting (in this case clapping) resulted in a period of diffuse attenuation, demonstrating a reactive record.

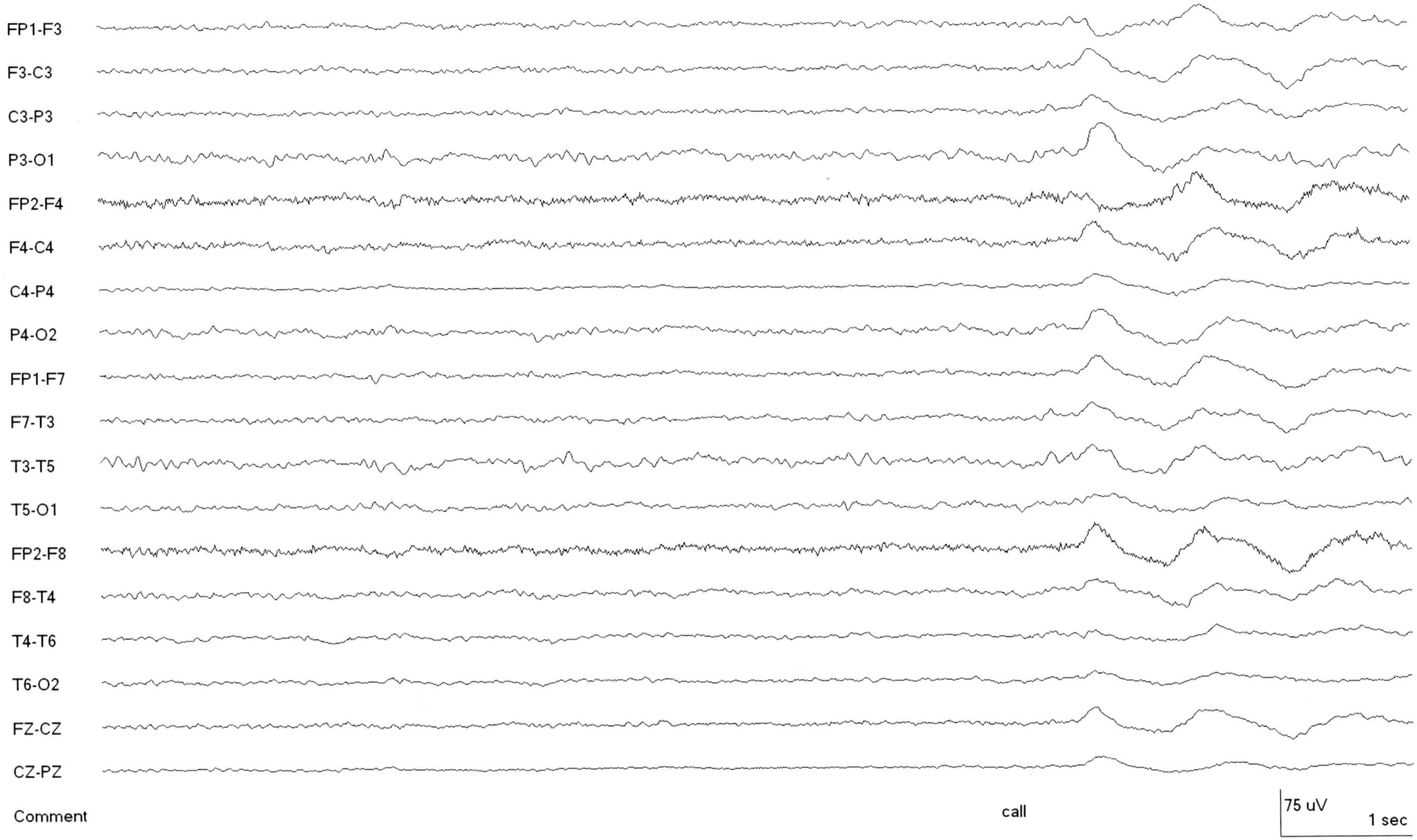

Figure 2.2 Reactivity in coma. The EEG in this 23-year-old comatose woman status post (s/p) traumatic brain injury shows generalized bursts of delta activity when called. Although the EEG demonstrates reactivity, clinically the patient was unchanged. Reactivity indicates a lighter level of coma.

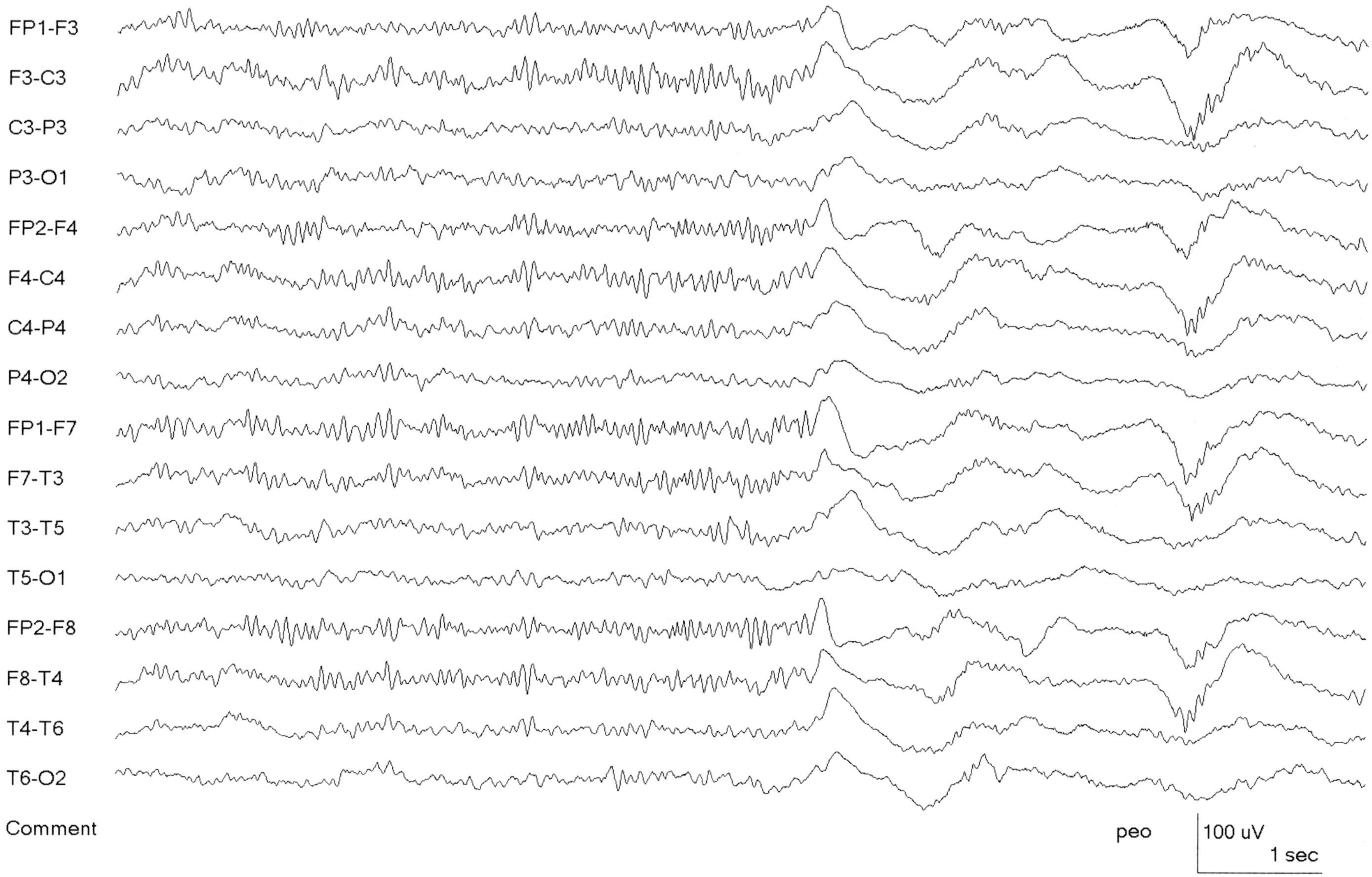

Figure 2.3 Reactivity. The EEG in this 31-year-old woman receiving propofol shows reactivity when eyes are passively opened. There is attenuation of faster background activity followed by bursts of higher amplitude delta activity.

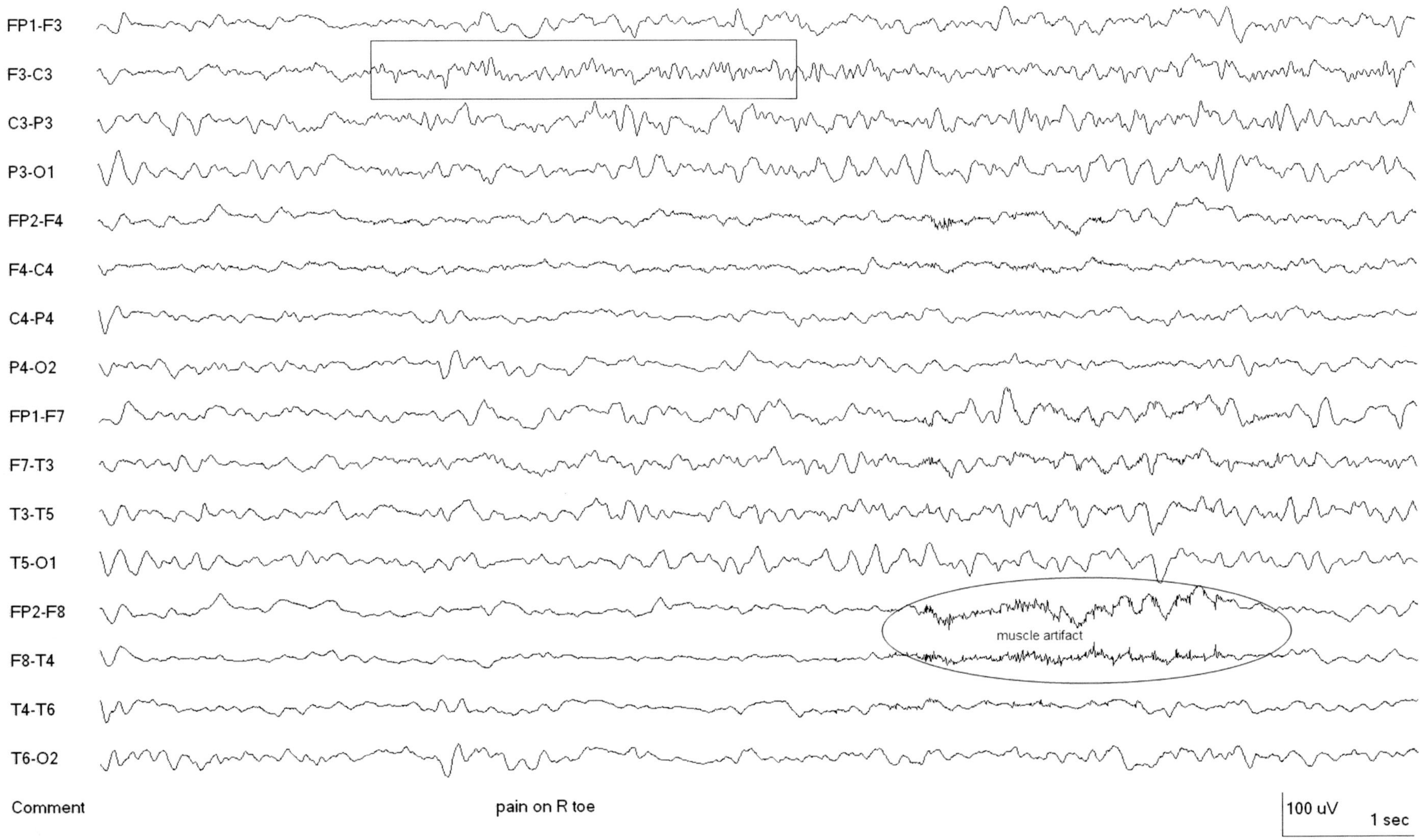

Figure 2.4 Unilateral reactivity. This 80-year-old woman suffered a right hemispheric stroke. The beginning of this EEG shows a mild asymmetry with attenuation in the right hemisphere. After painful stimulation of the right toe (labeled), there is an increase in faster frequency activity on the left (box), but the right hemisphere remains attenuated.

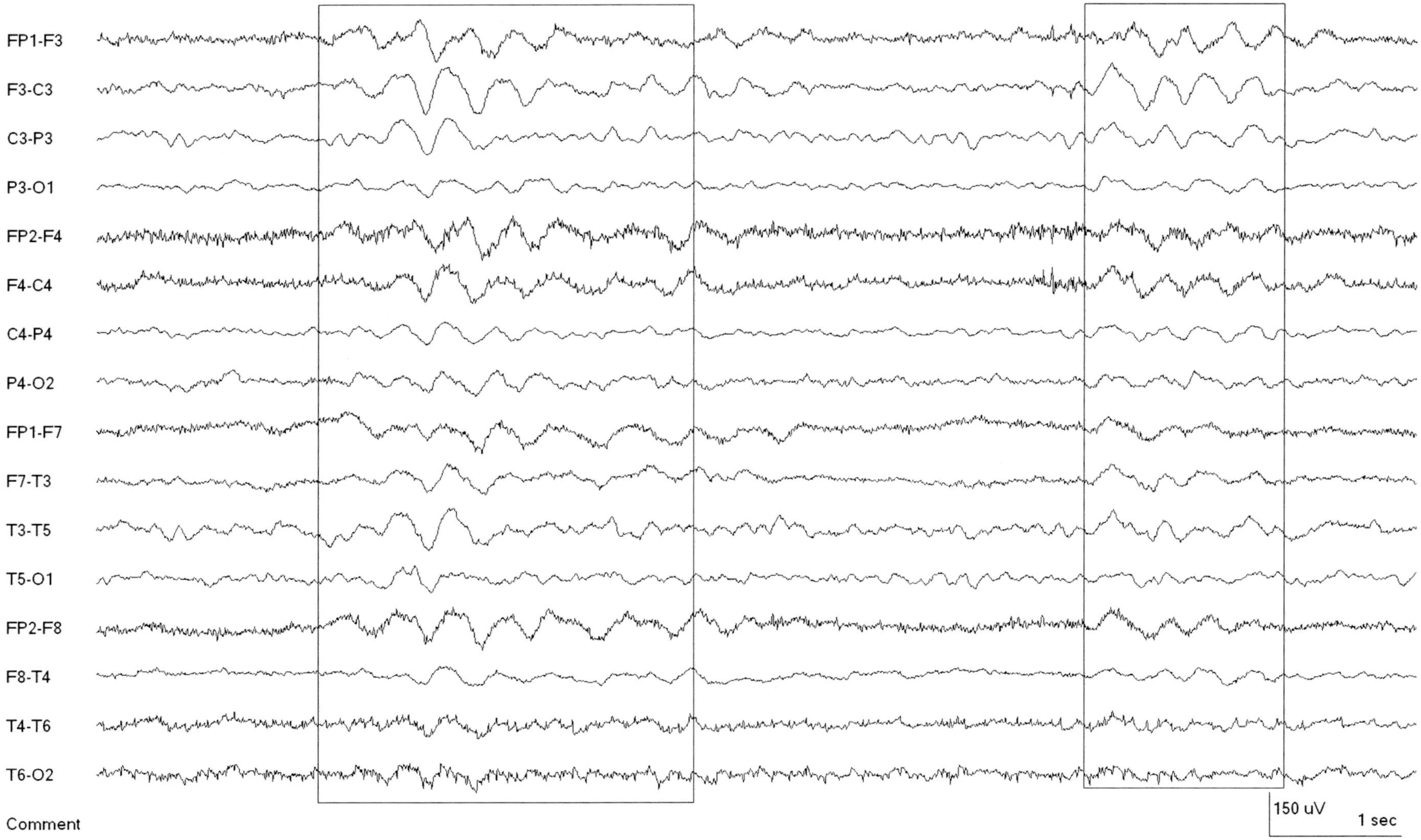

Figure 2.5 FIRDA versus artifact. (a) The EEG in this 61-year-old man shows several generalized bursts of frontal intermittent rhythmic delta activity (FIRDA) on a longitudinal bipolar montage. This is a nonspecific abnormality.

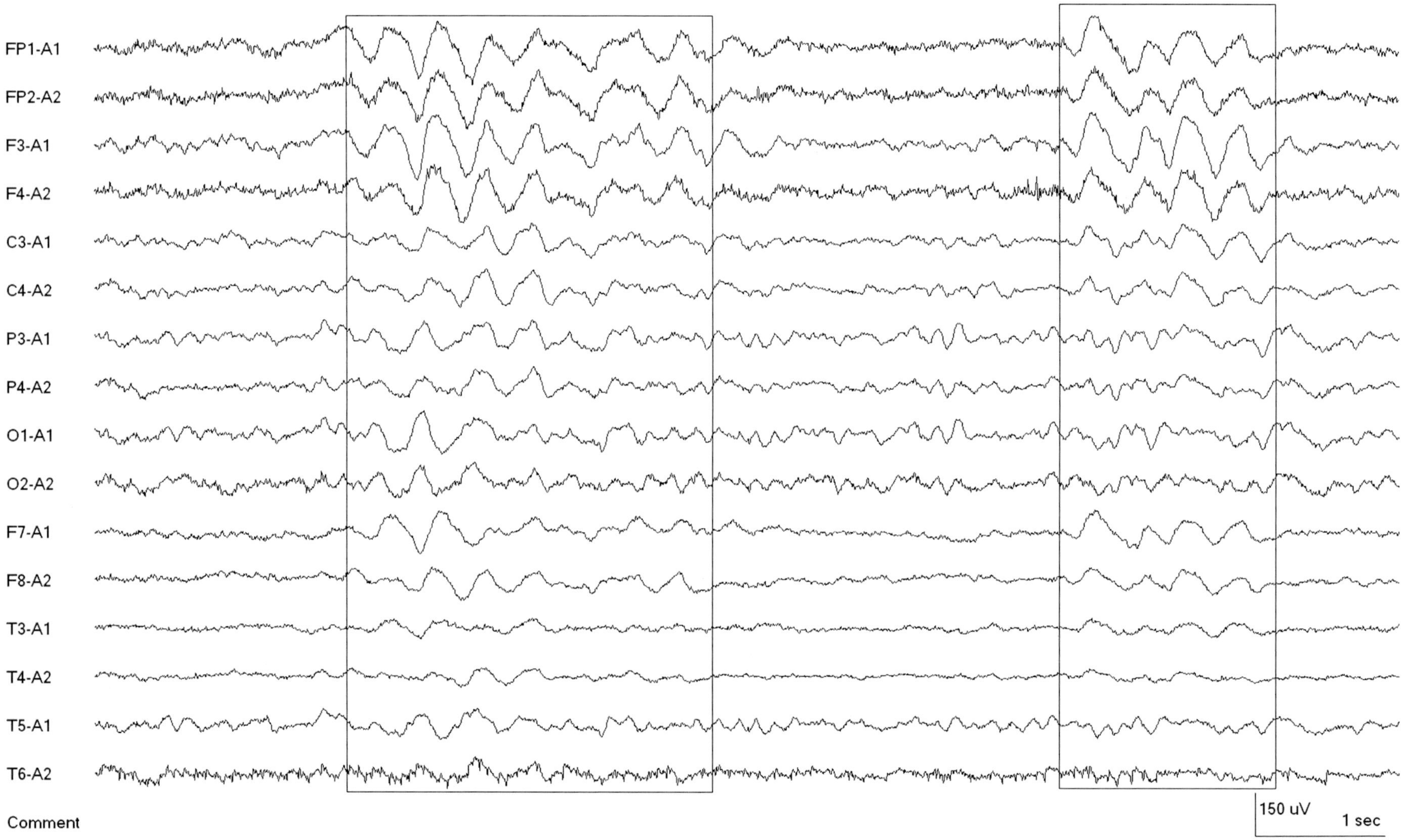

Figure 2.5 (*Continued*) (b) The same epoch reformatted to a referential montage to ipsilateral ears. The bursts of rhythmic delta are maximal anteriorly. The field indicates that this could not be vertical eye movements since complexes are not greater in Fp1 and Fp2 than they are in electrodes F3 and F4. However, it is possible that this could represent tongue movement (glossokinetic potential artifact, GKP) – see part c.

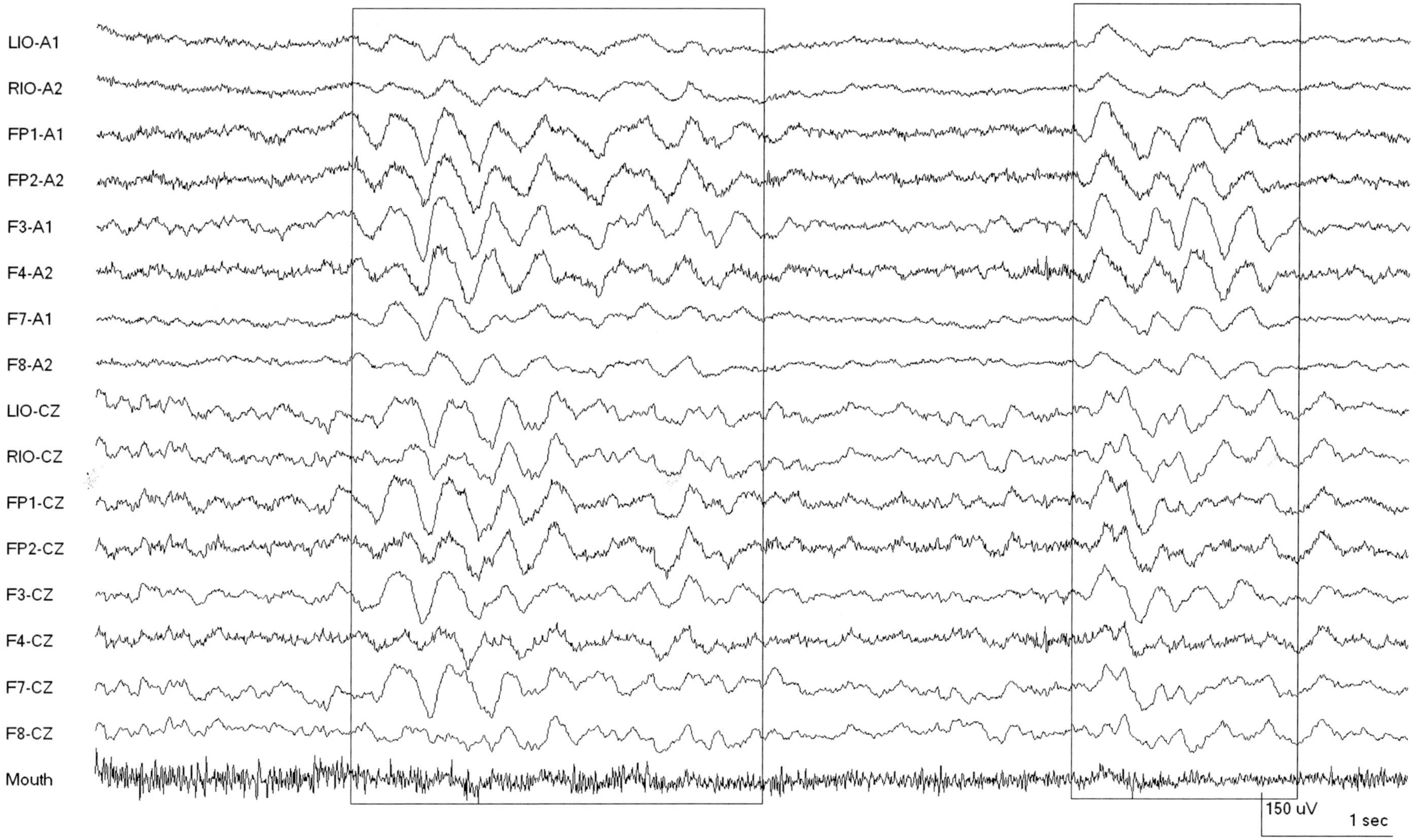

Figure 2.5 (*Continued*) (c) Additional electrodes have been placed below the eyes as well as electrodes placed above and below the mouth. The bursts of delta activity are in-phase between the inferior orbital electrodes (LIO and RIO) and electrodes Fp1 and Fp2. If they were vertical eye movements, the inferior orbital electrodes would always be out-of-phase with Fp1 and Fp2. Furthermore, if it were a glossokinetic potential artifact, the discharges would be of higher voltage in inferior orbital electrodes since they are closer to the tongue than are electrodes Fp1 and Fp2. In addition, electrodes placed about the mouth (last channel) would show the highest amplitude discharge if it were a tongue movement. As indicated, the bursts are not detected by these electrodes and are cerebral potentials, i.e. FIRDA.

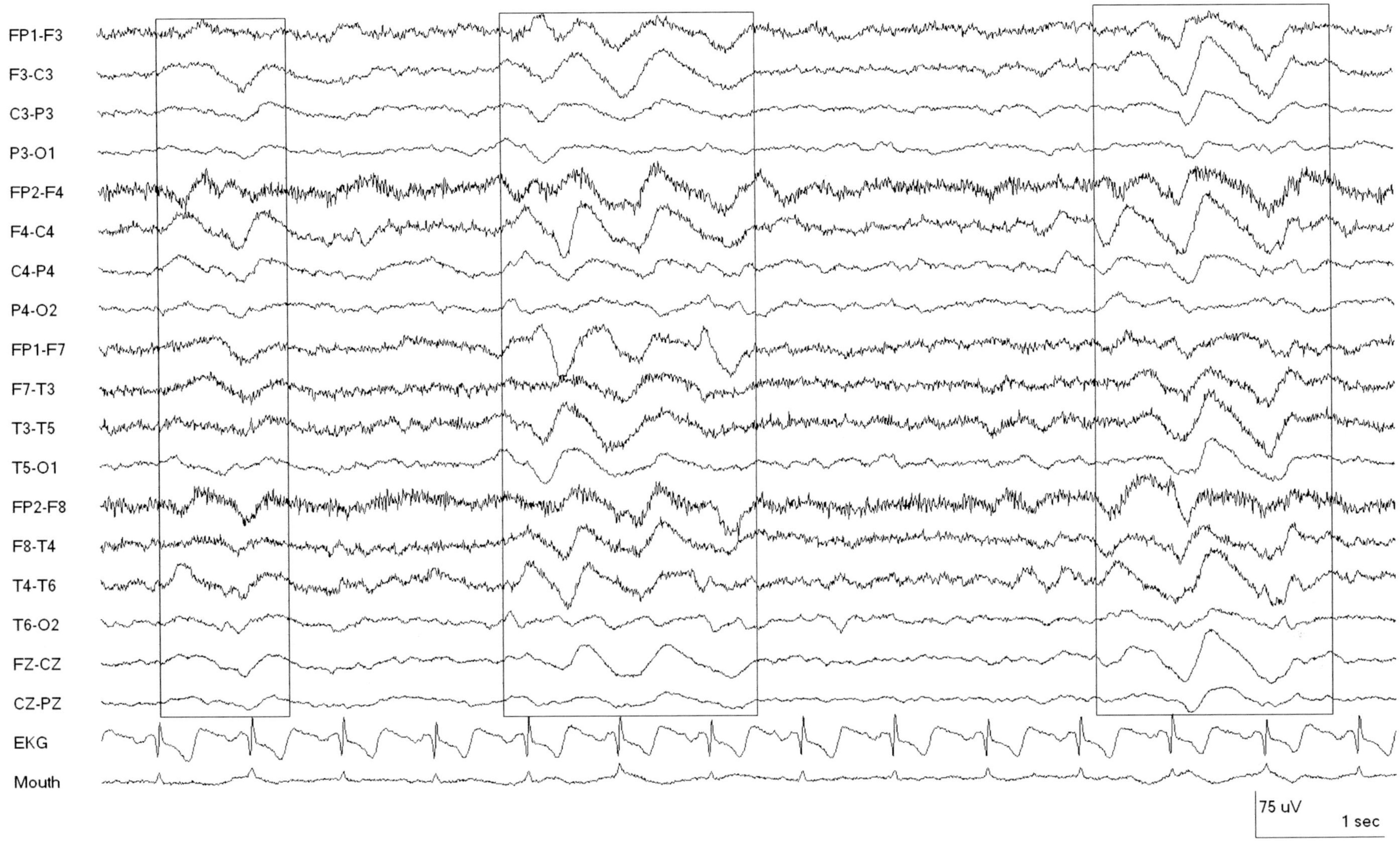

Figure 2.6 FIRDA. FIRDA (frontal intermittent rhythmic delta activity) is present in the EEG of this comatose 63-year-old woman s/p liver transplant. There is also diffuse background slowing.

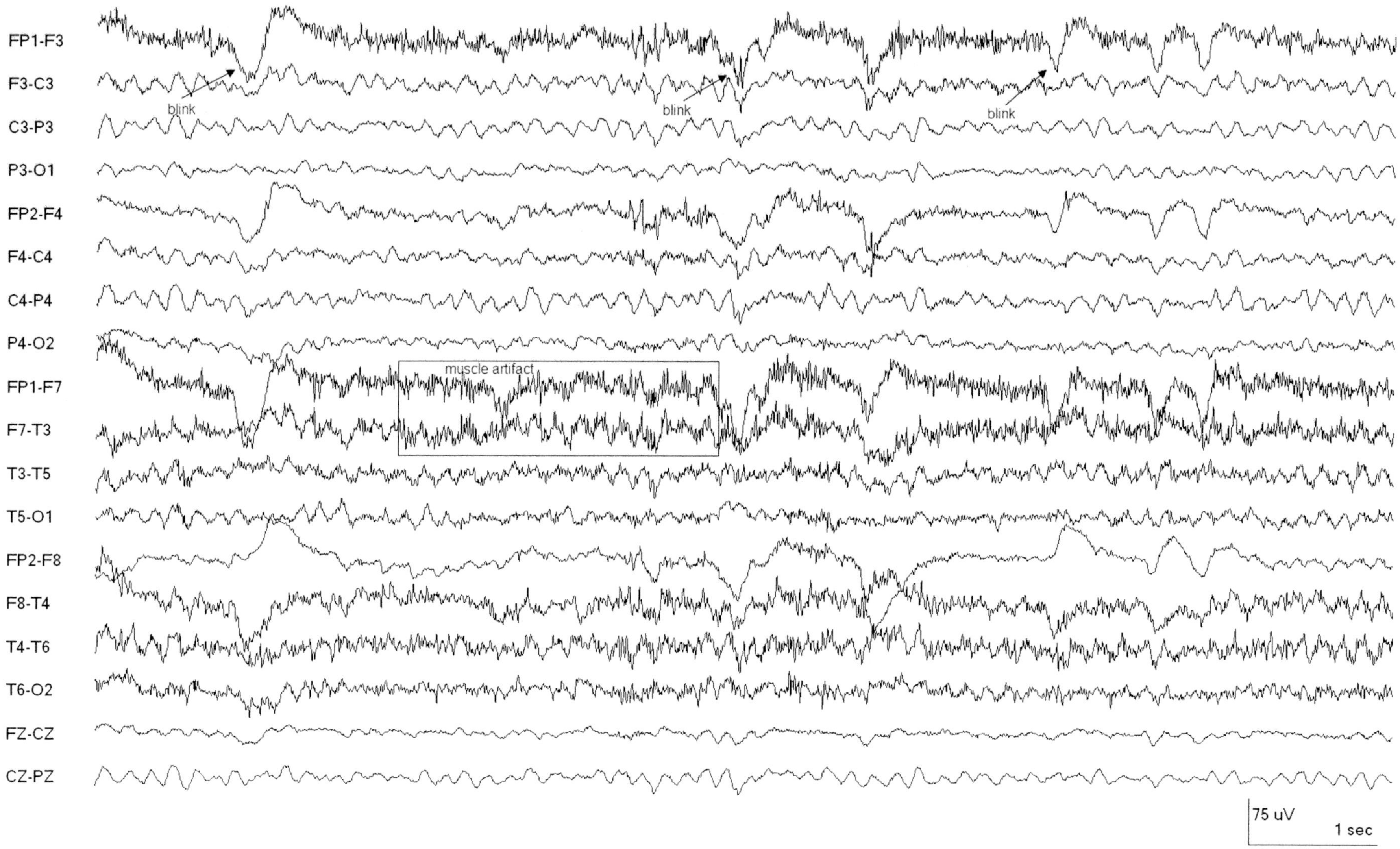

Figure 2.7 Mild diffuse slowing. The EEG in this 72-year-old man with renal failure shows mild diffuse slowing of background rhythms (mostly 6–7 Hz). The patient is awake, as evidenced by muscle artifact (especially at Fp1-F7 and F7-T3) and eye blinks (arrows).

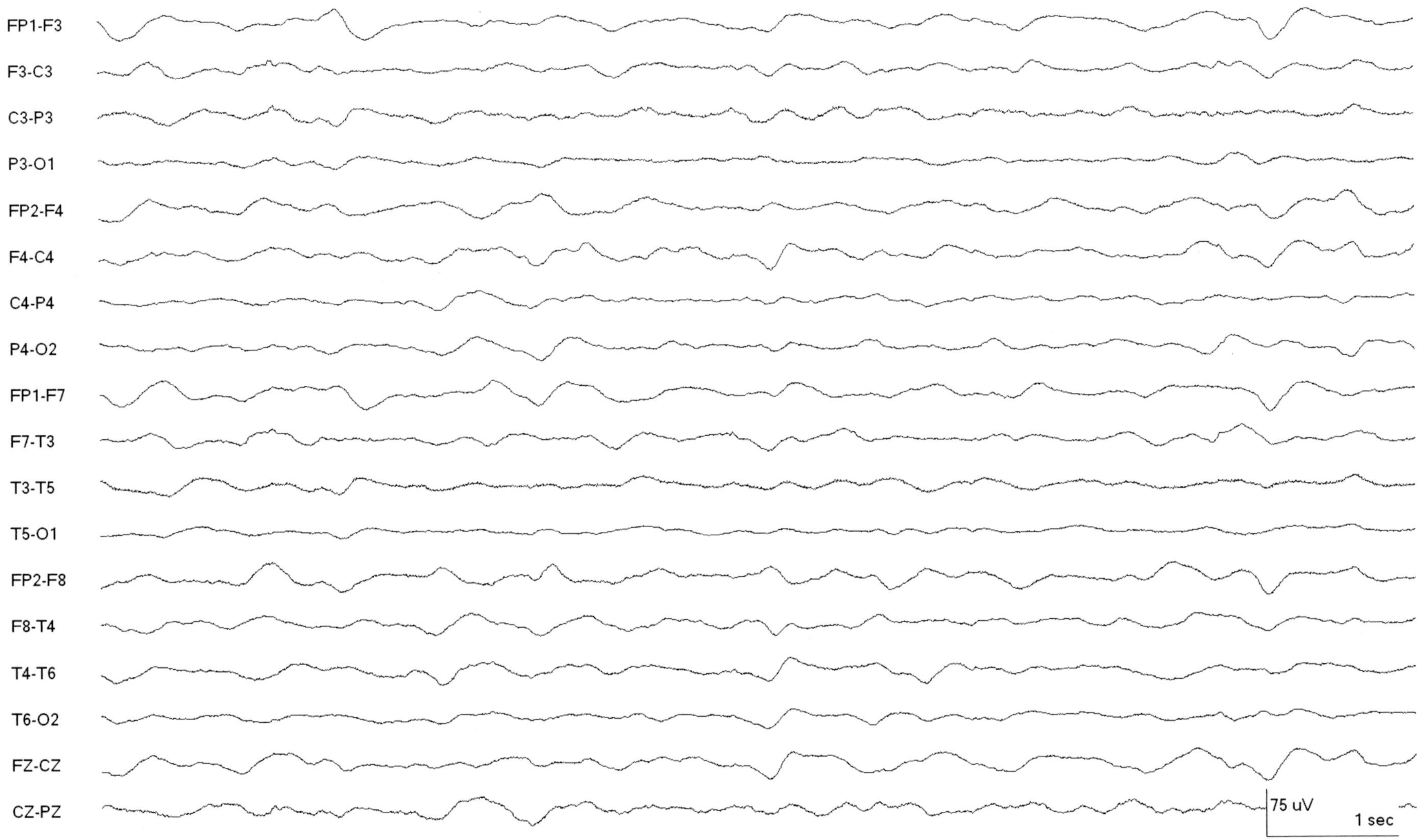

Figure 2.8 Diffuse slowing. The EEG in this 46-year-old man with hepatic encephalopathy shows marked diffuse symmetrical slowing and attenuation, with activity predominantly in the slow delta range along with absence of faster frequencies.

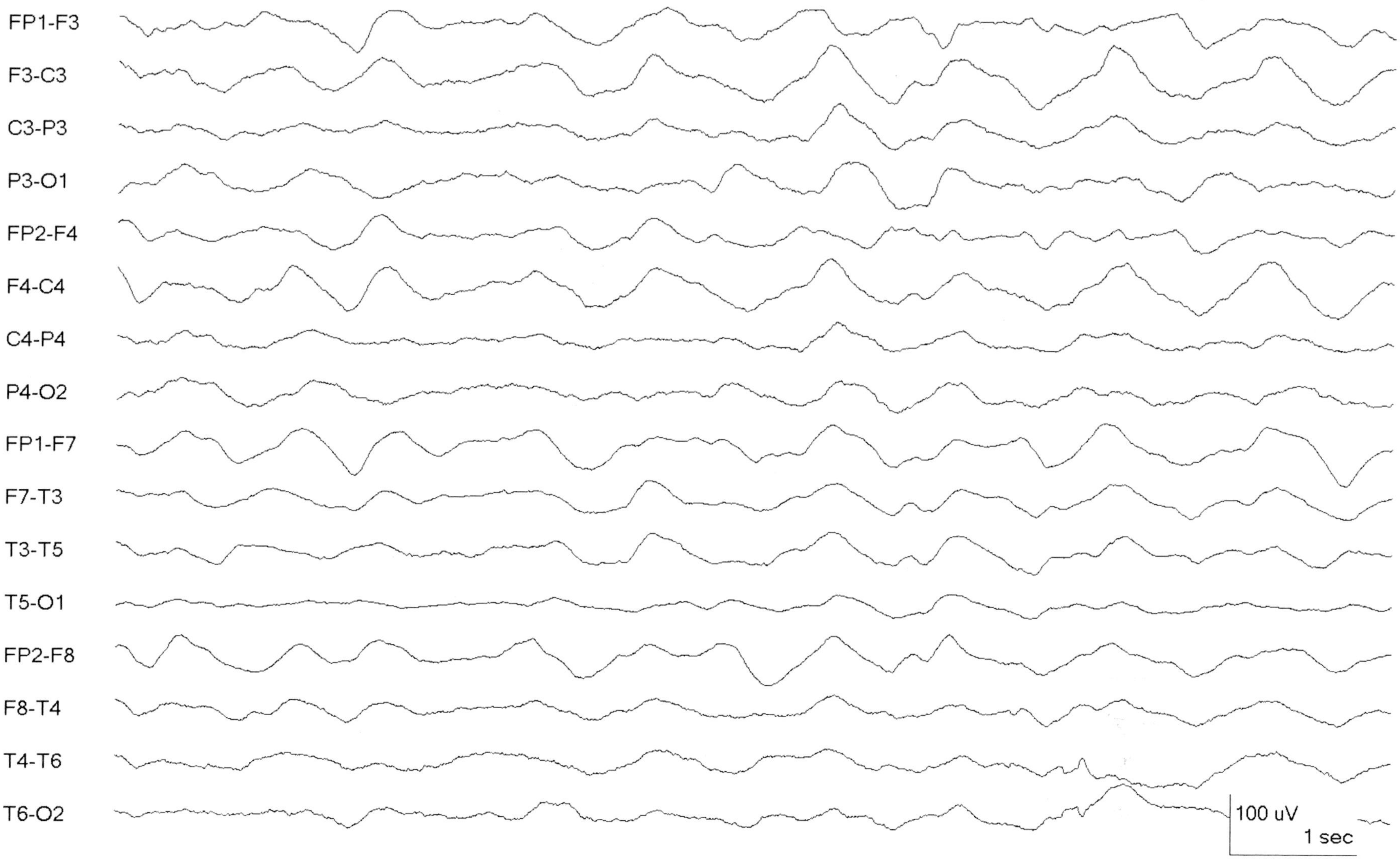

Figure 2.9 Diffuse slowing. The EEG in this 17-year-old comatose man involved in a motor vehicle accident shows marked diffuse slowing, predominantly in the 1–2 Hz (slow delta), and diffuse attenuation with no faster activity.

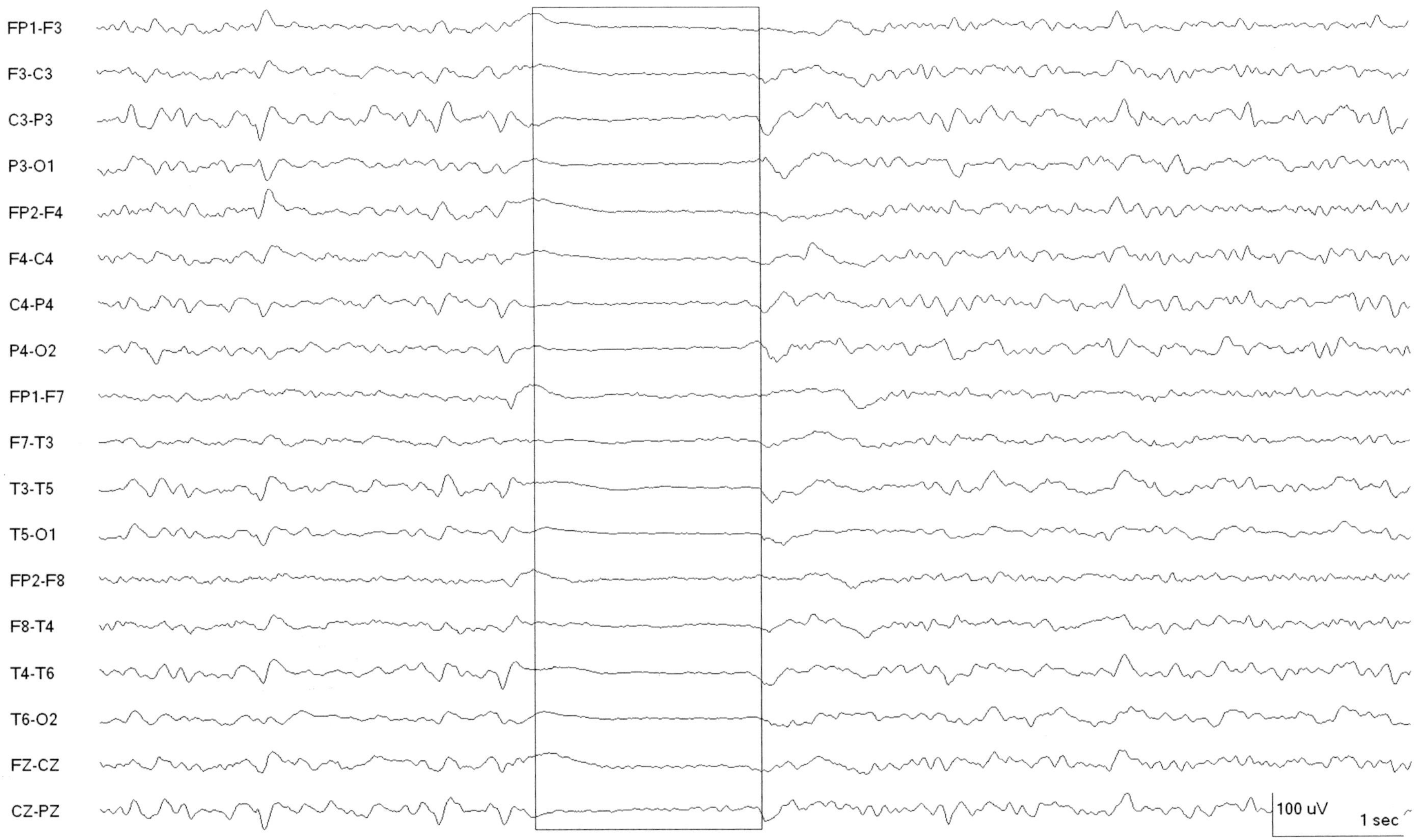

Figure 2.10 Intermittent suppression. The EEG in this 84-year-old woman shows a sudden 2 s period of suppression, not related to stimulation. She was receiving propofol. This is a nonspecific abnormality usually signifying moderate-to-severe encephalopathy.

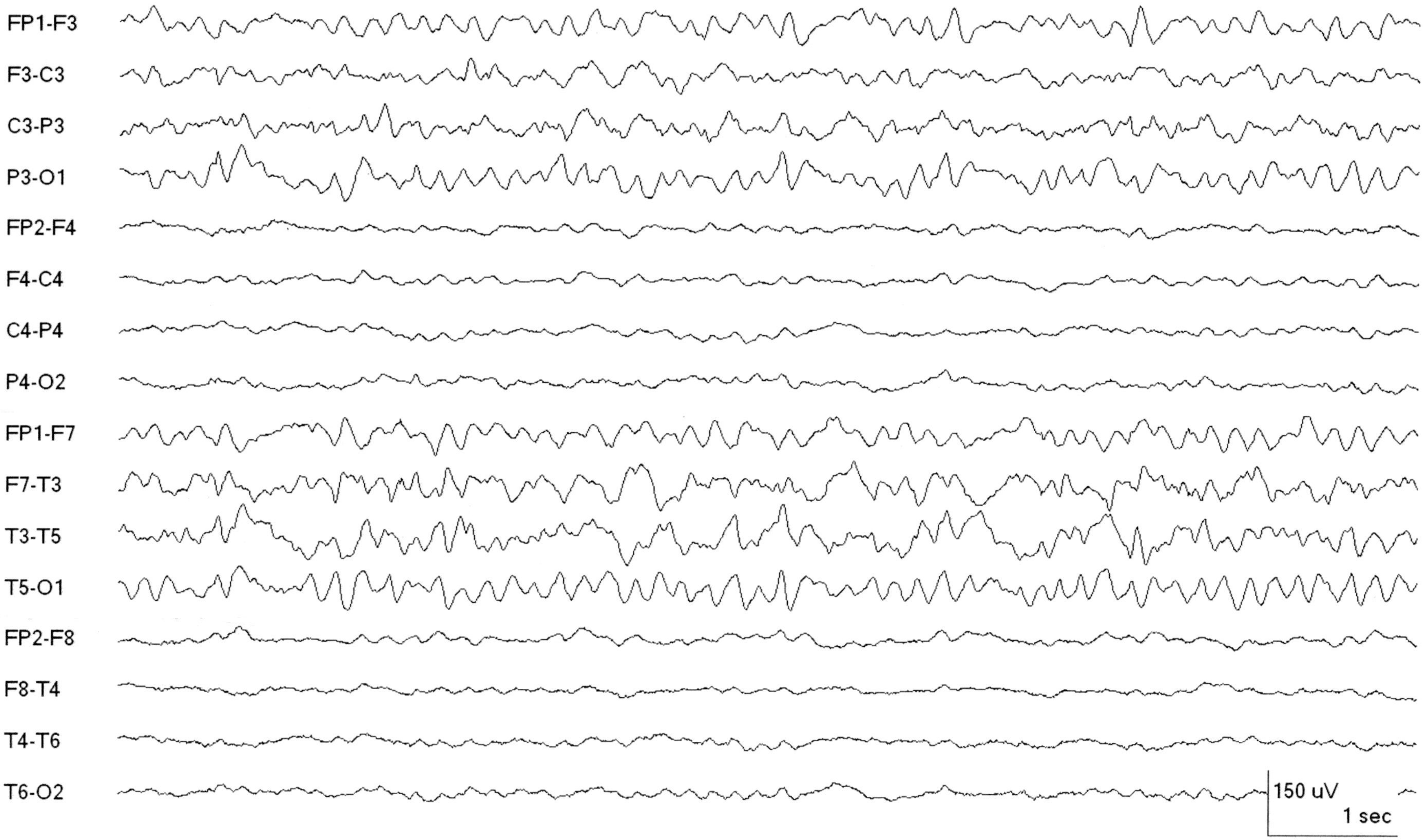

Figure 2.11 Unilateral attenuation. The EEG in this 48-year-old man shows marked hemispheric differences. Background activity is suppressed on the right. This could also be interpreted as increased voltage on the left and perhaps due to a skull defect; however, in this case it was due to a severe right cerebral contusion.

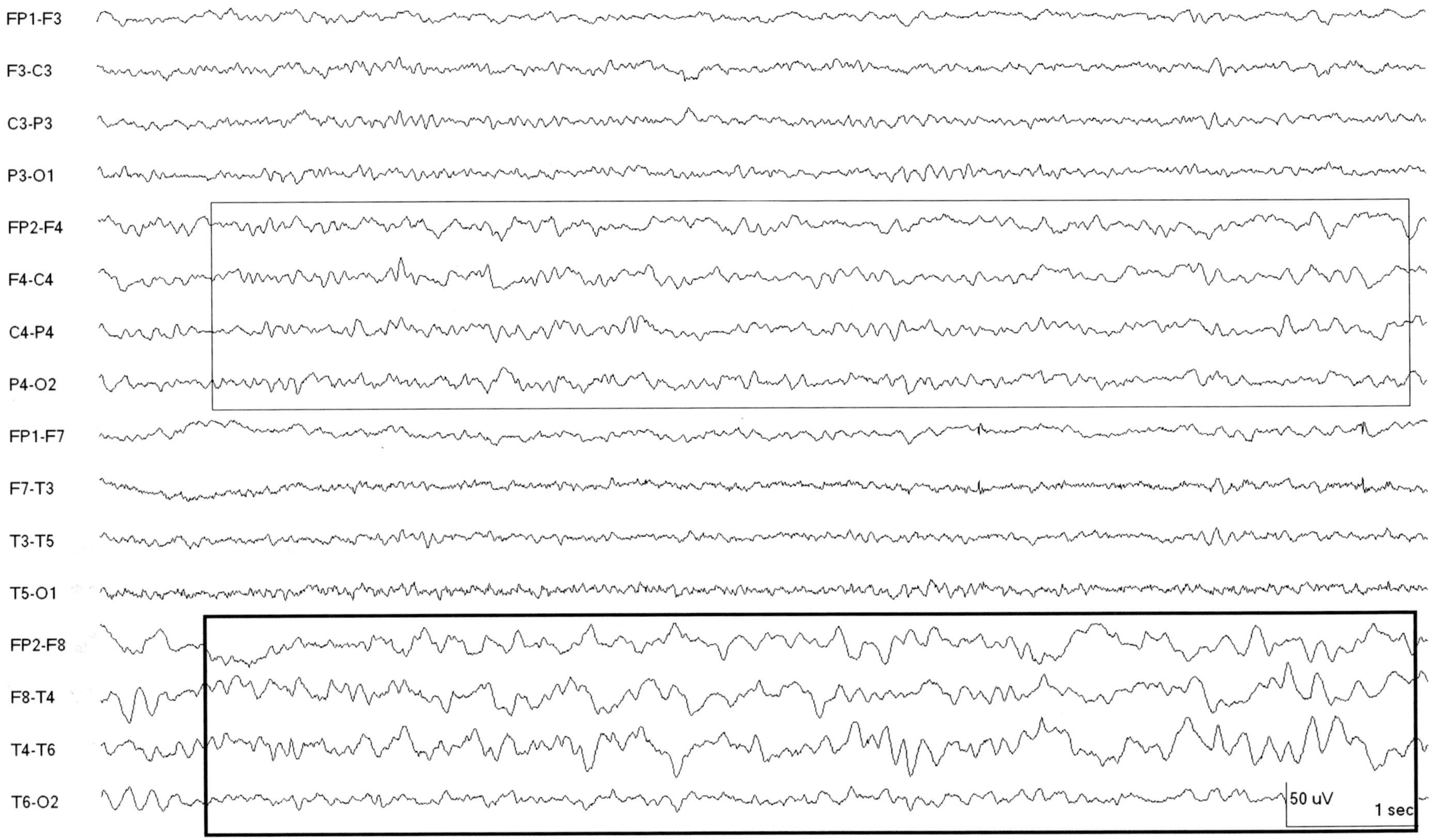

Figure 2.12 Unilateral slowing. This 40-year-old woman with a subarachnoid hemorrhage subsequently developed a right middle cerebral artery stroke. The EEG shows prominent slowing over the right side, most marked in the temporal region (box with thicker border), but also present in the parasagittal region (box with thinner border).

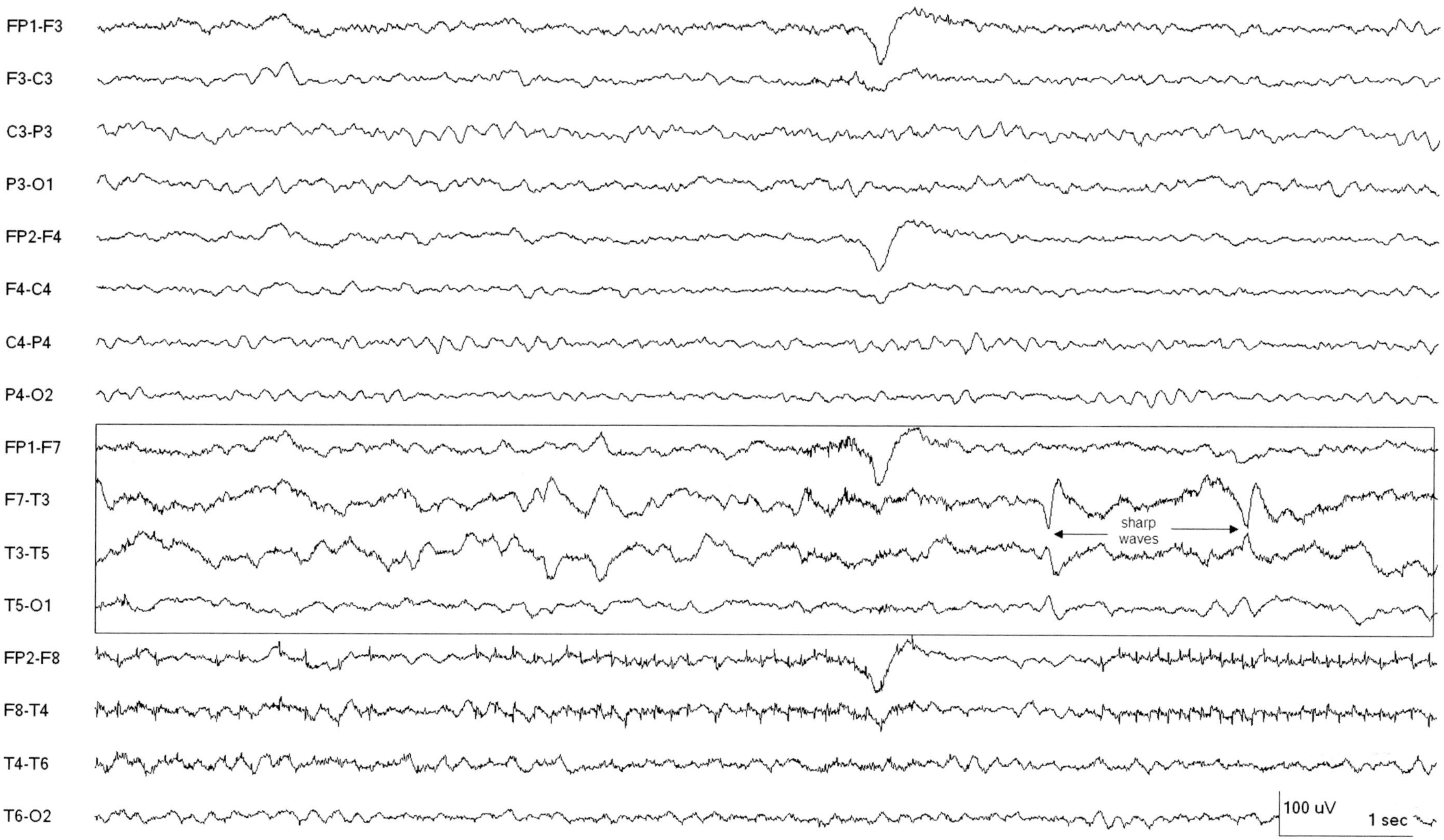

Figure 2.13 Temporal slowing and sharp waves. The EEG in this 55-year-old woman with a left-sided cerebral tumor shows prominent focal slowing, most marked in the left temporal region (box), as well as sharp waves (arrows) indicating epileptogenic potential, maximal in the mid-temporal area (electrode T3, where it is phase reversing on this bipolar recording).

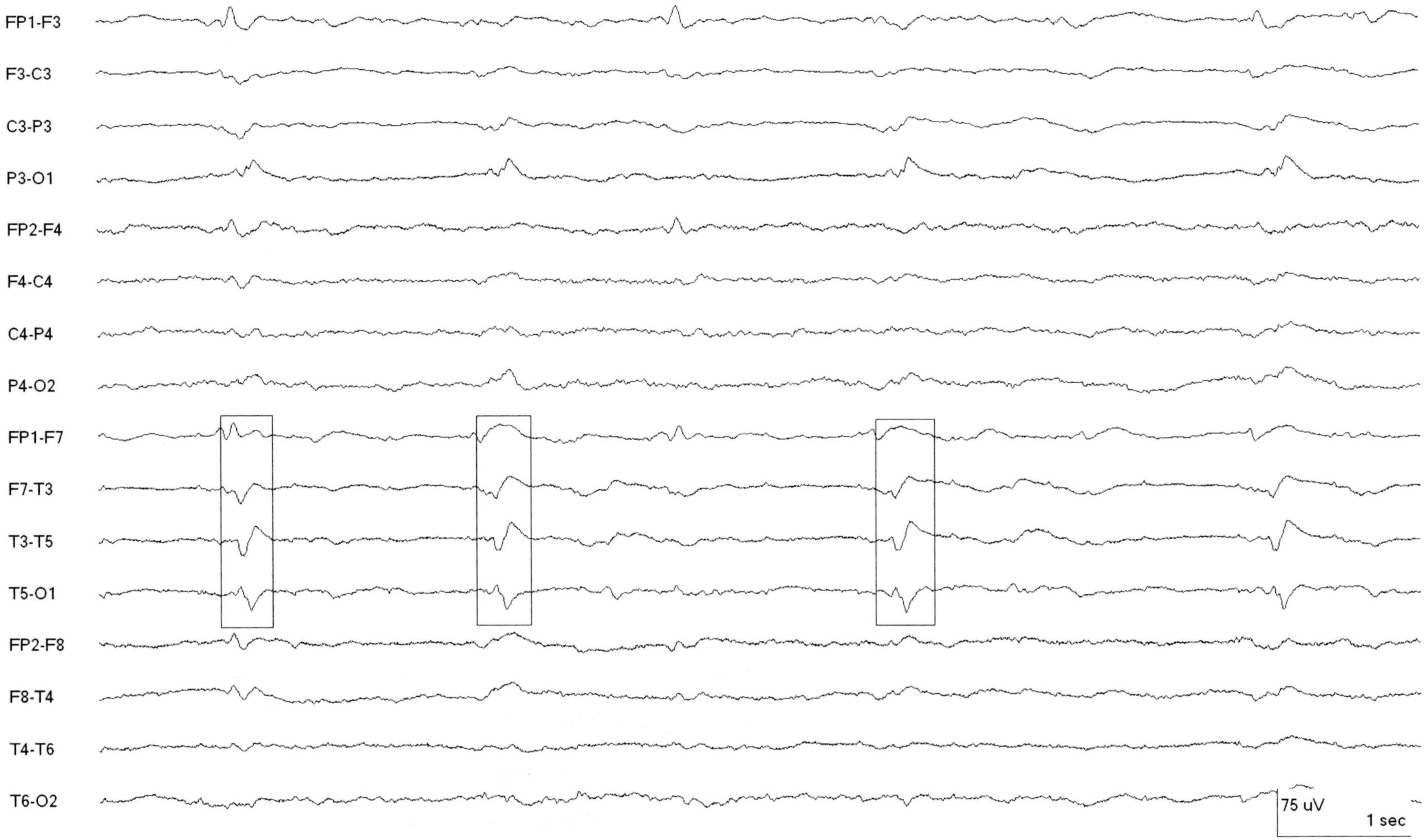

Figure 2.14 PLEDs. The EEG in this 66-year-old man with a history of a left hemispheric infarct was being evaluated for unresponsiveness following a generalized tonic–clonic seizure. The EEG shows left-sided PLEDs recurring every 1.5–3 s (0.3–0.75 discharges/s) and maximal in the left posterior temporal region (phase reversing at T5; boxes). The presence of PLEDs suggests a highly epileptogenic focus.

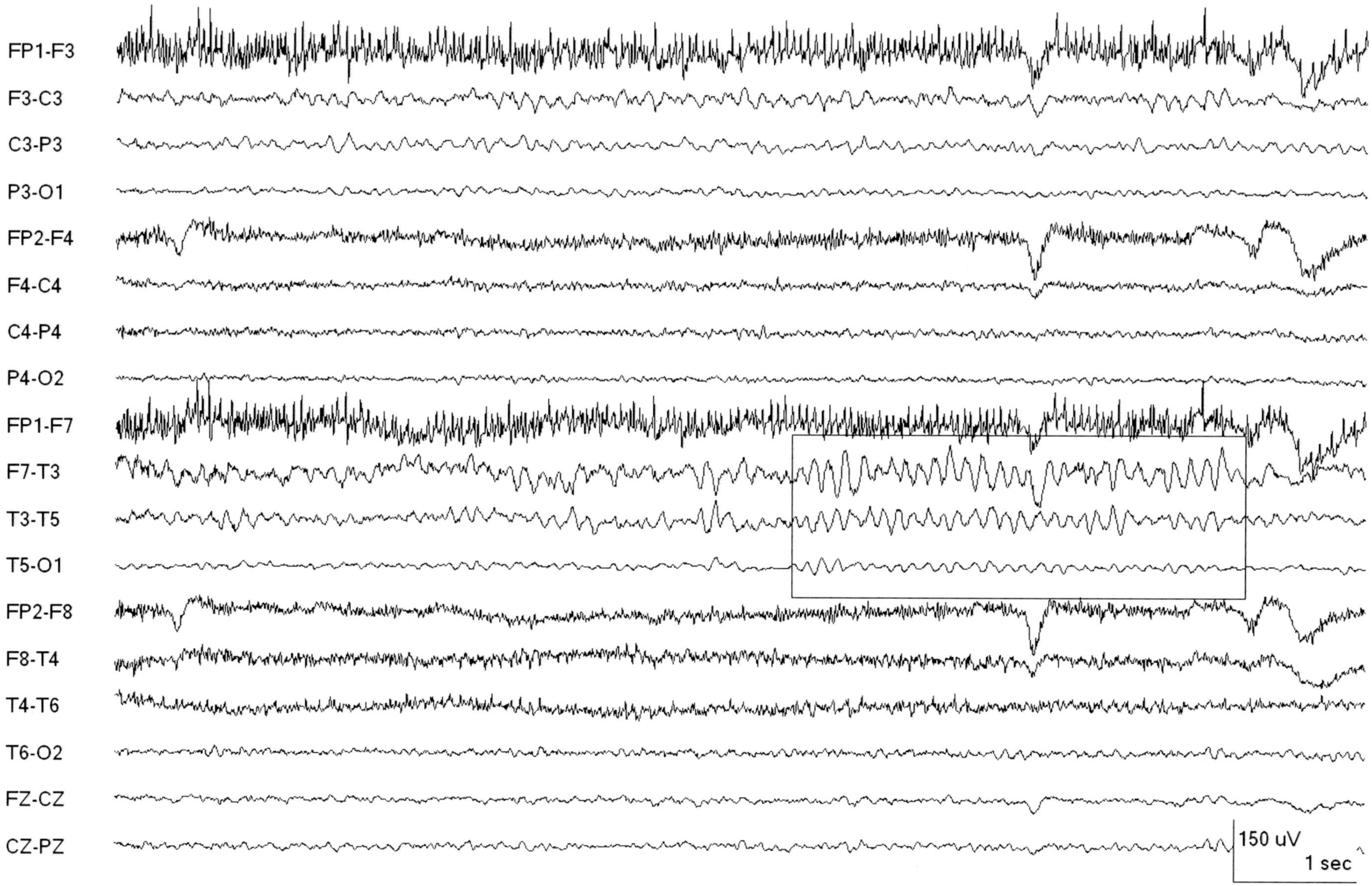

Figure 2.15 Breach rhythm. A 63-year-old woman s/p left frontal aneurysm clipping. This EEG shows higher amplitudes of faster frequencies on the left compared to the right, most prominent at T3 (left temporal; box). This is due to a skull defect on the left. In the presence of a skull defect (even a small one such as a skull fracture or burr hole), faster frequencies appear higher amplitude and often sharper, resulting in what is known as a breach rhythm or breach effect.

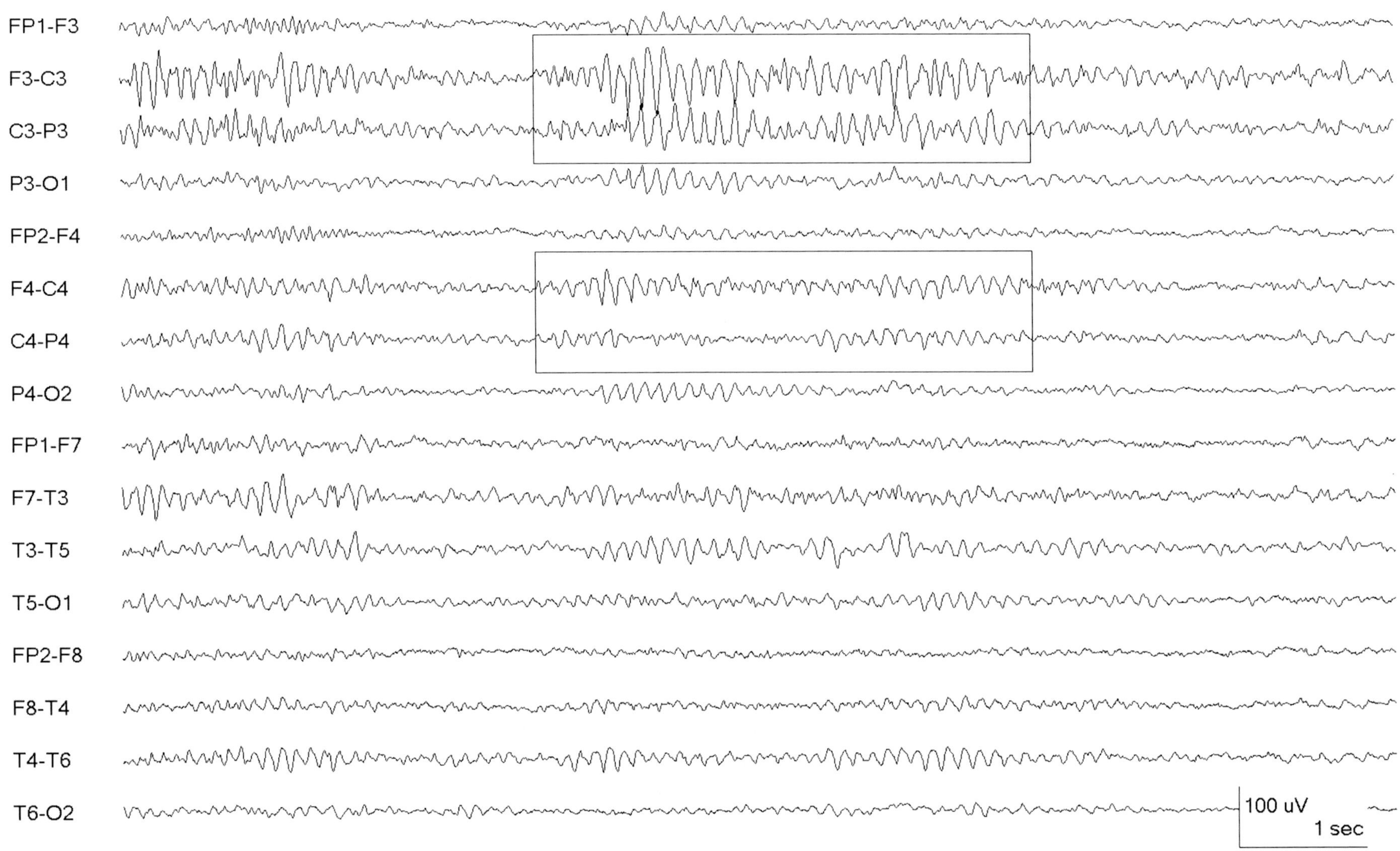

Figure 2.16 Breach rhythm. There is a marked asymmetry of background activity in central areas in this 75-year-old man with activity being of greater voltage on the left (C3 vs C4, boxes). The patient has had previous surgery in this area and this represents a breach rhythm due to the skull defect. Although at times this can be very spiky in appearance, this does not signify epileptogenic potential.

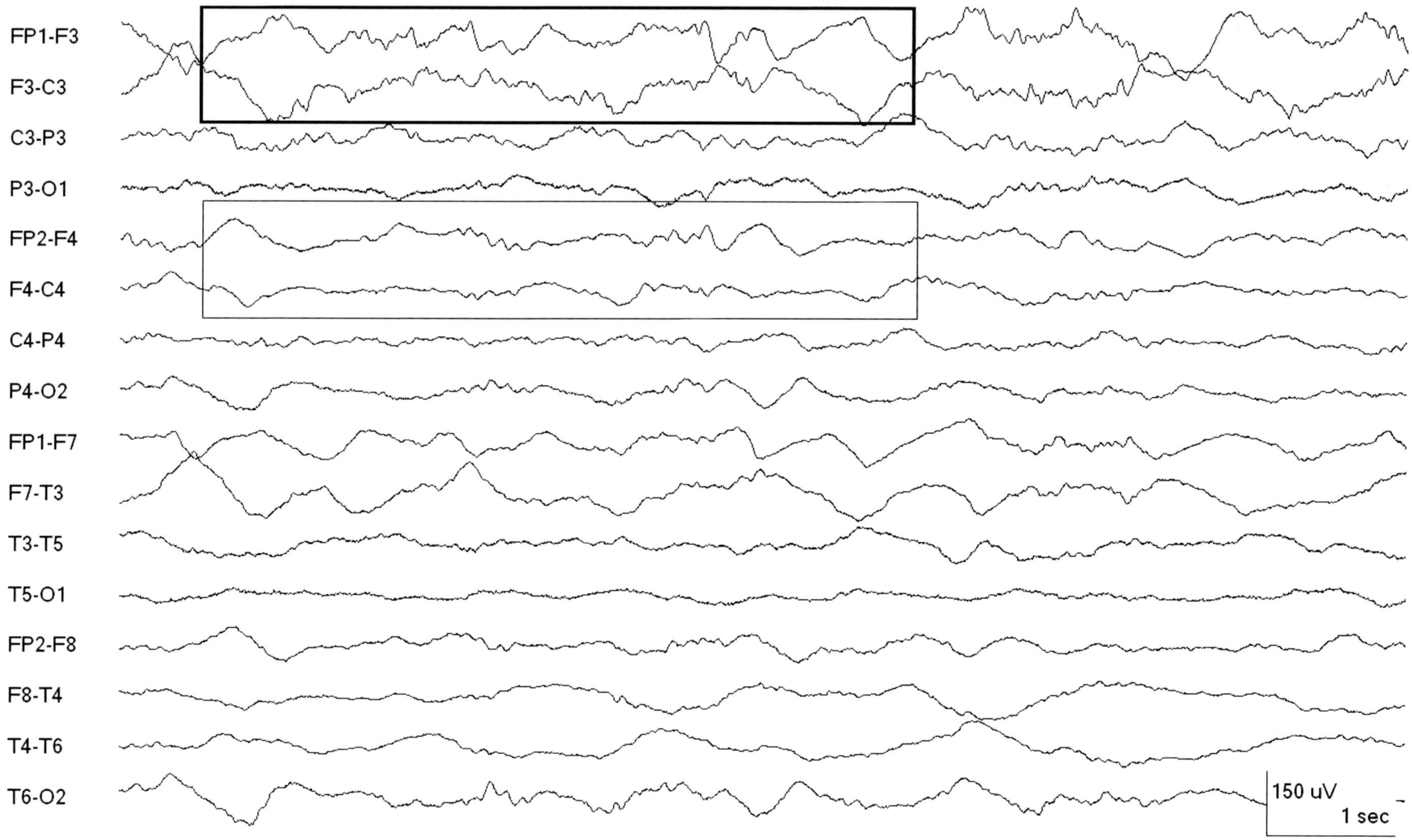

Figure 2.17 Diffuse slowing and breach. (a) The EEG in this 26-year-old comatose male s/p motor vehicle accident shows diffuse slowing. Background slowing is most marked anteriorly. It is of higher voltage on the left, as is the faster activity, especially at F3 (darker box; compare to F4, lighter box). The higher amplitude with faster activity on the left is due to his known left-sided skull defect (breach).

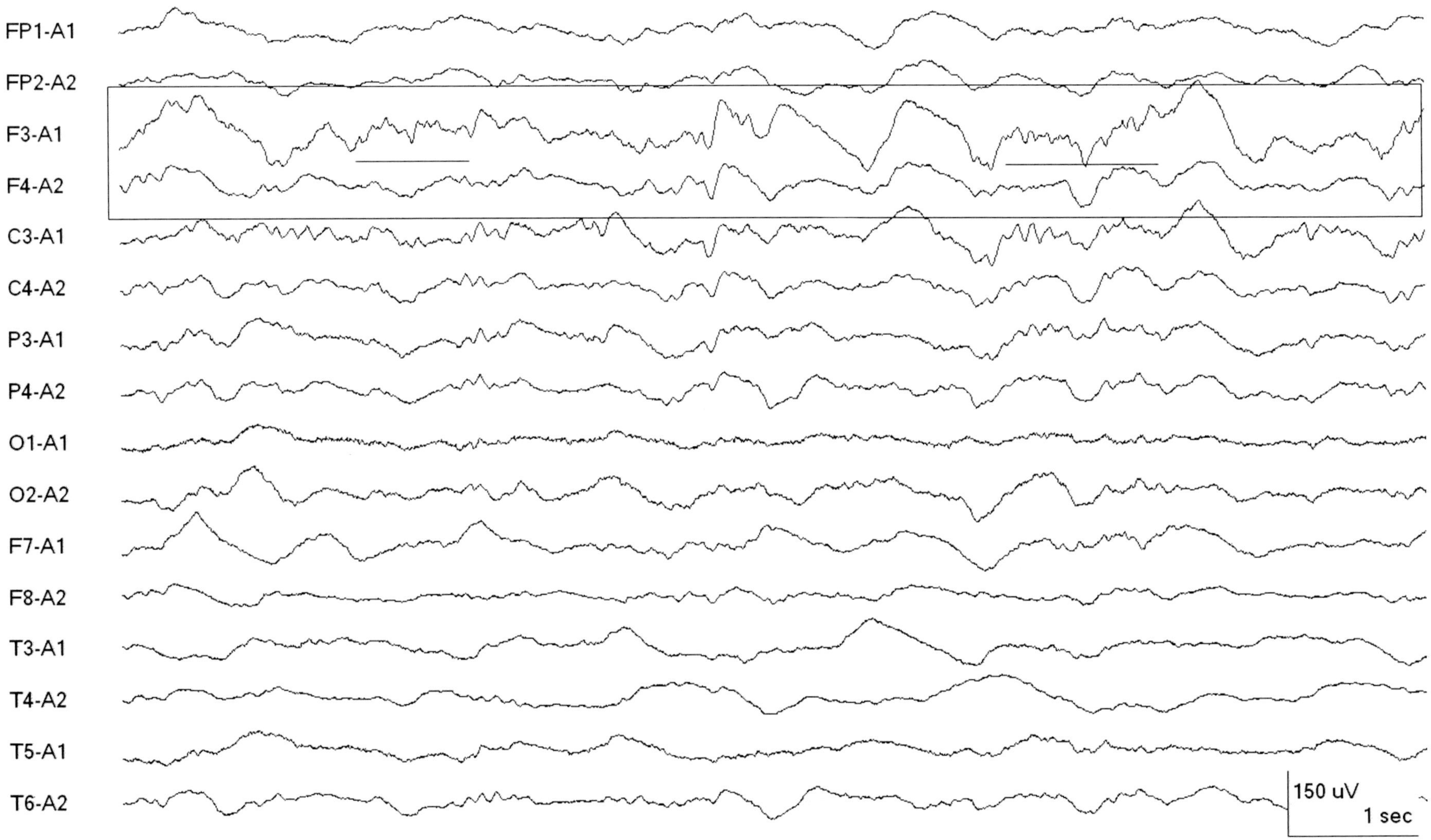

Figure 2.17 (*Continued*) (b) These hemispheric differences are well demonstrated in a reformatted referential montage to ipsilateral ears. The asymmetries are highlighted in the box with higher amplitude delta (slowing) on the left, indicating more severe underlying abnormality on the left and higher amplitude faster activity on the same side (marked by lines within the box) due to the skull defect.

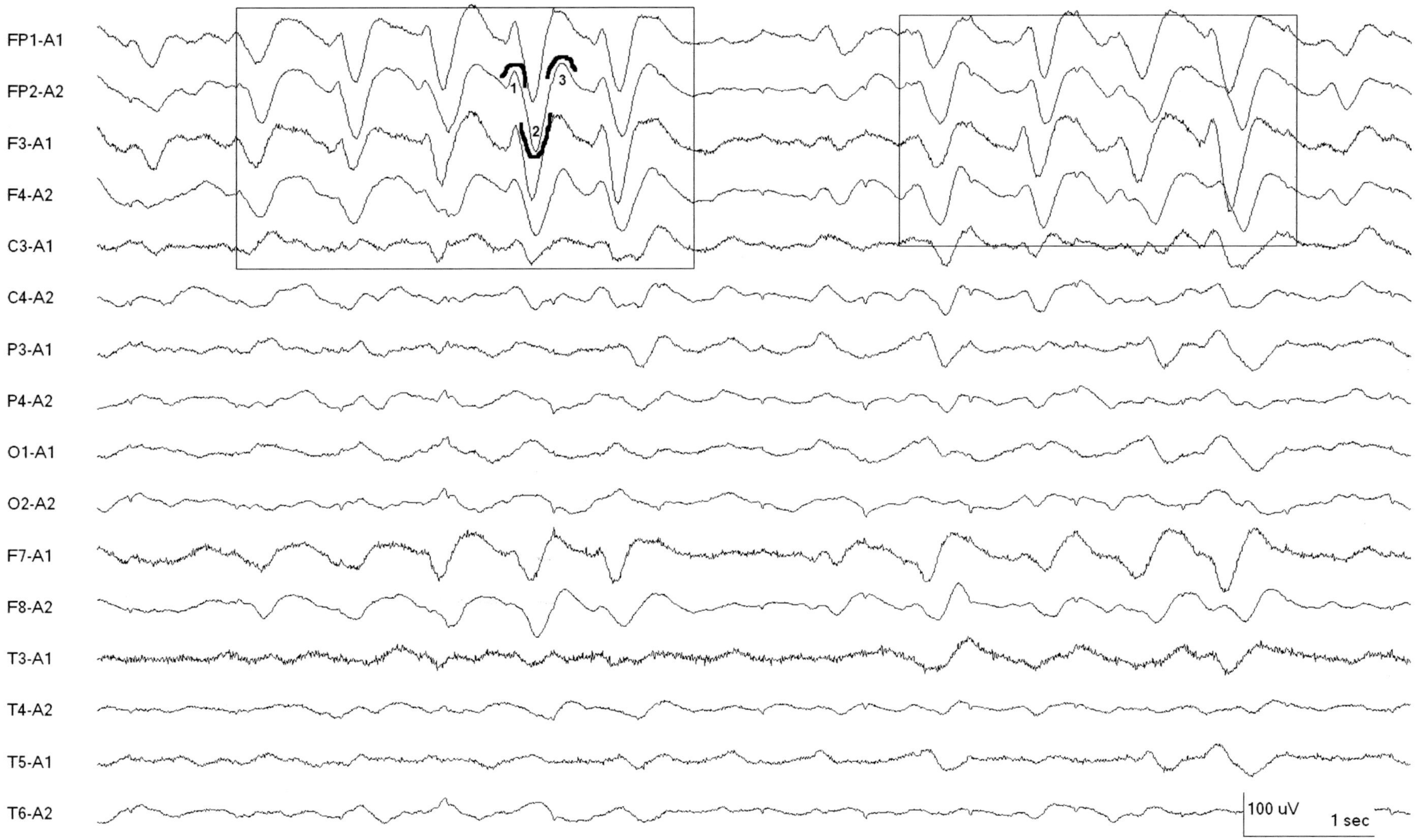

Figure 2.18 Triphasic waves. (a) Referential. The EEG in this 66-year-old woman awaiting a liver transplant shows clusters of triphasic waves at 1.5 per second (boxes). Note the typical frontal predominance, waxing and waning quality, and three phases of each discharge: small negativity (upgoing on this referential montage), then larger positivity (main component), followed by long slow negativity (see sample wave with all three phases labeled).

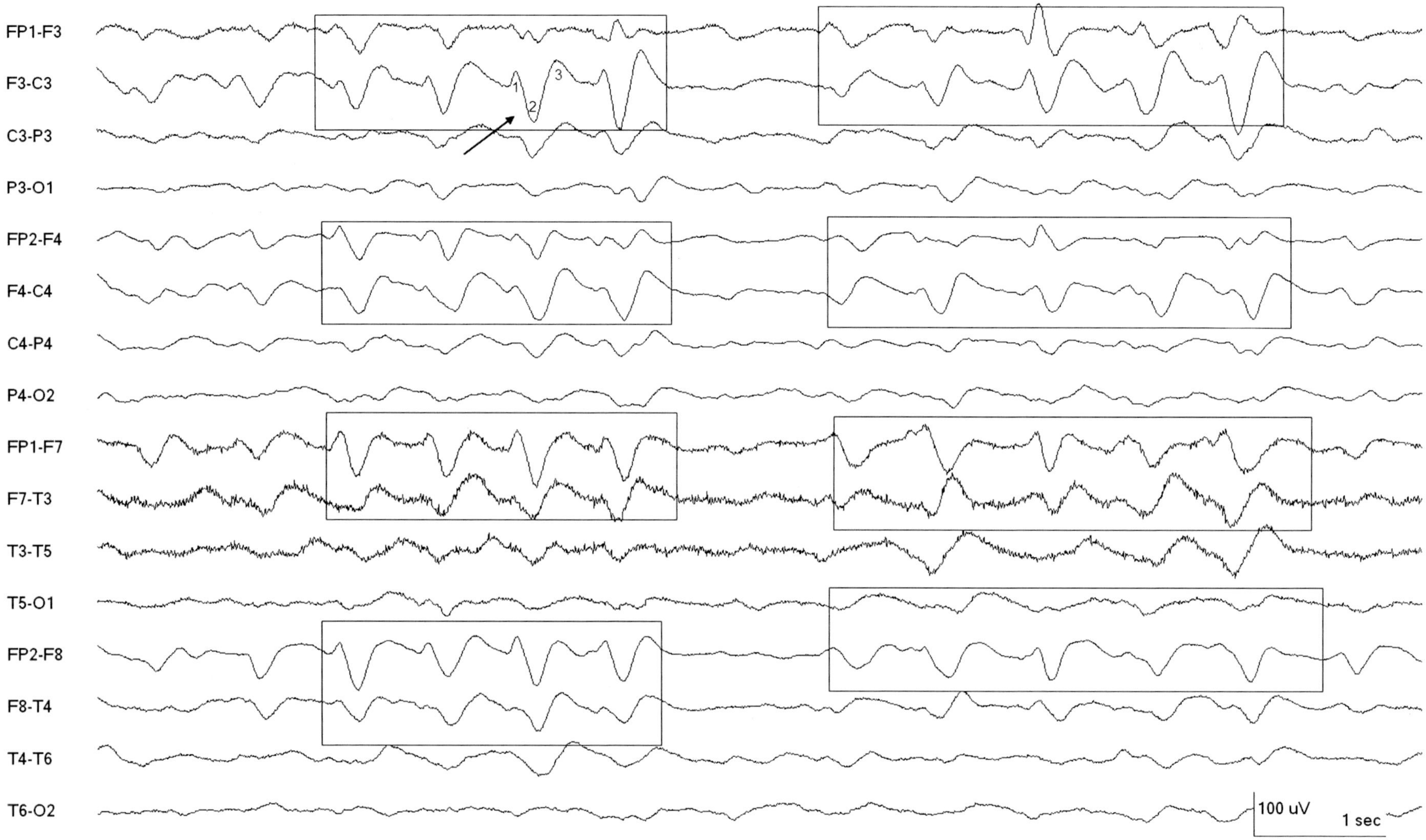

Figure 2.18 (*Continued*) (b) Bipolar.

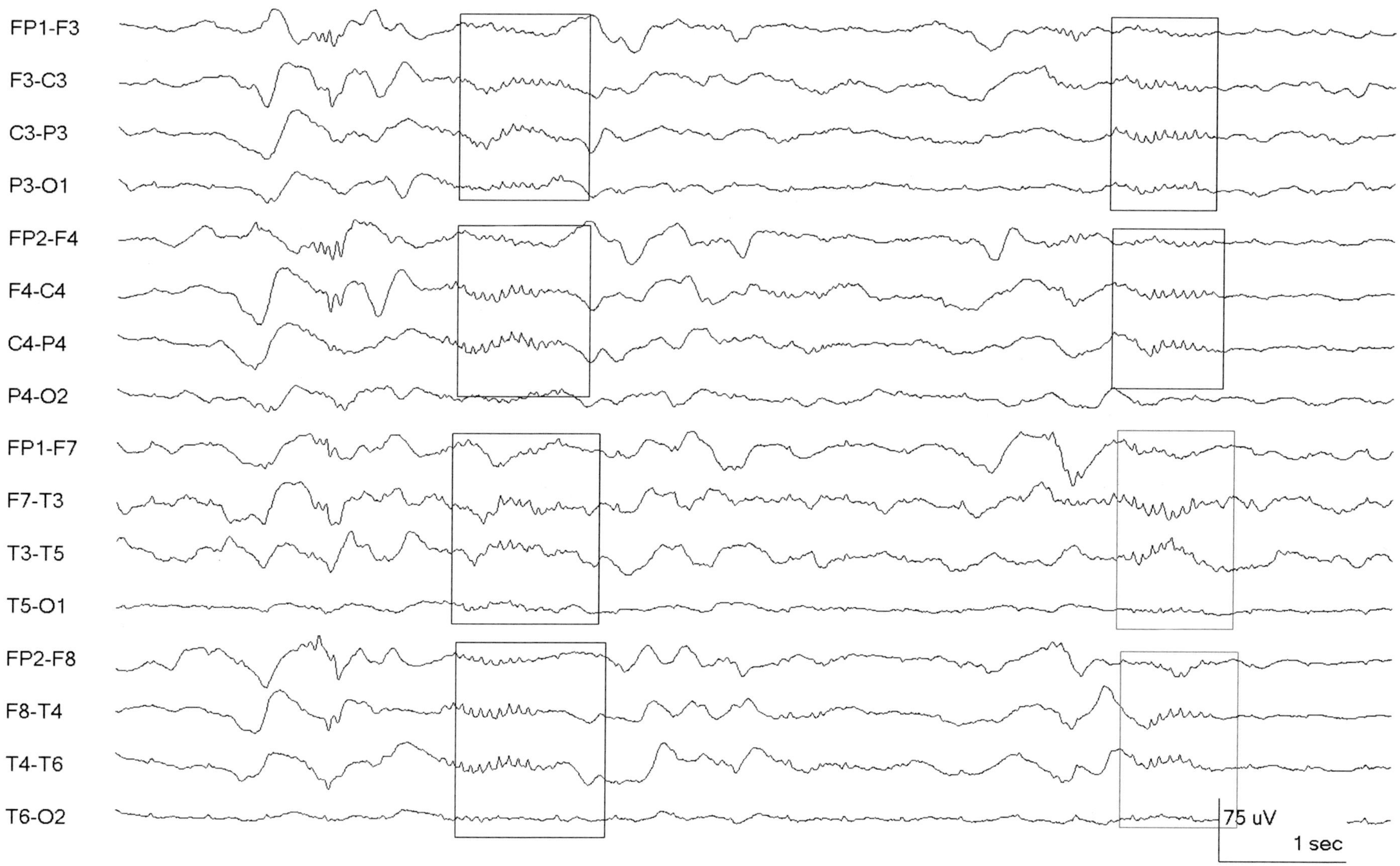

Figure 2.19 14 Hz positive spikes. (a) Bipolar. 14 Hz positive spikes are present in this 38-year-old comatose male with hepatic failure. Although this is a benign variant seen in drowsiness, it is also rarely seen in comatose patients with hepatic failure.

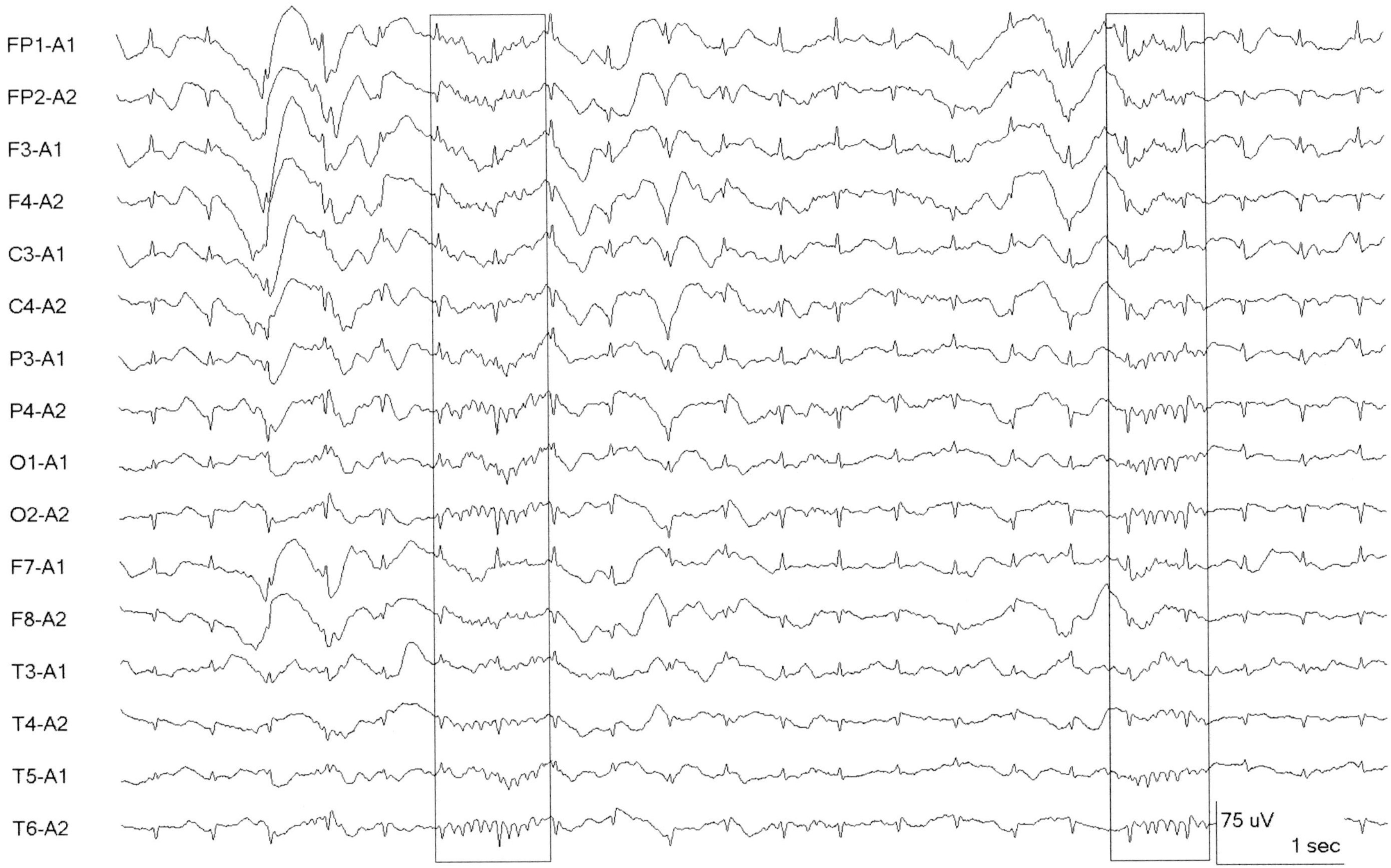

Figure 2.19 (*Continued*) (b) Referential. The epoch reformatted utilizing a referential montage to ipsilateral ears. These low-amplitude positive discharges (downgoing on this referential montage) are often maximal in the posterior temporal region (e.g. see T6 in this example within the boxes).

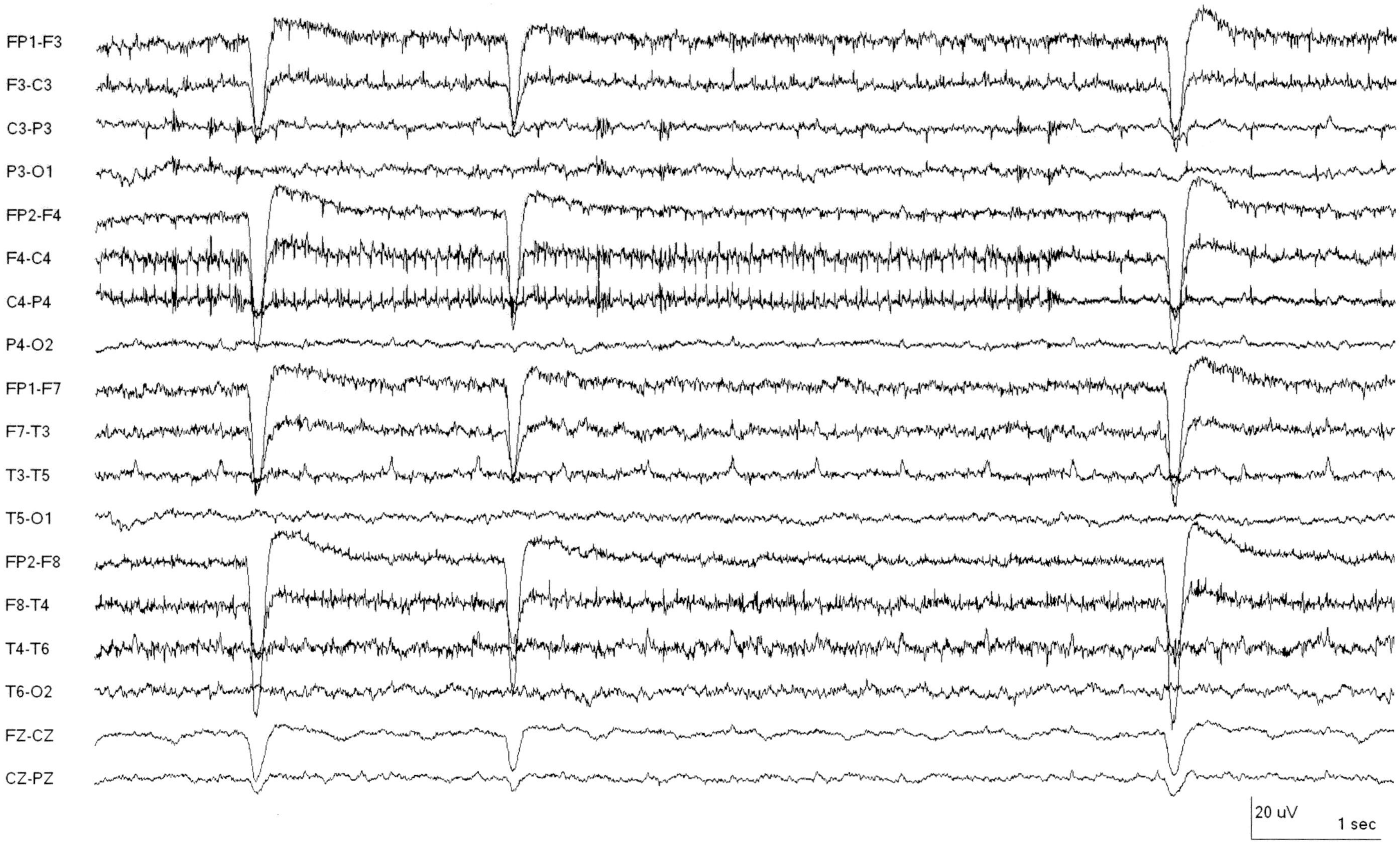

Figure 2.20 Diffuse attenuation. The EEG in this 48-year-old man in a vegetative state following a cardiac arrest shows marked suppression of background activity even at a high sensitivity (recorded at very high gain, note scale legend). Eye-blink artifacts are prominent as are muscle and EKG (especially at T3-T5); however, there is no definite cerebral activity.

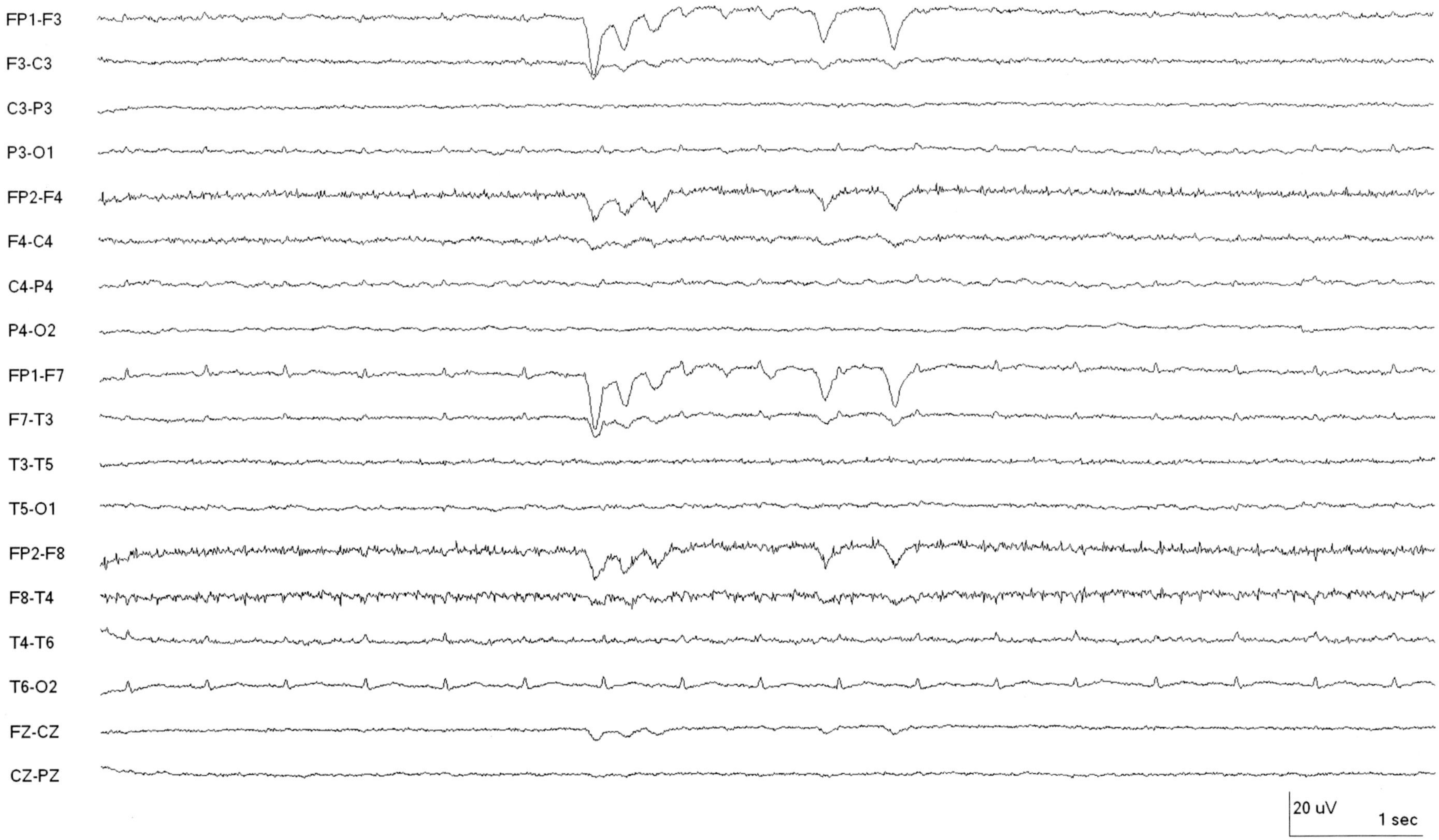

Figure 2.21 Diffuse attenuation. Similar to the previous figure, but with less muscle artifact. The EEG in this 44-year-old man in a persistent vegetative state (PVS) shows no evidence of definite cerebral activity despite very high gain (note scale legend). In the center of the epoch are several eye blinks. EKG artifact is present especially in T6-O2. Usually patients in a PVS show more EEG activity than this.

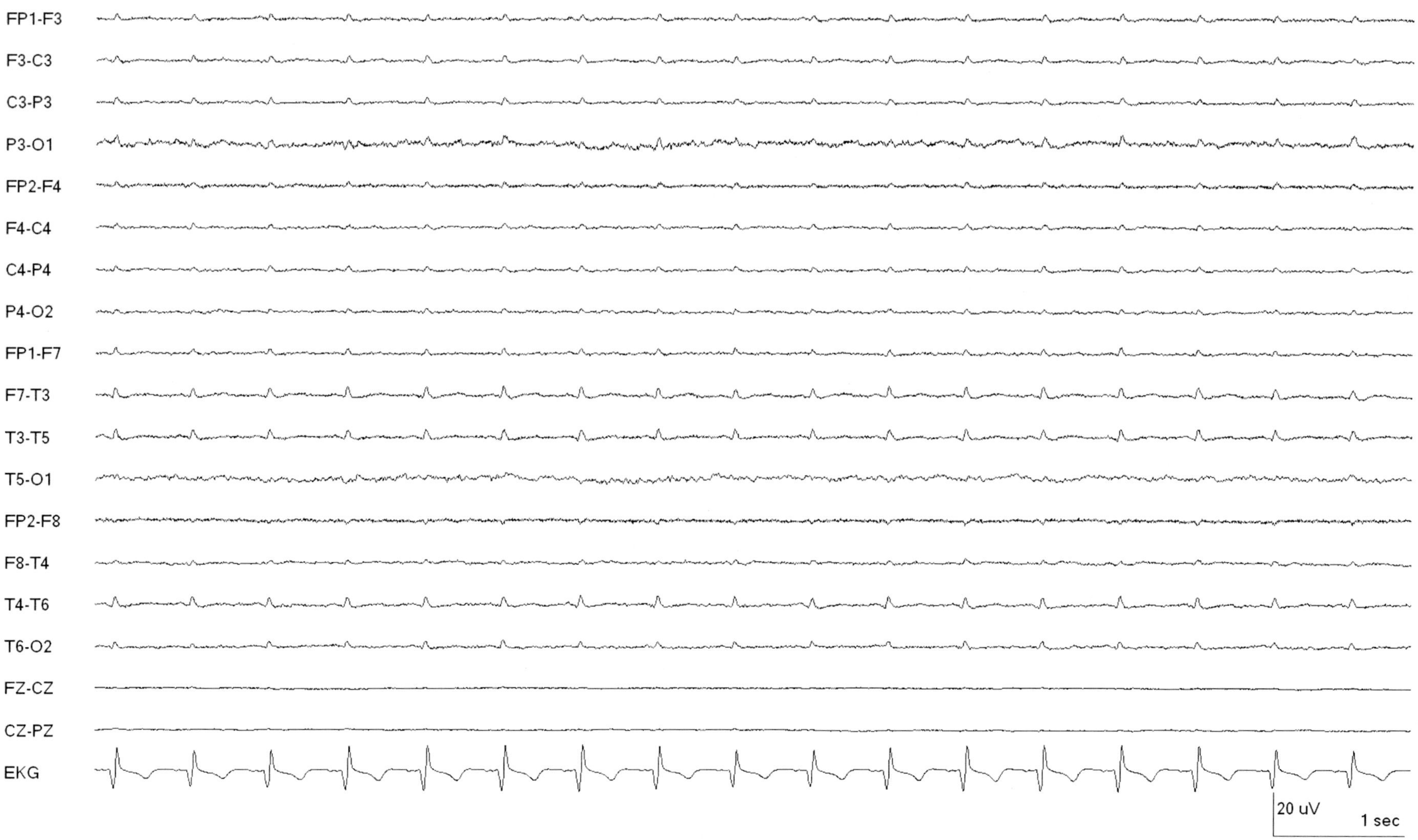

Figure 2.22 Electrocerebral inactivity. The EEG in this 50-year-old woman being evaluated for brain death demonstrates electrocerebral inactivity. There are strict guidelines for performing EEGs for this purpose (only done rarely in recent years) – see the American Clinical Neurophysiology Society guidelines regarding technical requirements for using EEG as part of the determination of brain death (in suggested reading list).

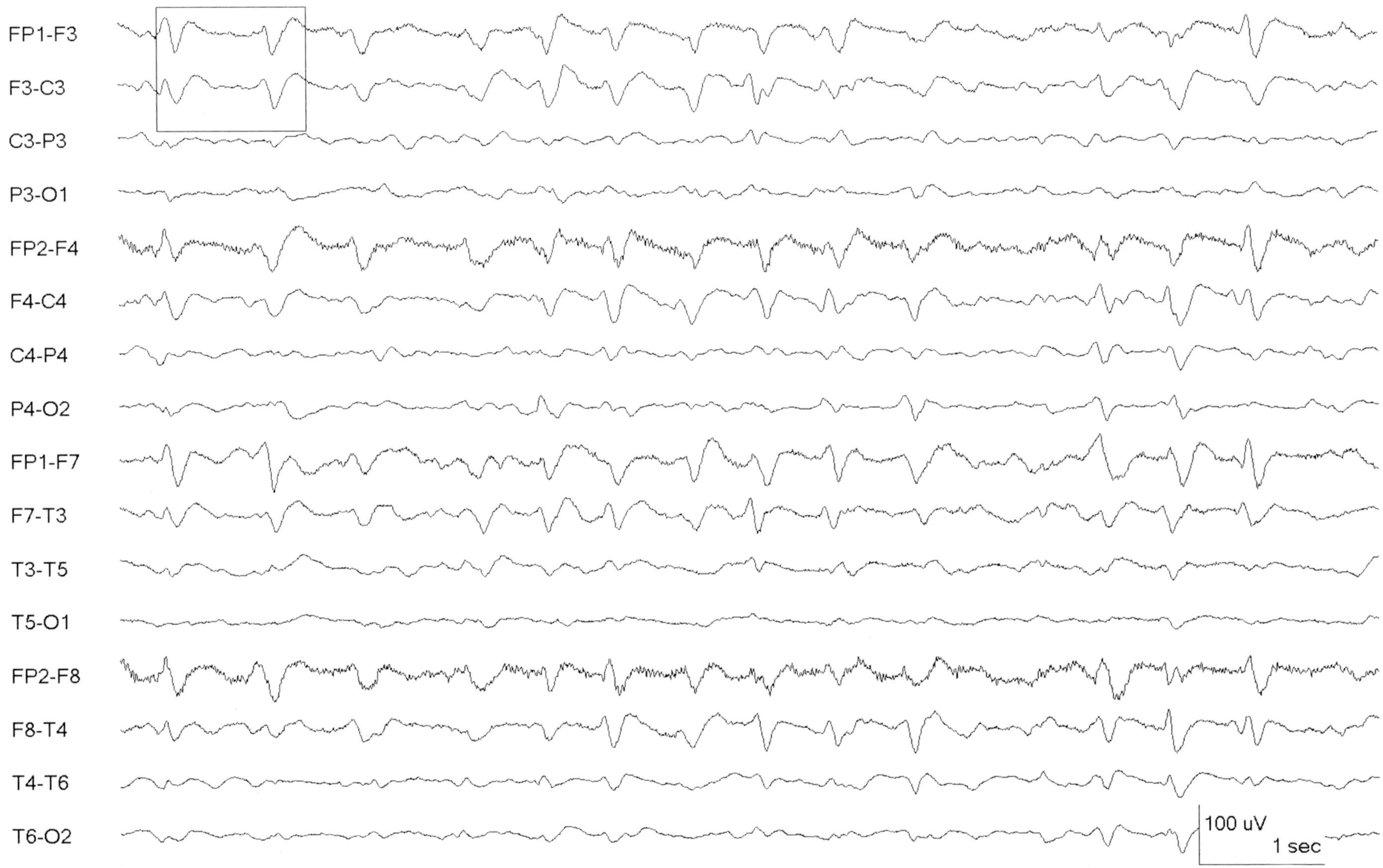

Figure 2.23 Generalized periodic discharges with triphasic morphology. (a) Bipolar. Waxing and waning generalized periodic discharges at 1–2 Hz with a triphasic morphology are present, maximal anteriorly, in this 72-year-old man s/p cardiac arrest.

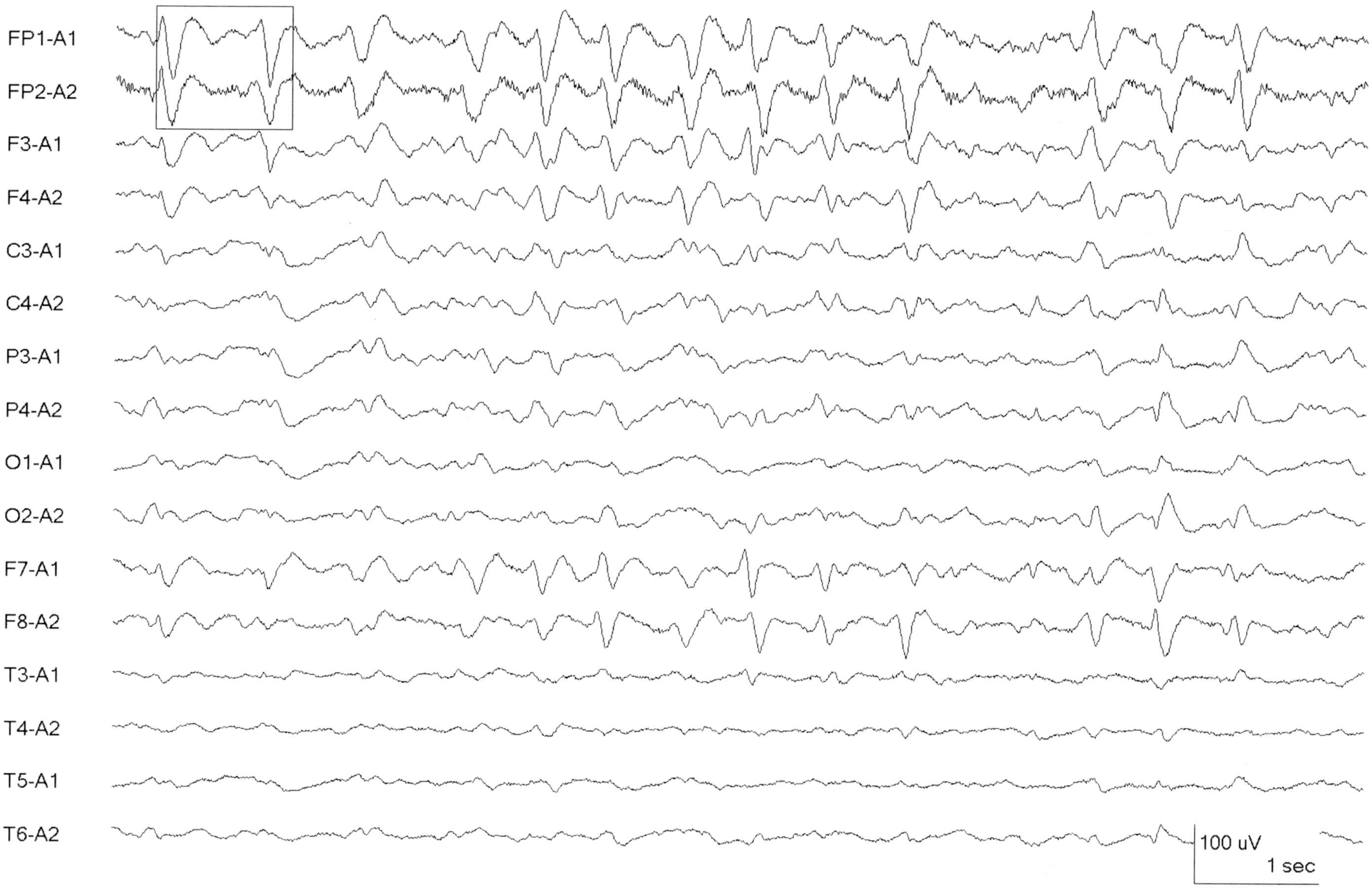

Figure 2.23 (*Continued*) (b) Referential. The epoch has been reformatted and is shown in a referential montage to ipsilateral ears.

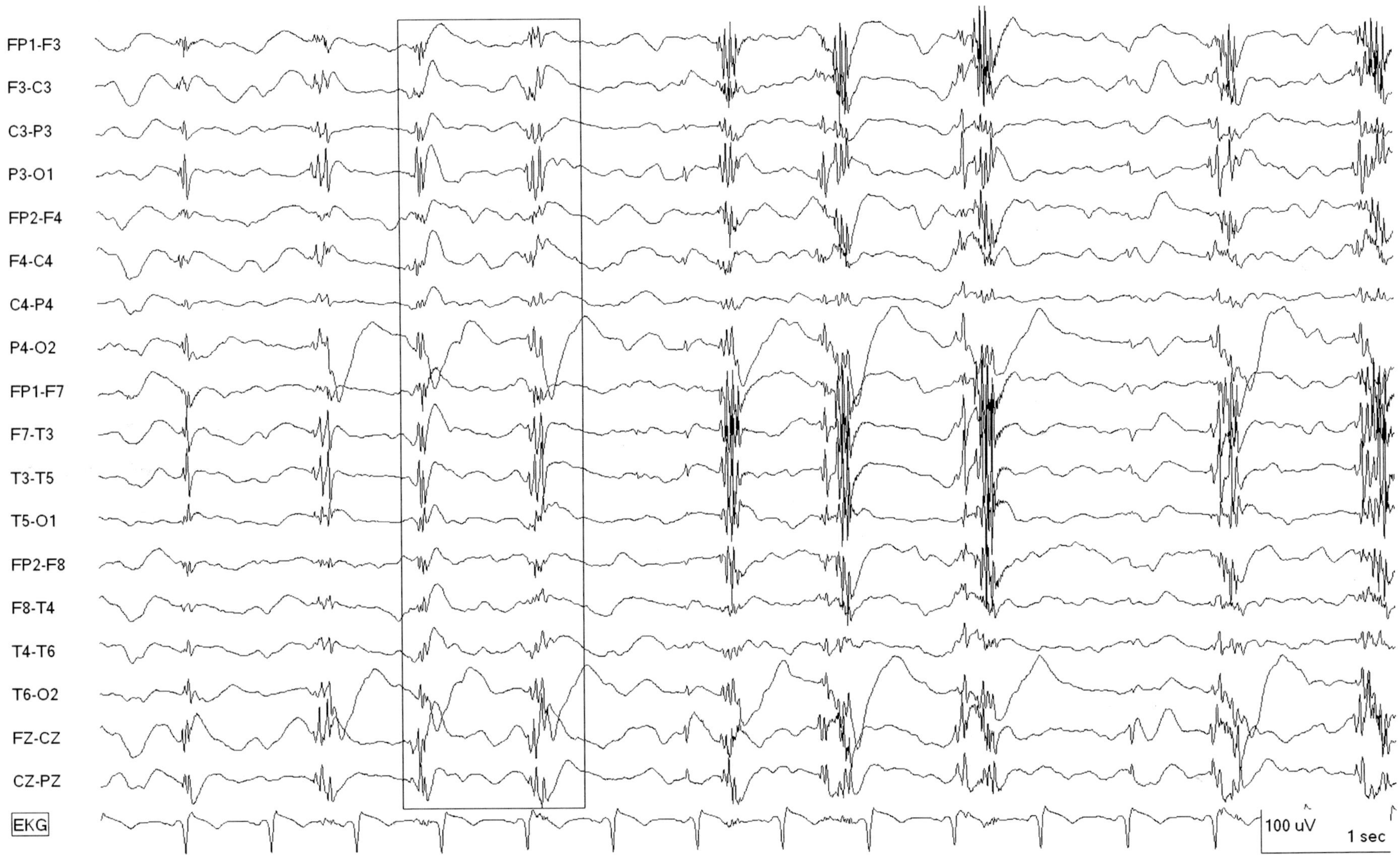

Figure 2.24 Myoclonic status epilepticus. The EEG in this 65-year-old man in myoclonic status epilepticus following an arrest shows repetitive generalized polyspikes (two examples are inside the box), maximal on the left, on a diffusely slow background.

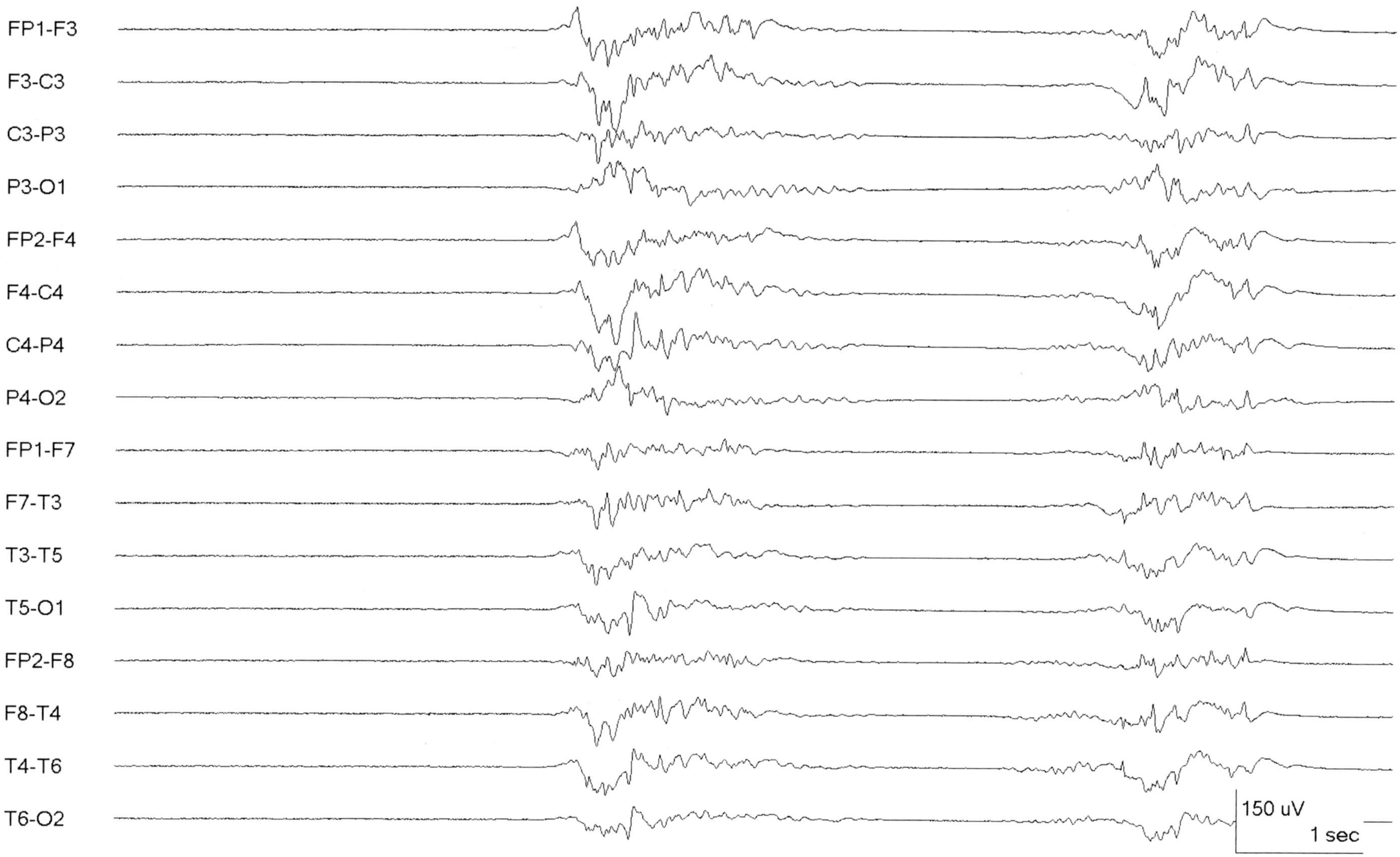

Figure 2.25 Suppression-burst. A suppression-burst pattern is present in this 55-year-old man s/p cardiac arrest.

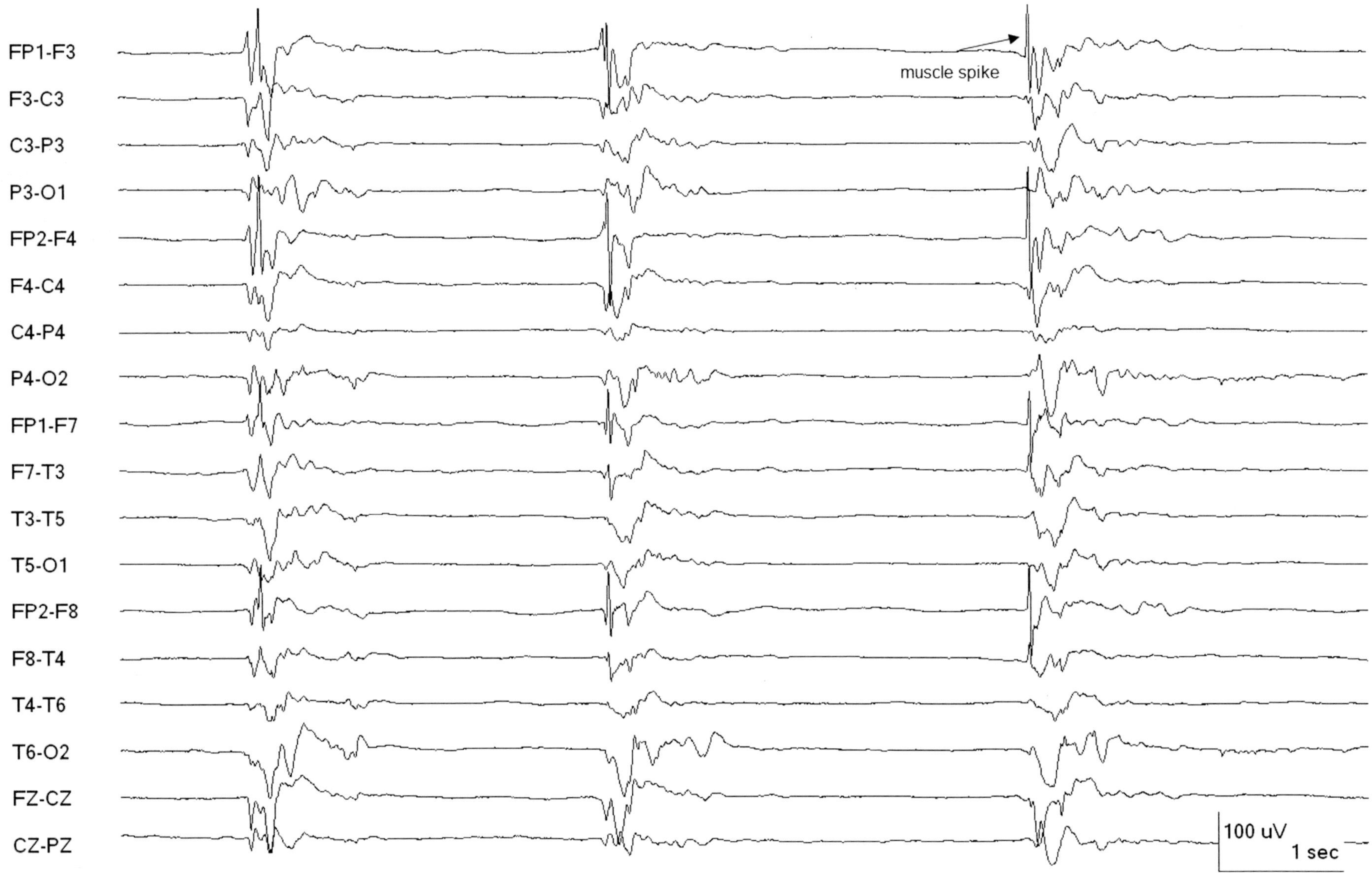

Figure 2.26 Suppression-burst plus muscle artifact. (a) The EEG in this 66-year-old woman shows a suppression-burst pattern likely with superimposed muscle spikes (arrow). The latter are prominent in the Fp1 and Fp2 electrodes but not in midline electrodes (Fz, Cz and Pz), which are usually free of muscle artifact. The patient was in myoclonic status epilepticus post arrest.

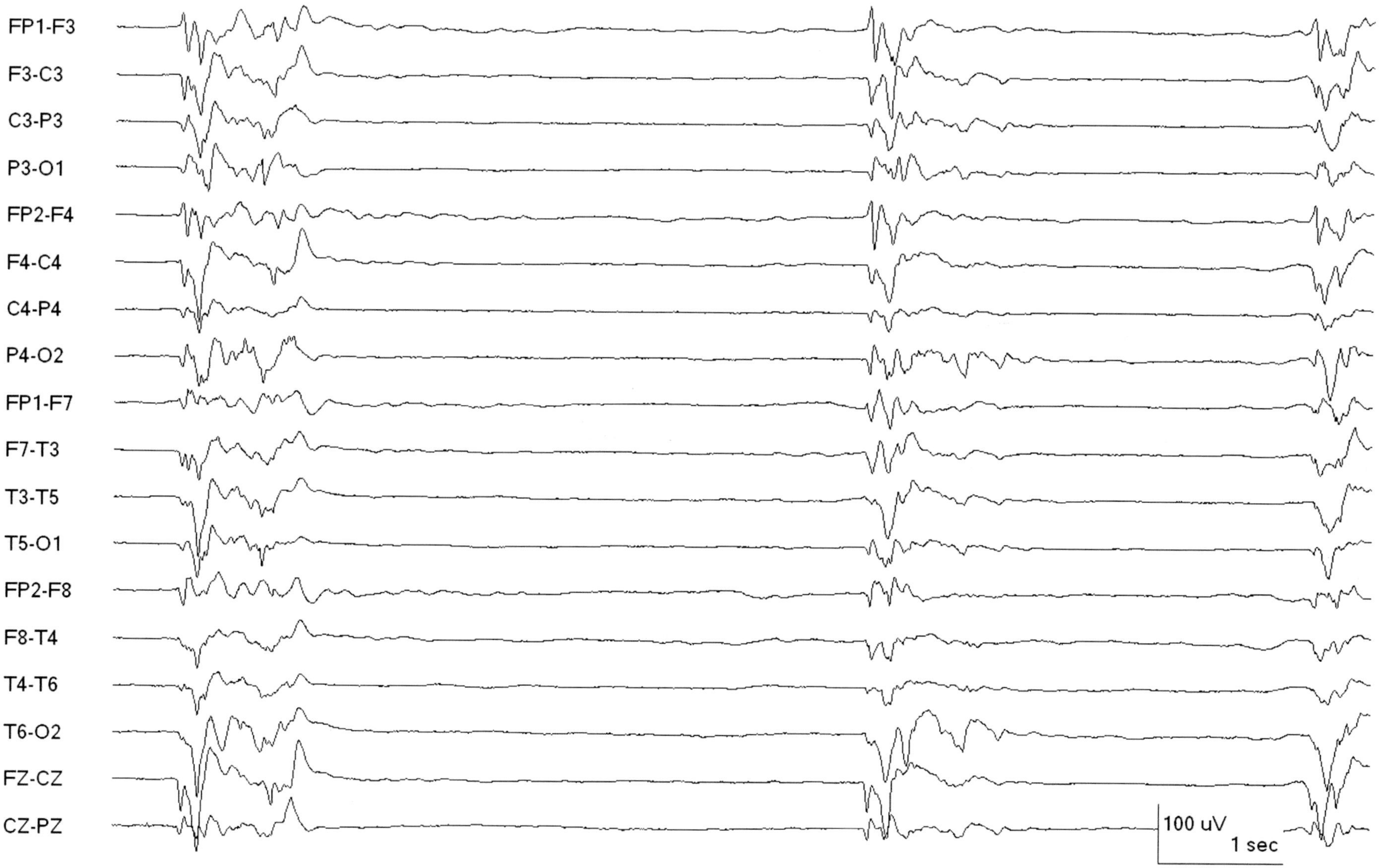

Figure 2.26 (*Continued*) (b) Following the administration of vecuronium (a paralytic), the pattern persists confirming that these bursts represent brain activity; muscle artifact is no longer present.

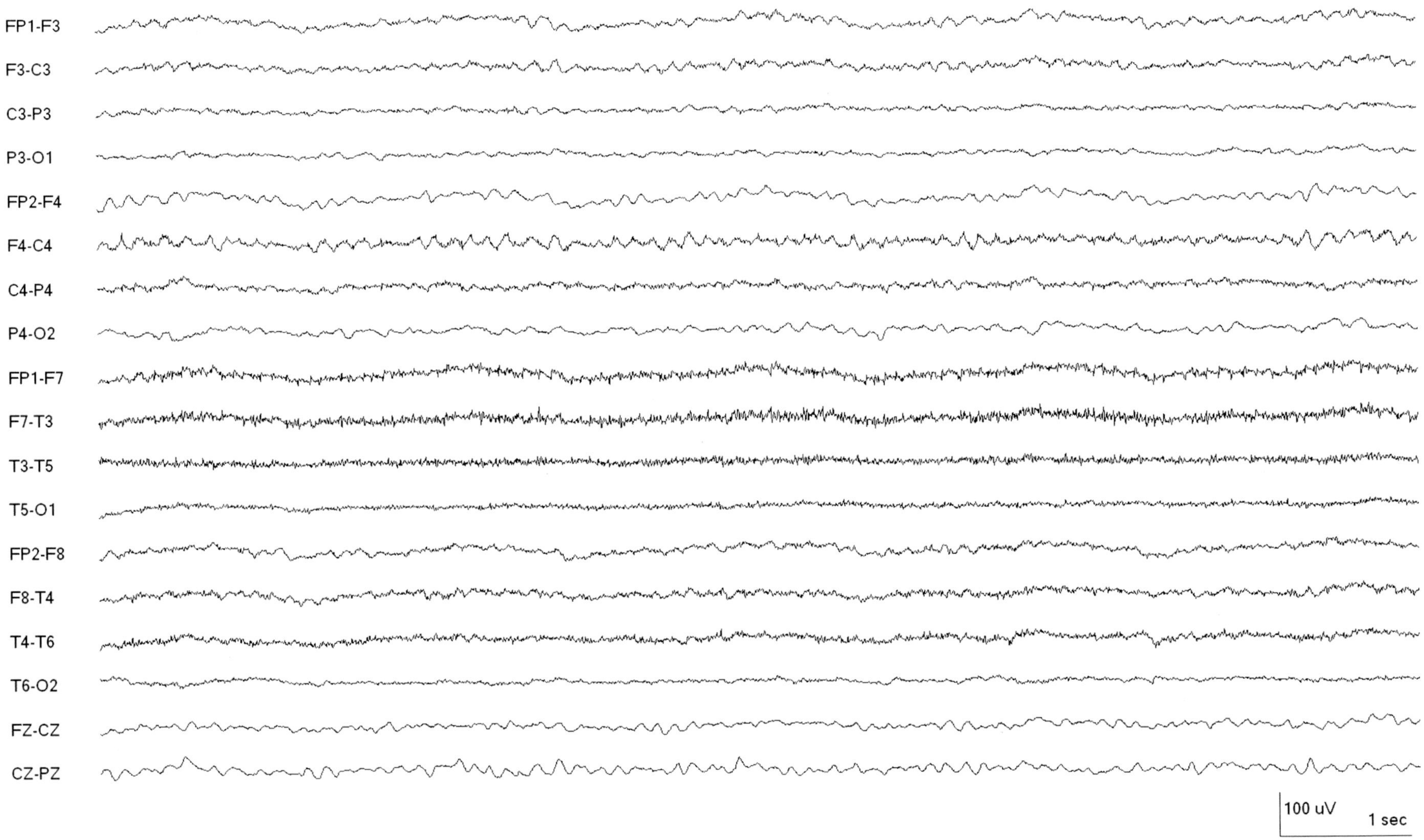

Figure 2.27 Alpha coma. The EEG in this 42-year-old comatose man with a history of an arrest 1 day previously shows an alpha coma pattern with continuous, frontally predominant and monomorphic 8 Hz activity. The pattern was nonreactive.

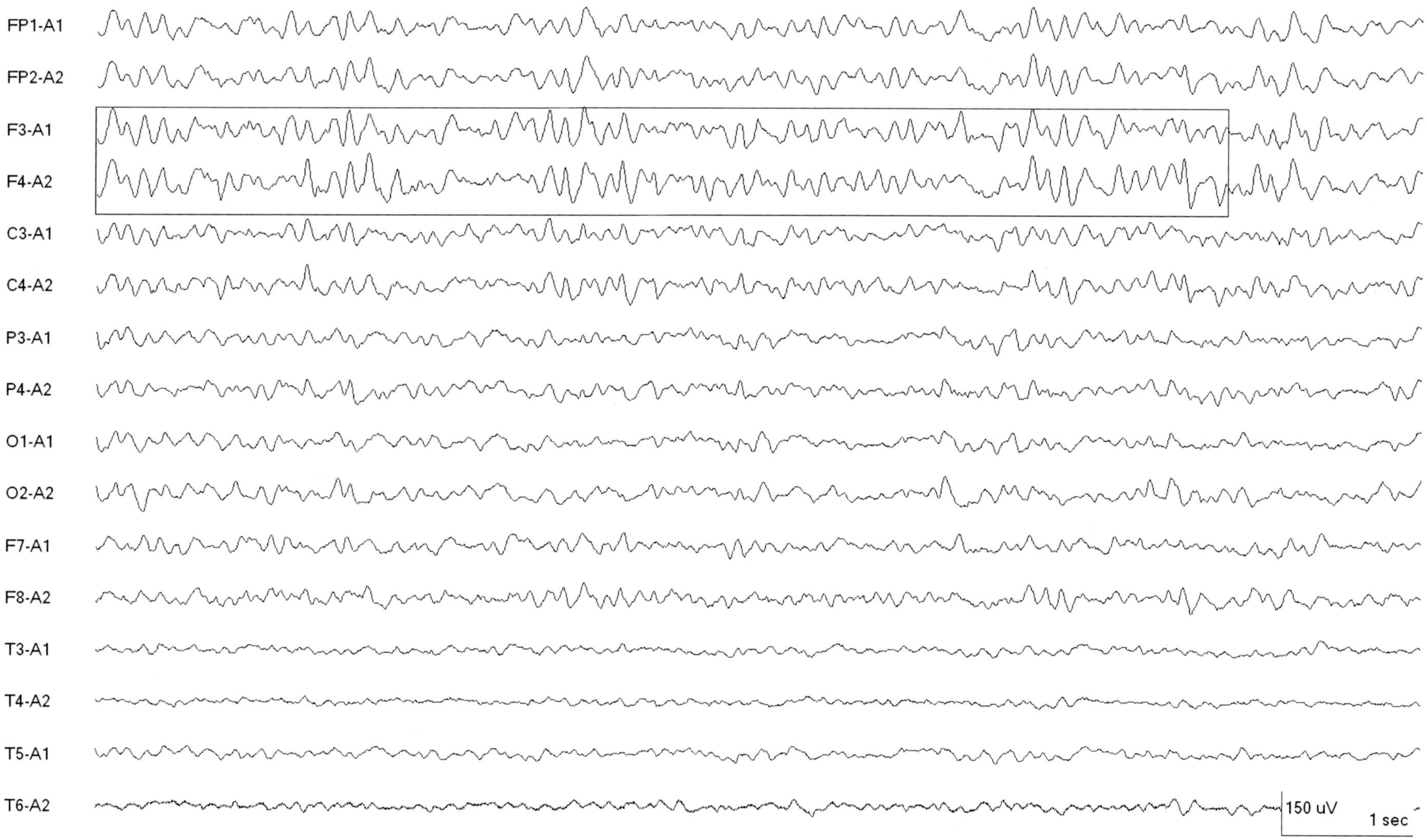

Figure 2.28 Diffuse slowing. Diffuse slowing of background activity predominantly in the alpha–theta range is present, maximal anteriorly, in this 44-year-old woman with hepatic failure secondary to an acetaminophen overdose.

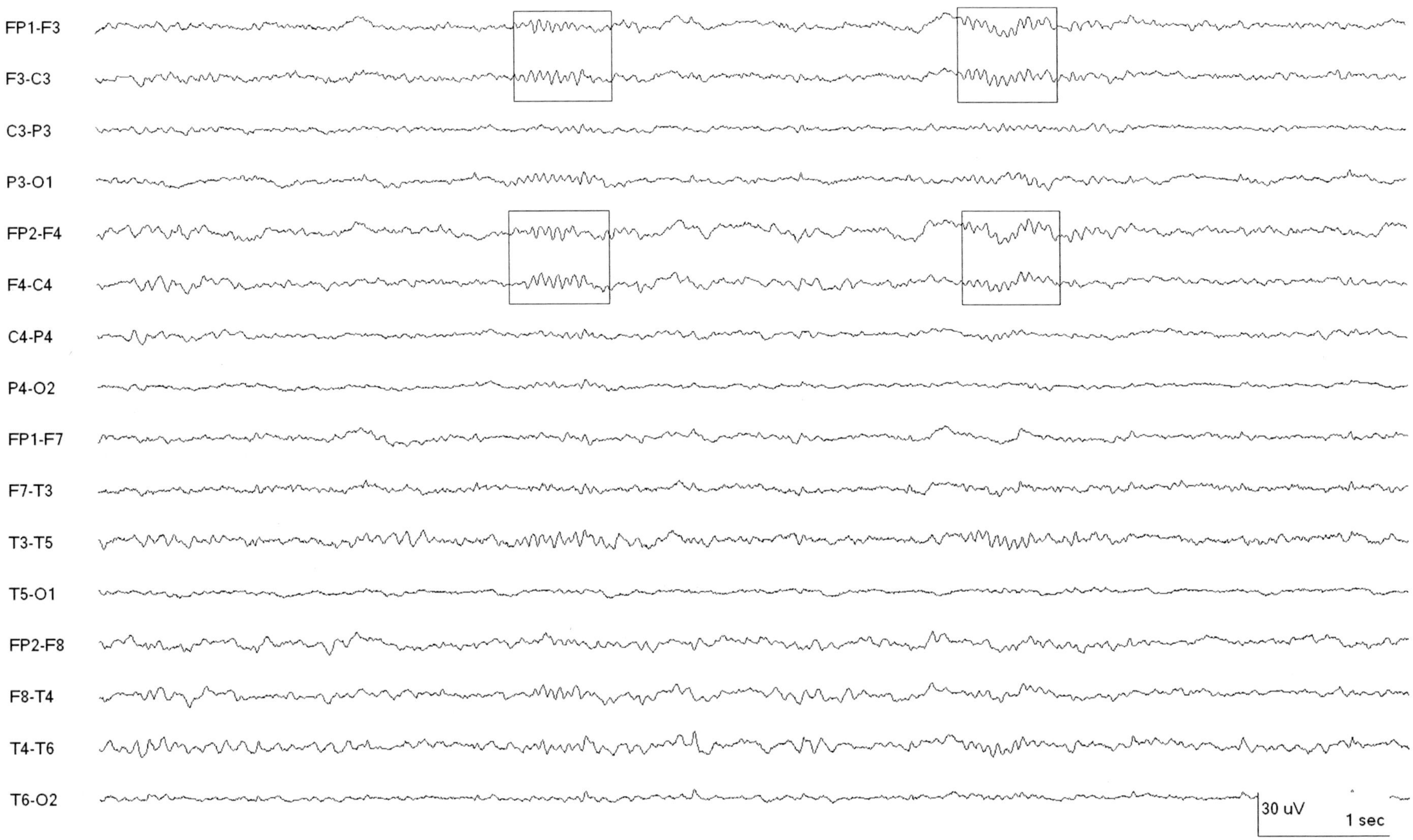

Figure 2.29 Spindle coma. The EEG in this 61-year-old comatose man with a subarachnoid hemorrhage shows sleep spindles consistent with a spindle coma pattern. This pattern resembles normal sleep but the patient cannot be awakened.

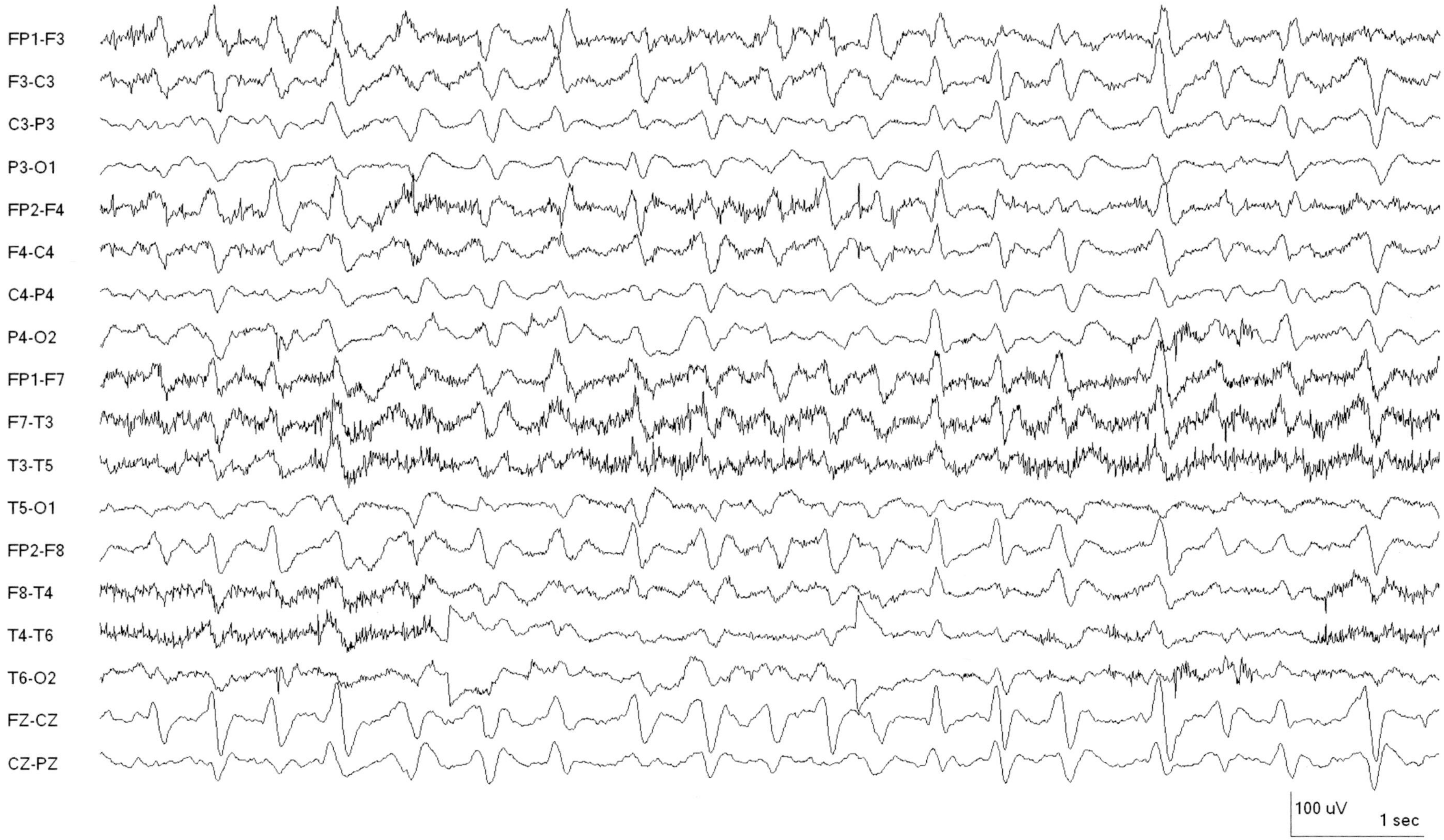

Figure 2.30 Nonconvulsive status epilepticus vs. triphasic waves. (a) This EEG of a 75-year-old man with altered mental status and renal failure shows generalized periodic discharges at 2–3 Hz, sometimes with triphasic morphology. It was felt that the patient may have been in nonconvulsive status due to cefepime intake (recently discontinued).

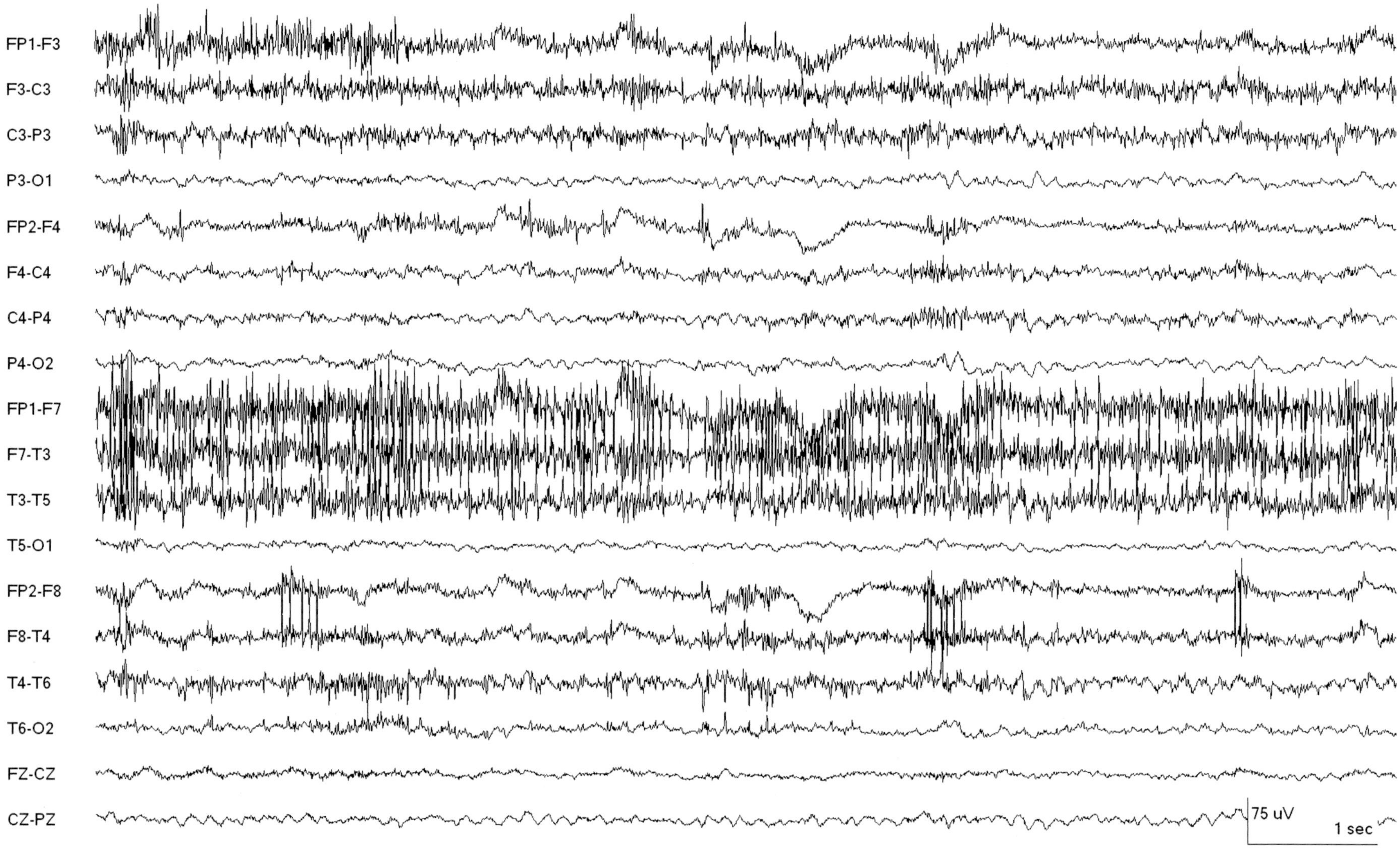

Figure 2.30 (*Continued*) (b) The following day, the EEG was considerably improved, as was the patient. His renal function, however, was unchanged.

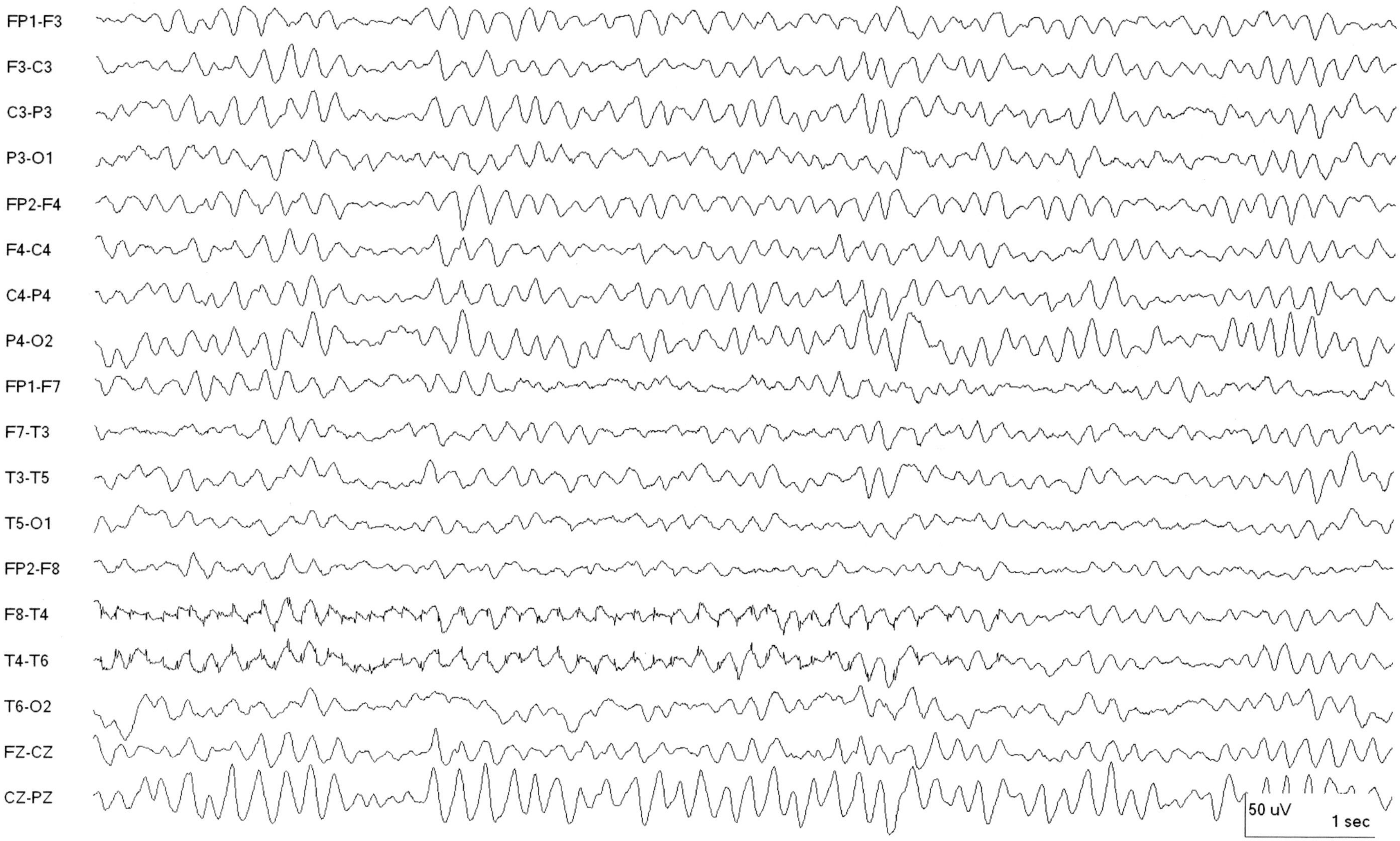

Figure 2.31 Propofol effect and nonconvulsive status. (a) The EEG in this 46-year-old man on propofol for refractory status epilepticus shows diffuse activity, predominantly in the theta range.

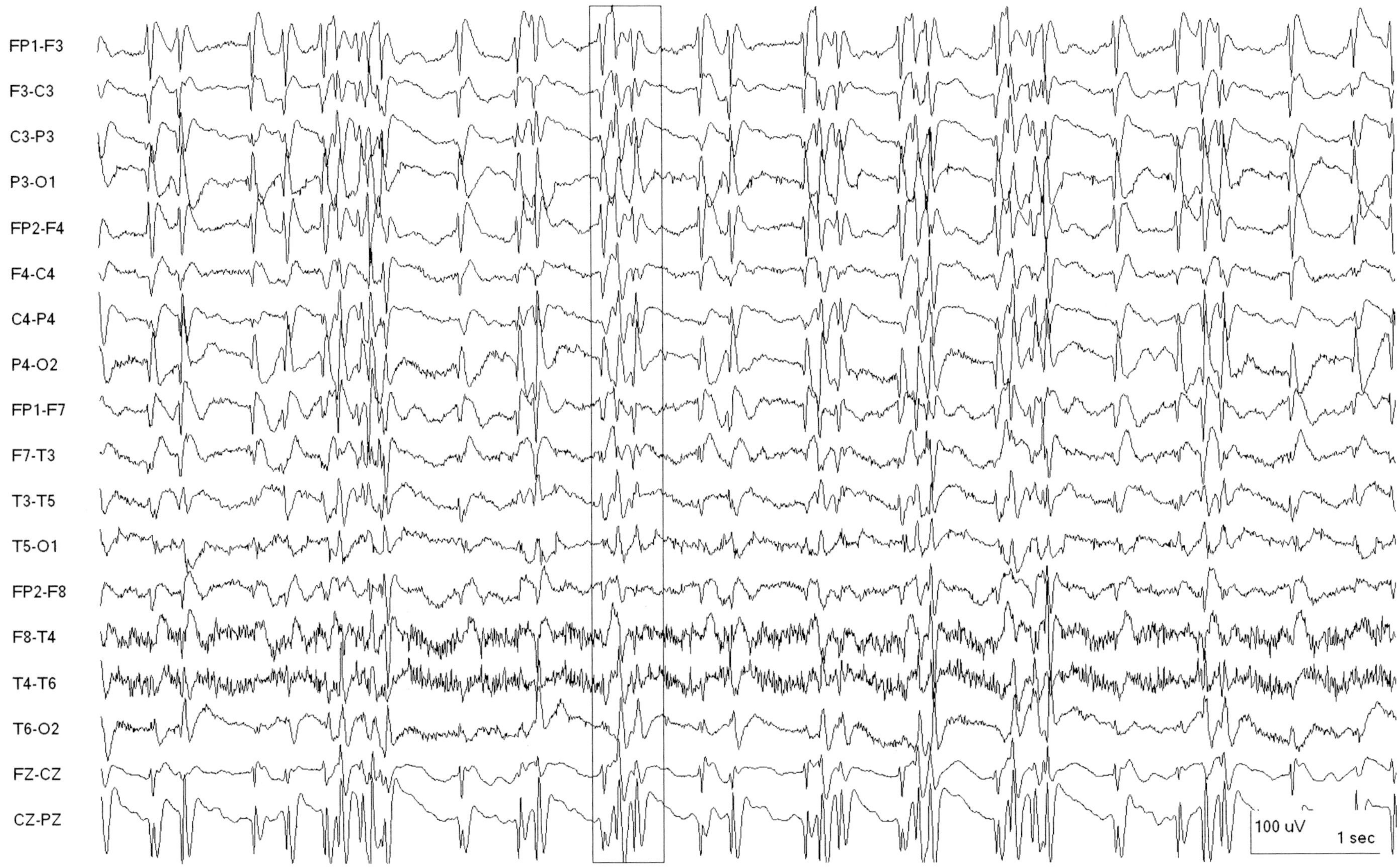

Figure 2.31 (*Continued*) (b) Later that day when propofol was stopped, the EEG resumed its prior appearance with bursts of generalized spikes and polyspikes (box) consistent with electrographic status epilepticus (nonconvulsive in this case).

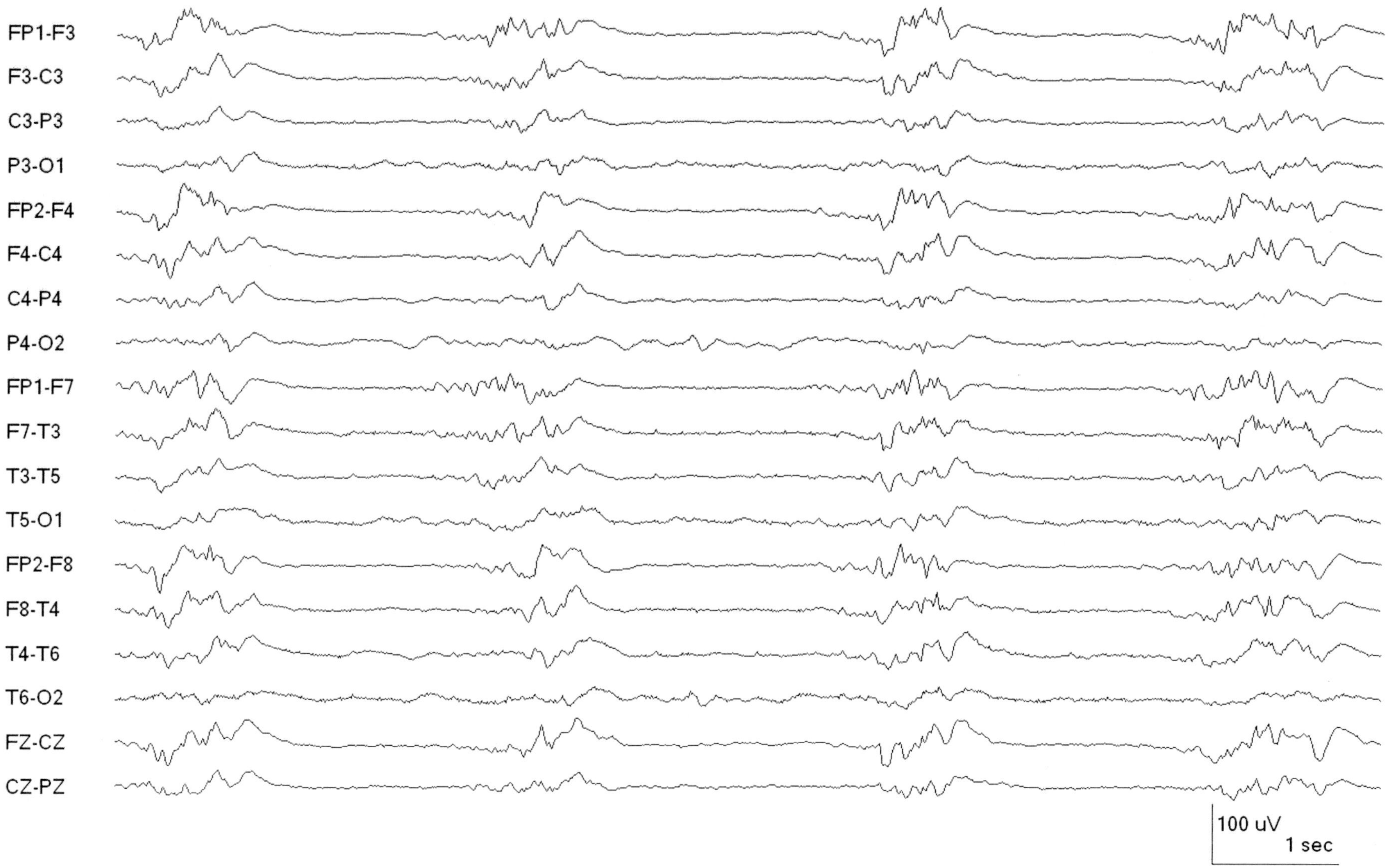

Figure 2.32 Barbiturate-induced suppression-burst. (a) A suppression-burst pattern in a 65-year-old man undergoing a carotid endarterectomy. The patient had been given pentobarbital prior to intubation.

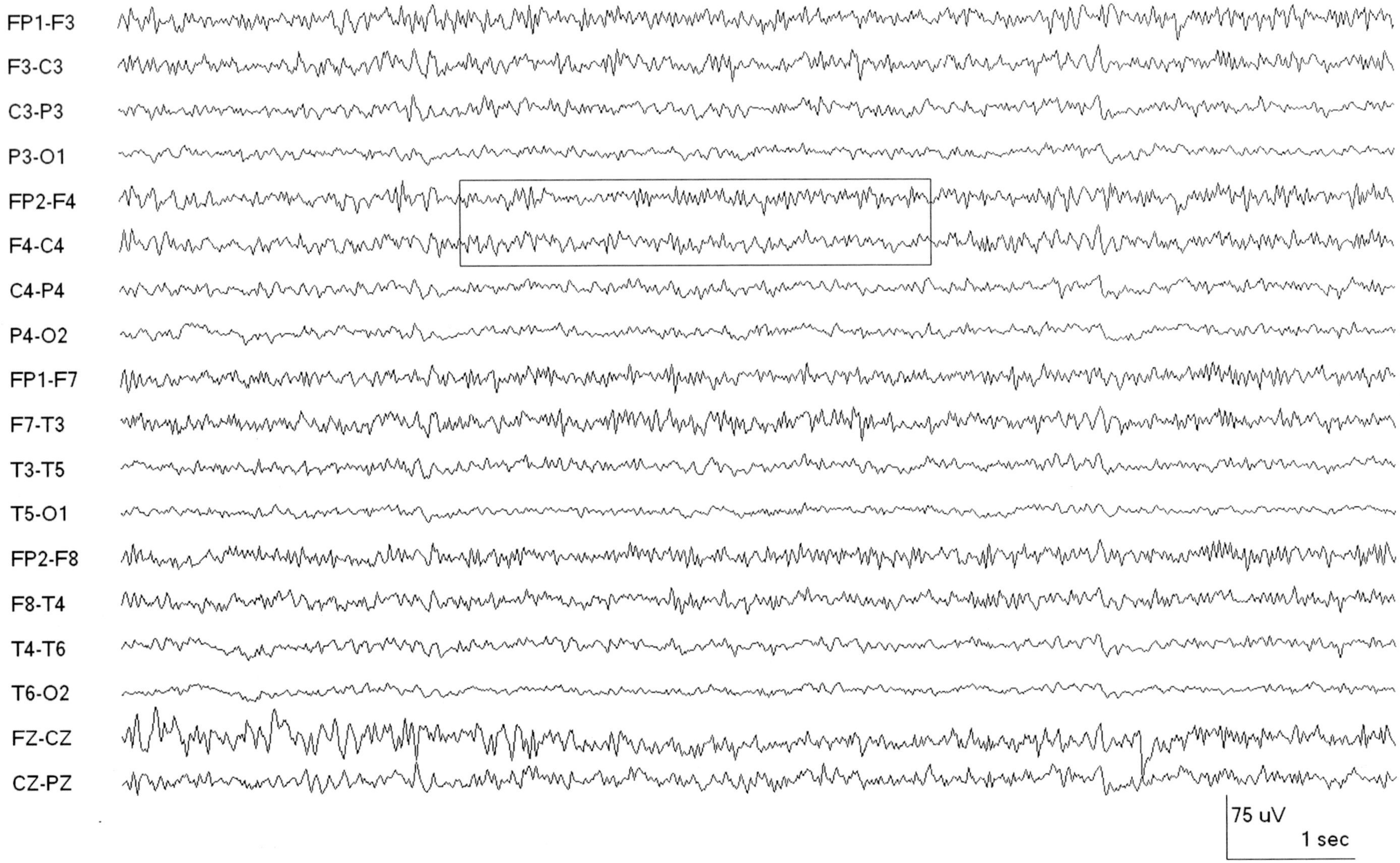

Figure 2.32 (*Continued*) (b) Later in the tracing, the EEG shows a lighter level of coma. The background is now continuous with diffuse beta activity (some alpha as well), more prominent anteriorly (as in box).

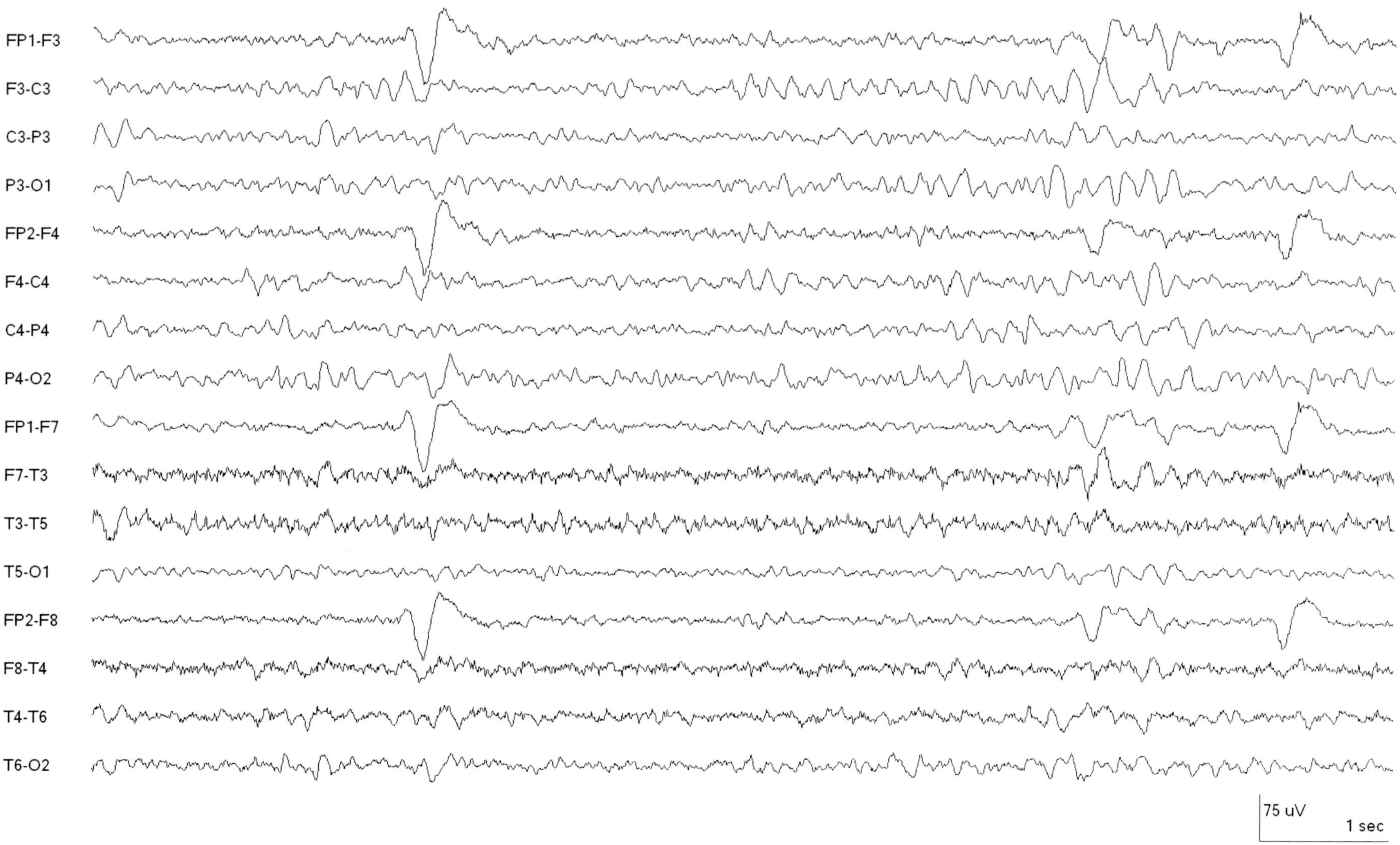

Figure 2.33 Phenytoin toxicity. The EEG in this 28-year-old woman with phenytoin toxicity shows mild diffuse slowing of background rhythms with excess theta activity and occasional bursts of slowing.

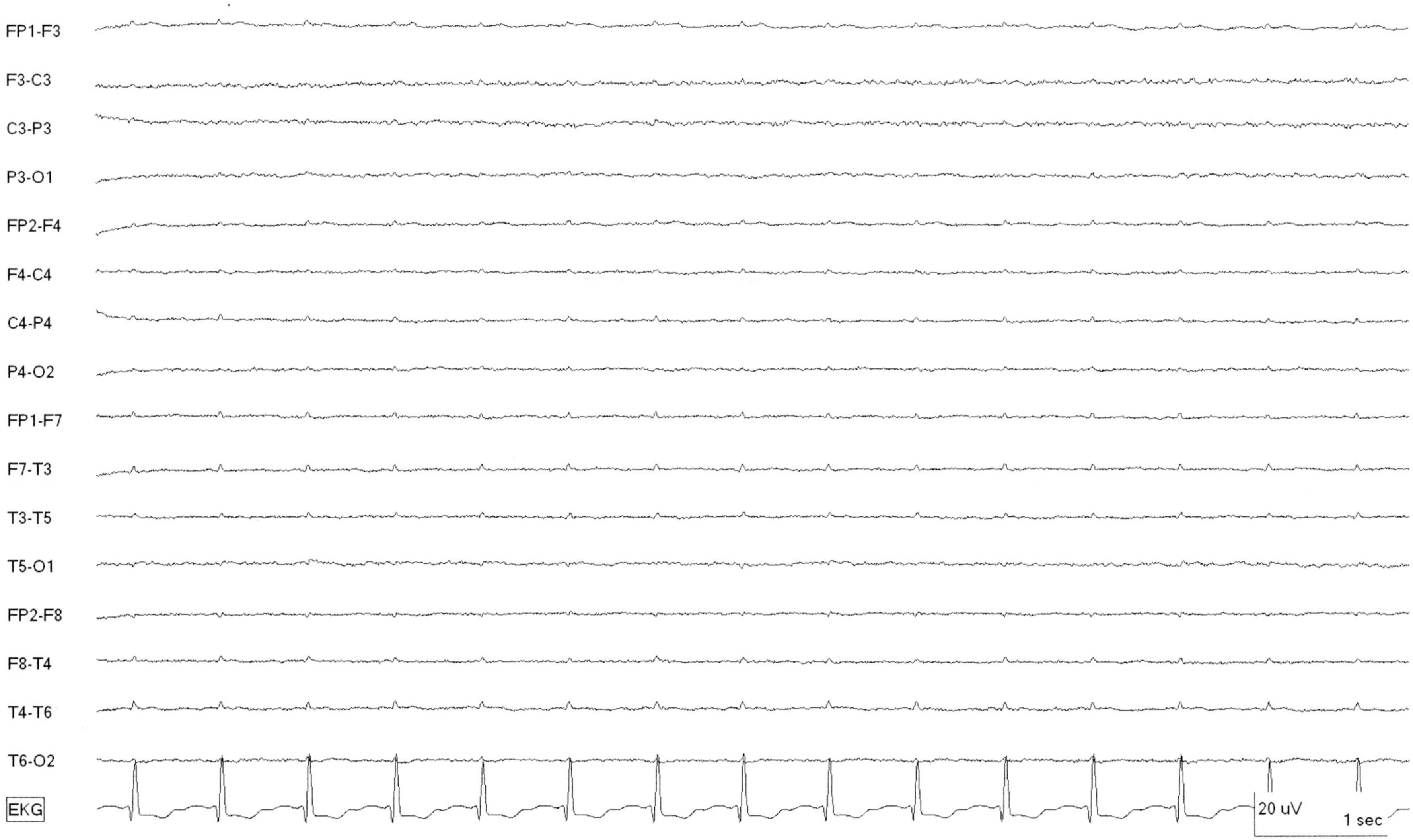

Figure 2.34 Electrocerebral inactivity due to barbiturates. (a) The EEG in this 30-year-old woman in a pentobarbital-induced coma shows no evidence of cerebral activity despite the high gain.

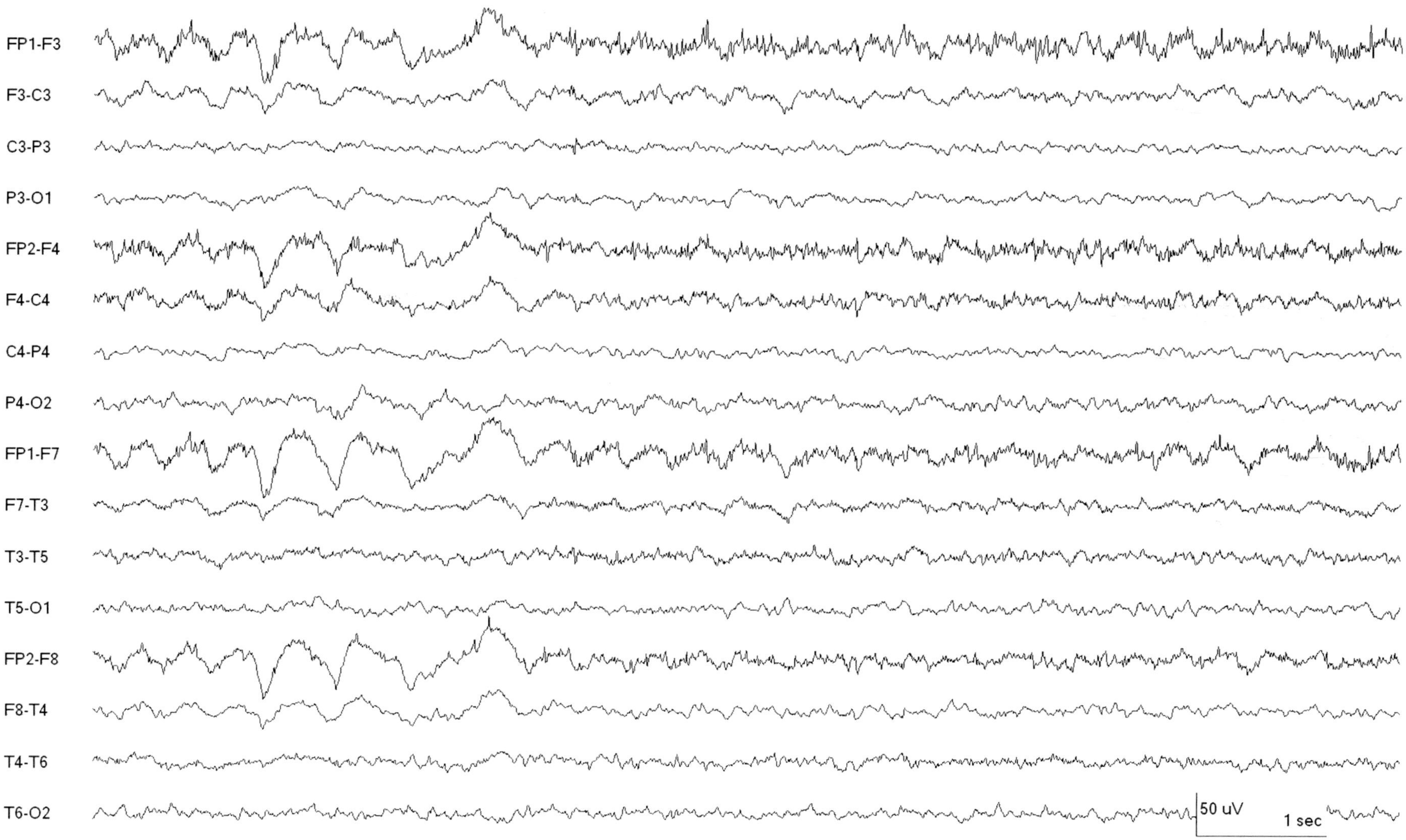

Figure 2.34 (*Continued*) (b) Several days later, following discontinuation of pentobarbital, there is now cerebral activity. The EEG is diffusely slow, including bursts of higher amplitude frontally predominant delta (first several seconds).

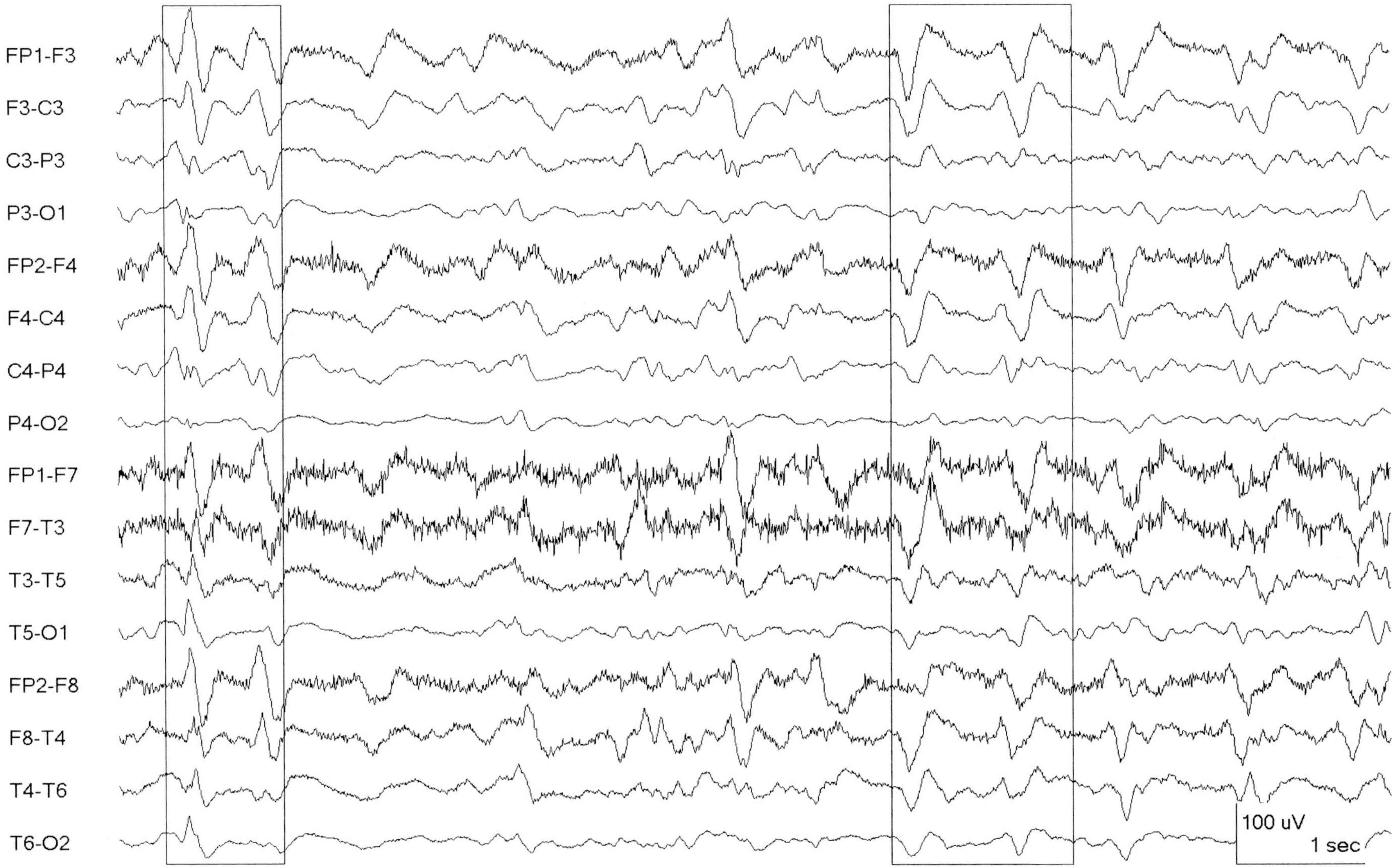

Figure 2.35 Baclofen toxicity. The EEG in this 87-year-old woman being evaluated for a confusional state shows generalized biphasic and triphasic waveforms, sometimes quasiperiodic at approximately 1 per second (boxes). The patient was being treated with baclofen. Mental status cleared following the discontinuation of this medication and the EEG improved.

3 Seizures and status epilepticus

Seizures are quite common in the intensive care unit (ICU), particularly in patients with acute or chronic brain injuries. The prevalence of seizures in those undergoing continuous EEG monitoring (generally for 24 h or more) ranges from 8% in those without prior seizures and with no subtle signs of seizures to 48% after convulsive status epilepticus to more than 50% in those who are comatose in a neurological ICU. Most studies of acute brain injury (including traumatic brain injury, intracerebral hemorrhage and subarachnoid hemorrhage) show a prevalence of seizures of 15–40%. It is clear from many studies now that the majority of seizures in the critically ill are nonconvulsive and can therefore only be diagnosed via EEG. Seizures appear to be an independent predictor of worse outcome in multiple populations.

Seizures in the critically ill with encephalopathy tend to be of slower frequencies, lasting longer and have less clearly defined onset, evolution and offset than seizures in awake patients. Thus, they can be more difficult to recognize, both visually and via computer-based detection. In general, there must be clear evolution in frequency, morphology or location of an ongoing EEG pattern to be sure it represents seizure activity. However, in prolonged nonconvulsive seizures, the evolution can be subtle or absent. Differentiating between ictal and interictal is often quite difficult, if not impossible (see Chapter 4).

Figure list

Figure 3.1 Nonconvulsive status epilepticus, focal.

Figure 3.2 Nonconvulsive status epilepticus, generalized.

Figure 3.3 Nonconvulsive status epilepticus, pre- and post-treatment.

Figure 3.4 Focal seizure.

Figure 3.5–3.6 PLEDs evolving into focal seizure.

Figure 3.7–3.8 Focal seizures.

Figure 3.9 Nonconvulsive status epilepticus vs. triphasic waves.

Figure 3.10 Nonconvulsive status epilepticus, generalized.

Suggested reading

Brenner, R.P. (2002) Is it status? *Epilepsia* **43**(Suppl 3), 103–113.

Brenner, R.P. (2004) EEG in convulsive and nonconvulsive status epilepticus. *Journal of Clinical Neurophysiology* **21**, 319–331.

Chong, D.J. and Hirsch, L.J. (2005) Which EEG patterns warrant treatment in the critically ill? Reviewing the evidence for treatment of periodic epileptiform discharges and related patterns. *Journal of Clinical Neurophysiology* **22**, 79–91.

Atlas of EEG in Critical Care Lawrence J. Hirsch and Richard P. Brenner

Claassen, J., Mayer, S.A., Kowalski, R.G. *et al.* (2004) Detection of electrographic seizures with continuous EEG monitoring in critically ill patients. *Neurology* **62**, 1743–1748.

DeLorenzo, R.J., Waterhouse, E.J., Towne, A.R. *et al.* (1998) Persistent nonconvulsive status epilepticus after the control of convulsive status epilepticus. *Epilepsia* **39**, 833–840.

Drislane, F.W. Blum, A.S. and Schomer, D.L. (1999) Focal status epilepticus: clinical features and significance of different EEG patterns. *Epilepsia* **40**, 1254–1260.

Granner, M.A. and Lee, S.I. (1994) Nonconvulsive status epilepticus: EEG analysis in a large series. *Epilepsia* **35**, 42–47.

Jette, N., Claassen, J., Emerson, R.G. *et al.* (2006) Frequency and predictors of nonconvulsive seizures during continuous electroencephalographic monitoring in critically ill children. *Archives of Neurology* **63**, 1750–1755.

Jirsch, J. and Hirsch, L.J. (2007) Nonconvulsive seizures: Developing a rational approach to the diagnosis and management in the critically ill population. *Clinical Neurophysiology* **118**, 1660–1670.

Jordan, K.G. (1993) Continuous EEG and evoked potential monitoring in the neuroscience intensive care unit. *Journal of Clinical Neurophysiology* **10**, 445–475.

Jordan, K.G. (1995) Neurophysiologic monitoring in the neuroscience intensive care unit. *Neurological Clinics* **13**, 579–626.

Kaplan, P.W. (1999) Assessing the outcomes in patients with nonconvulsive status epilepticus: nonconvulsive status epilepticus is underdiagnosed, potentially overtreated, and confounded by comorbidity. *Journal of Clinical Neurophysiology* **16**, 341–52; discussion 353.

Kaplan, P.W. (2006) The EEG of status epilepticus. *Journal of Clinical Neurophysiology* **23**, 221–229.

Kaplan, P.W. (2007) EEG criteria for nonconvulsive status epilepticus. *Epilepsia* **48** (Suppl 8), 39–41.

Lowenstein, D.H. and Aminoff, M.J. (1992) Clinical and EEG features of status epilepticus in comatose patients. *Neurology* **42**, 100–104.

Nei, M., Lee, J.M., Shanker, V.L. and Sperling, M.R. (1999) The EEG and prognosis in status epilepticus. *Epilepsia* **40**, 157–163.

Pandian, J.D., Cascino, G.D., So, E.L. *et al.* (2004) Digital video-electroencephalographic monitoring in the neurological-neurosurgical intensive care unit: Clinical features and outcome. *Archives of Neurology* **61**, 1090–1094.

Privitera, M., Hoffman, M., Moore, J.L. *et al.* (1994) EEG detection of nontonic-clonic status epilepticus in patients with altered consciousness. *Epilepsy Research* **18**, 155–166.

Towne, A.R., Waterhouse, E.J., Boggs, J.G. *et al.* (2000) Prevalence of nonconvulsive status epilepticus in comatose patients. *Neurology* **54**, 340–345.

Vespa, P.M., Nuwer, M.R., Nenov, V. *et al.* (1999) Increased incidence and impact of nonconvulsive and convulsive seizures after traumatic brain injury as detected by continuous electroencephalographic monitoring. *Journal of Neurosurgery* **91**, 750–760.

Vespa, P.M., O'Phelan, K., Shah, M. *et al.* (2003) Acute seizures after intracerebral hemorrhage: a factor in progressive midline shift and outcome. *Neurology* **60**, 1441–1446.

Young, G.B., Jordan, K.G. and Doig, G.S. (1996) An assessment of nonconvulsive seizures in the intensive care unit using continuous EEG monitoring: An investigation of variables associated with mortality. *Neurology* **47**, 83–89.

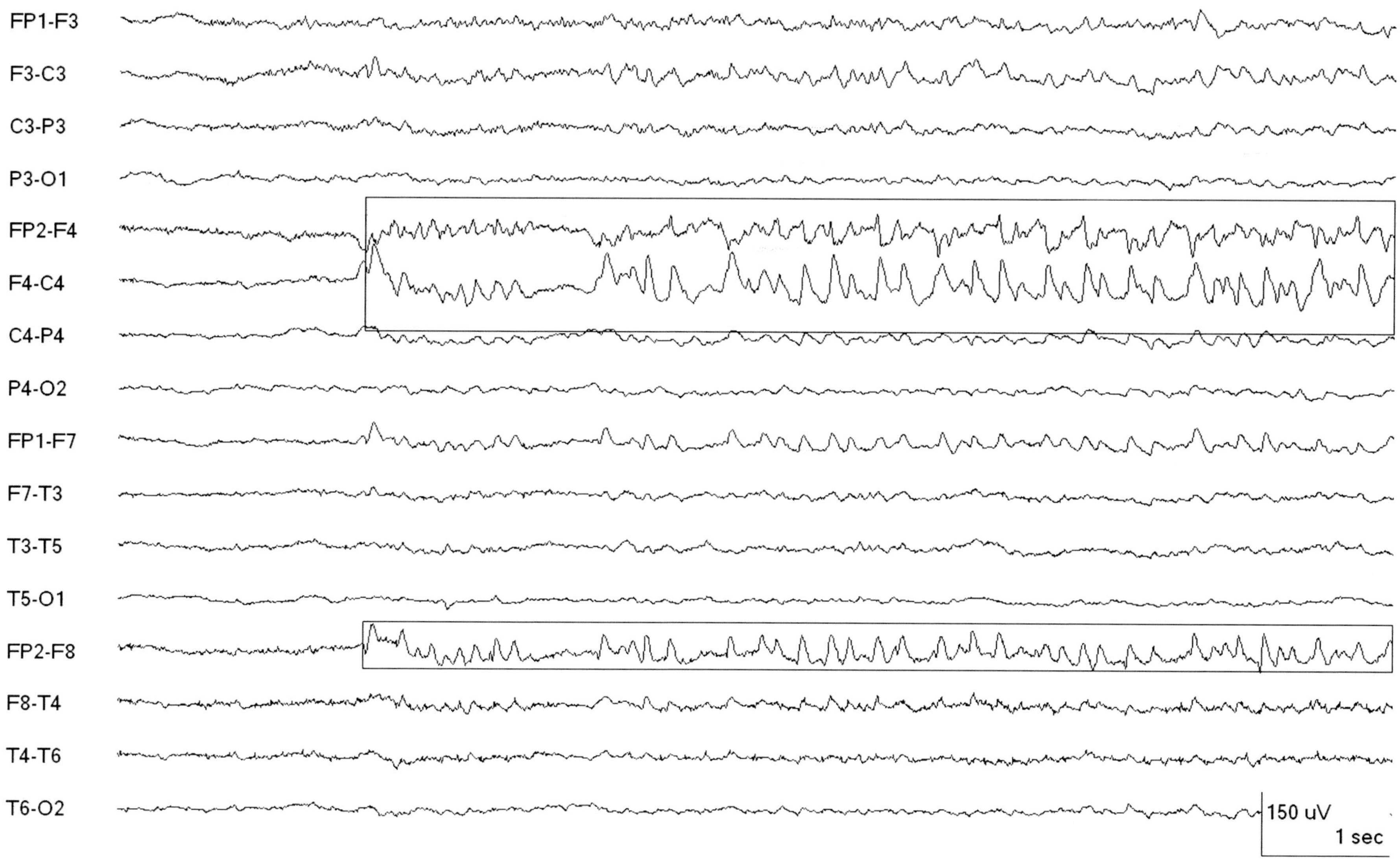

Figure 3.1 Nonconvulsive seizures and status epilepticus, focal. (a) This 49-year-old woman with a history of head trauma, seizures and strokes was being evaluated for decreased mental status. During the recording, she had repetitive right-sided electrographic seizures beginning in the right frontal region (highlighted) and was in focal (also known as partial) nonconvulsive status epilepticus.

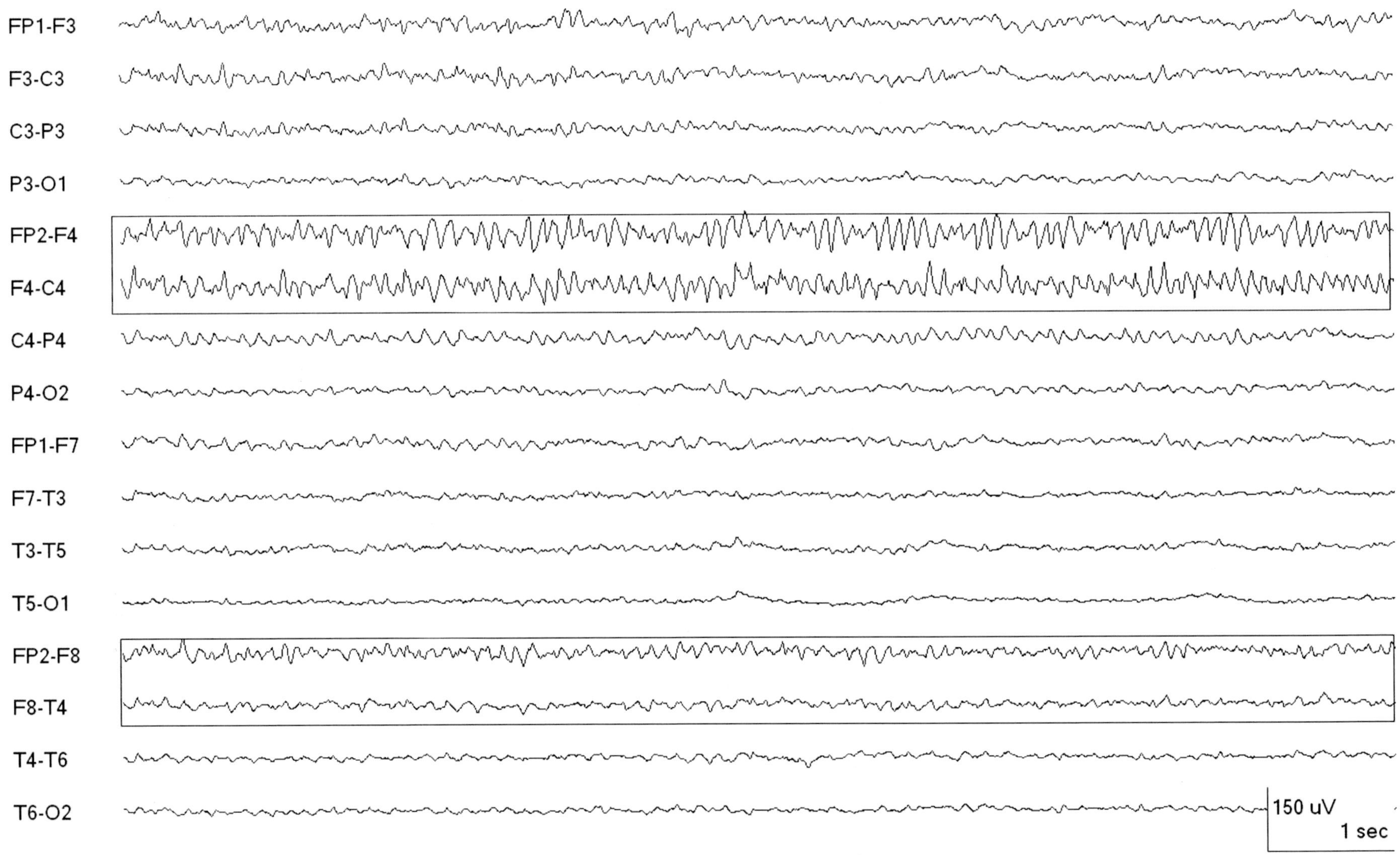

Figure 3.1 (*Continued*) (b) Thirty seconds later, the discharge has become faster, thus demonstrating evolution in frequency and morphology and therefore unequivocally ictal. The frequency in this sample is predominantly in the alpha range.

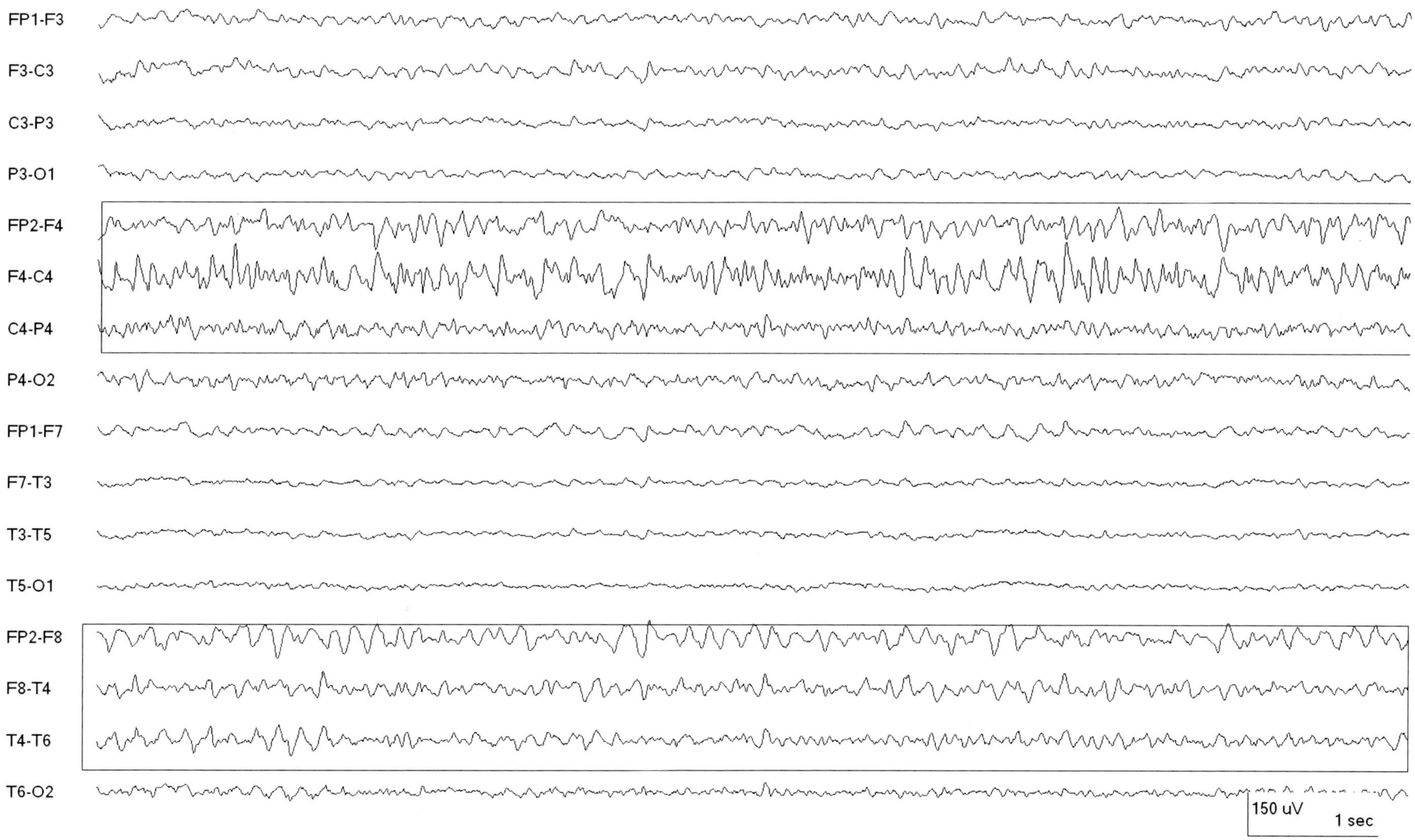

Figure 3.1 (*Continued*) (c) Four minutes later, the discharge continues, becoming more widespread and slower, thus demonstrating evolution in location and further evolution in frequency and morphology. There were no associated movements.

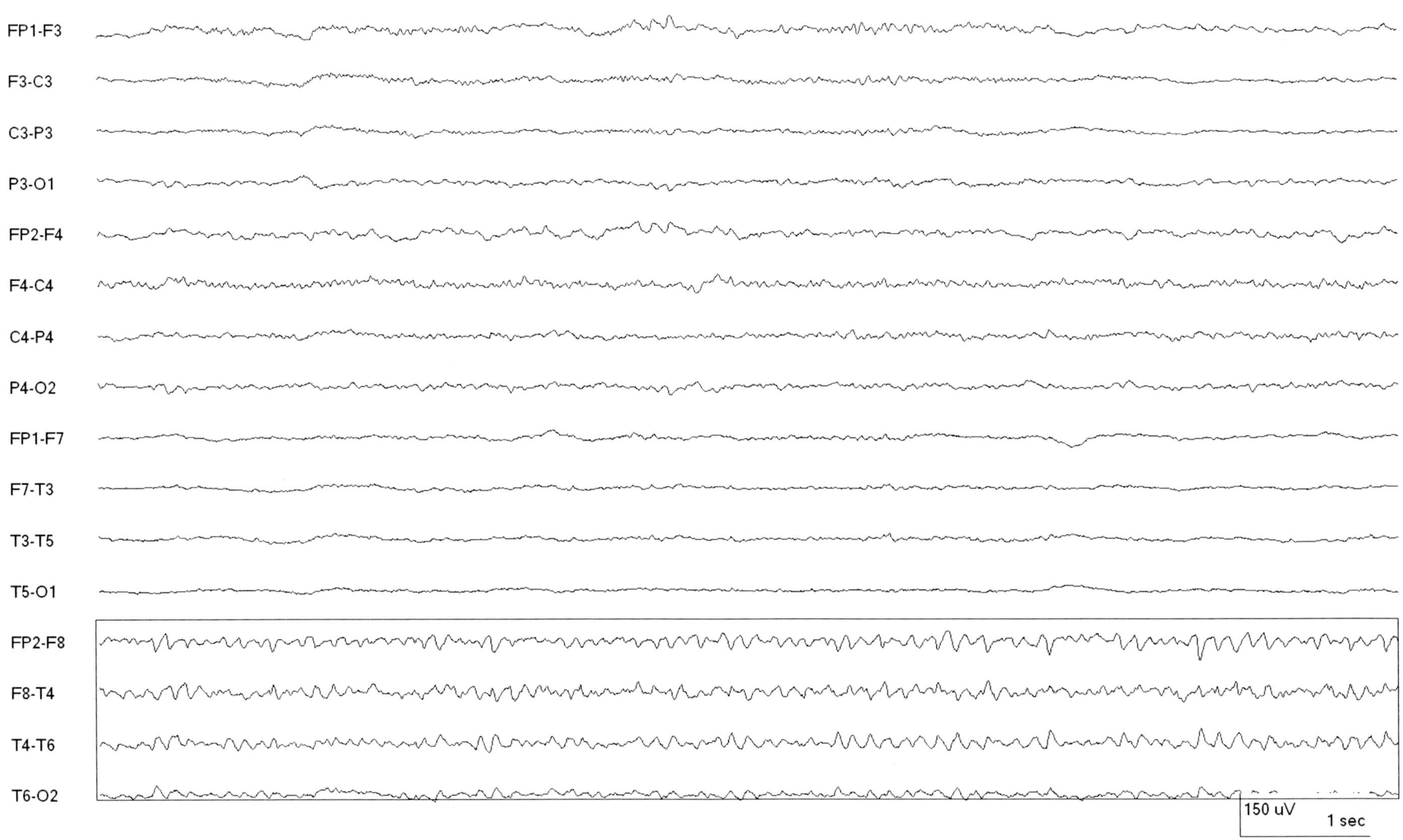

Figure 3.1 (*Continued*) (d) The discharge is now in the right temporal region only. The patient was given intravenous lorazepam.

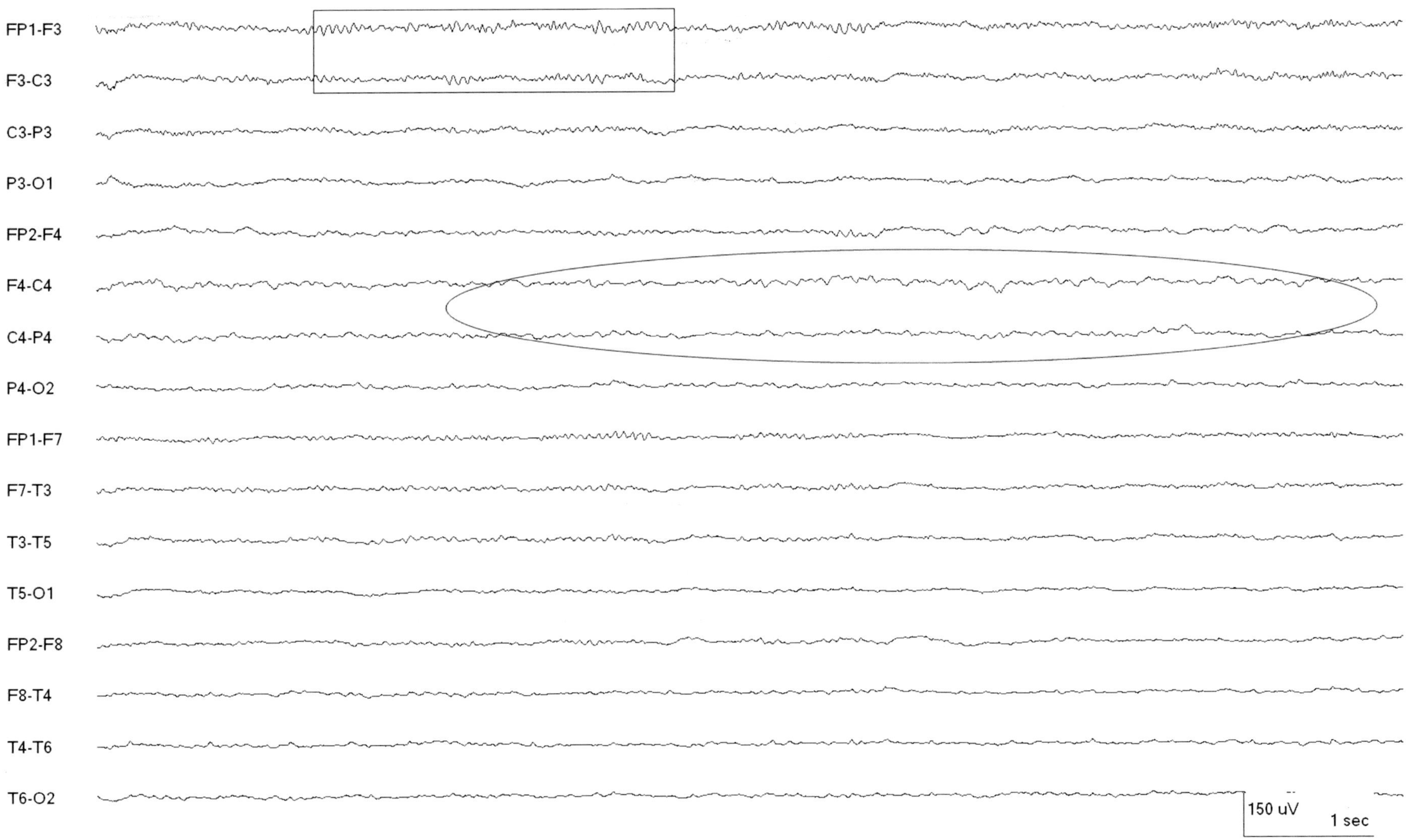

Figure 3.1 (*Continued*) (e) The discharge ceased after the administration of lorazepam. Beta activity (likely from the benzodiazepine) is present, but predominantly over the left hemisphere (box) (i.e. attenuated on the right – see ellipse – suggesting cortical dysfunction on the right, as is commonly seen postictally); mild focal slowing (suggesting dysfunction including subcortical white matter) can also be appreciated in the right parasagittal region (ellipse).

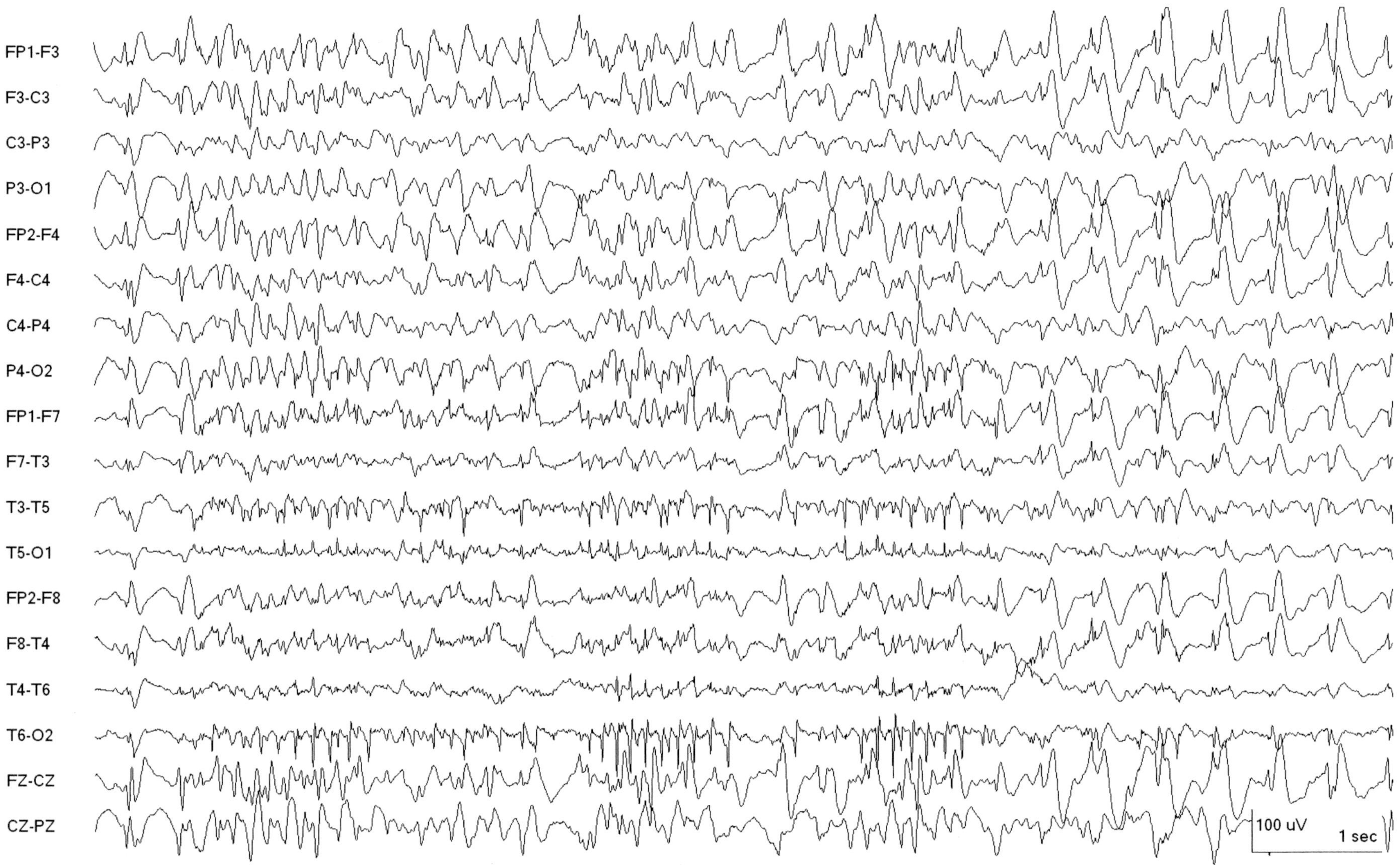

Figure 3.2 Nonconvulsive status epilepticus, generalized. (a) Bipolar. This EEG in a 44-year-old man with a history of mental retardation and seizures shows generalized epileptiform abnormalities, irregular and fast (varying from 3 to >8 Hz), slowing down in the last few seconds to 2.5–3 Hz, when it develops a spike-wave morphology. The patient was in nonconvulsive status epilepticus.

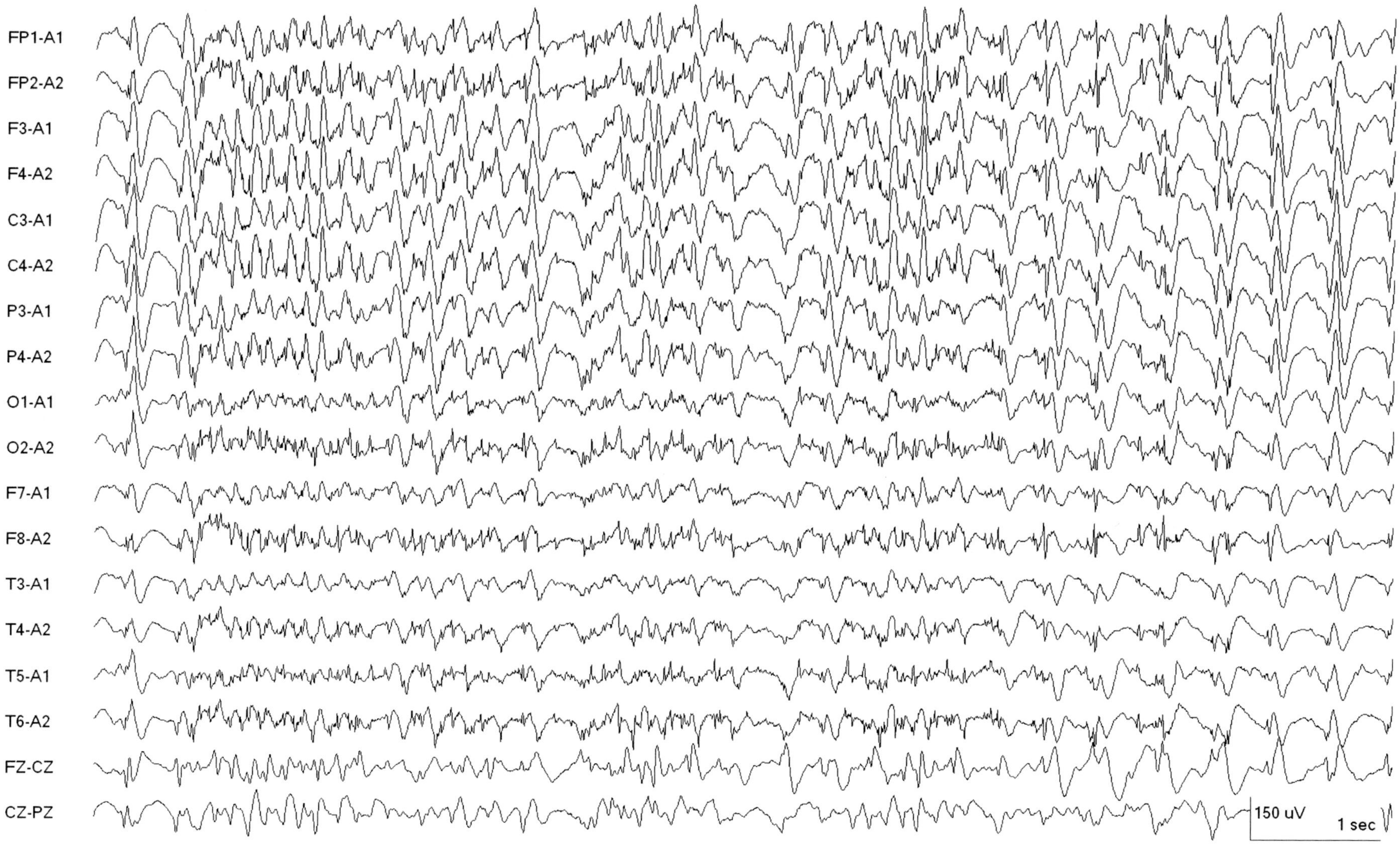

Figure 3.2 (*Continued*) (b) Referential. The epoch has been reformatted utilizing a referential montage to ipsilateral ears.

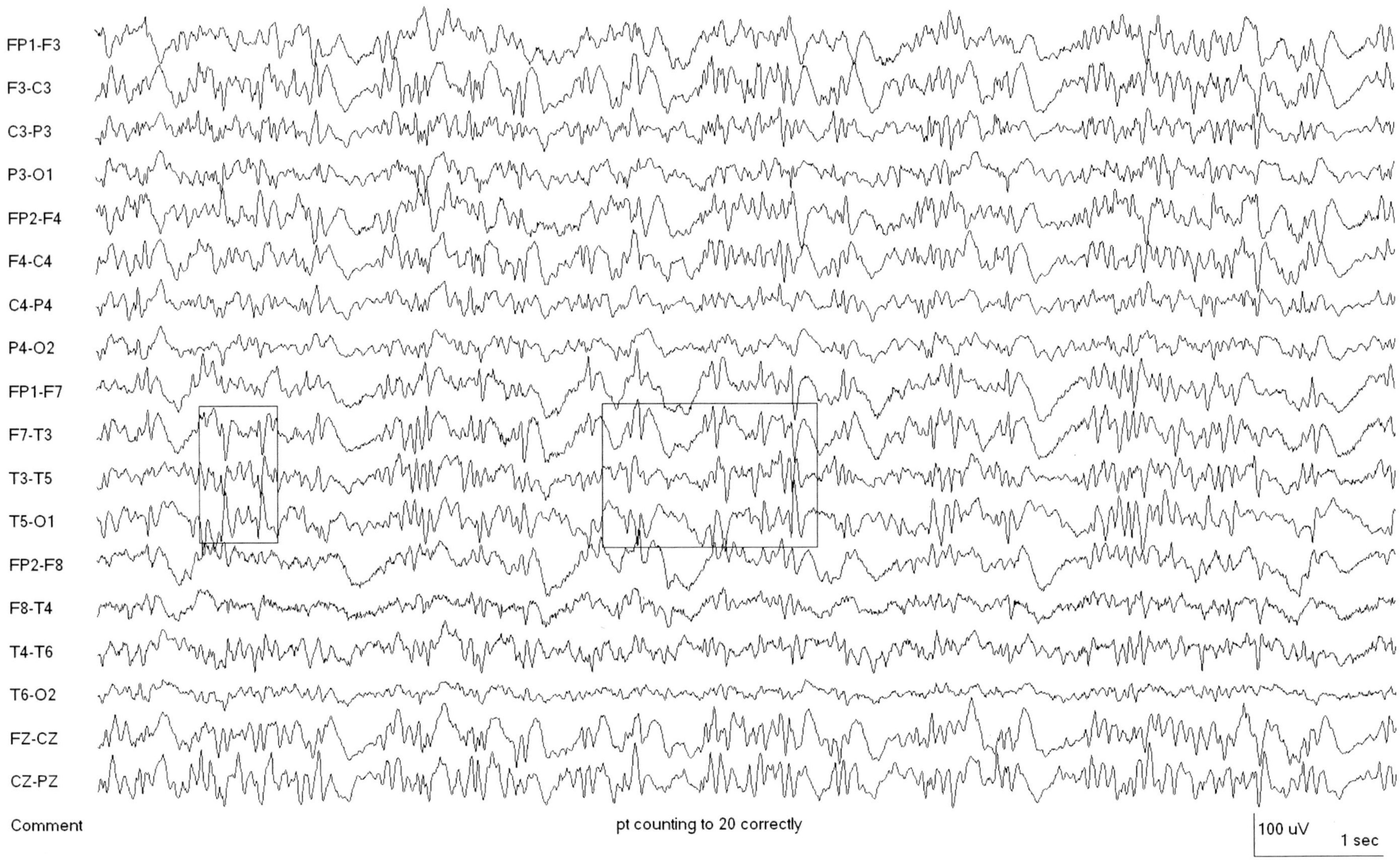

Figure 3.3 Nonconvulsive status epilepticus. (a) This 20-year-old man was in nonconvulsive status epilepticus (NCSE) associated with continual, widespread epileptiform activity. The patient was able to answer many questions correctly, although he was frequently slow in his responses.

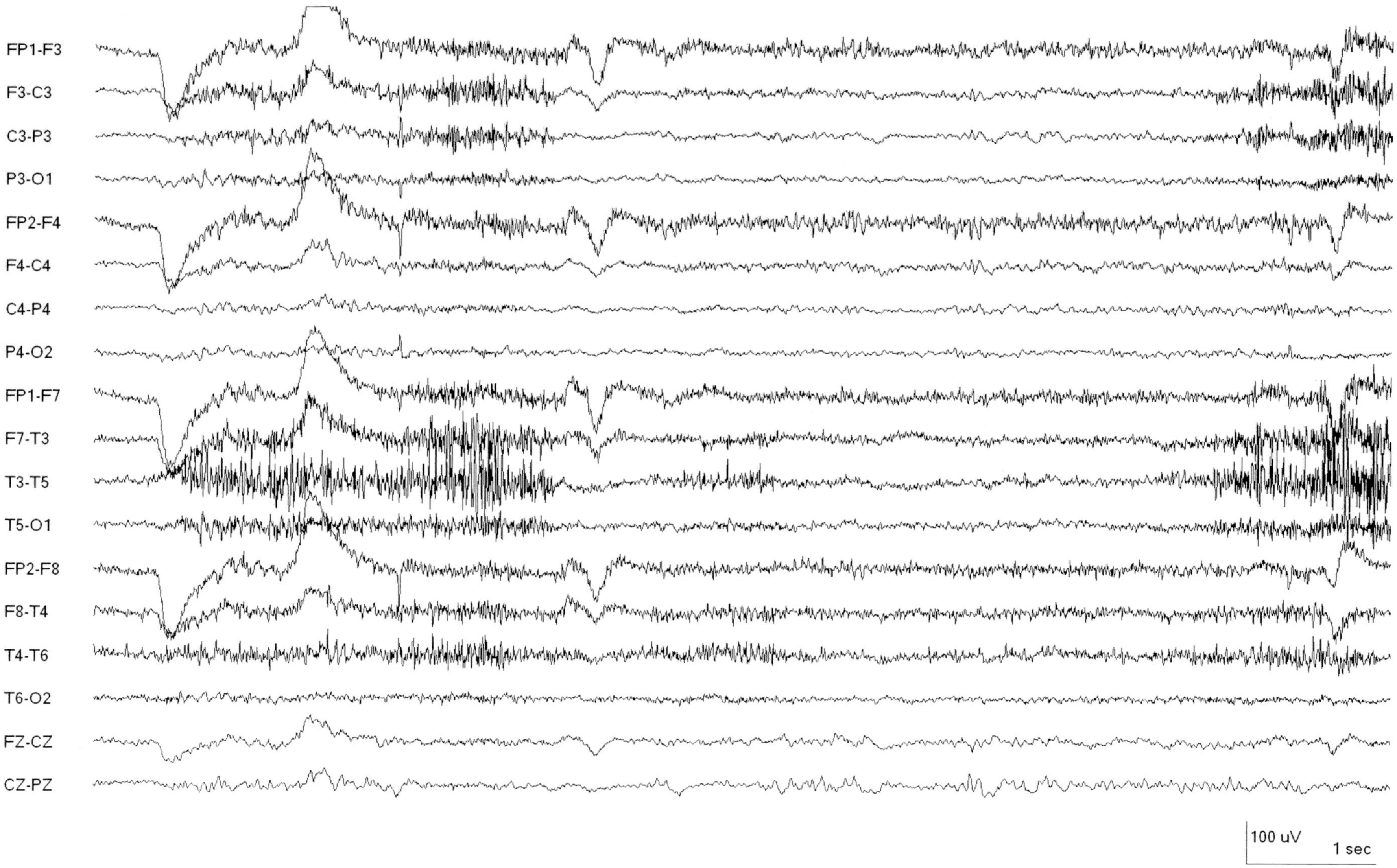

Figure 3.3 (*Continued*) (b) His clinical state and EEG improved following the administration of lorazepam confirming the diagnosis of NCSE.

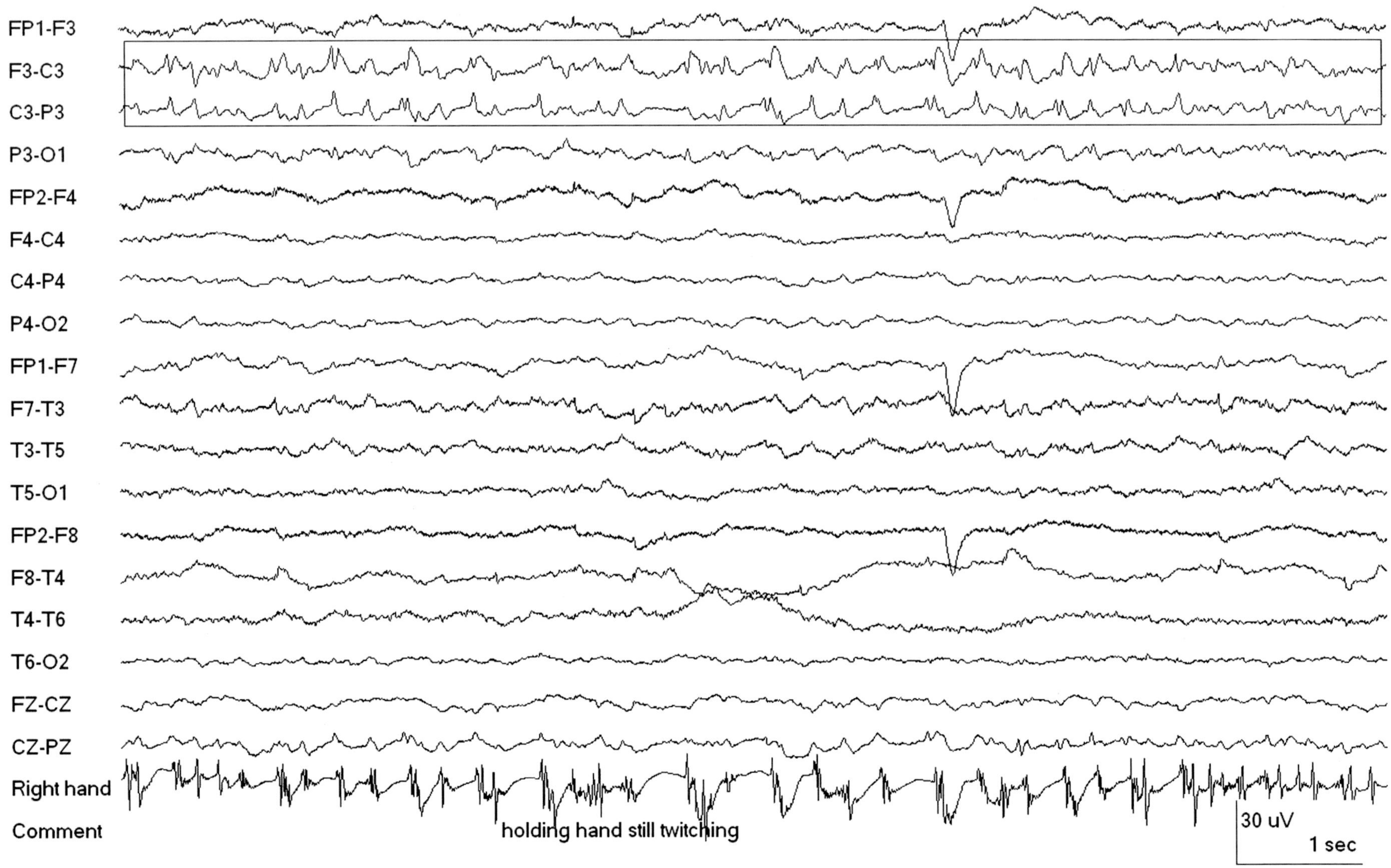

Figure 3.4 Focal seizure. This 33-year-old woman with acute hepatic failure had focal seizures characterized by twitching movements of the right hand; see the last channel, which is an electrode on the right hand and shows muscle contractions during the twitching. Repetitive spikes and sharp waves are present in the left central area, irregular but recurring at 3–5 per second. This is a clinical and electrographic focal seizure from the left Rolandic region.

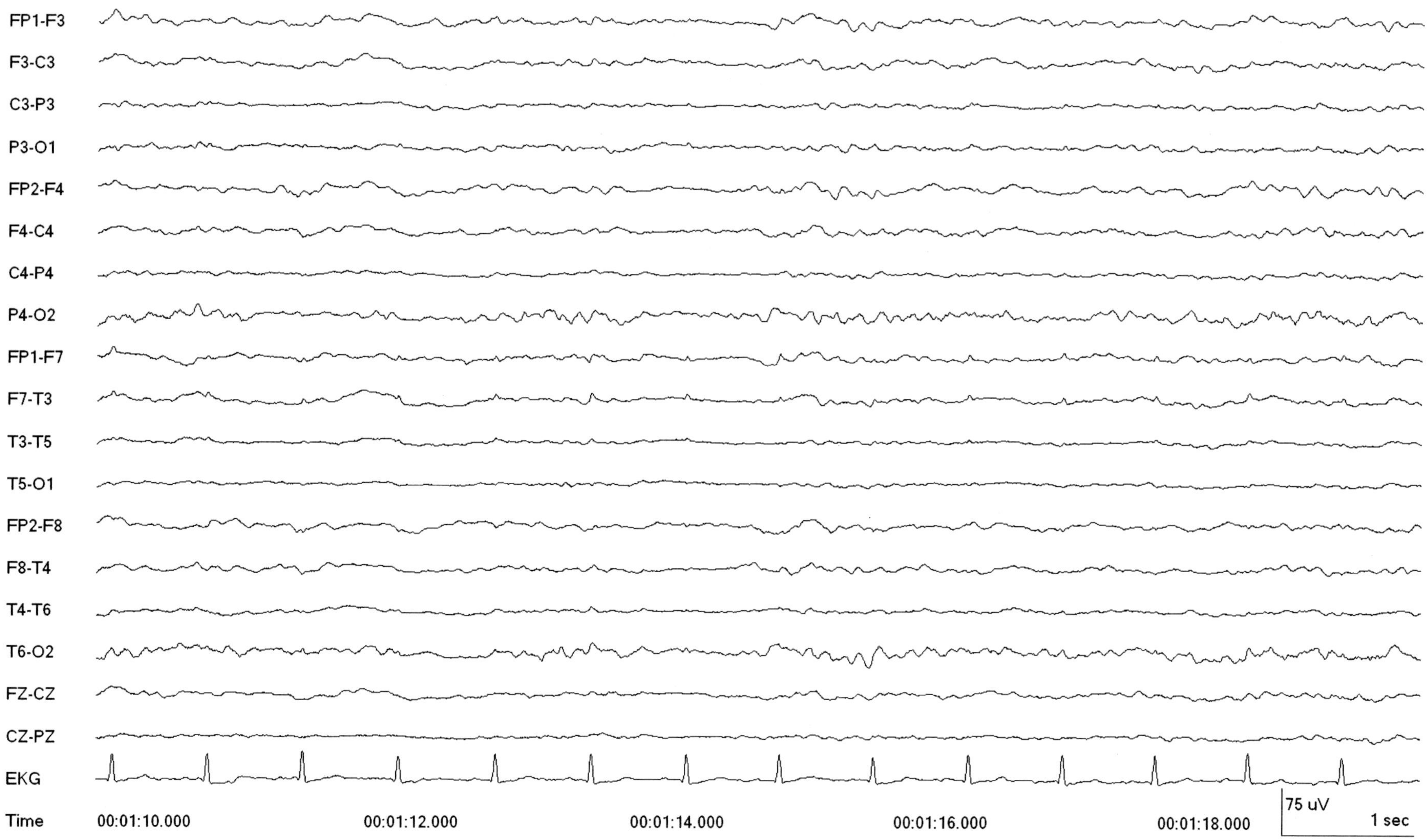

Figure 3.5 PLEDs evolving into focal seizure. (a). The baseline EEG in this 82-year-old woman with a history of acute renal failure, being evaluated for seizures, shows diffuse slowing of background activity.

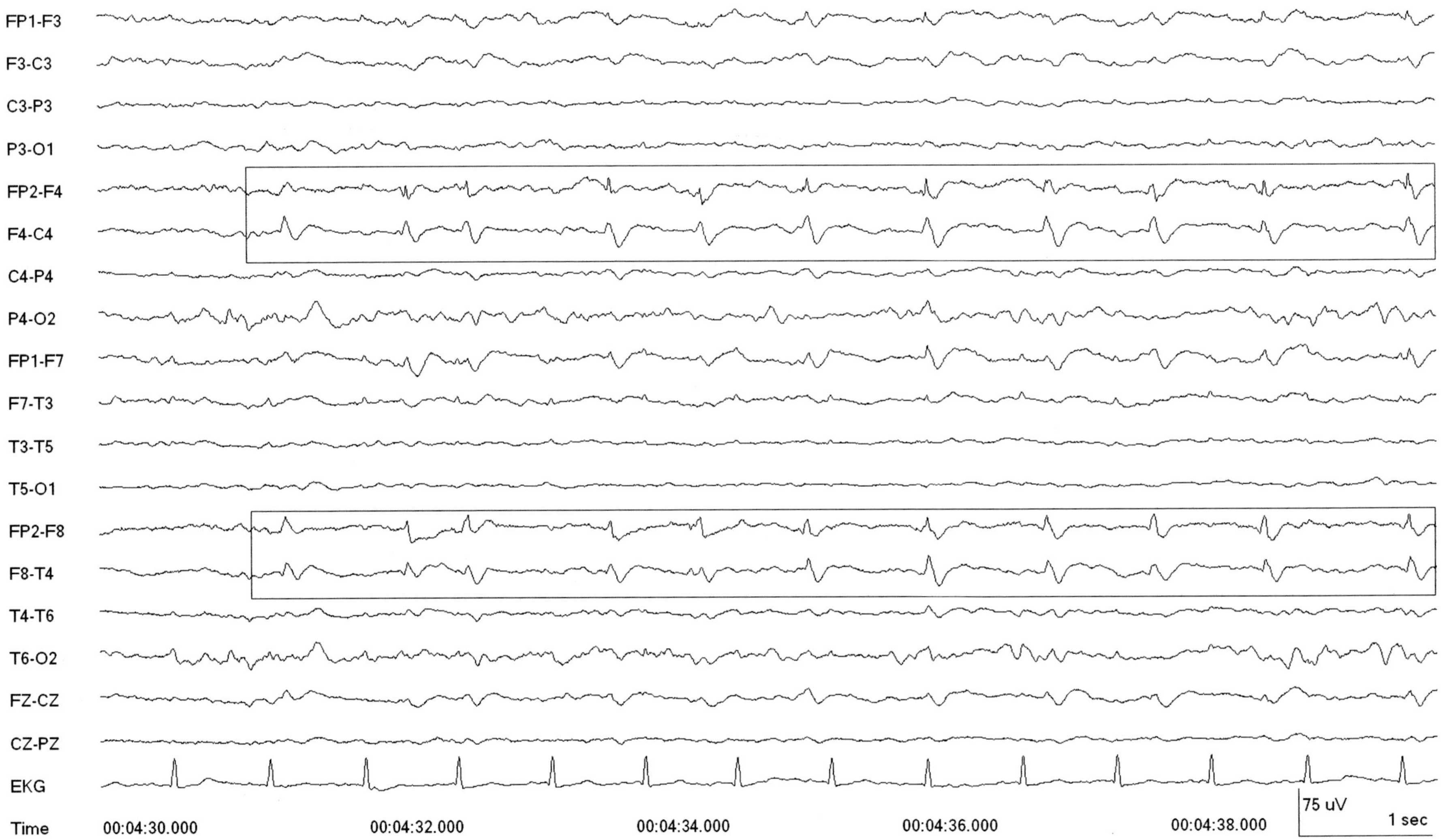

Figure 3.5 (*Continued*) (b) Right frontal periodic lateralized epileptiform discharges (PLEDs) at approximately 1 Hz begin to appear, maximal at F4 and F8 (boxes).

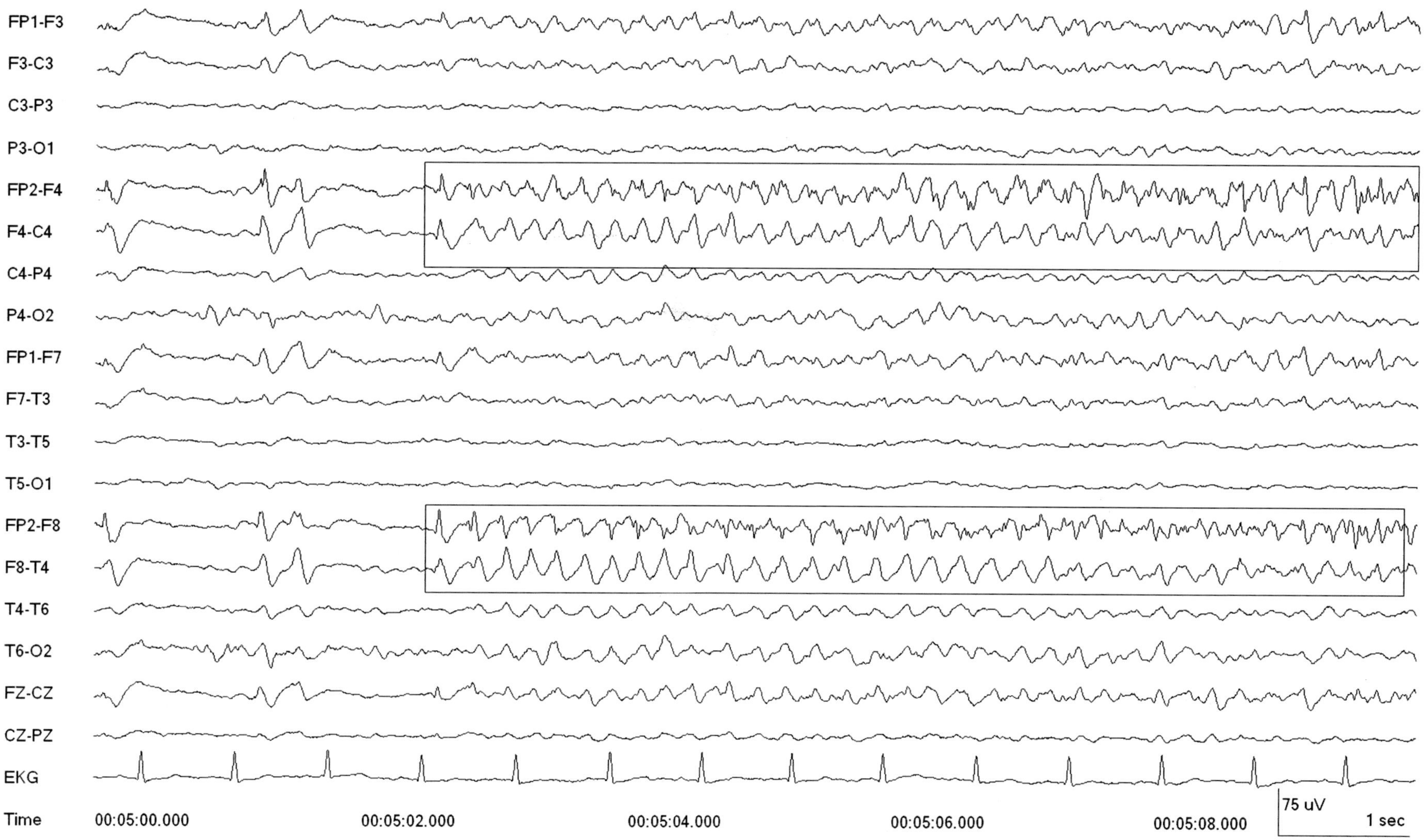

Figure 3.5 (*Continued*) (c) The PLEDs are then replaced by an electrographic seizure that begins with rhythmic sharply contoured theta (boxes).

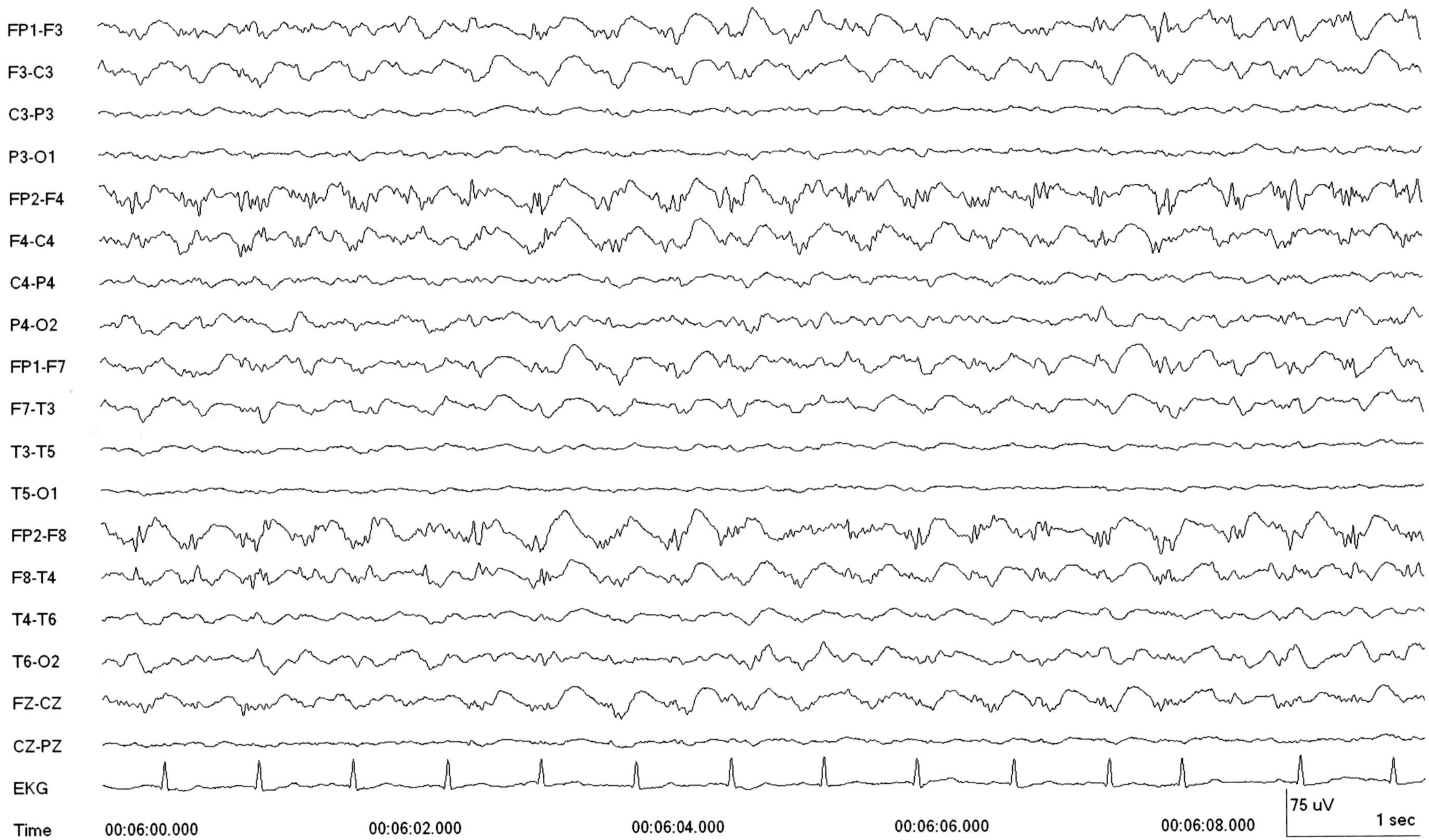

Figure 3.5 (*Continued*) (d) The ictal discharge has evolved in frequency from theta to delta, now consisting of rhythmic approximately 2.5 Hz activity with superimposed sharply contoured beta at F4 and F8. It has also spread to involve more of the left hemisphere now, though remaining maximal on the right.

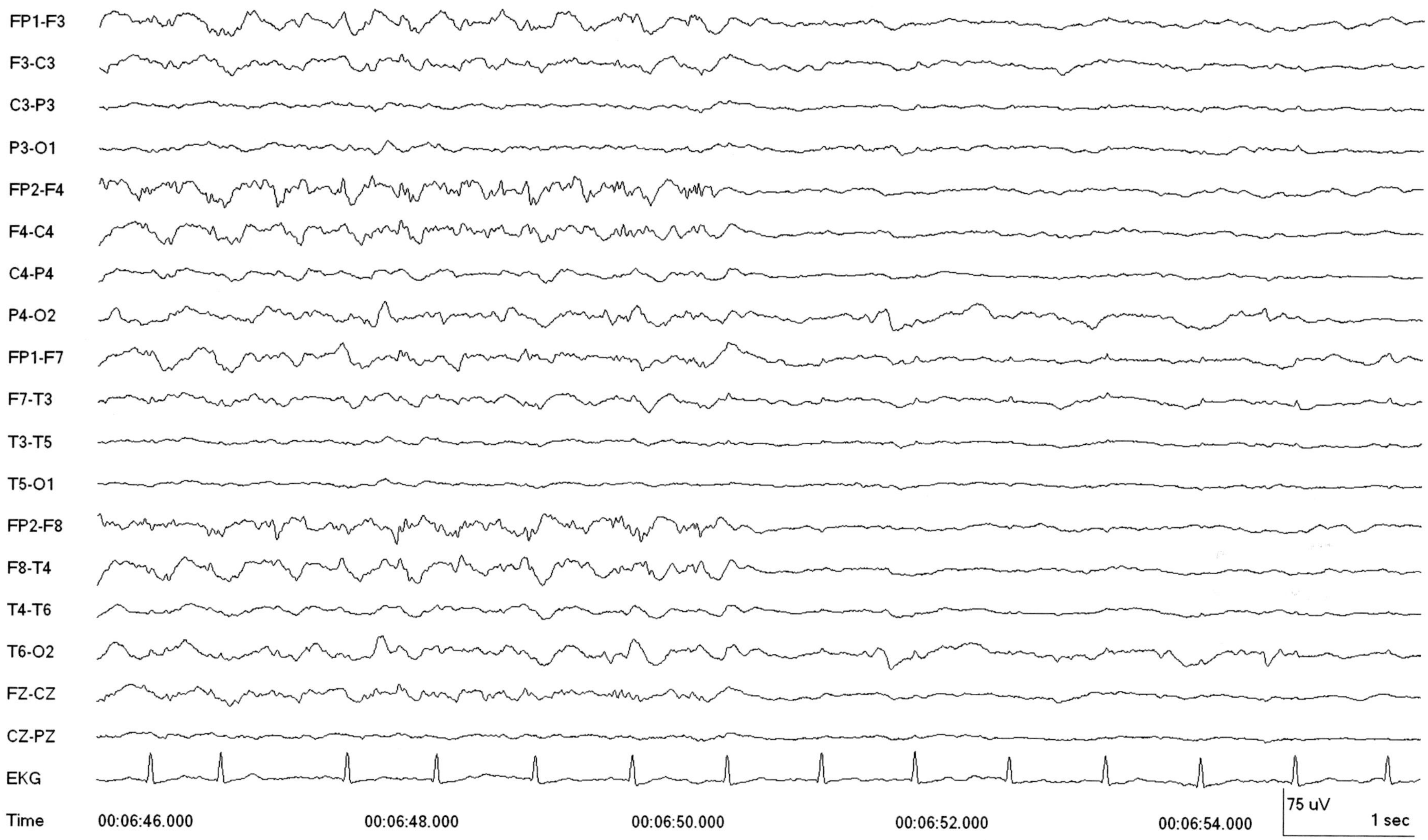

Figure 3.5 (*Continued*) (e) The seizure ends abruptly in the middle of this page.

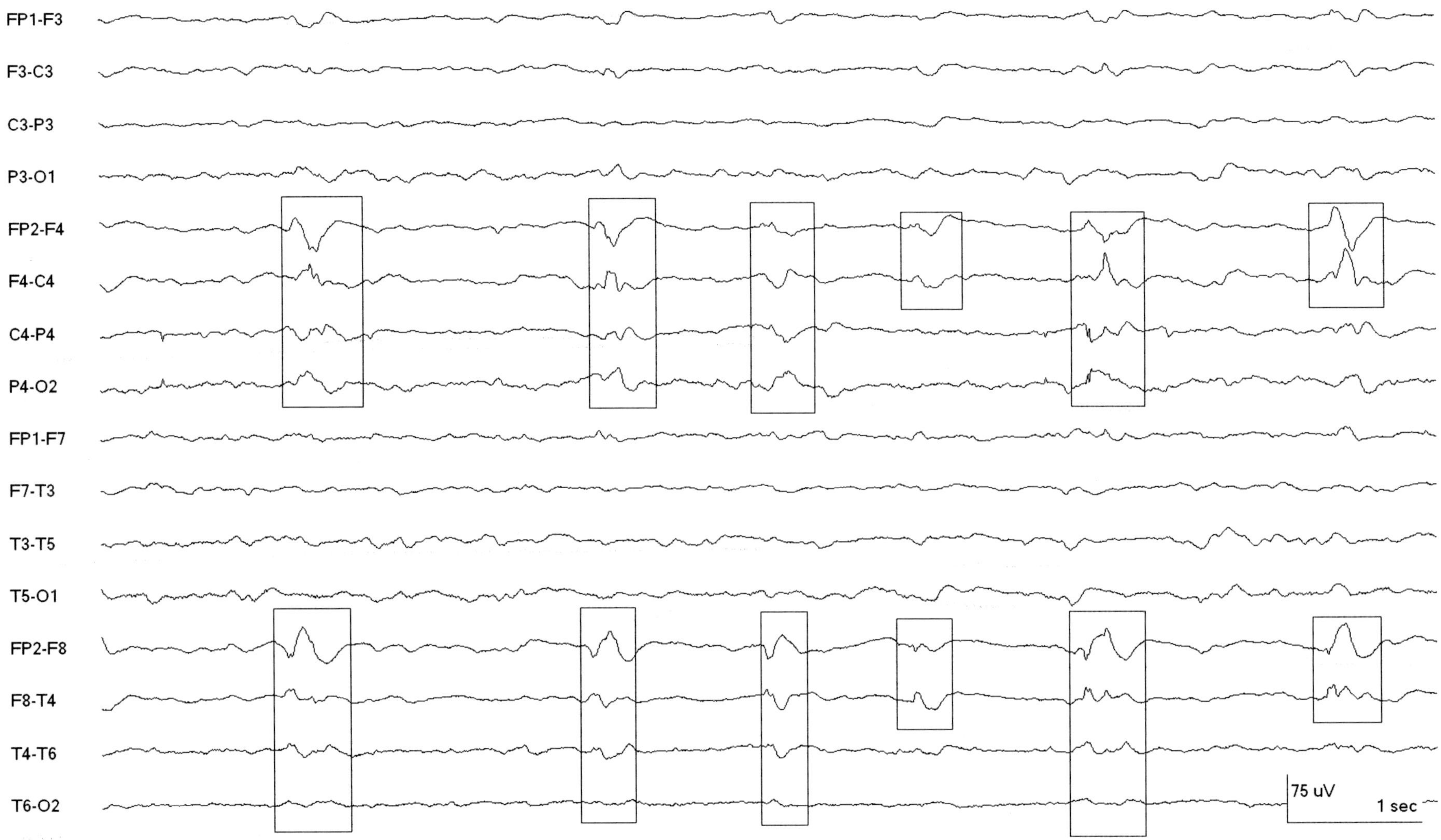

Figure 3.6 PLEDs evolving into focal seizure. (a) First of four consecutive 10 s epochs from a 57-year-old woman status post (s/p) right 'strokectomy' (resection of necrotic area within a large infarct) and evacuation of right subdural hematoma. This sample shows blunt approximately 0.5 Hz right-sided periodic discharges; these still qualify as 'PLEDs' even though the discharges are not frankly 'epileptiform'.

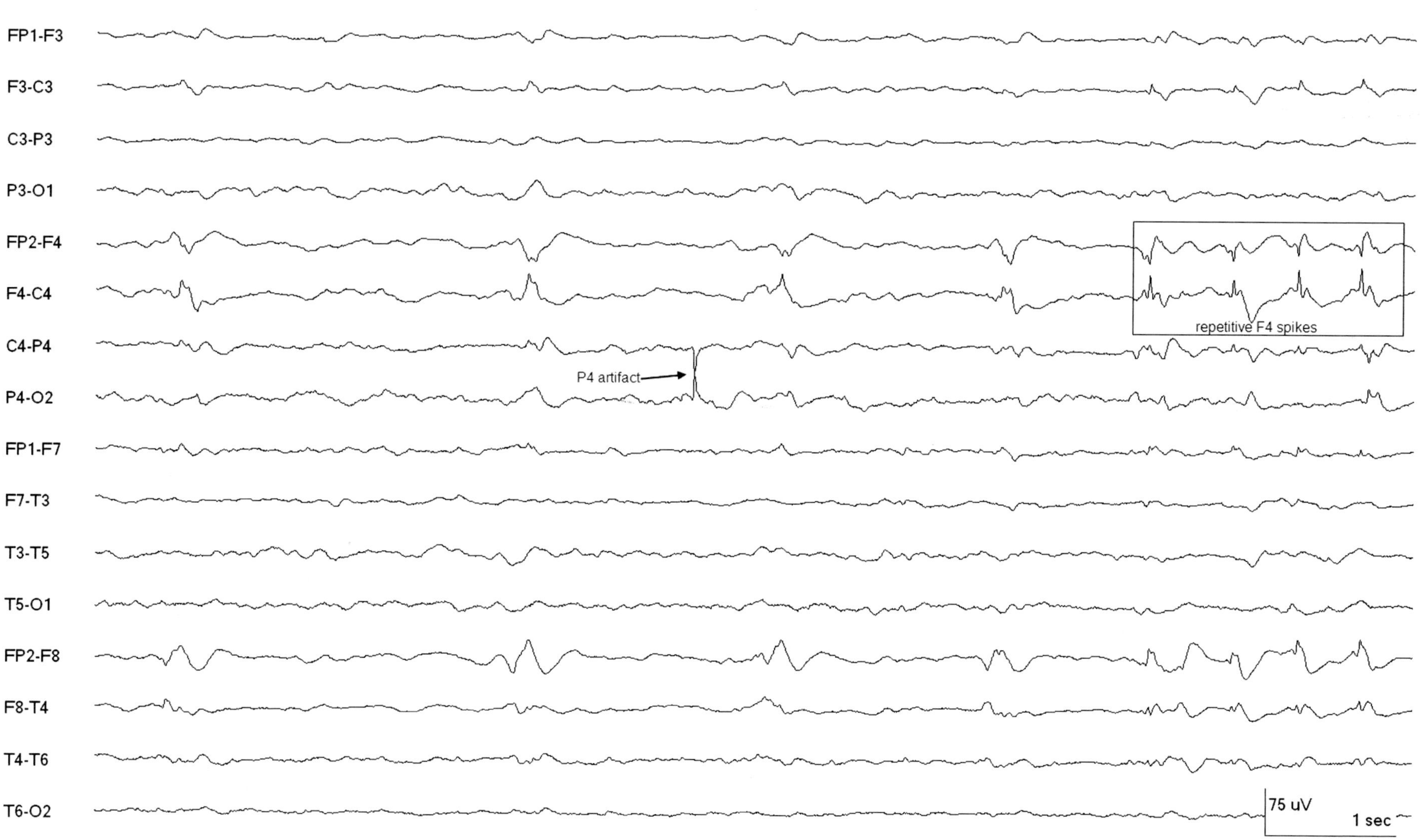

Figure 3.6 (*Continued*) (b) Ten seconds later, the discharges have changed morphologically, particularly toward the end of the sample, now consisting of faster repetitive spikes, maximal at electrode F4 (box). There is also an electrode artifact at P4 (arrow; note lack of field: seen only in channels with P4).

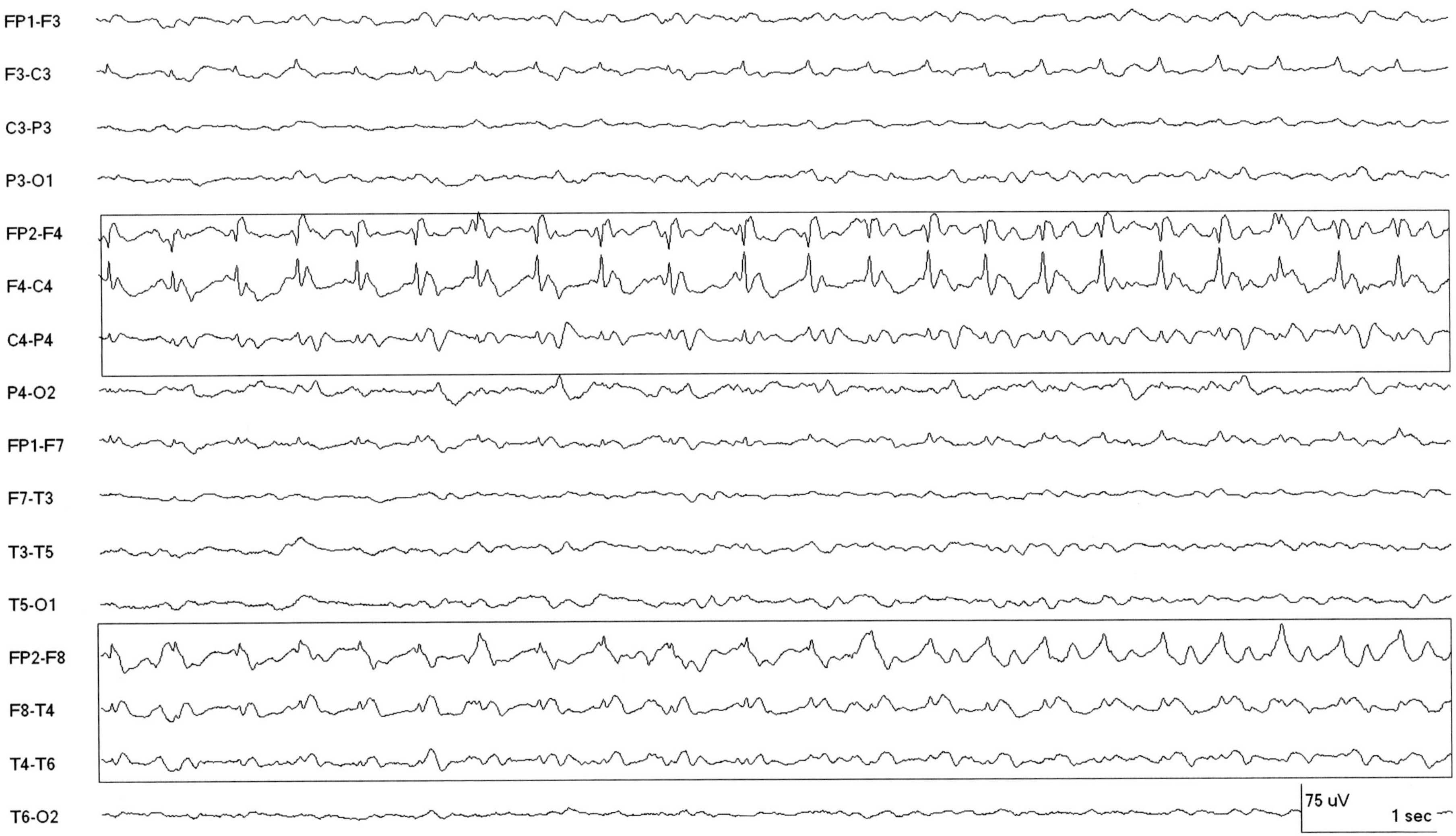

Figure 3.6 (*Continued*) (c) Ten seconds later, the discharge becomes more widespread over the right hemisphere, faster (now up to three per second), and with slowly evolving morphology.

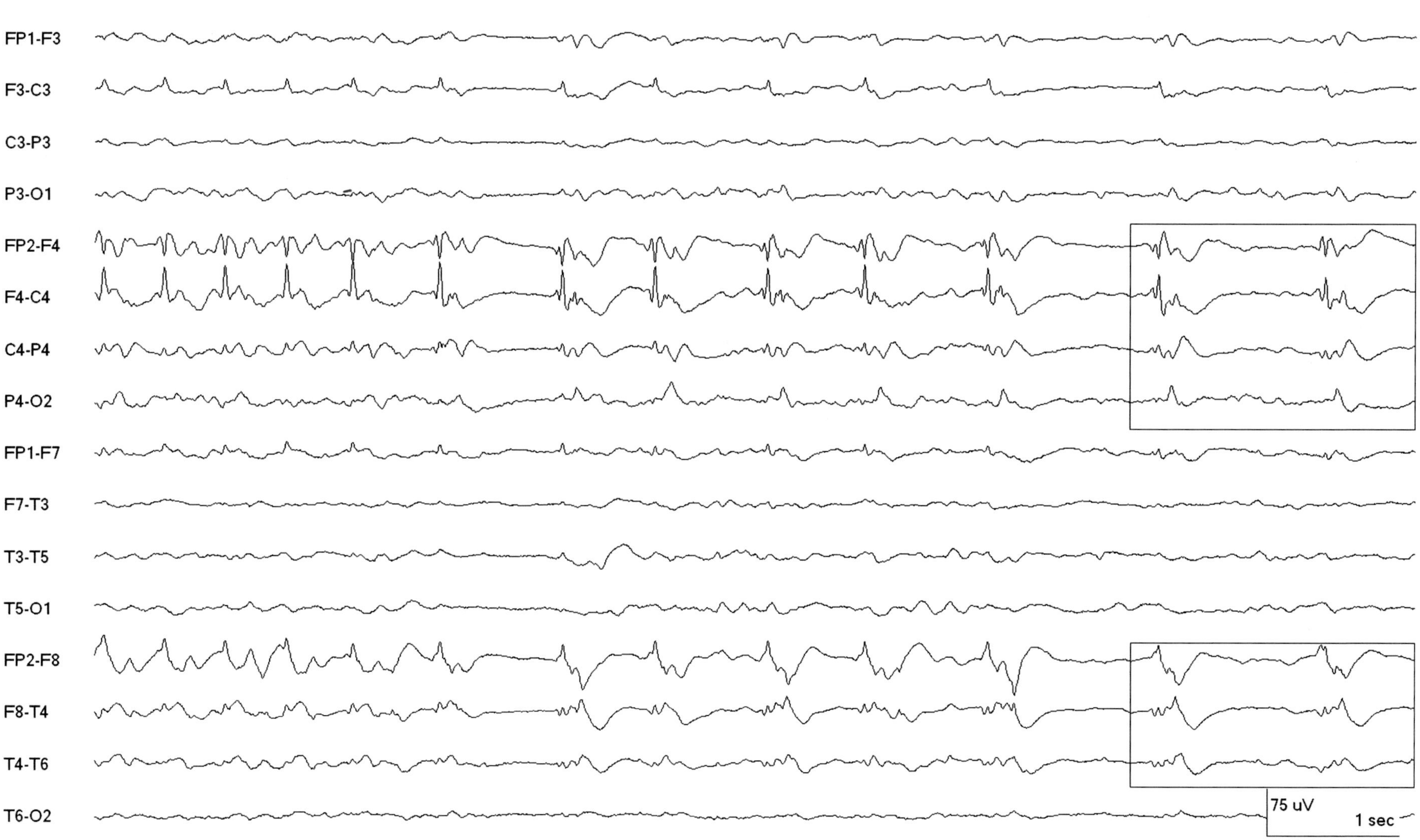

Figure 3.6 (*Continued*) (d) The discharge is slowing and breaking up 10 s later, returning to PLEDs in the last few seconds.

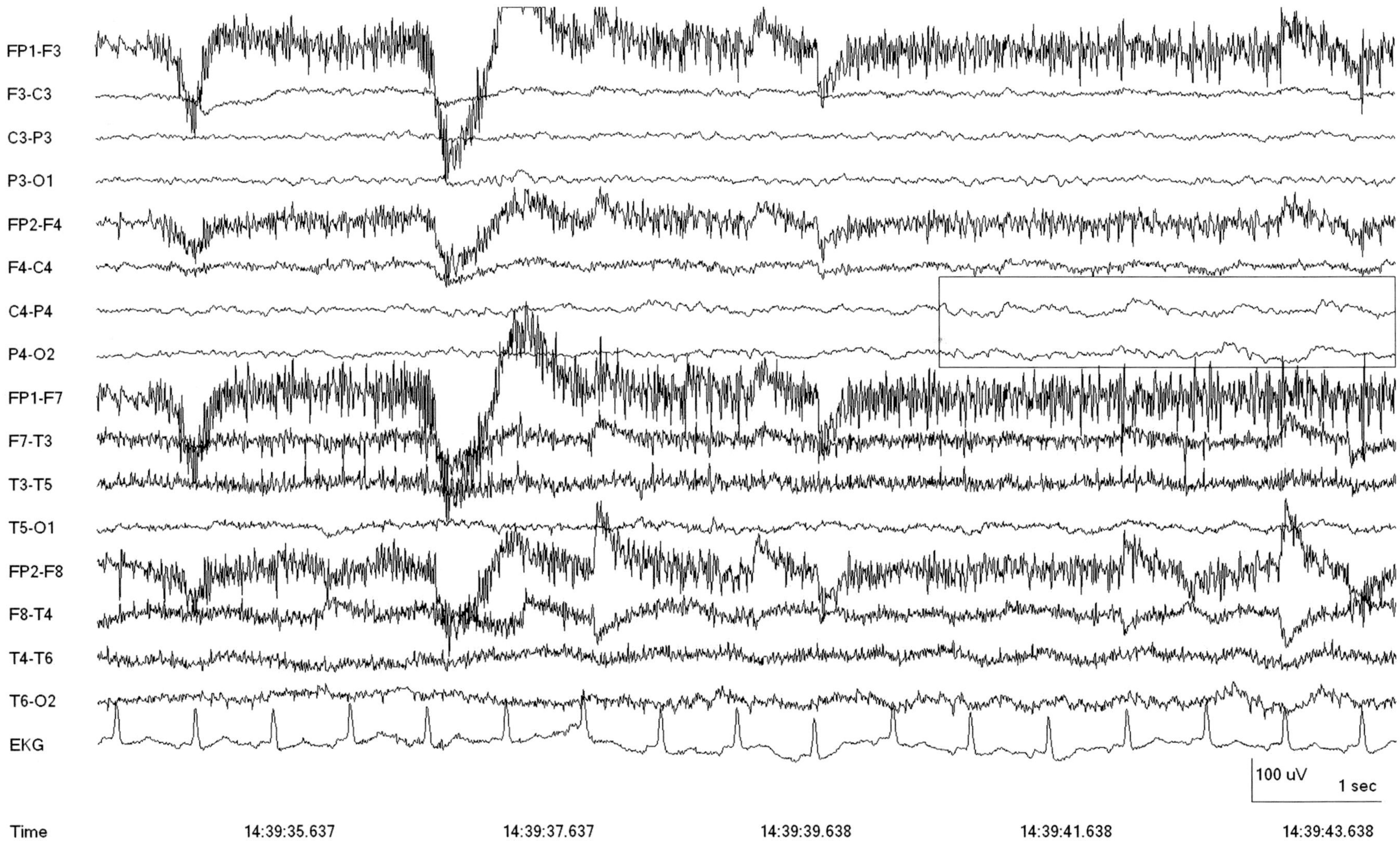

Figure 3.7 Focal seizure. (a) This EEG is from a 22-year-old man s/p lung and heart transplant. The patient had a right-sided subdural hematoma evacuated 10 days prior to this EEG. One hour before the onset of the recording, the patient had a focal motor seizure involving the left face and eye. There is mild focal slowing in the right posterior head region (box).

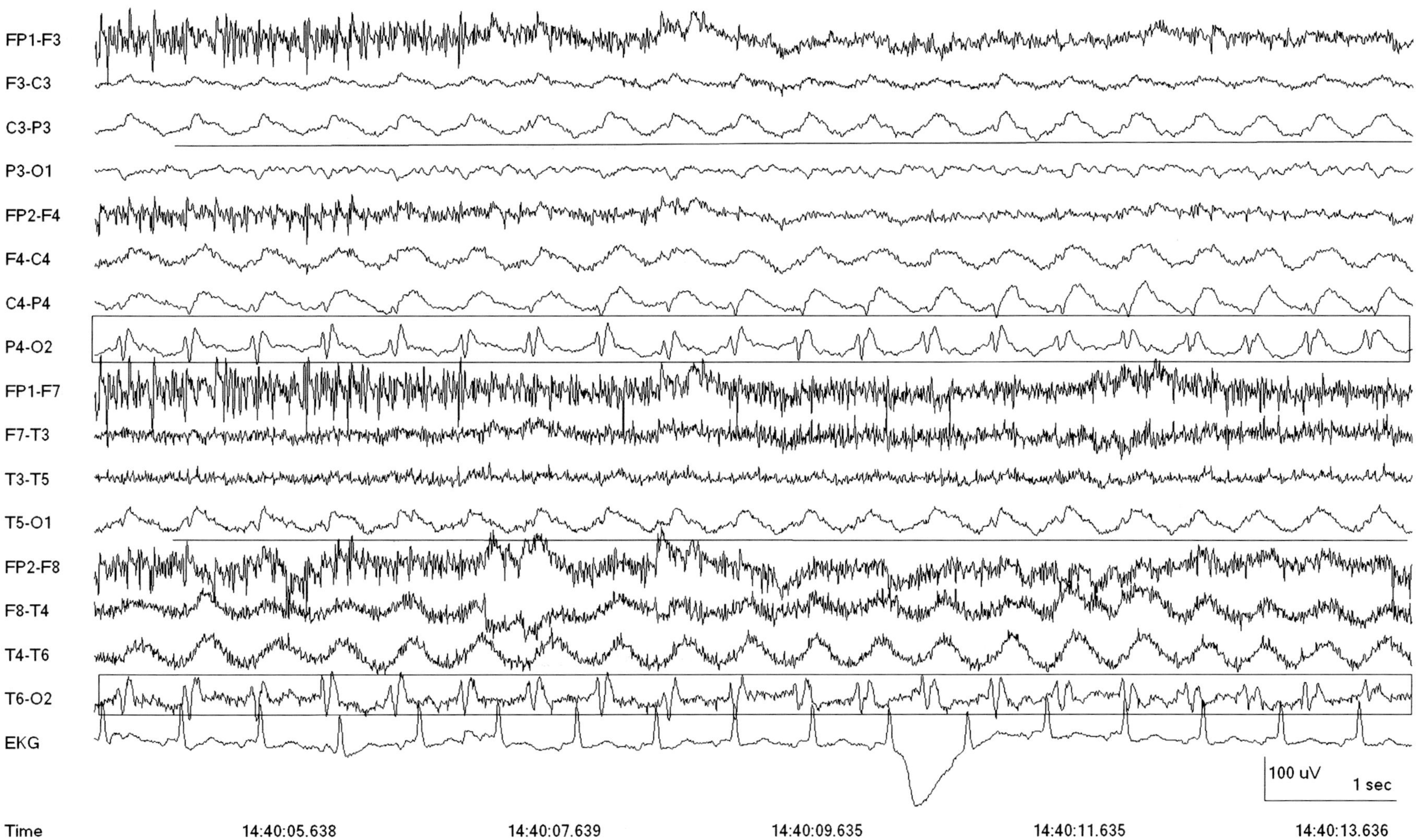

Figure 3.7 (*Continued*) (b) Thirty seconds later, spike-and-wave discharges are present at two per second in the right posterior head region (boxes) with synchronous rhythmic delta present over homologous areas on the left (underlined). The electrocardiogram (EKG) channel confirms that this is not EKG or pulse artifact.

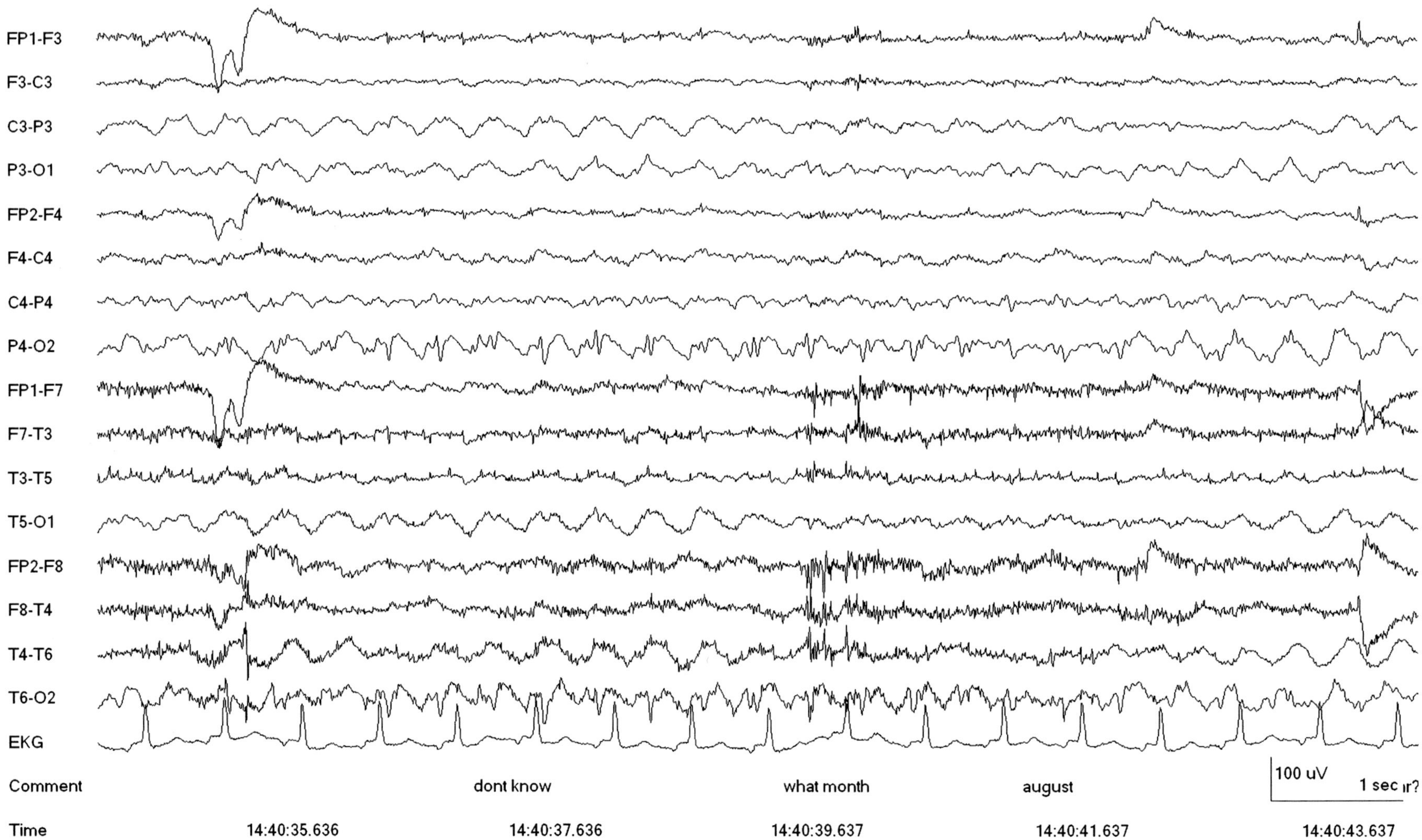

Figure 3.7 (*Continued*) (c) The discharge continues 30 s later, at which time the patient was answering questions. There is clear evolution, with the ictal discharge, still maximal in the posterior right hemisphere, becoming lower amplitude and faster, and changing in morphology.

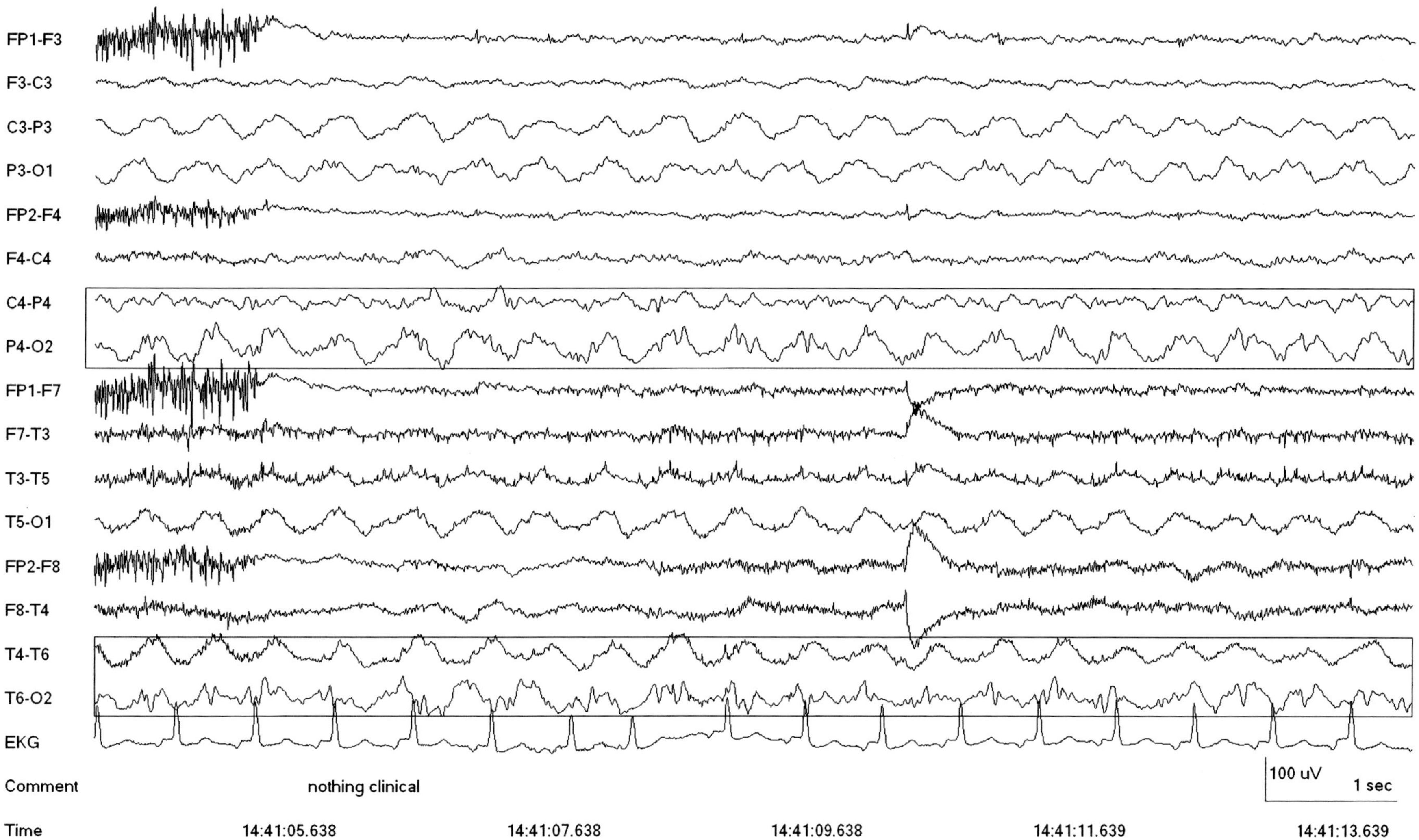

Figure 3.7 (*Continued*) (d) Thirty seconds later, the discharges are still present, although now becoming slower and changing somewhat in morphology. The pattern now consists of rhythmic delta with superimposed fast activity (boxes).

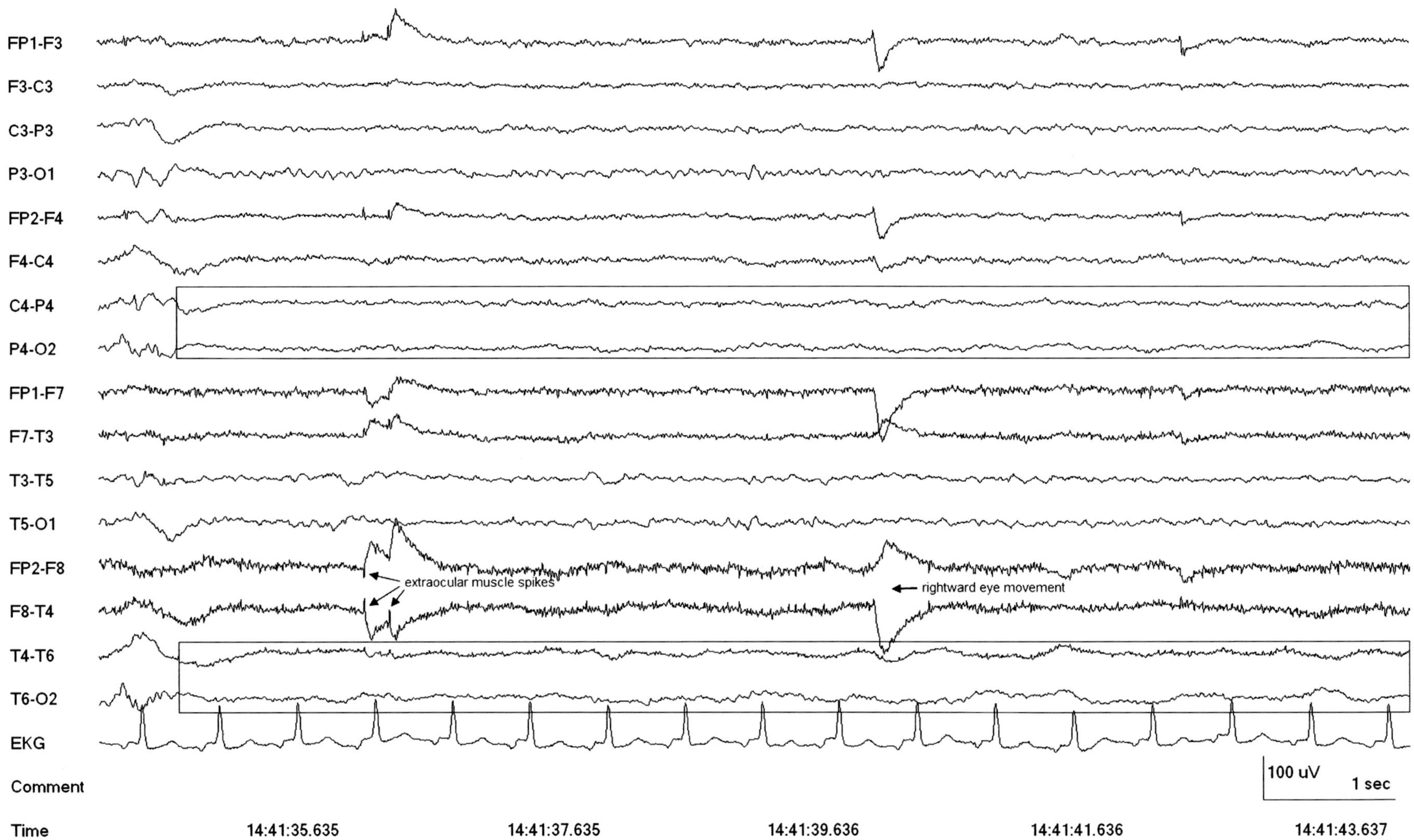

Figure 3.7 (*Continued*) (e) It is no longer present 30 seconds later. There appears to be attenuation of faster activity in the same area that had the maximal ictal discharge (boxes), probably postictal attenuation of cortical activity, though this should be confirmed in a referential recording.

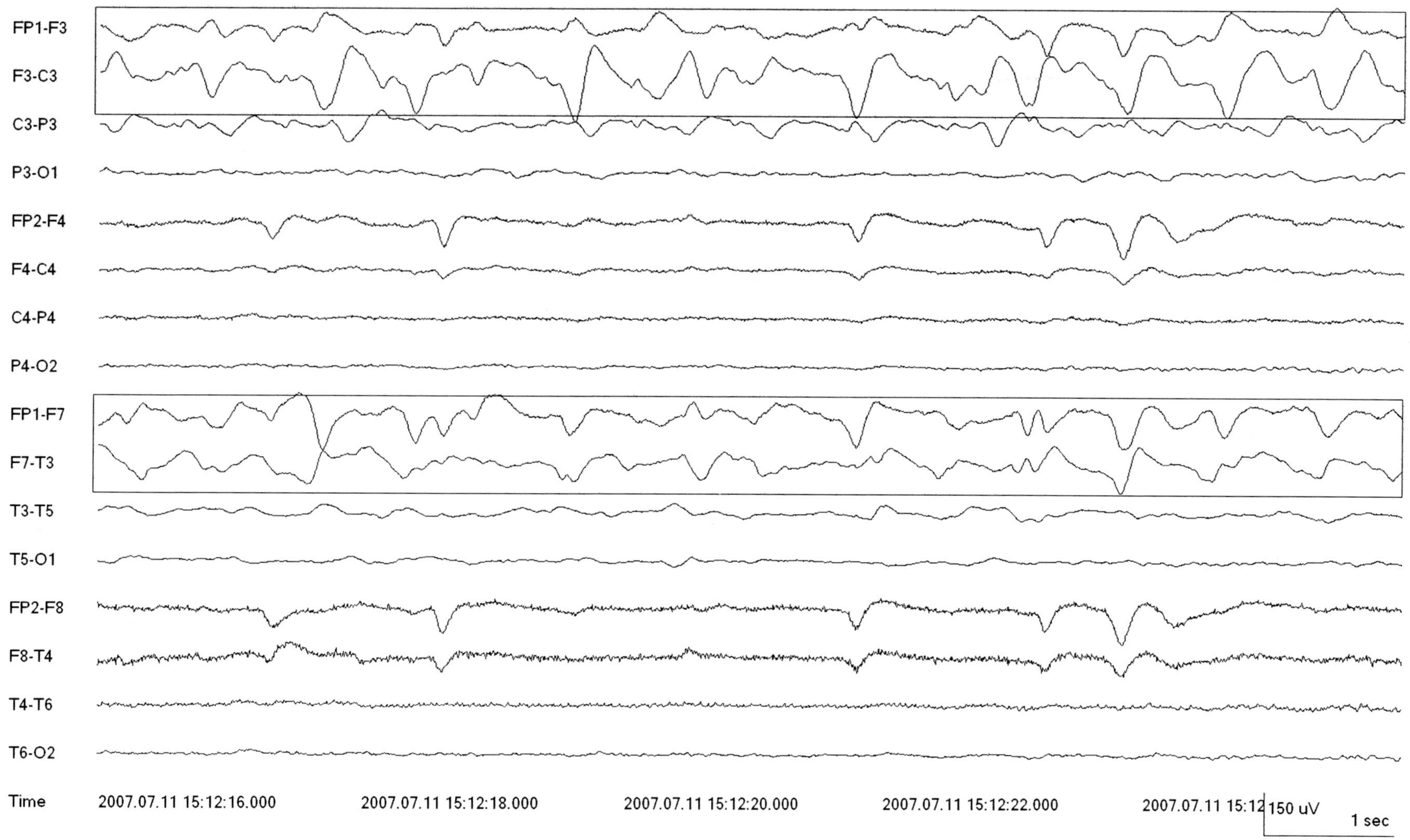

Figure 3.8 Focal motor seizure. (a) The baseline EEG in this 49-year-old woman s/p left-sided 'strokectomy' and cranioplasty shows high-voltage irregular delta activity, sometimes sharply contoured, in the left fronto-temporal region (boxes).

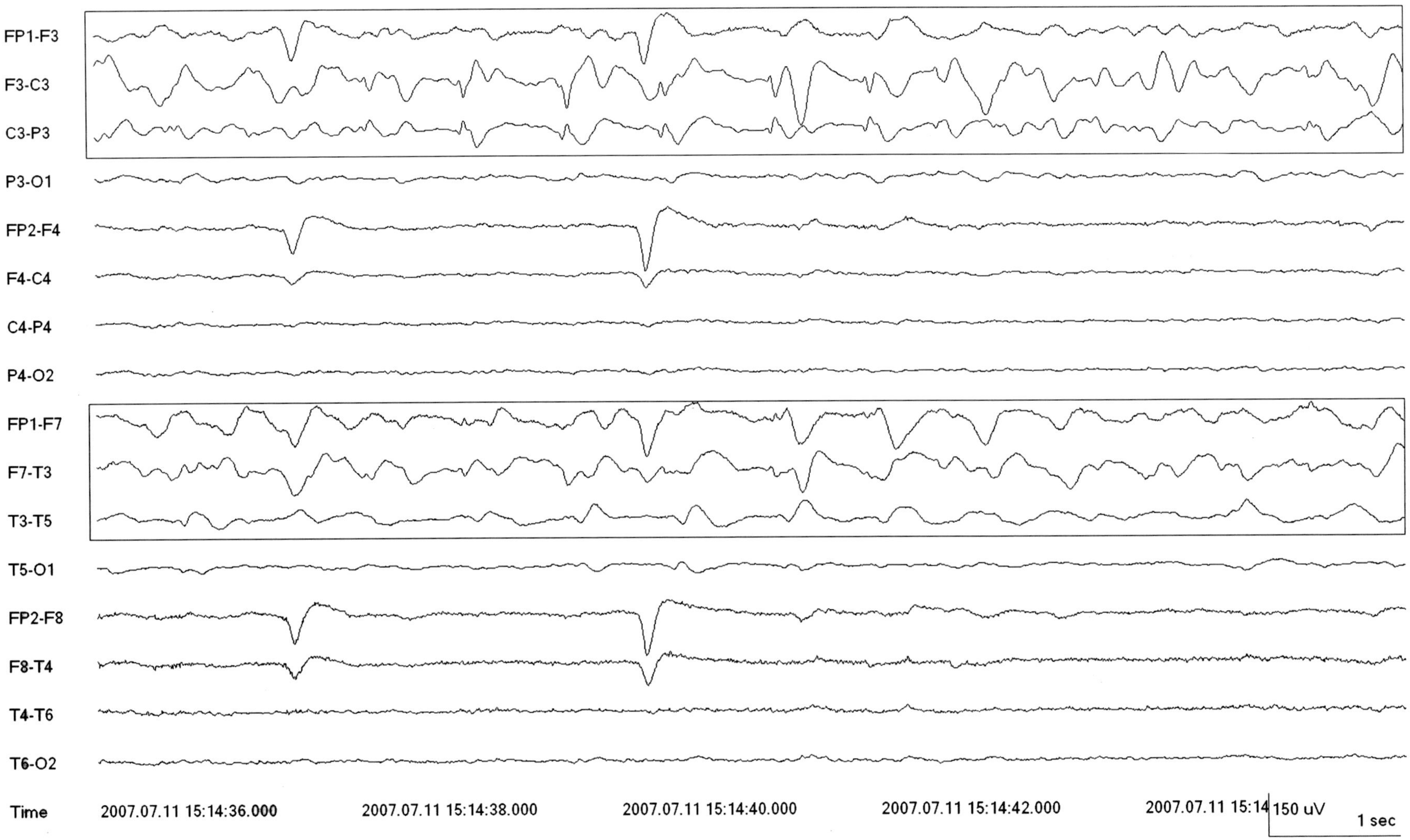

Figure 3.8 (*Continued*) (b) The left-sided seizure begins to slowly evolve, becoming faster with intermixed epileptiform discharges.

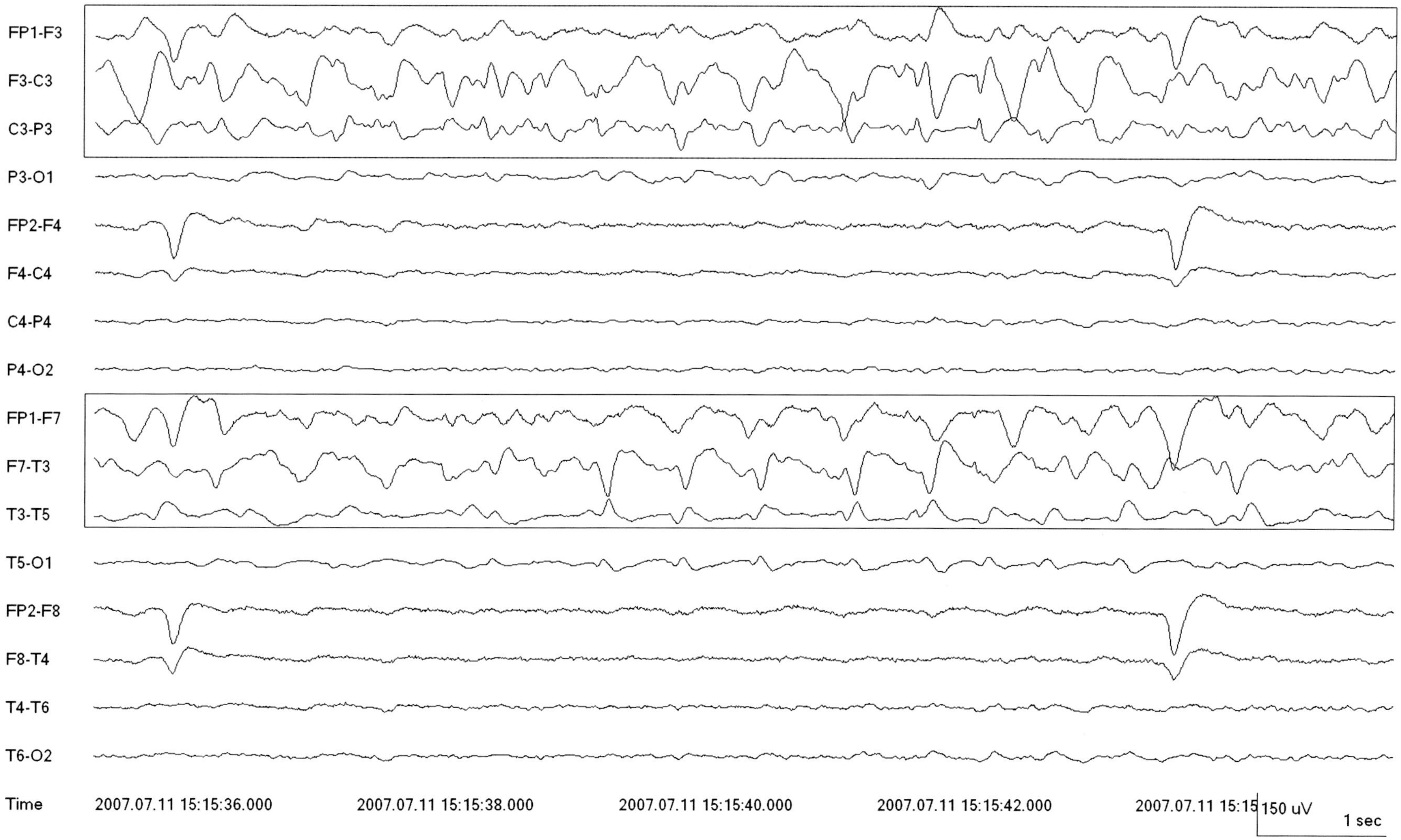

Figure 3.8 (*Continued*) (c). Slow evolution continues.

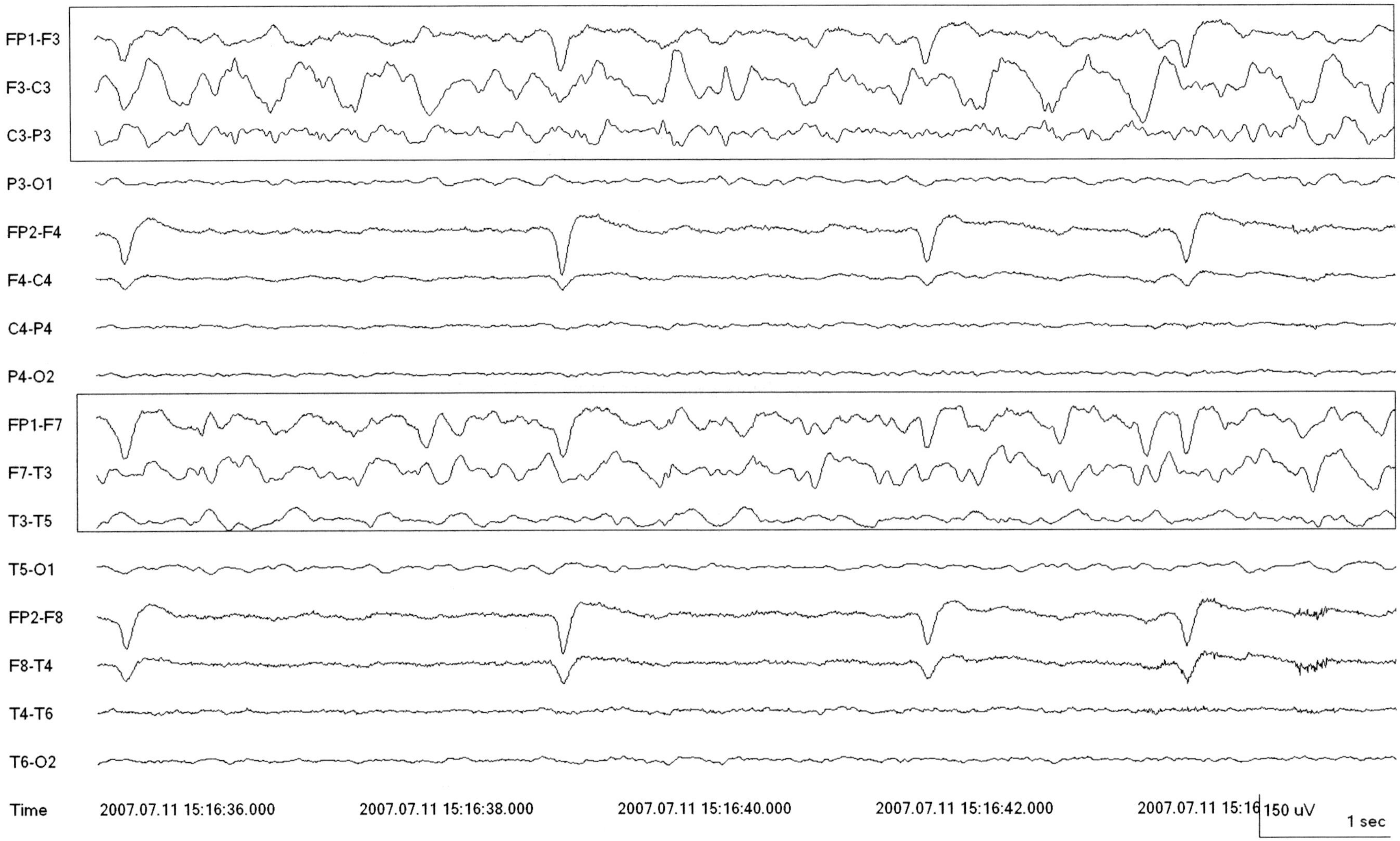

Figure 3.8 (*Continued*) (d) Slow evolution continues, now lower amplitude and faster.

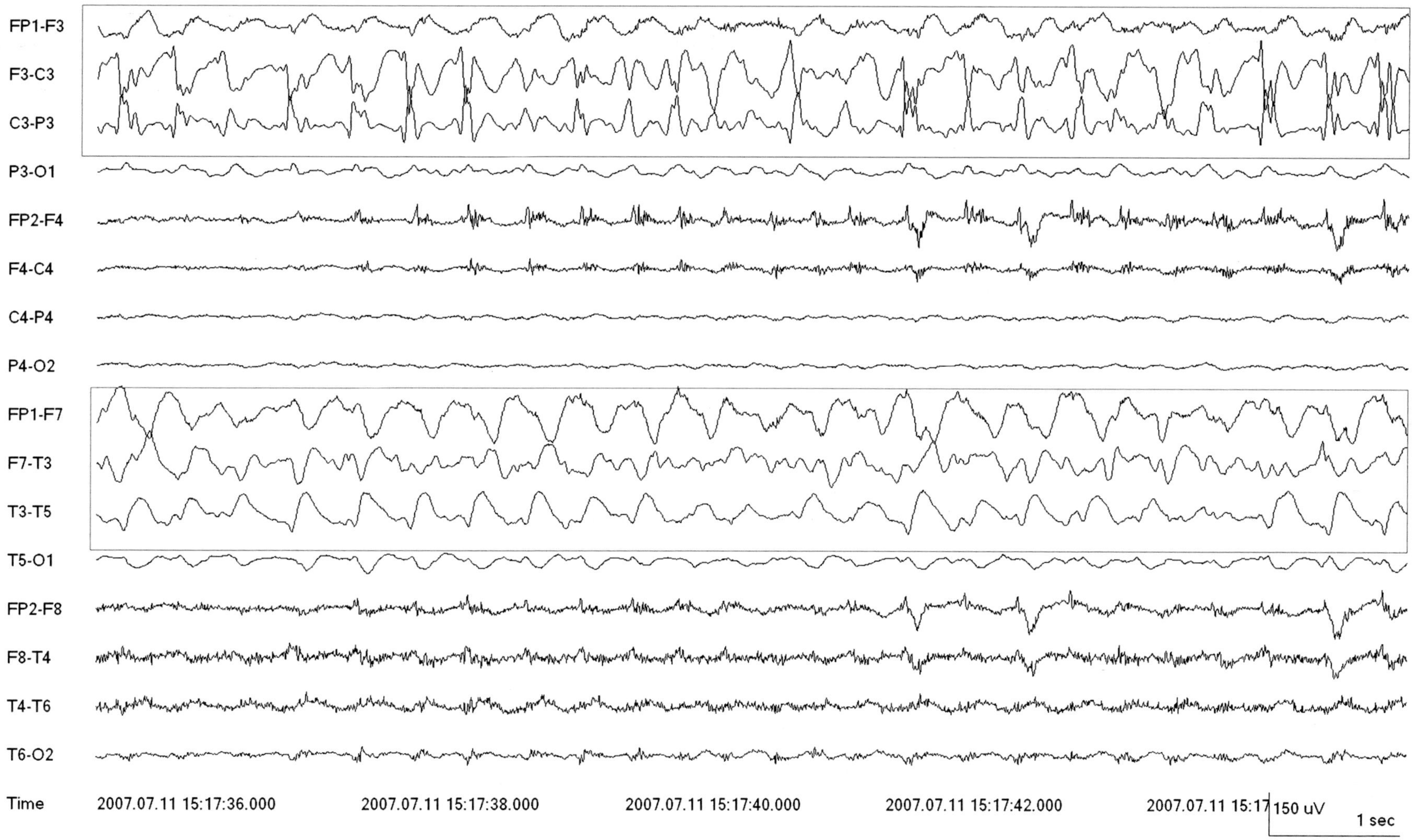

Figure 3.8 (*Continued*) (e) Evolution continues, now with repetitive spikes in the left central area that become more widespread and associated with head jerking to the right and extension of the right arm and leg. Low-amplitude right-sided muscle artifact begins to appear, probably due to face/scalp muscle contraction on that side (contralateral to the ictal discharge).

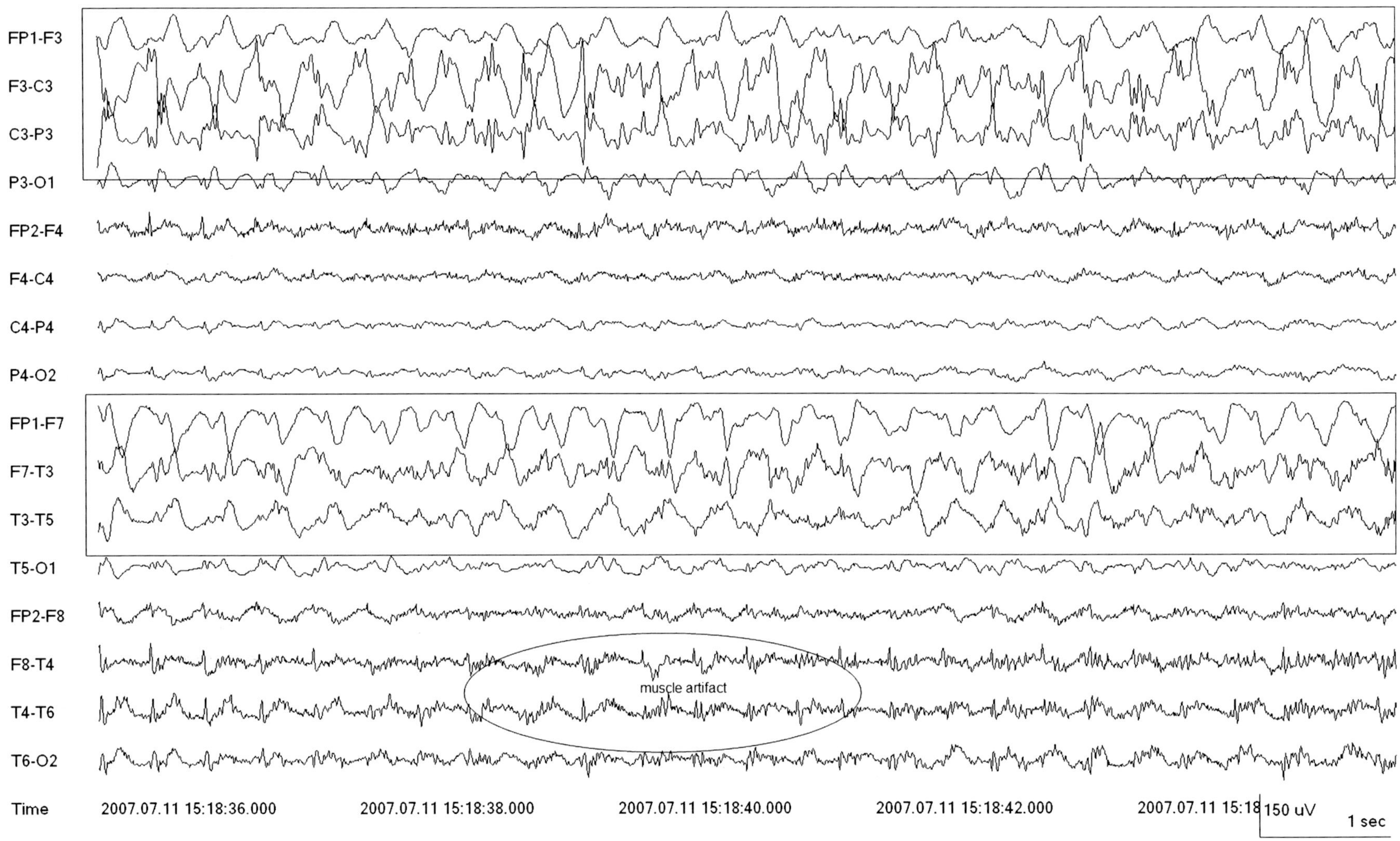

Figure 3.8 (*Continued*) (f) Muscle artifact on the right increases, now with repetitive higher amplitude muscle artifact from clonic jerking of the right face and scalp muscles. The ictal pattern on the left continues to evolve, higher amplitude, sharper and faster (boxes).

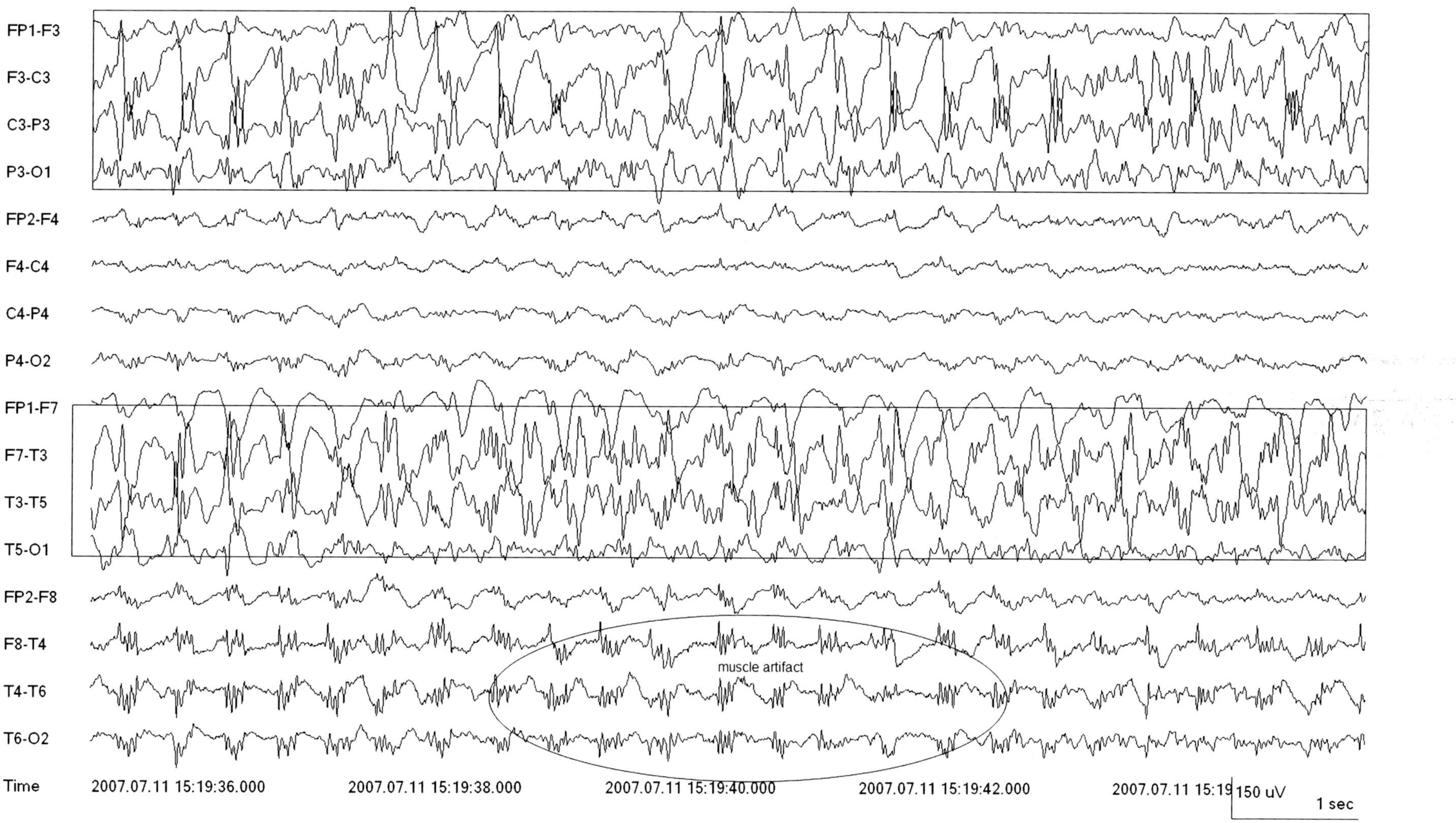

Figure 3.8 (*Continued*) (g) The clinical and electrographic seizure continues.

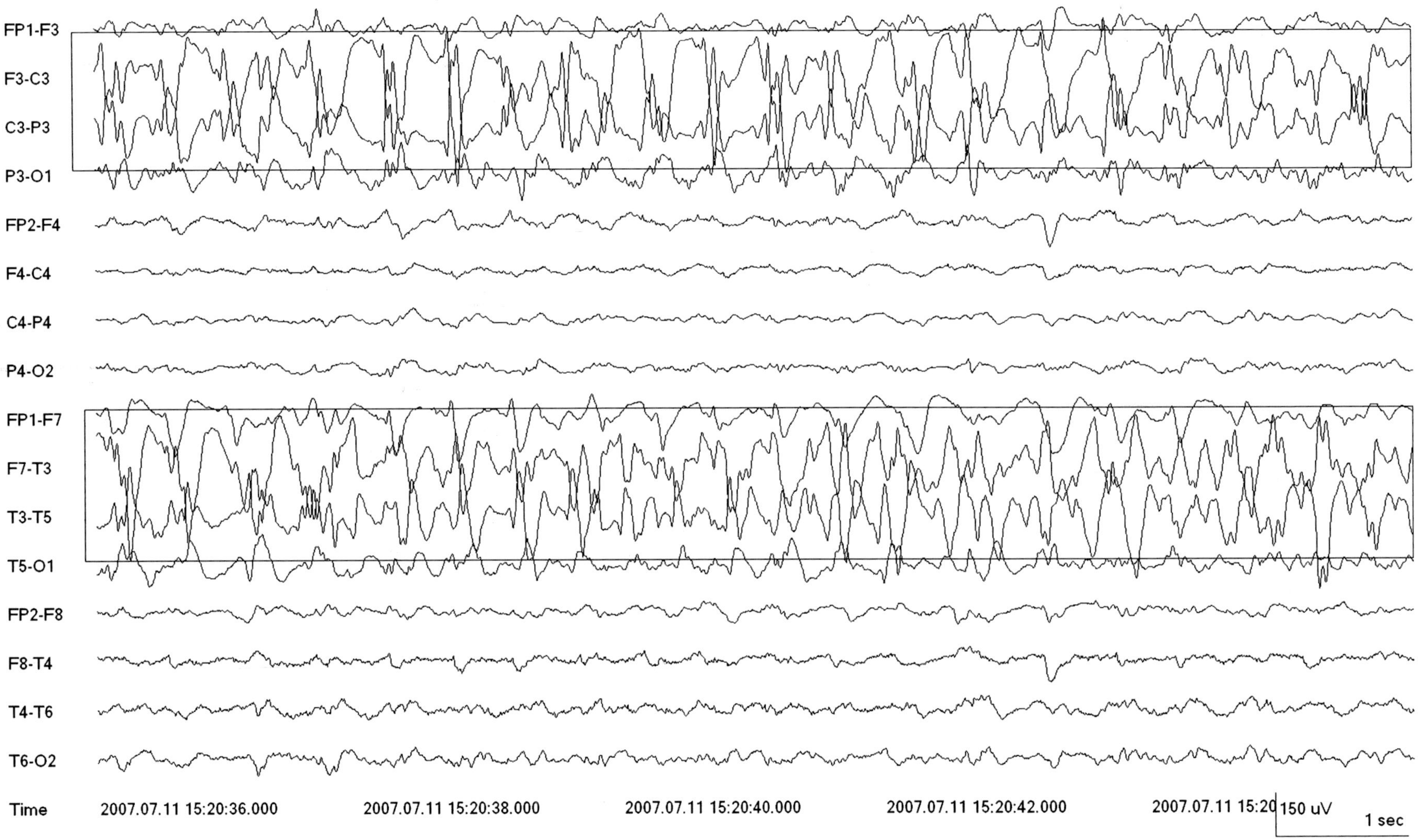

Figure 3.8 (*Continued*) (h) The seizure continues.

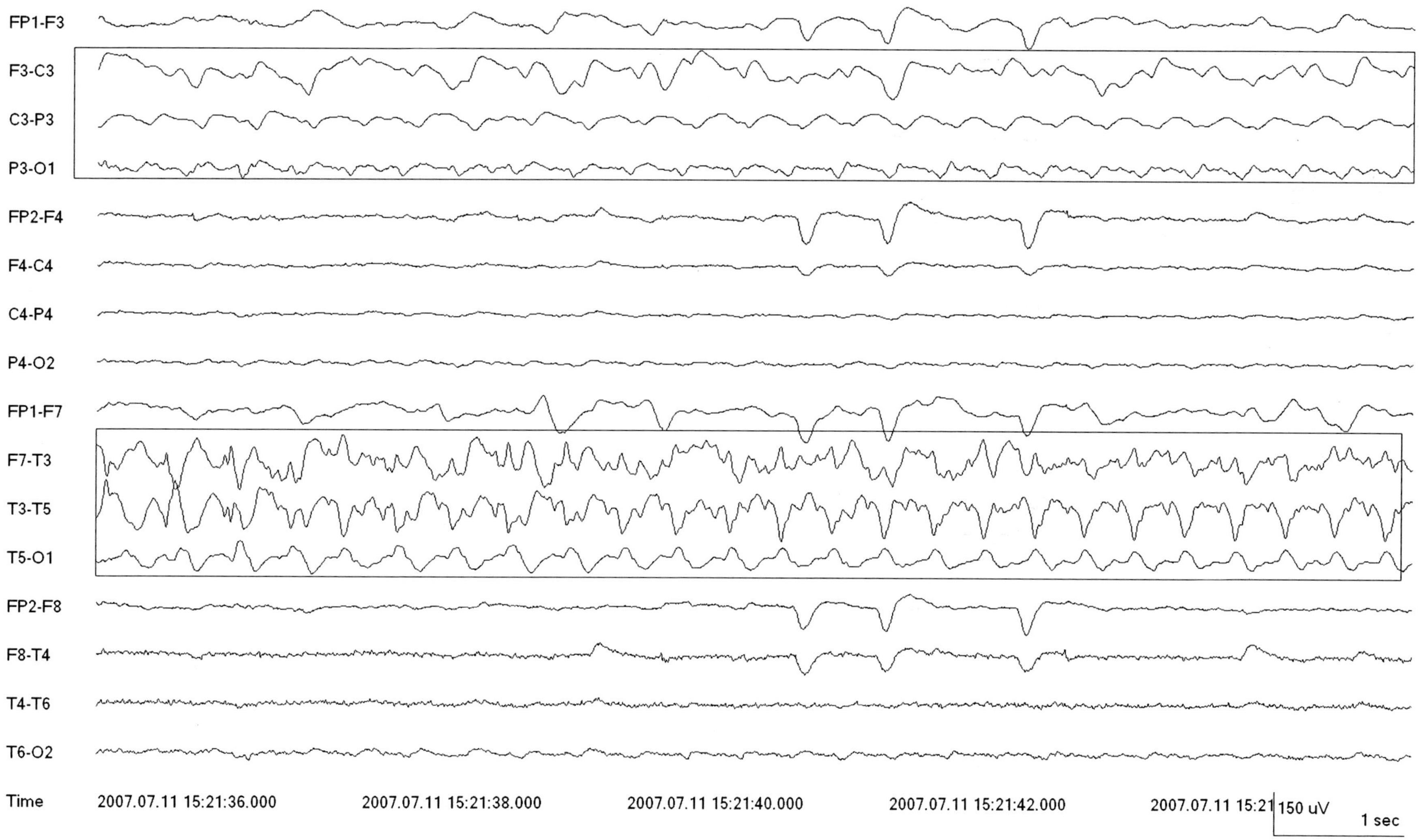

Figure 3.8 (*Continued*) (i) The ictal discharge ceases in the parasagittal region, but continues in the left temporal region.

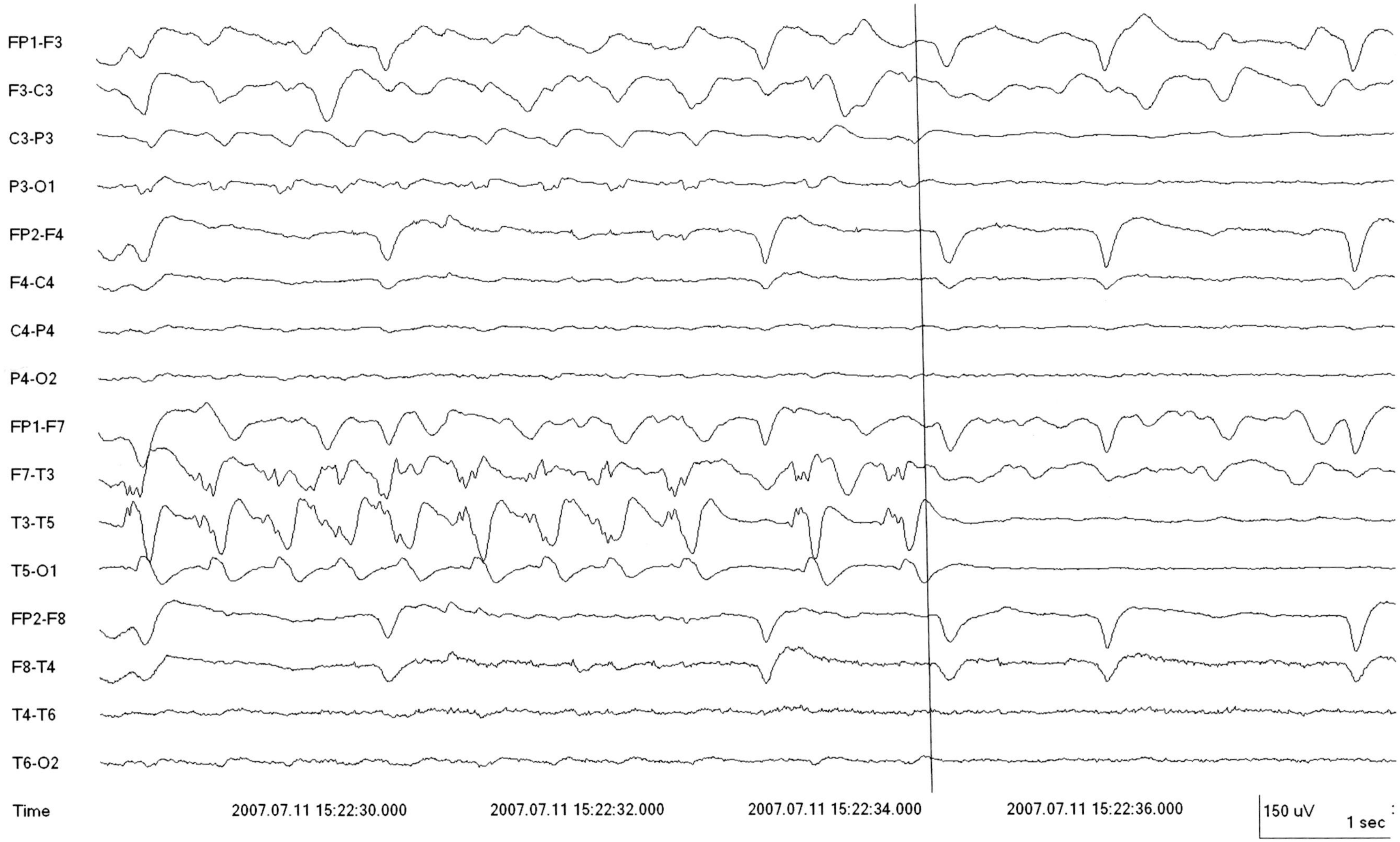

Figure 3.8 (*Continued*) (j) The seizure ends after a total of 8 min.

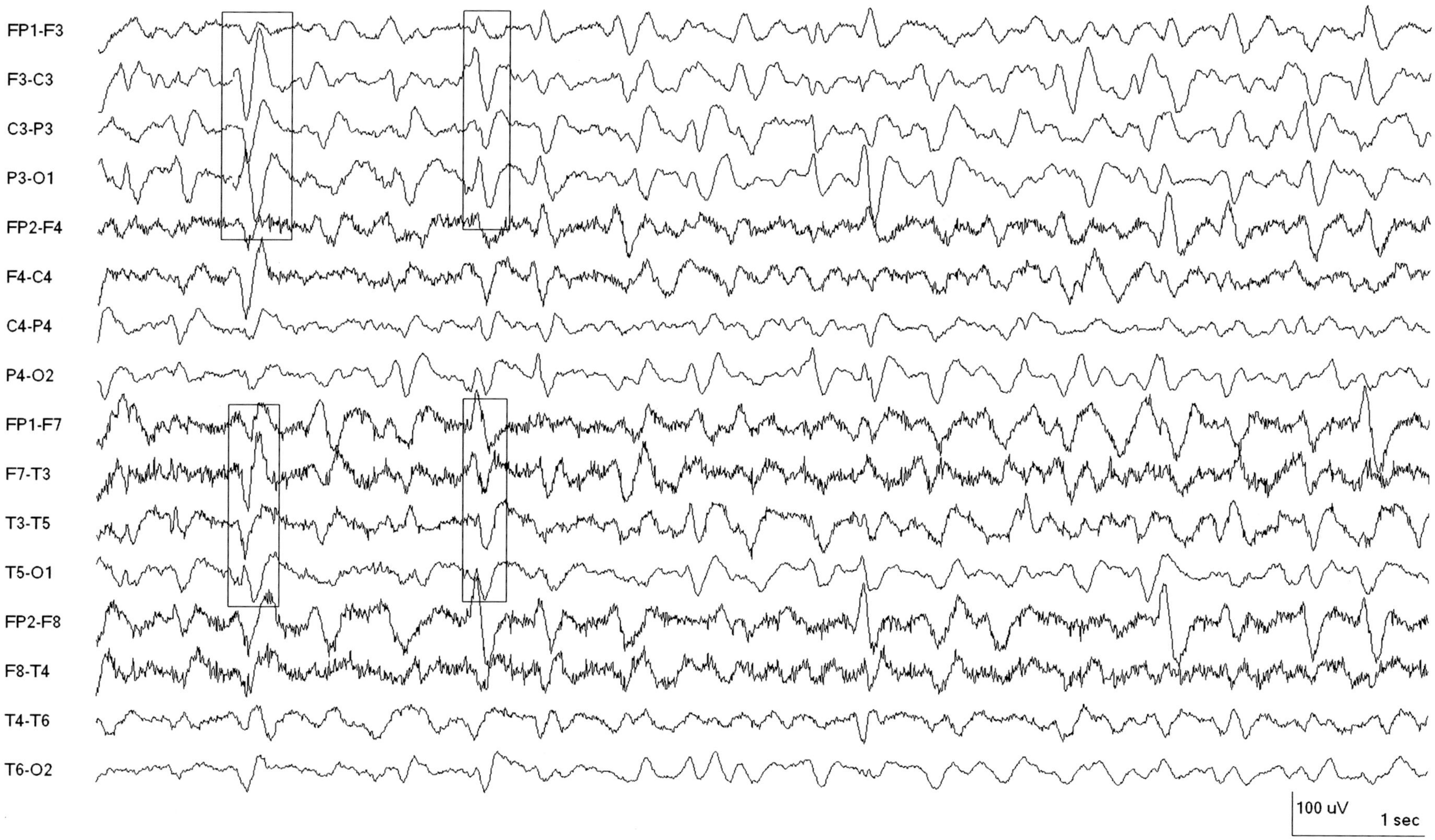

Figure 3.9 Nonconvulsive status epilepticus. (a) This EEG is from an 83-year-old woman with acute renal failure who suddenly became unresponsive. It shows high-voltage sharp waves (some highlighted), often biphasic or triphasic in configuration and frequently of higher voltage on the left and superimposed on a semirhythmic, slow background. Occasionally, these were periodic with a frequency of 2 Hz. The discharges did not change following application of auditory or painful stimuli. It was felt that the patient may have been in nonconvulsive status and she was given 2 mg of lorazepam.

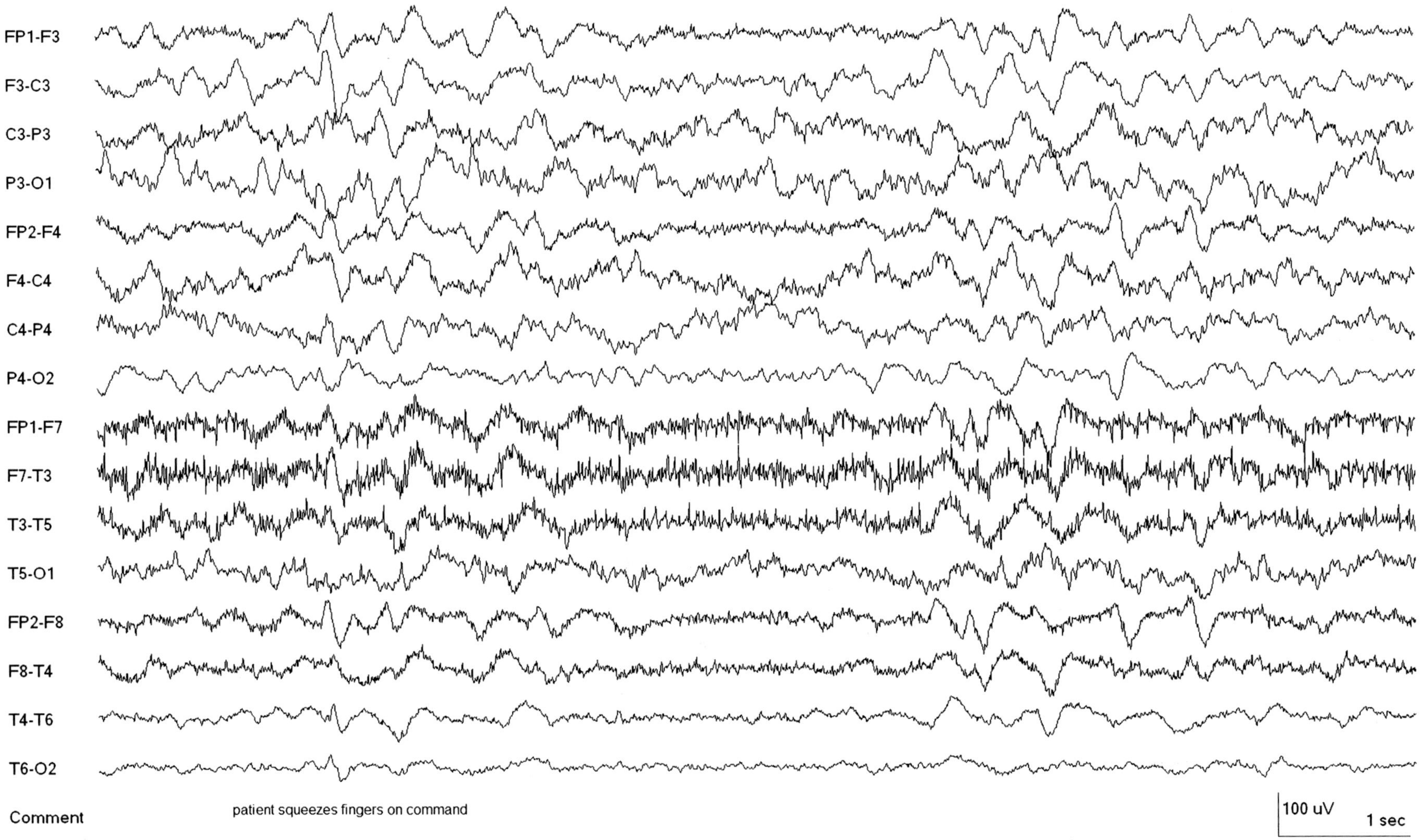

Figure 3.9 (*Continued*) (b) The EEG improved following treatment. The patient awakened and later in the recording was following commands and attempting to speak. The clinical improvement confirmed the diagnosis of nonconvulsive status epilepticus (NCSE). If the EEG had improved like this but the patient did not improve, no conclusion could have been reached regarding the presence or absence of NCSE, as other patterns such as triphasic waves often resolve with benzodiazepines as well.

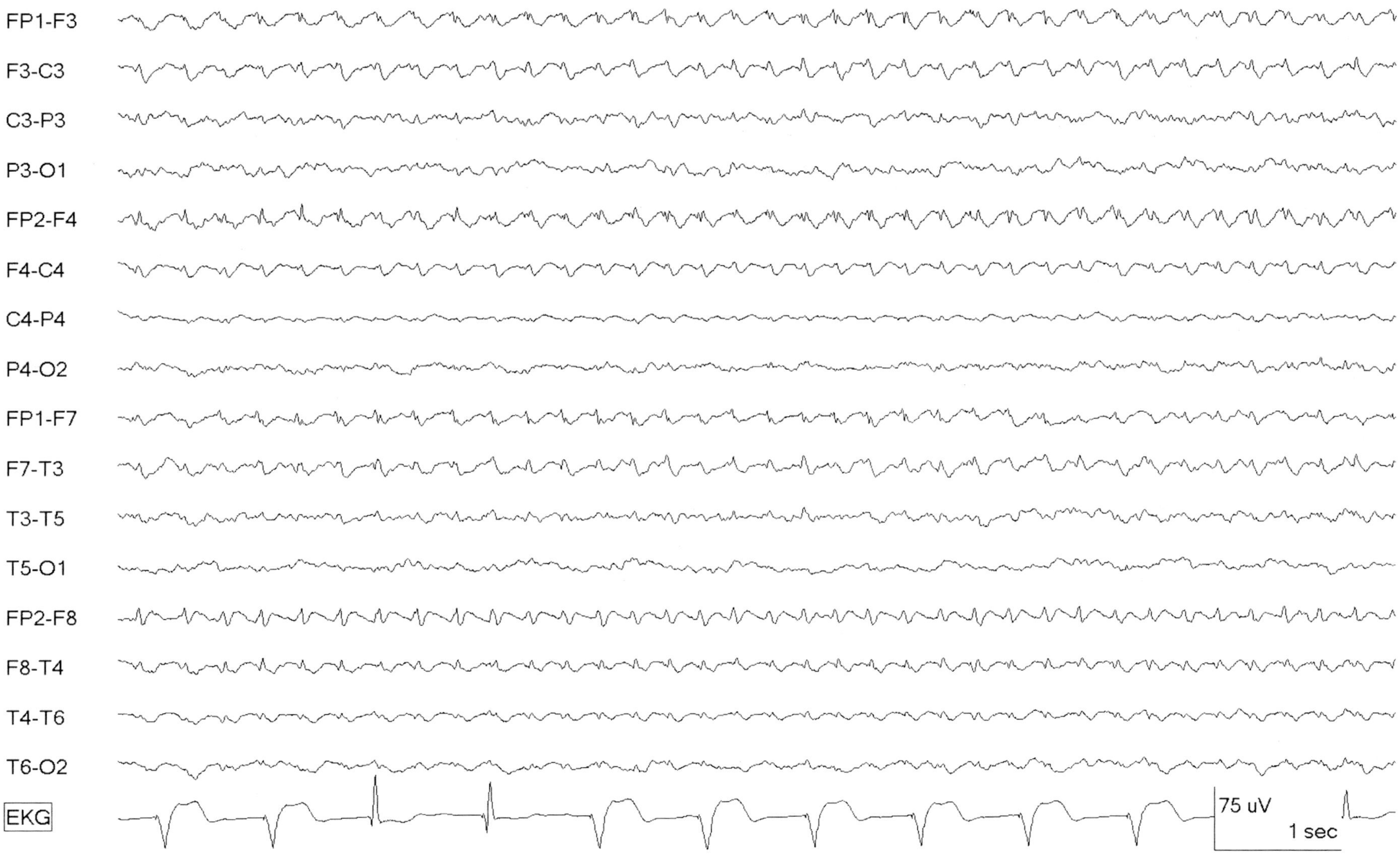

Figure 3.10 Generalized nonconvulsive status epilepticus. This 82-year-old man with recent head trauma is in generalized nonconvulsive status epilepticus. Rhythmic discharges are present diffusely at 3–4 per second, maximal anteriorly, where there is a spike-wave morphology.

4 Periodic discharges and other controversial EEG patterns

4.1 PLEDs, BIPLEDs, GPEDs and triphasic waves

Periodic epileptiform discharges are common in the intensive care unit (ICU) setting. When lateralized, they are known as periodic lateralized epileptiform discharges (PLEDs). These consist of lateralized complexes usually recurring every 1–2 s. The complexes often (but not always) consist of sharp waves or spikes that may be followed by a slow wave. The clinical picture associated with PLEDs is usually obtundation, focal seizures and focal neurological signs. The majority of patients with PLEDs will have seizures during the acute stage of illness. Although clearly ictal in some cases, PLEDs are usually considered an interictal pattern or on an unstable ictal–interictal continuum; however, this is controversial and some feel they are often ictal. When a patient with PLEDs has a seizure, a new pattern usually appears, typically consisting of faster rhythmic activity. Acute stroke is the most common etiology of PLEDs, although any acute brain injury that tends to cause seizures can manifest as PLEDs. Most patients with herpes simplex encephalitis develop PLEDs, maximal in temporal region(s) and often consisting of prolonged complexes (approximately 0.5 s) recurring every 1–4 s; however, this pattern is certainly not specific for this diagnosis. Regardless of etiology, PLEDs are usually a transient phenomenon. With time (days–weeks), discharges tend to decrease in amplitude, the repetition rate decreases and ultimately discharges cease.

Bilateral independent PLEDs (BIPLEDs) are less common, are associated with worse mental status (usually coma) and worse outcome than unilateral PLEDs, and are also highly associated with seizures during the acute illness.

When periodic discharges are generalized, they are known as generalized periodic epileptiform discharges (GPEDs). These can be seen in a variety of settings including in postanoxic coma (when the background is often flat between discharges), after convulsive status epilepticus, with metabolic disorders, in Creutzfeldt-Jacob disease, during Hashimoto encephalopathy, from medication toxicity (e.g. baclofen, lithium, ifosfamide and cefepime) and in end-stage Alzheimer disease. Like PLEDs, GPEDs are highly associated with seizures, although a bit less compared to PLEDs. Although not well studied, more than half of patients with GPEDs seem to have definite seizures during the acute illness.

Triphasic waves are a type of generalized periodic discharge. They were initially described in hepatic encephalopathy, but can occur in any toxic/metabolic encephalopathy. They have also been termed as 'blunt spike and wave', which describes their appearance. They tend to recur at one or two per second and wax and wane throughout a recording, partly dependent on level of alertness. Nonconvulsive status epilepticus can appear quite similar. Although some have suggested specific features that are more common in patients with metabolic encephalopathy rather than seizures, almost all of these studies suffer from lack of a gold standard

Atlas of EEG in Critical Care Lawrence J. Hirsch and Richard P. Brenner

for making the final diagnosis. It is clear that in a given individual, EEG alone often cannot distinguish between triphasic waves of metabolic encephalopathy and nonconvulsive seizures. Unfortunately, both resolve with benzodiazepines as well. Thus, only clinical improvement with benzodiazepines can be used to prove the presence of nonconvulsive status epilepticus. It is almost impossible to disprove it.

4.2 SIRPIDs

With the advent of continuous video-EEG recordings in the ICU, it became apparent that alerting stimuli (suction, exam, noise, pain) in encephalopathic patients commonly elicit highly epileptiform patterns such as periodic discharges, rhythmic delta or unequivocally evolving electrographic seizures. They can be focal or generalized. This was termed stimulus-induced periodic, rhythmic or ictal discharges (SIRPIDs). The duration and prominence of the pattern often correlate with the duration and degree of stimulation, and the pattern can usually be reproduced with further stimulation (after allowing return to the non-stimulated background). This is usually a purely electrographic finding with no obvious clinical accompaniment, although some patients will have clinical seizures as well; these are typically focal motor, as other types would be very difficult to detect. The exact clinical, therapeutic and prognostic significance of SIRPIDs remains undefined.

4.3 Standardized nomenclature

The Critical Care Monitoring Committee of the American Clinical Neurophysiology Society has proposed standardized nomenclature for rhythmic and periodic EEG patterns encountered in the ICU.

The committee has attempted to develop standardized terminology for the patterns discussed above, as well as other controversial patterns seen in the critically ill in order to allow scientific study. The nomenclature has undergone several rounds of revisions. The latest version (June 2009) is included in this book as an appendix. Furthermore, the proposed term that would be used for each pattern shown in this chapter is given at the end of the corresponding figure legend.

Figure List

Figure 4.1–4.3 GPEDs.

Figure 4.4 PLEDs-plus.

Figure 4.5 PLEDs.

Figure 4.6 PLEDs and seizure.

Figure 4.7–4.9 PLEDs.

Figure 4.10–4.11 BIPLEDs.

Figure 4.12 SIRPIDs: GPEDs.

Figure 4.13 SIRPIDs: rhythmic delta.

Figure 4.14–4.17 SIRPIDs: triphasic waves vs. nonconvulsive status.

Figure 4.18 Stimulus-induced focal seizure with clinical correlate.

Suggested reading

Brenner, R.P. and Schaul, N. (1990) Periodic EEG patterns: classification, clinical correlation, and pathophysiology. *Journal of Clinical Neurophysiology* **7**, 249–267.

Chong, D.J. and Hirsch, L.J. (2005) Which EEG patterns warrant treatment in the critically ill? Reviewing the evidence for treatment of periodic epileptiform discharges and related patterns. *Journal of Clinical Neurophysiology* **22**, 79–91.

de la Paz, D. and Brenner, R.P. (1981) Bilateral independent periodic lateralized epileptiform discharges. Clinical significance. *Archives of Neurology* **38**, 713–715.

Foley, J.M., Watson, C.W. and Adams, R.D. (1950) Significance of the electroencephalographic changes in hepatic coma. *Transactions of the American Neurological Associations* **75**, 161–164.

Fountain, N.B. and Waldman, W.A. (2001) Effects of benzodiazepines on triphasic waves: Implications for nonconvulsive status epilepticus. *Journal of Clinical Neurophysiology* **18**, 345–352.

Garcia-Morales, I., Garcia, M.T., Galan-Davila, L. *et al.* (2002) Periodic lateralized epileptiform discharges: etiology, clinical aspects, seizures, and evolution in 130 patients. *Journal of Clinical Neurophysiology* **19**, 172–177.

Garzon, E., Fernandes, R.M. and Sakamoto, A.C. (2001) Serial EEG during human status epilepticus: evidence for PLED as an ictal pattern. *Neurology* **57**, 1175–1183.

Hirsch, L.J. and Rampal, N. (2008) Gilman S, (ed.), *MedLink Neurology*. MedLink Corporation, San Diego. Available at www.medlink.com (August 2007; last updated July 2008).

Hirsch, L.J., Claassen, J., Mayer, S.A. *et al.* (2004) Stimulus-induced rhythmic, periodic, or ictal discharges (SIRPIDs): A common EEG phenomenon in the critically ill. *Epilepsia* **45**, 109–123.

Hirsch, L.J., Pang, T., Claassen, J. *et al.* (2008) Focal motor seizures induced by alerting stimuli in critically ill patients. *Epilepsia* **49**, 968–973.

Husain, A.M., Mebust, K.A. and Radtke, R.A. (1999) Generalized periodic epileptiform discharges: Etiologies, relationship to status epilepticus, and prognosis. *Journal of Clinical Neurophysiology* **16**, 51–58.

Kaplan, P.W. and Birbeck, G. (2006) Lithium-induced confusional states: nonconvulsive status epilepticus or triphasic encephalopathy? *Epilepsia* **47**, 2071–2074.

Klass, D.W. (1990) Principles in the differentiation of atypical spike-waves and triphasic waves. *American Journal of EEG Technology* **30**, 313–314.

Lai, C.W. and Gragasin, M.E. (1988) Electroencephalography in herpes simplex encephalitis. *Journal of Clinical Neurophysiology* **5**, 87–103.

Martinez-Rodriguez, J.E., Barriga, F.J., Santamaria, J. *et al.* (2001) Nonconvulsive status epilepticus associated with cephalosporins in patients with renal failure. *American Journal of Medicine*; **111**, 115–119.

Pohlmann-Eden, B., Hoch, D.B., Cochius, J.I. *et al.* (1996) Periodic lateralized epileptiform discharges – a critical review. *Journal of Clinical Neurophysiology* **13**, 519–530.

Primavera, A., Audenino, D. and Cocito, L. (2002) Ifosfamide encephalopathy and nonconvulsive status epilepticus. *Canadian Journal of Neurological Science* **29**, 180–183.

Rae-Grant, A., Blume, W., Lau, C. *et al.* (1987) The electroencephalogram in Alzheimer-type dementia. A sequential study correlating the electroencephalogram with psychometric and quantitative pathologic data. *Archives of Neurology*; **44**, 50–54.

Reiher, J., Rivest, J., Grand'Maison, F. *et al.* (1991) Periodic lateralized epileptiform discharges with transitional rhythmic discharges: association with seizures. *Electroencephalography in Clinical Neurophysiology* **78**, 12–17.

Treiman, D.M., Walton, N.Y. and Kendrick, C. (1990) A progressive sequence of electroencephalographic changes during generalized convulsive status epilepticus. *Epilepsy Research* **5**, 49–60.

Yemisci, M., Gurer, G., Saygi, S. *et al.* (2003) Generalised periodic epileptiform discharges: clinical features, neuroradiological evaluation and prognosis in 37 adult patients. *Seizure* **12**, 465–472.

Zak, R., Solomon, G., Petito, F. *et al.* (1994) Baclofen-induced generalized nonconvulsive status epilepticus. *Annals of Neurology* **36**, 113–114.

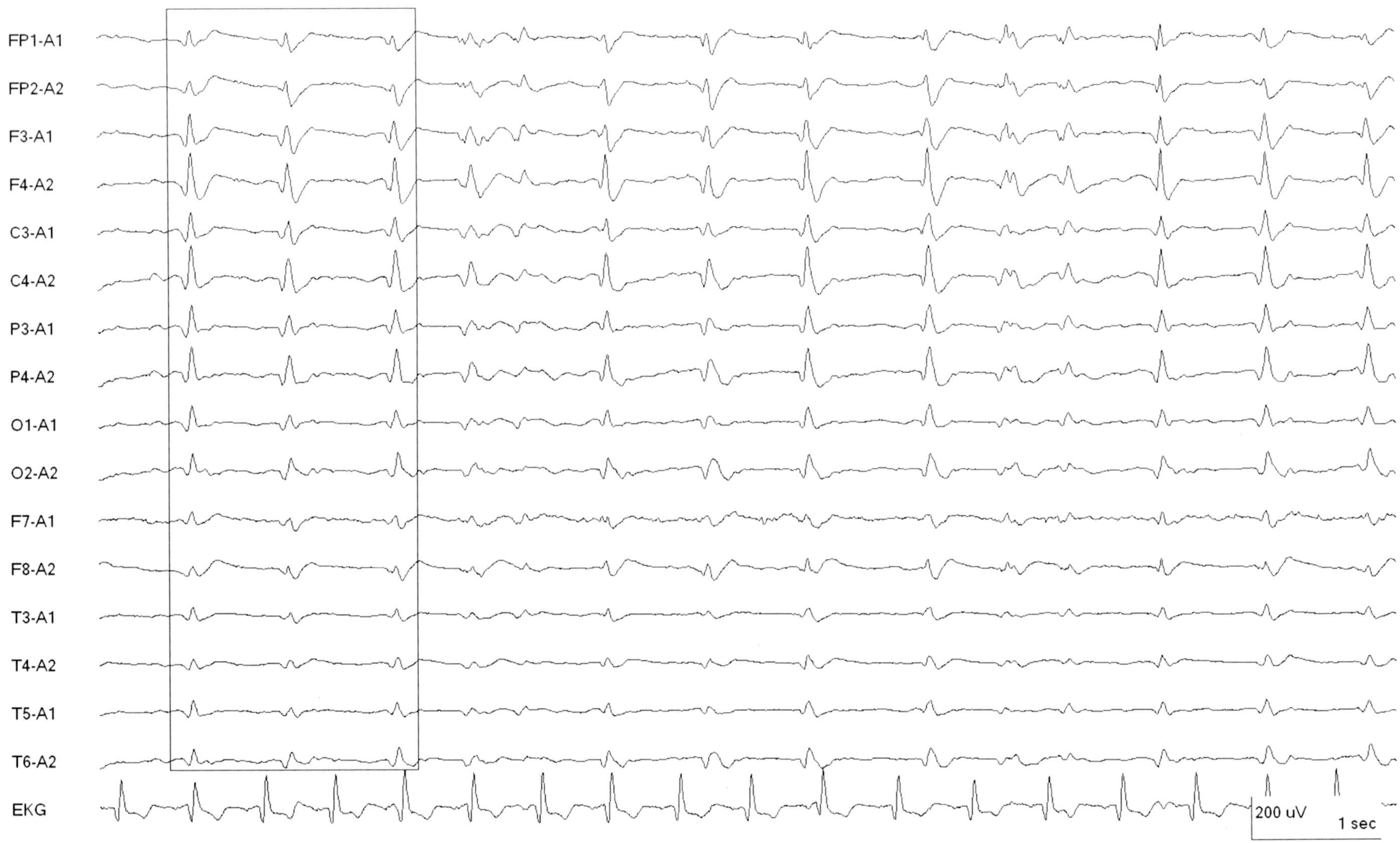

Figure 4.1 Generalized periodic epileptiform discharges (GPEDs). GPEDs are present in this 33-year-old man status post (s/p) motor vehicle accident and anoxia. The first three discharges are included in the box. American Clinical Neurophysiology Society (ACNS) proposal name: GPDs.

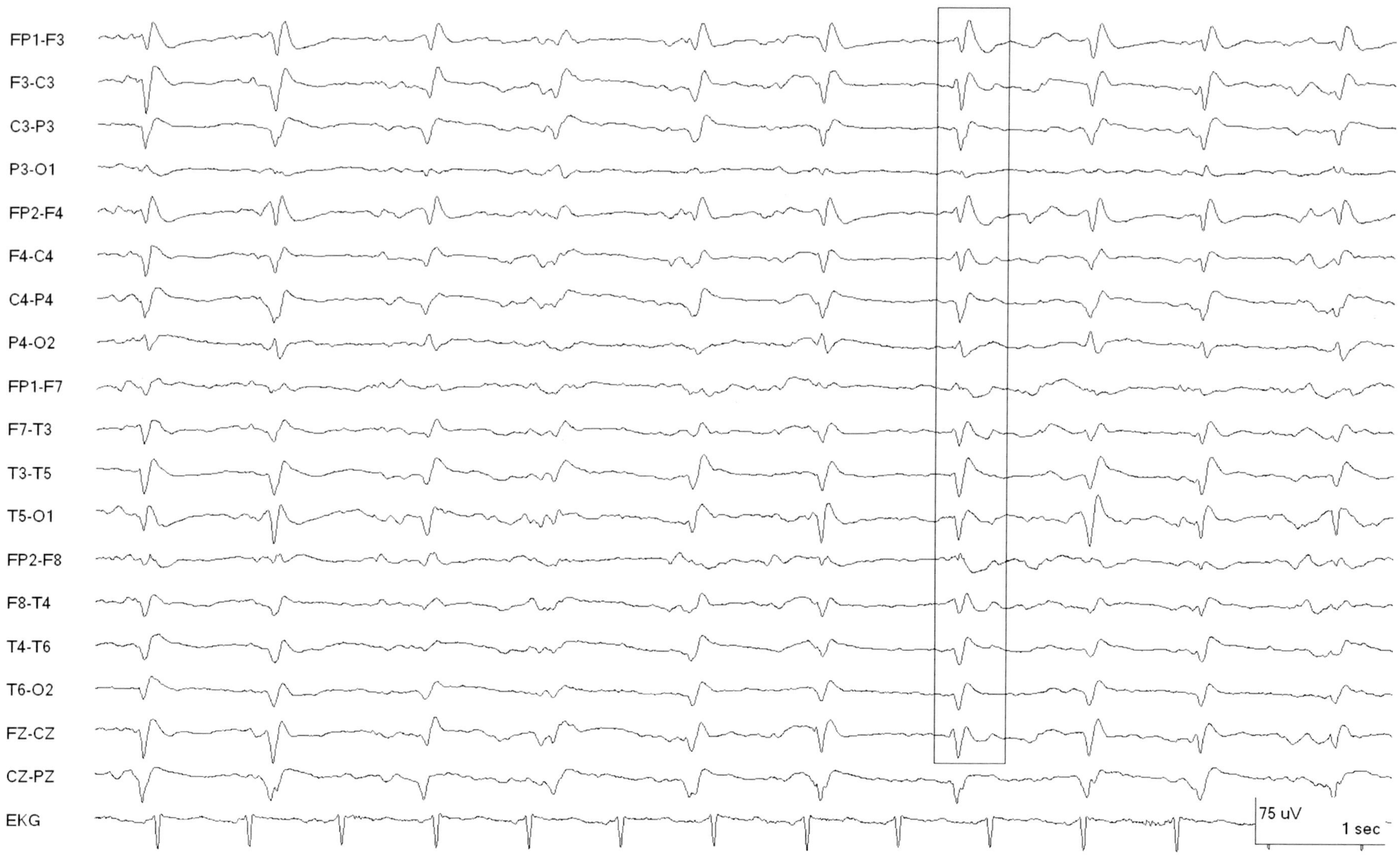

Figure 4.2 GPEDs. The EEG in this 45-year-old man shows GPEDs. The patient was receiving propofol and had been in status epilepticus. Note the triphasic morphology (one example in box), which is not rare in seizure-related GPEDs despite the traditional teaching that they suggest metabolic encephalopathy.

ACNS proposal name: GPDs (with triphasic morphology).

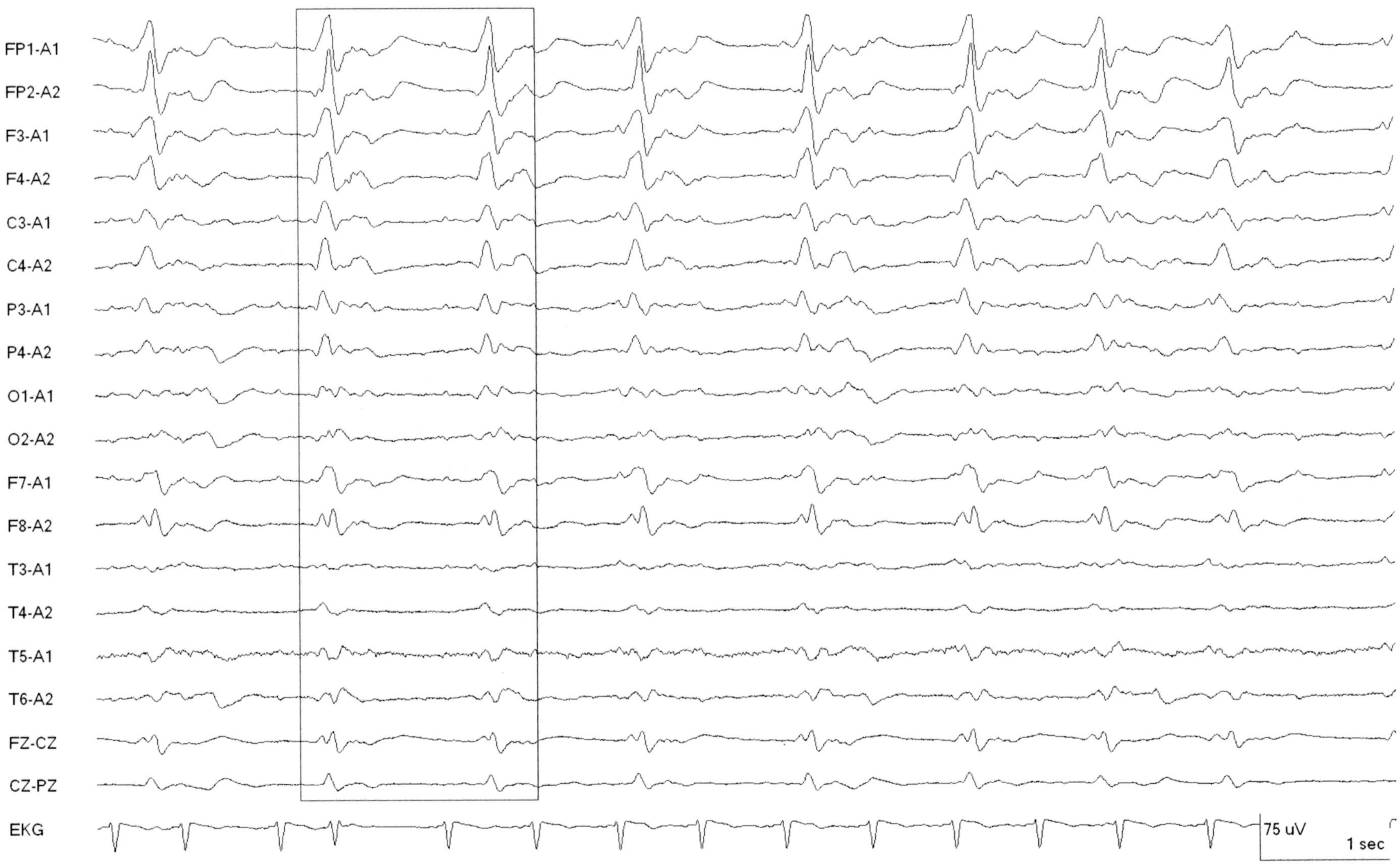

Figure 4.3 GPEDs. GPEDs are present in this 75-year-old comatose woman at just under 1 per second. Two discharges are present in the box. As is typical, they are frontally predominant.

ACNS proposal name: GPDs (frontally predominant).

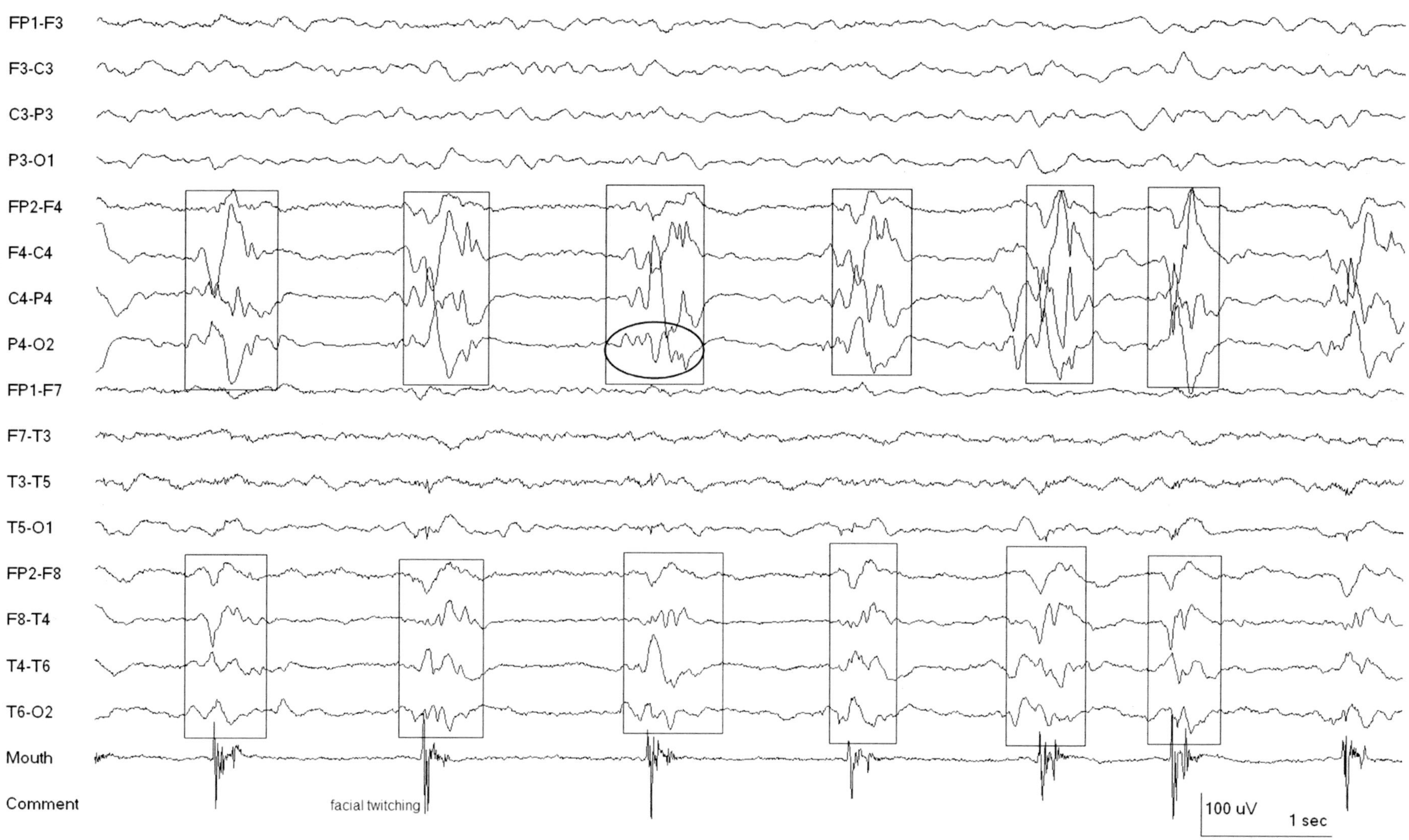

Figure 4.4 Periodic lateralized epileptiform discharges (PLEDs), ictal. The EEG in this 79-year-old man with herpes simplex encephalitis shows right-sided PLEDs (boxes) associated with movements of the left side of the face (note electromyogram (EMG) channel labeled 'Mouth' showing the face twitching with each discharge). The low-amplitude rhythmic discharges seen with each complex (one example at P4-O2 highlighted with ellipse) would make this qualify as PLEDs-plus. In this case, these are clearly ictal PLEDs, not interictal, given the clinical correlate.

ACNS proposal name: LPDs+.

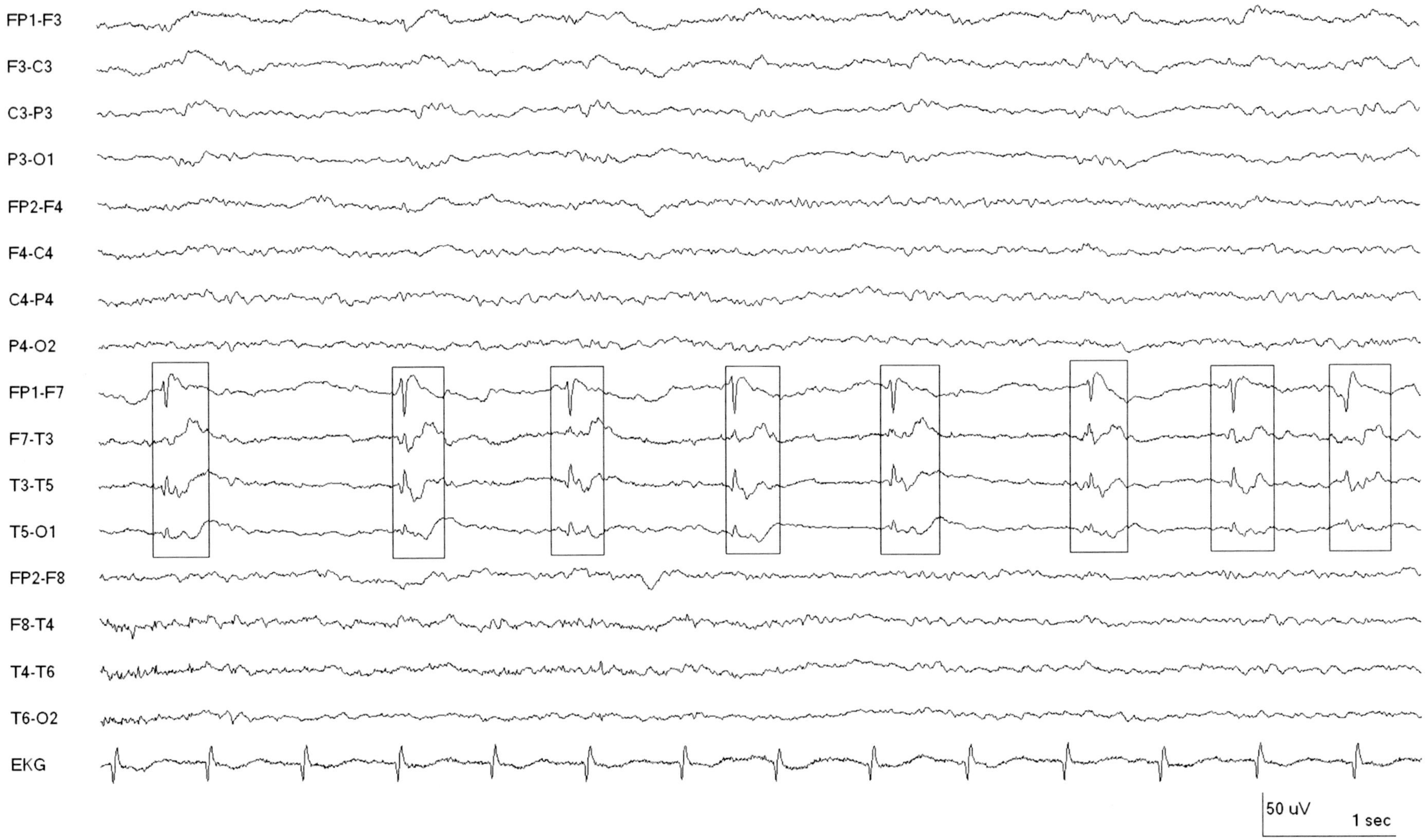

Figure 4.5 PLEDs. The EEG in this 64-year-old man demonstrates PLEDs (boxes), maximal in the left temporal region, usually at electrode F7. The patient had new onset seizures and a stroke 6 months before. The discharges have a spike-like configuration in this example.

ACNS proposal name: LPDs.

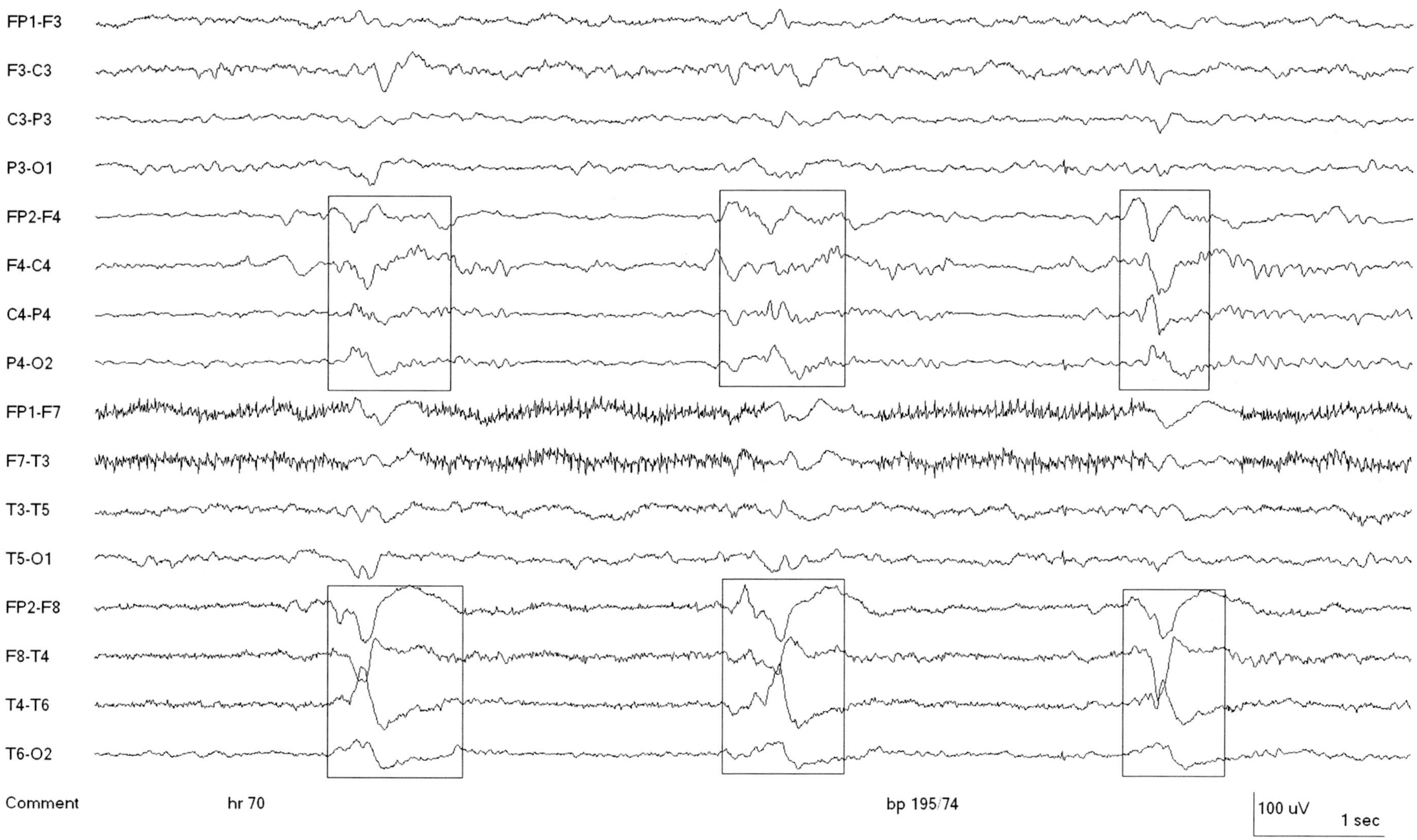

Figure 4.6 PLEDs, then focal seizure. (a) Right-sided PLEDs (boxes) are present in this 87-year-old woman with herpes simplex encephalitis (HSE). Note that each discharge is not actually epileptiform (i.e. not a spike or sharp wave) but is primarily a delta wave, perhaps sharply contoured. This is typical of HSE and does not change the high correlation with seizures. This is also one of the reasons the 'E' for epileptiform was dropped in the new ACNS nomenclature.

ACNS proposal name: LPDs.

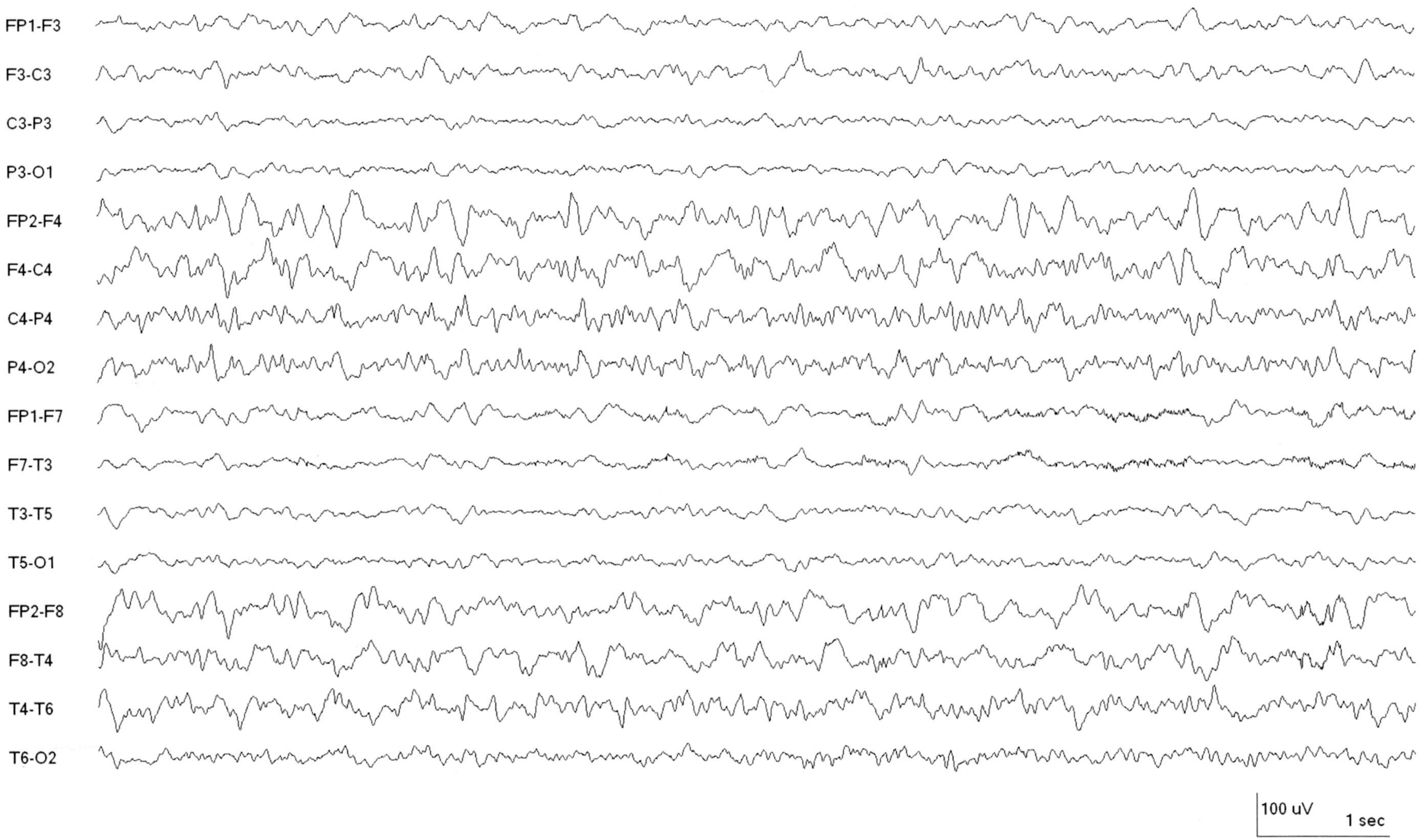

Figure 4.6 (*Continued*) (b) A sample taken later in the same recording shows that the PLEDs have been replaced by a focal electrographic seizure involving the entire right hemisphere in this sample. This rather common occurrence of PLEDs being replaced by a completely different seizure pattern has been used to support the widely held impression that PLEDs are usually interictal rather than ictal.

ACNS proposal name: not applicable; would still be termed a seizure.

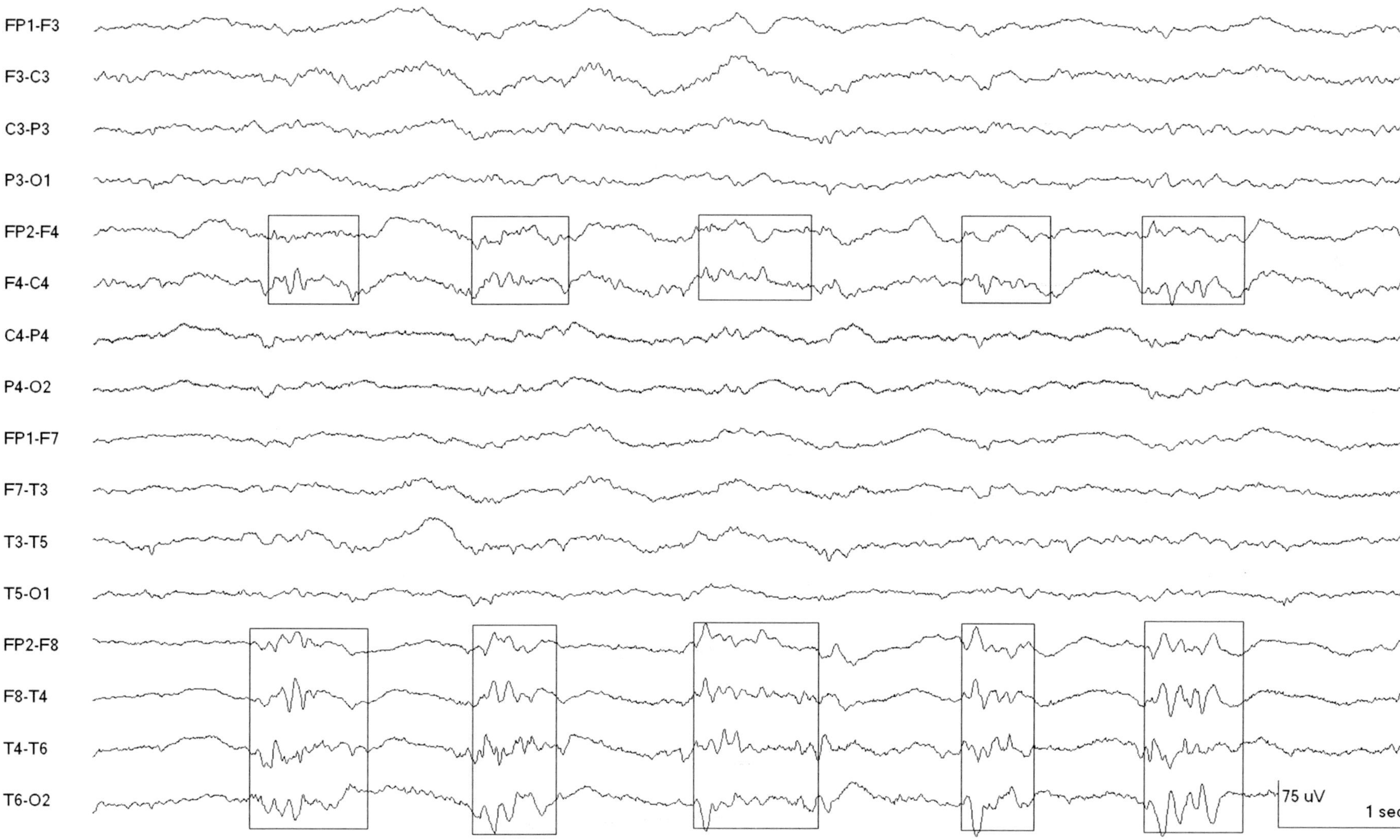

Figure 4.7 PLEDs. The EEG in this 21-year-old woman with lupus demonstrates probable right-sided PLEDs. The complexes consist of brief groups of alpha frequency activity. This is another example in which each discharge is not epileptiform; however, the periodicity makes this likely to be a highly epileptogenic pattern (i.e. highly associated with seizures).

ACNS proposal name: LPDs or unilateral discontinuous background.

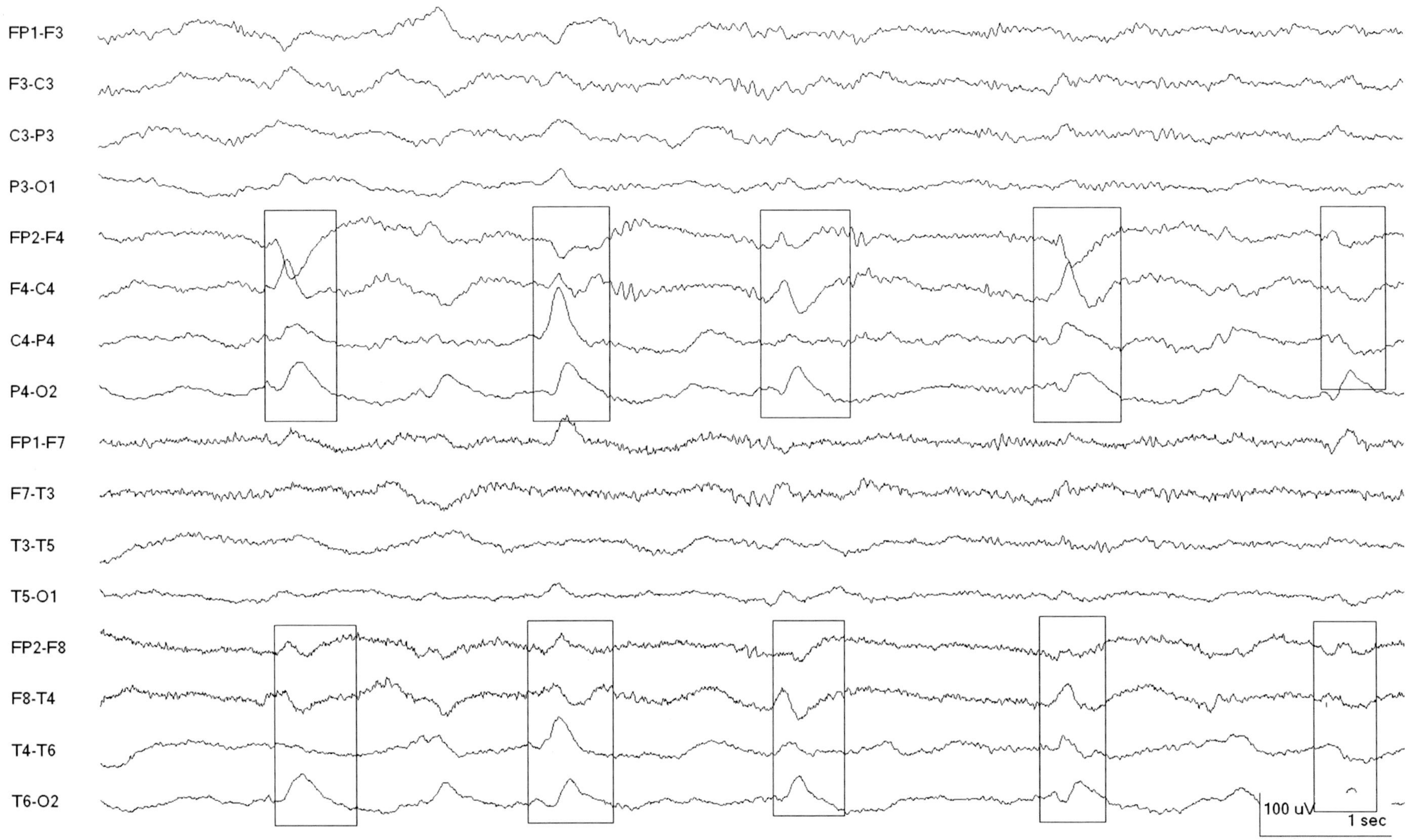

Figure 4.8 PLEDs. The EEG in this 26-year-old man shows PLEDs consisting of broad quasi-periodic slow waves over the right hemisphere. The patient had two tonic-clonic seizures the evening before the EEG. See comments in Figure 4.6.

ACNS proposal name: LPDs.

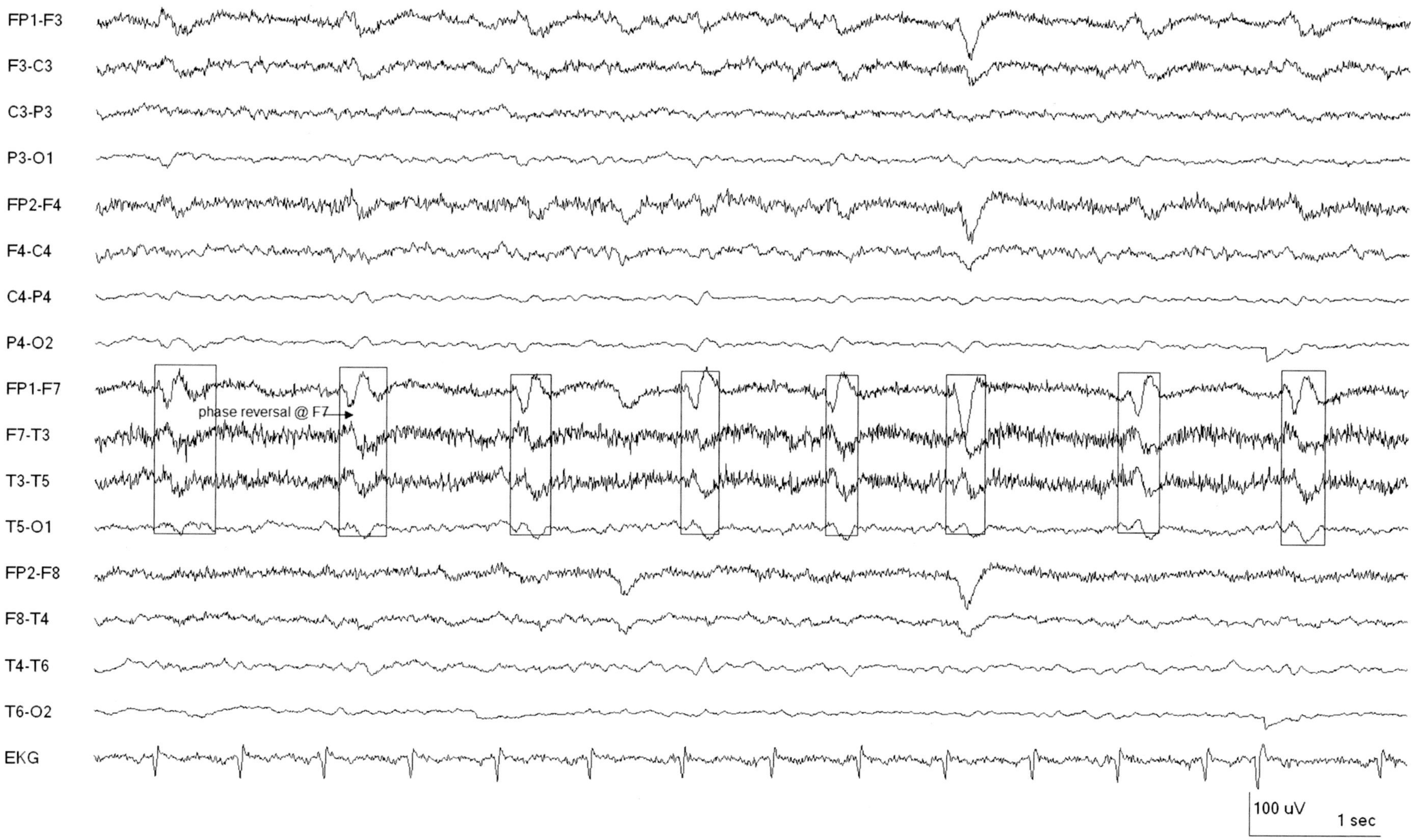

Figure 4.9 PLEDs. Left-sided PLEDs, maximal at electrode F7, are present in this 54-year-old woman.

ACNS proposal name: LPDs.

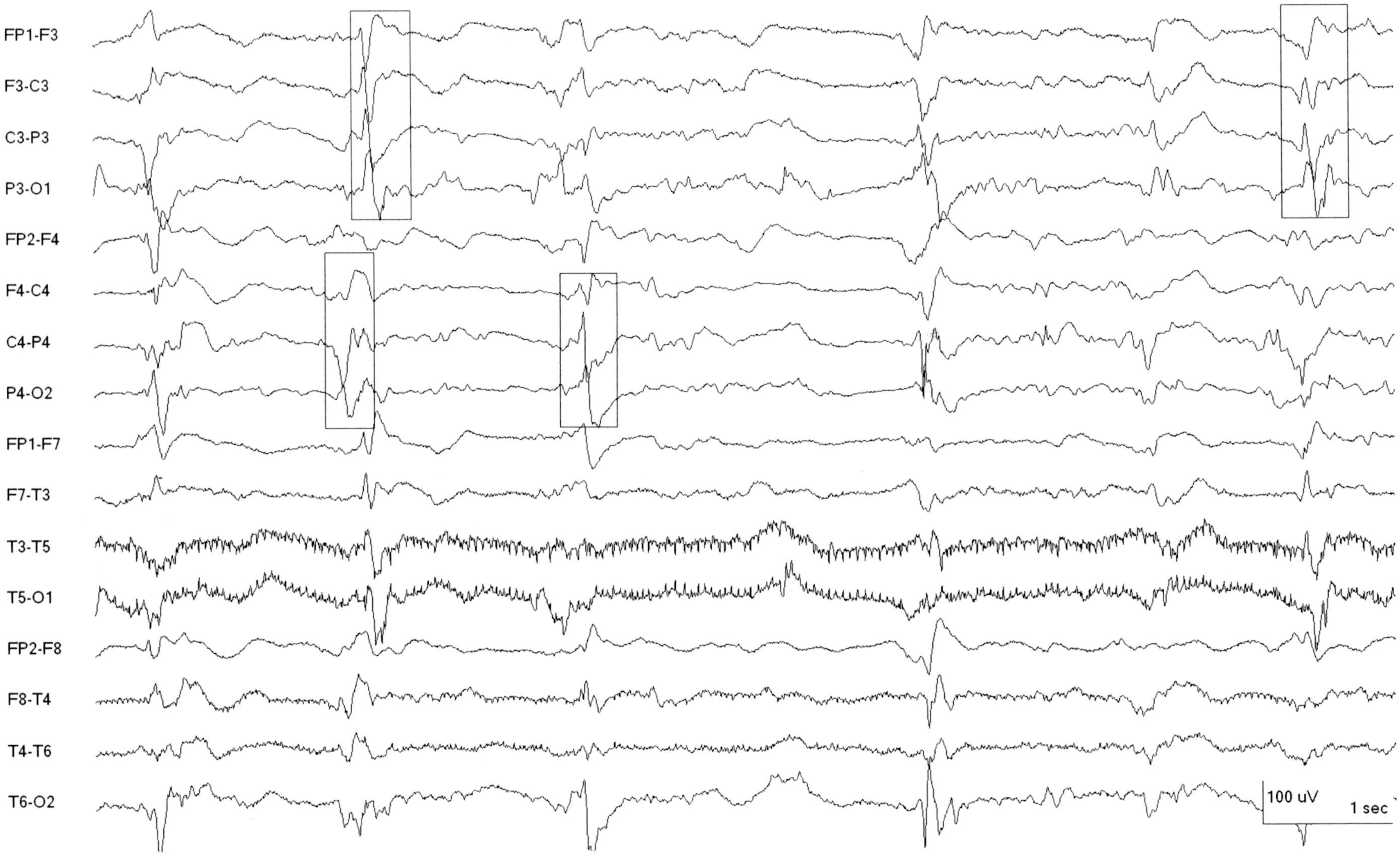

Figure 4.10 BIPLEDs. Widely spaced (<1 per second) BIPLEDs are present in this 21-year-old woman with mental retardation, chromosomal abnormalities and seizures (two discharges are highlighted on each side). The patient became unresponsive after having generalized seizures. Note that there are periodic discharges (PLEDs) occurring in each hemisphere independent of each other.

ACNS proposal name: BIPDs.

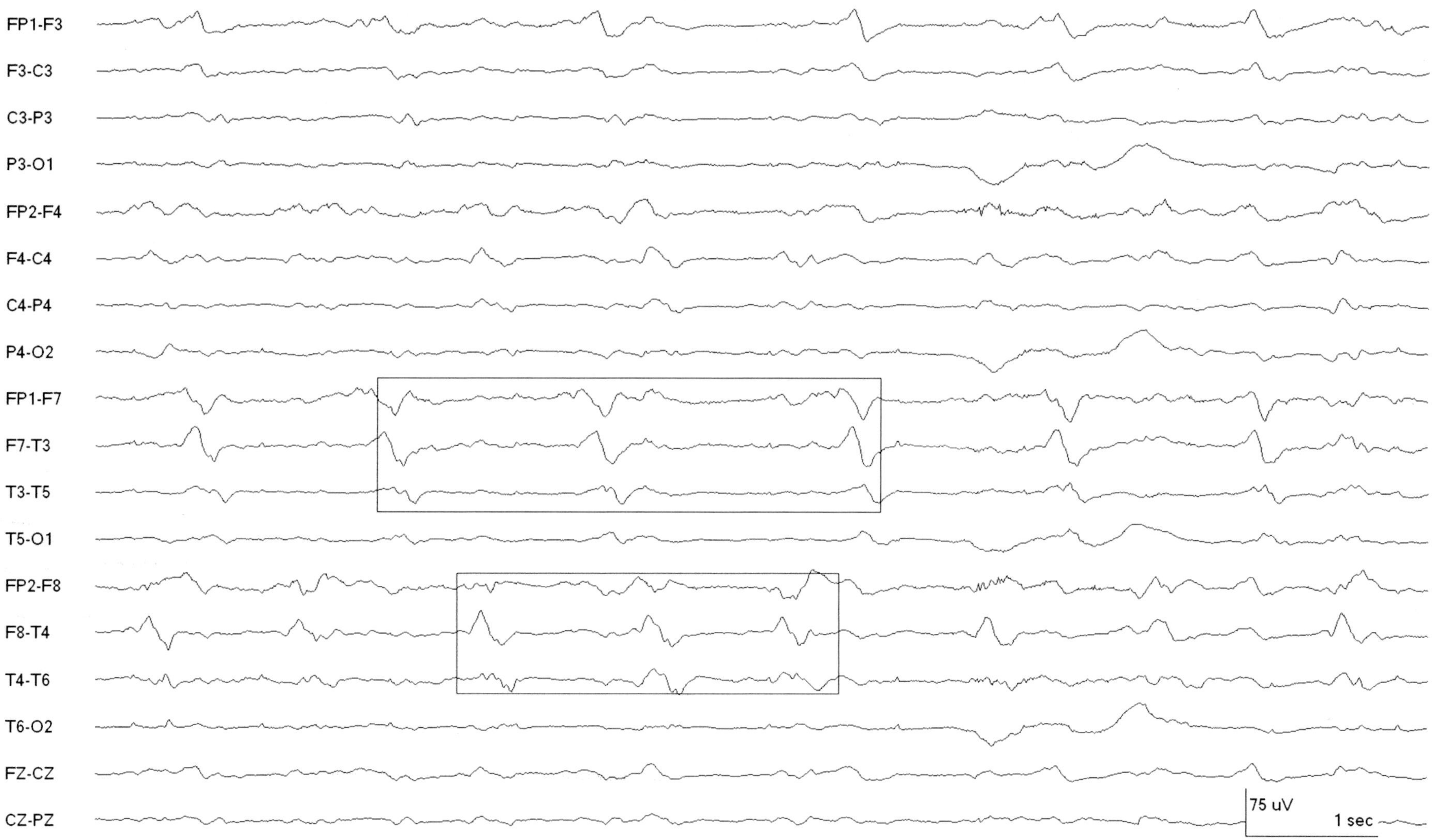

Figure 4.11 BIPLEDs. The EEG in this 75-year-old comatose woman shows BIPLEDs (three discharges on each side are boxed). The patient had a cardiac arrest the day before.

ACNS proposal name: BIPDs.

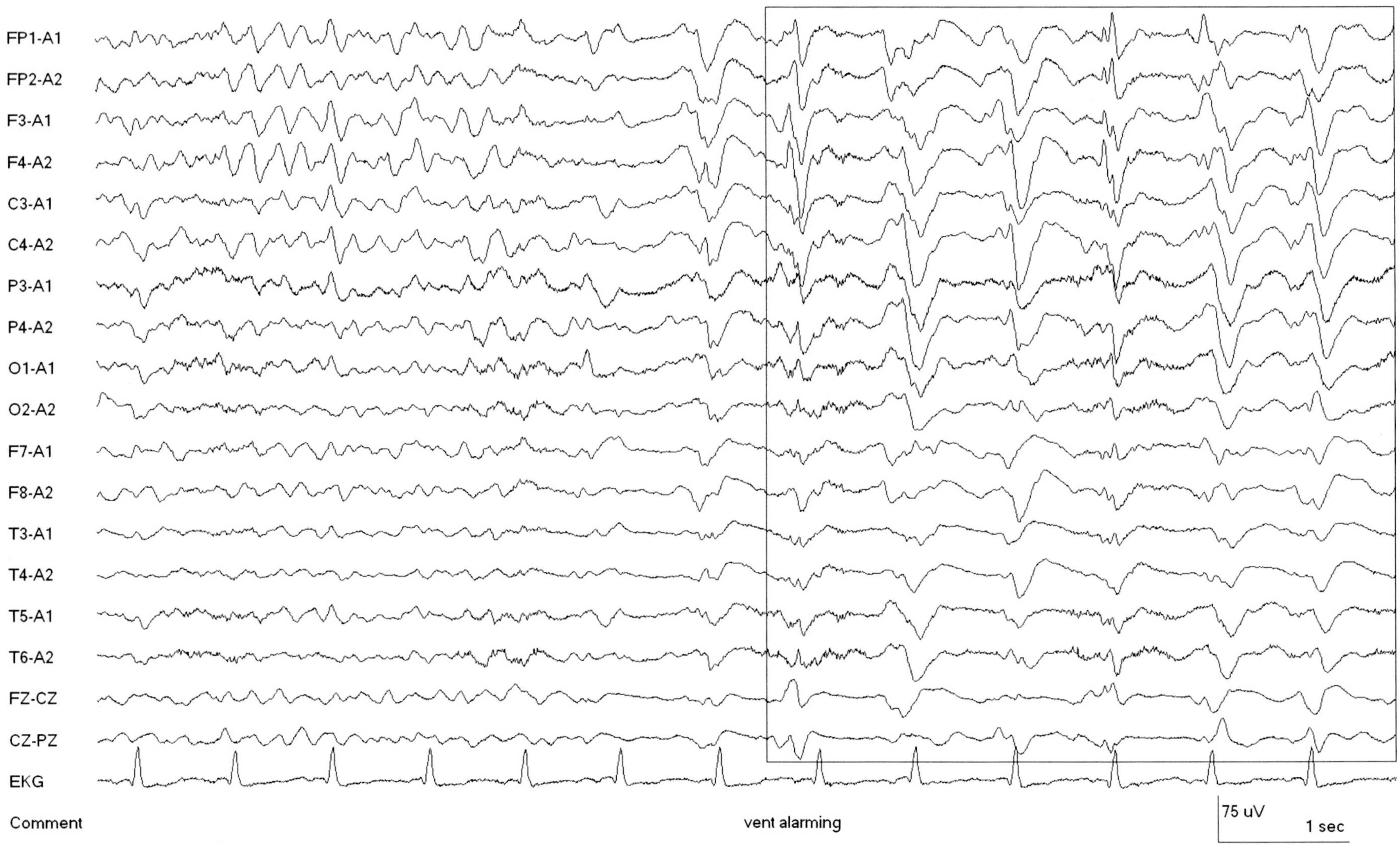

Figure 4.12 GPEDs and stimulus-induced rhythmic, periodic or ictal discharges (SIRPIDs). SIRPIDs are present in this 62-year-old comatose man. The patient had become unresponsive following abdominal surgery. There is a change in the EEG following alerting stimulation with the appearance of GPEDs (box).

ACNS proposal name: SI-GPDs.

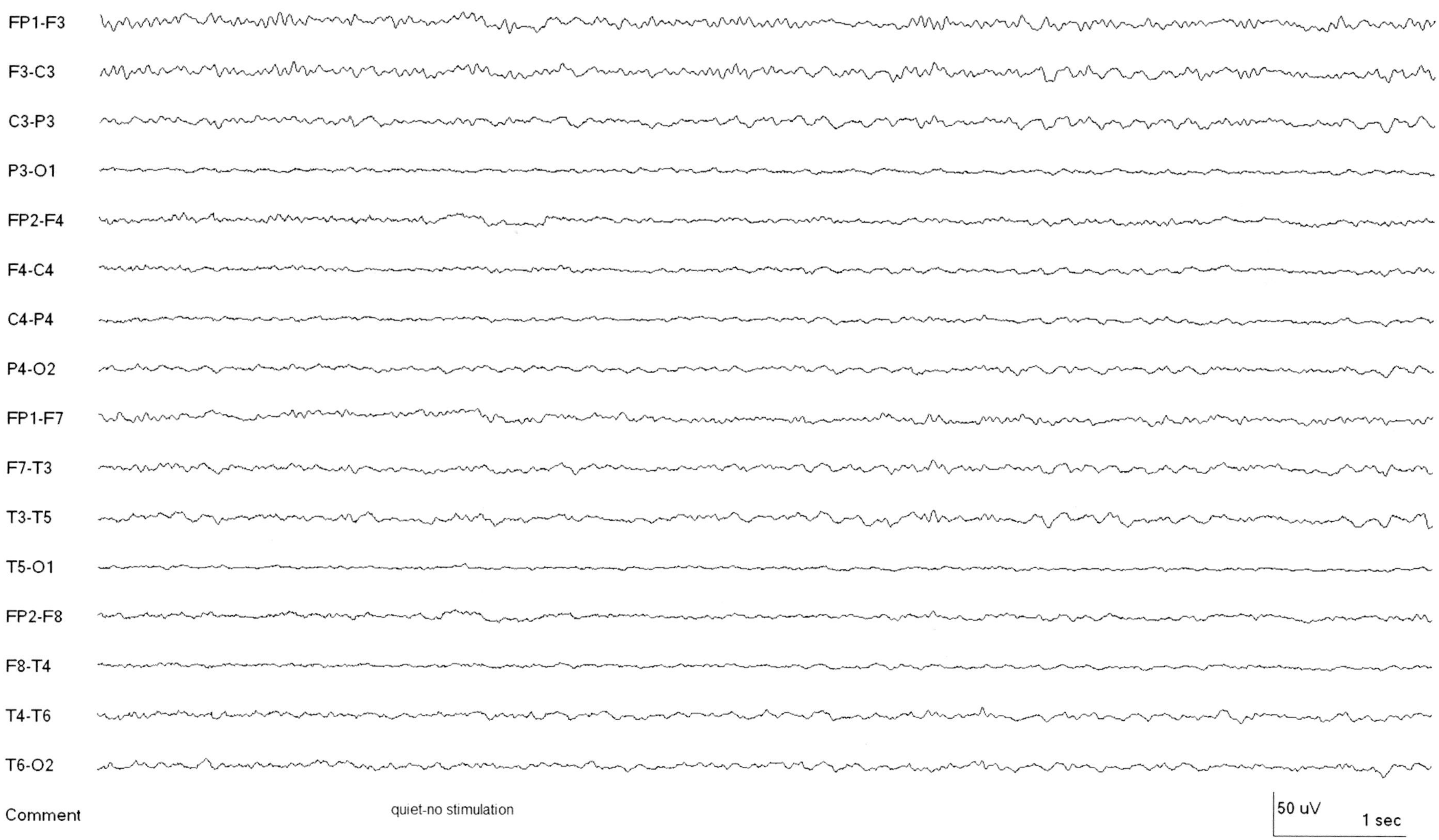

Figure 4.13 Rhythmic delta and SIRPIDs. (a) The initial EEG in this 36-year-old comatose woman s/p cardiac arrest shows low-voltage background activity with beta activity present anteriorly and of higher voltage on the left. Background rhythms are otherwise predominantly in the theta range.

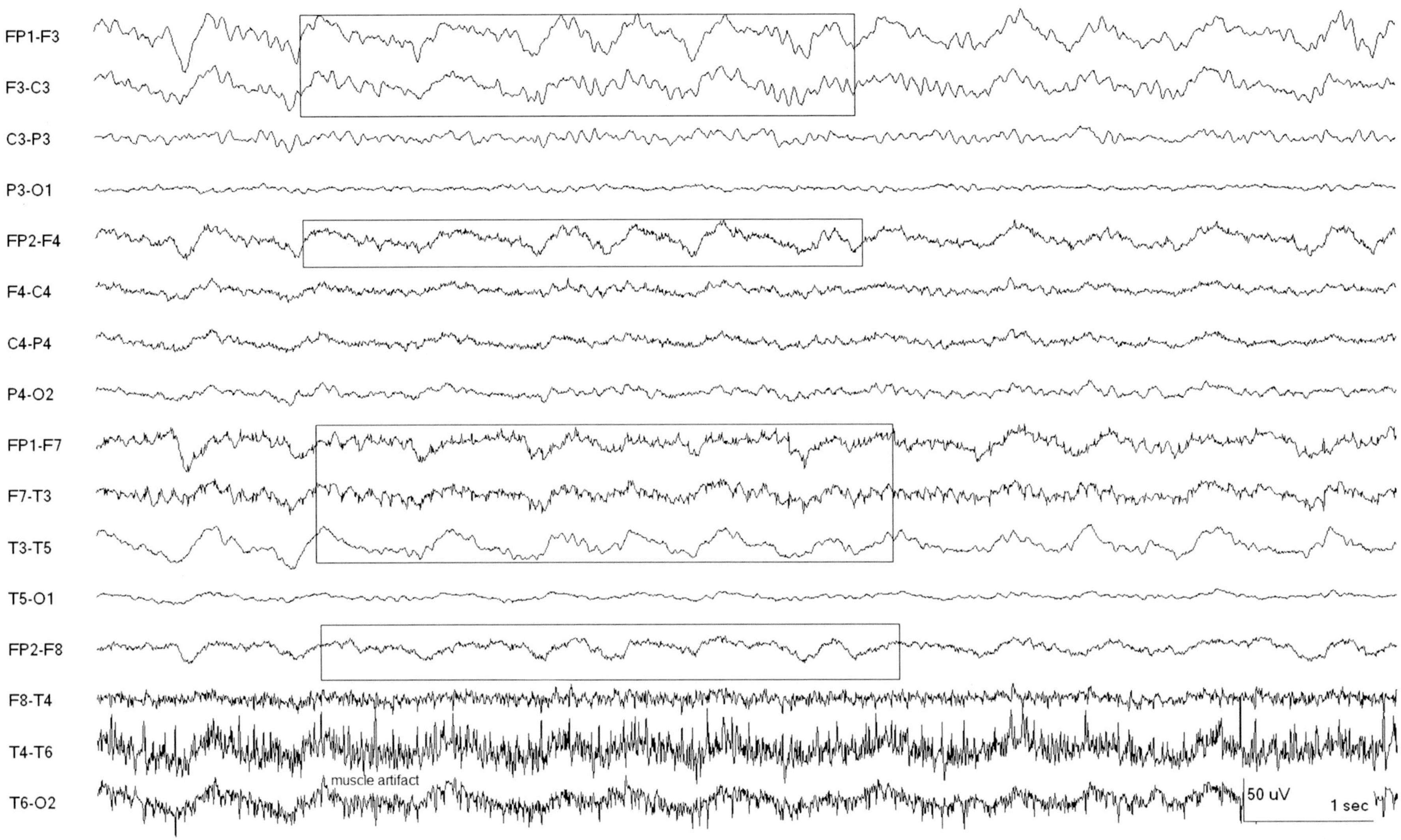

Figure 4.13 (*Continued*) (b) Following painful stimulation, SIRPIDs, consisting of rhythmic delta activity in this case, are present bilaterally. ACNS proposal name: SI-GRDA.

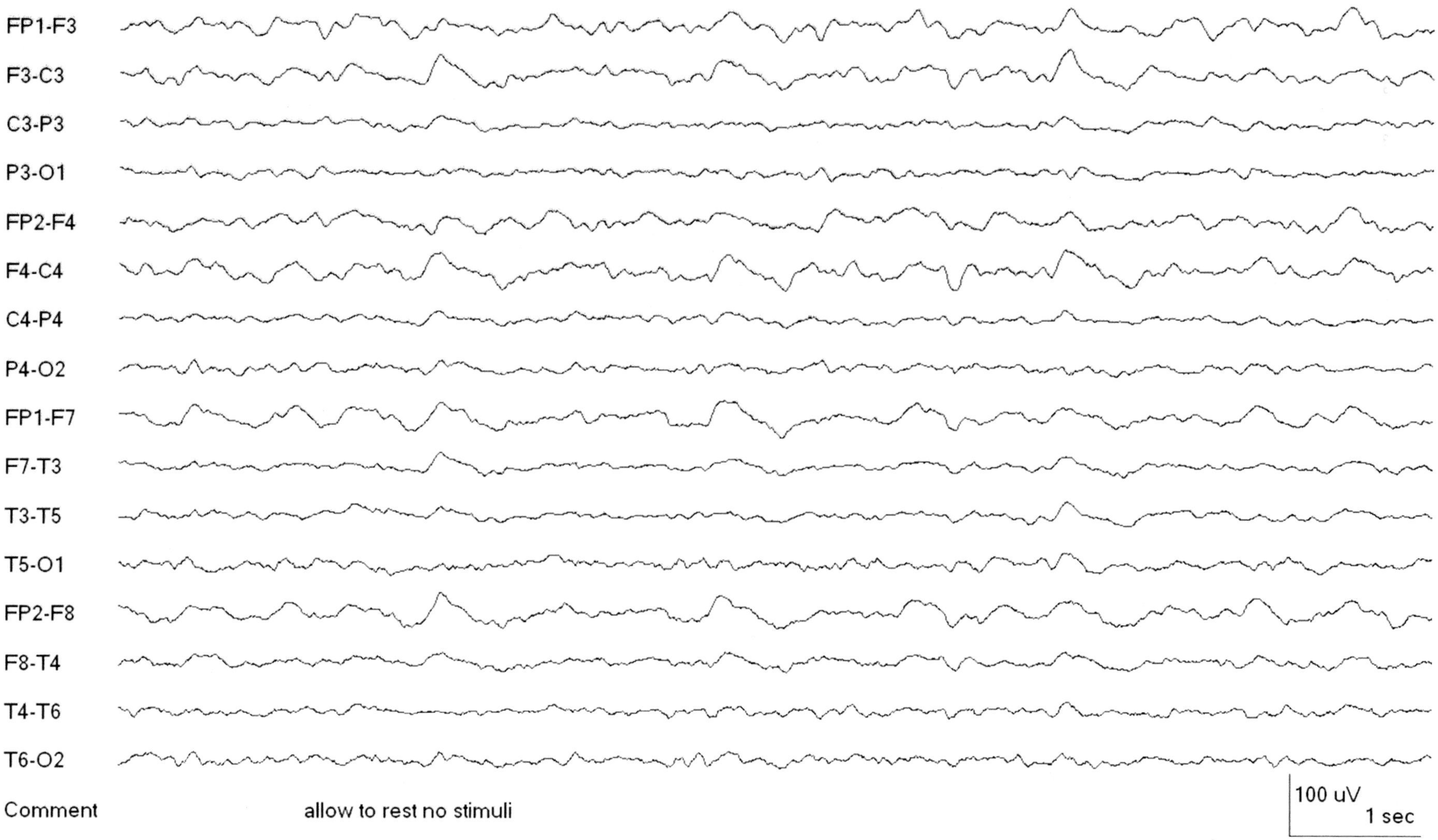

Figure 4.14 SIRPIDs: GPEDs vs. triphasic waves vs. seizure. (a) The baseline (nonstimulated) EEG in this 61-year-old man with listeria meningitis and normal renal and hepatic function shows diffuse slowing of background activity with delta activity prominent anteriorly.

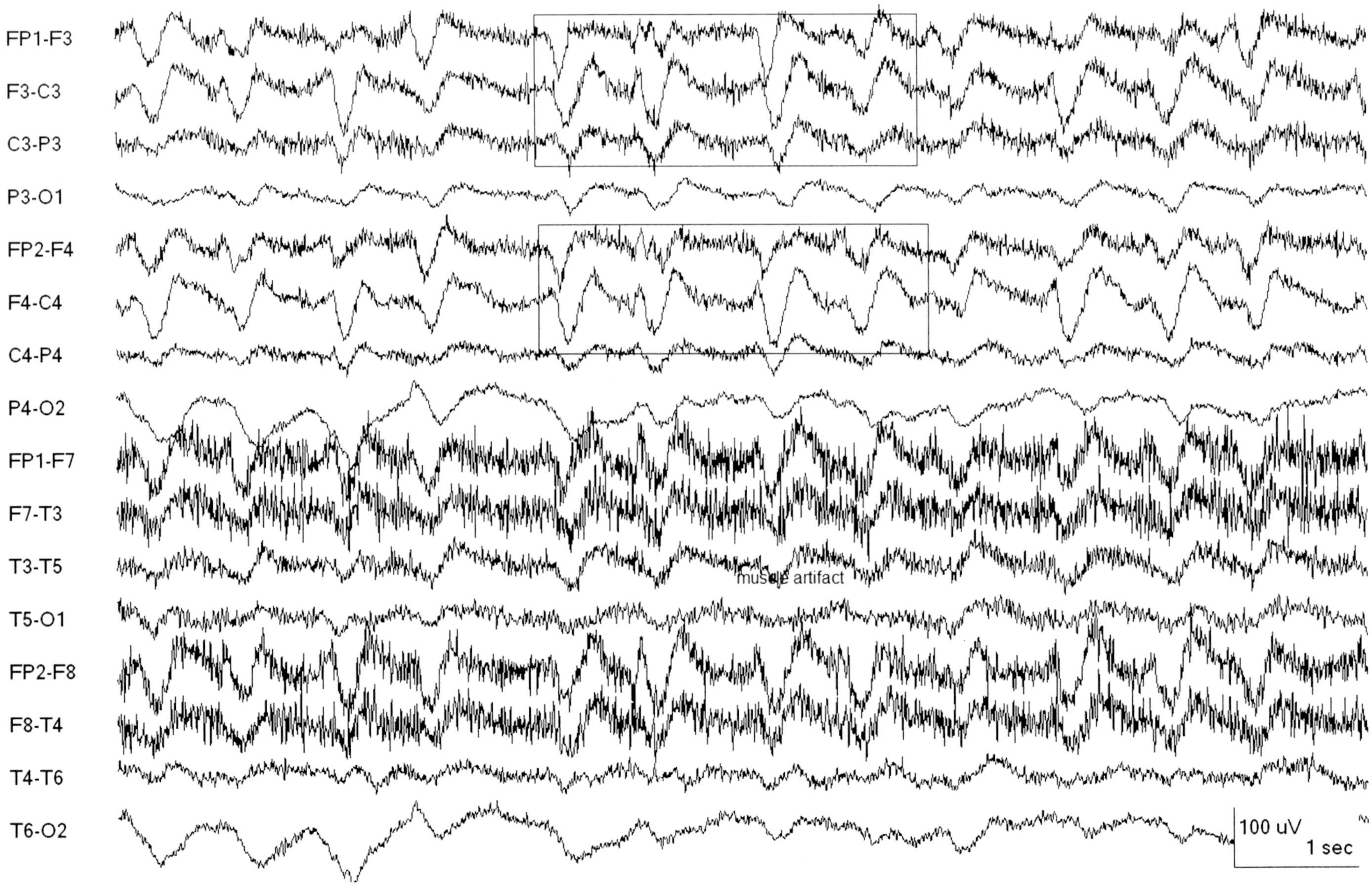

Figure 4.14 (*Continued*) (b) Following painful stimulation there is a generalized periodic pattern fluctuating in frequency between 1 and 2 Hz, usually with a triphasic morphology, and on a semirhythmic, slow background. Four discharges are in the boxes. This is an example of SIRPIDs and is a *potentially* ictal pattern. Note the much greater muscle artifact after stimulation.

ACNS proposal name: SI-GPDs+, fluctuating, with triphasic morphology.

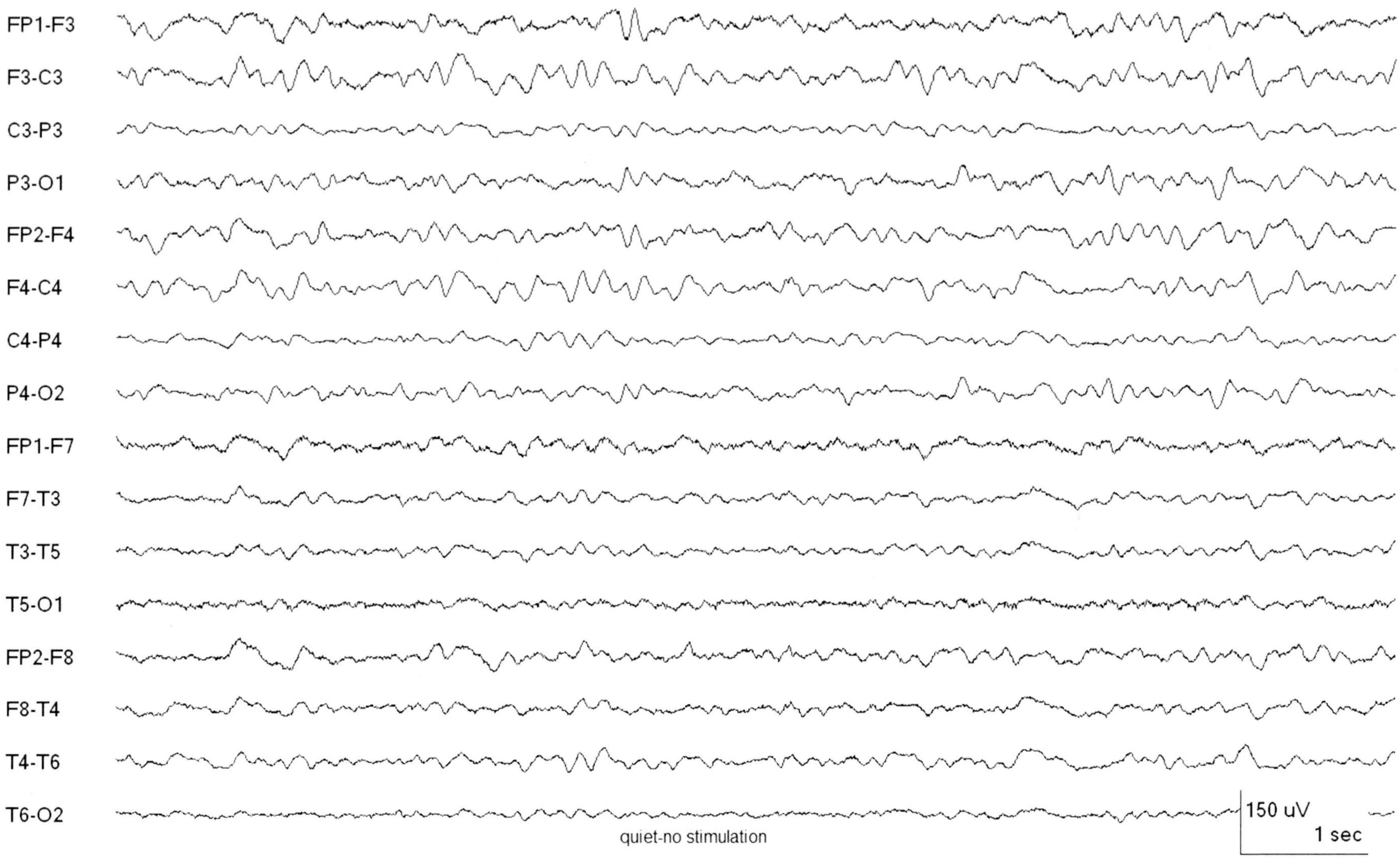

Figure 4.15 SIRPIDs: GPDs vs. triphasic waves vs. seizure. (a) The EEG in this 52-year-old woman shows diffuse slowing predominantly in the theta range when the patient was not stimulated.

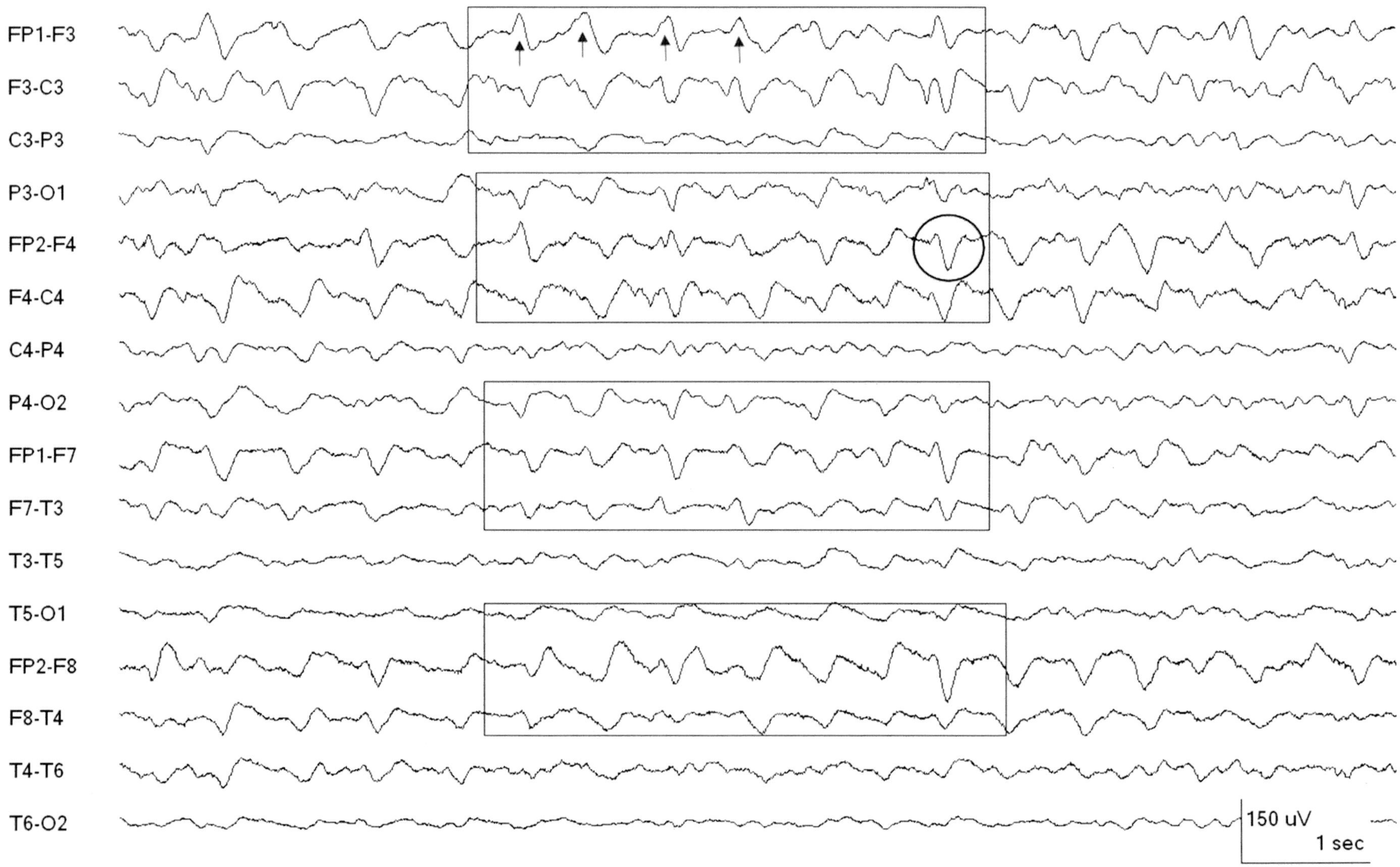

Figure 4.15 (*Continued*) (b) Following stimulation, generalized periodic discharges at approximately two per second are seen (boxes, with four discharges in a row marked with arrows), sometimes with triphasic morphology (example circled), maximal anteriorly, with a semirhythmic slow background. This pattern is potentially ictal or on the ictal–interictal continuum, but can also be seen in metabolic encephalopathy. EEG alone cannot reliably distinguish between these possibilities.

ACNS proposal name: SI-GPDs+, with triphasic morphology.

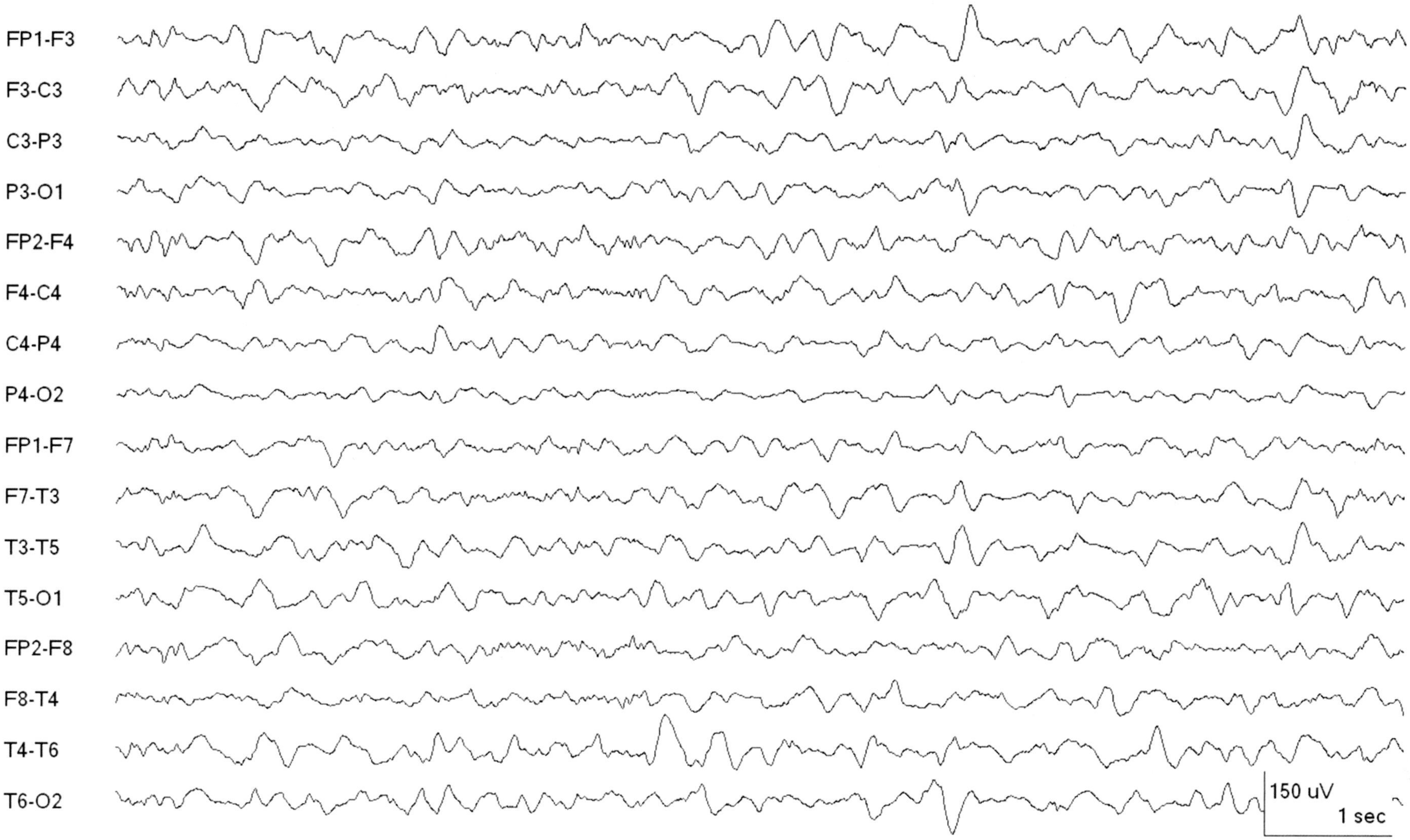

Figure 4.16 GPEDs and SIRPIDs. (a) The first tracing in this 75-year-old comatose woman with end-stage renal disease on dialysis and receiving cefepime shows diffuse slowing of background rhythms predominantly in the theta and delta range.

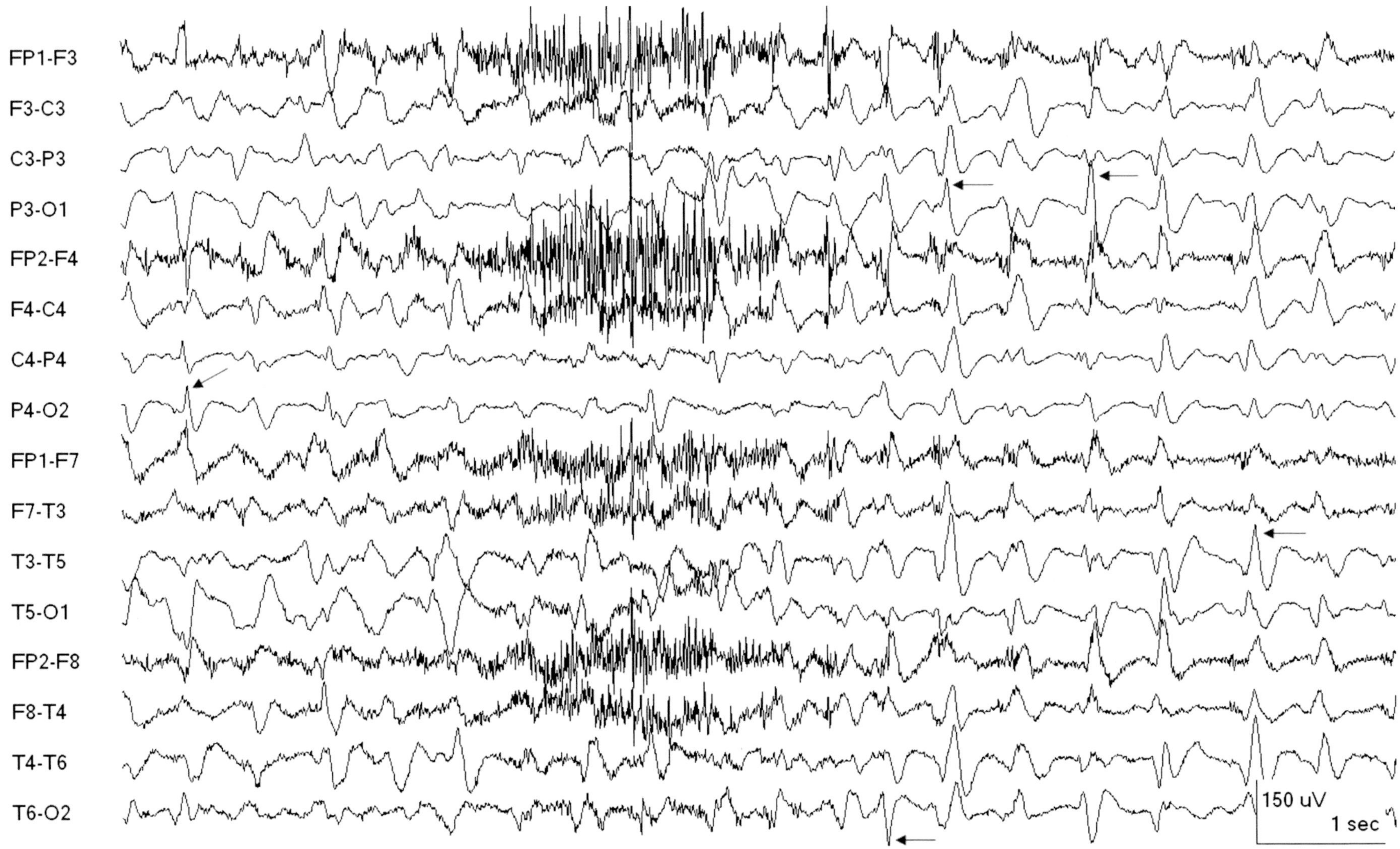

Figure 4.16 (*Continued*) (b) Following stimulation, there are generalized periodic sharp waves (GPEDs) occurring at a rate of approximately 2 Hz, but with some variability. This is another example of SIRPIDs. We would consider this pattern on the ictal–interictal continuum and treat it as such; however, it remains possible that it is unrelated to seizures. The high amplitude and sharp morphology of many of the discharges (several marked with arrows) makes this more likely to be related to seizures.

ACNS proposal name: SI-GPDs.

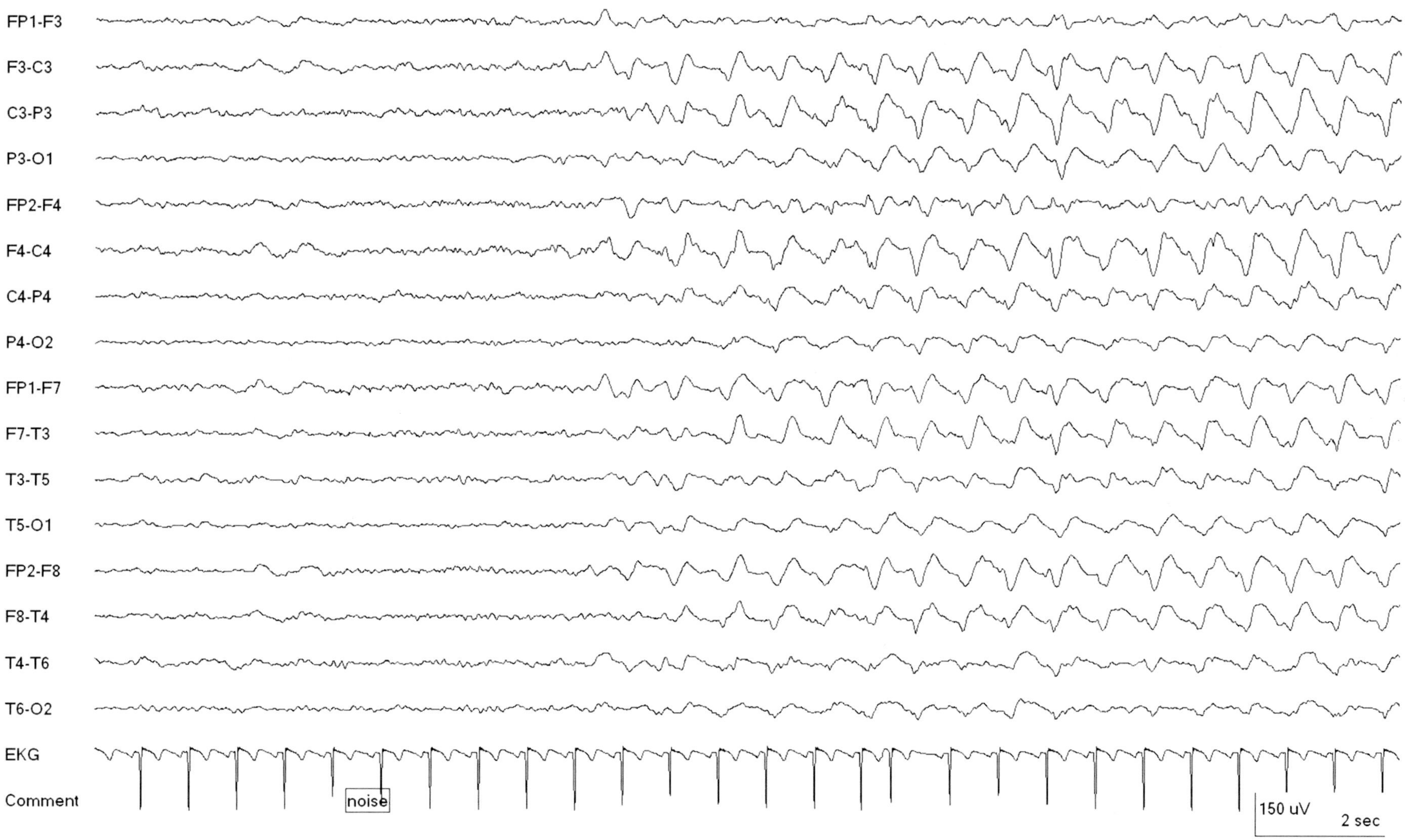

Figure 4.17 SIRPIDs, possibly ictal. (a) Following stimulation of this 65-year-old woman with recent seizures being evaluated for decreased mental status, there is a widespread rhythmic pattern that could be described as either sharply contoured rhythmic delta activity or periodic discharges, and that sometimes resembles triphasic waves. Note this is a compressed EEG at slower 'paper' speed.

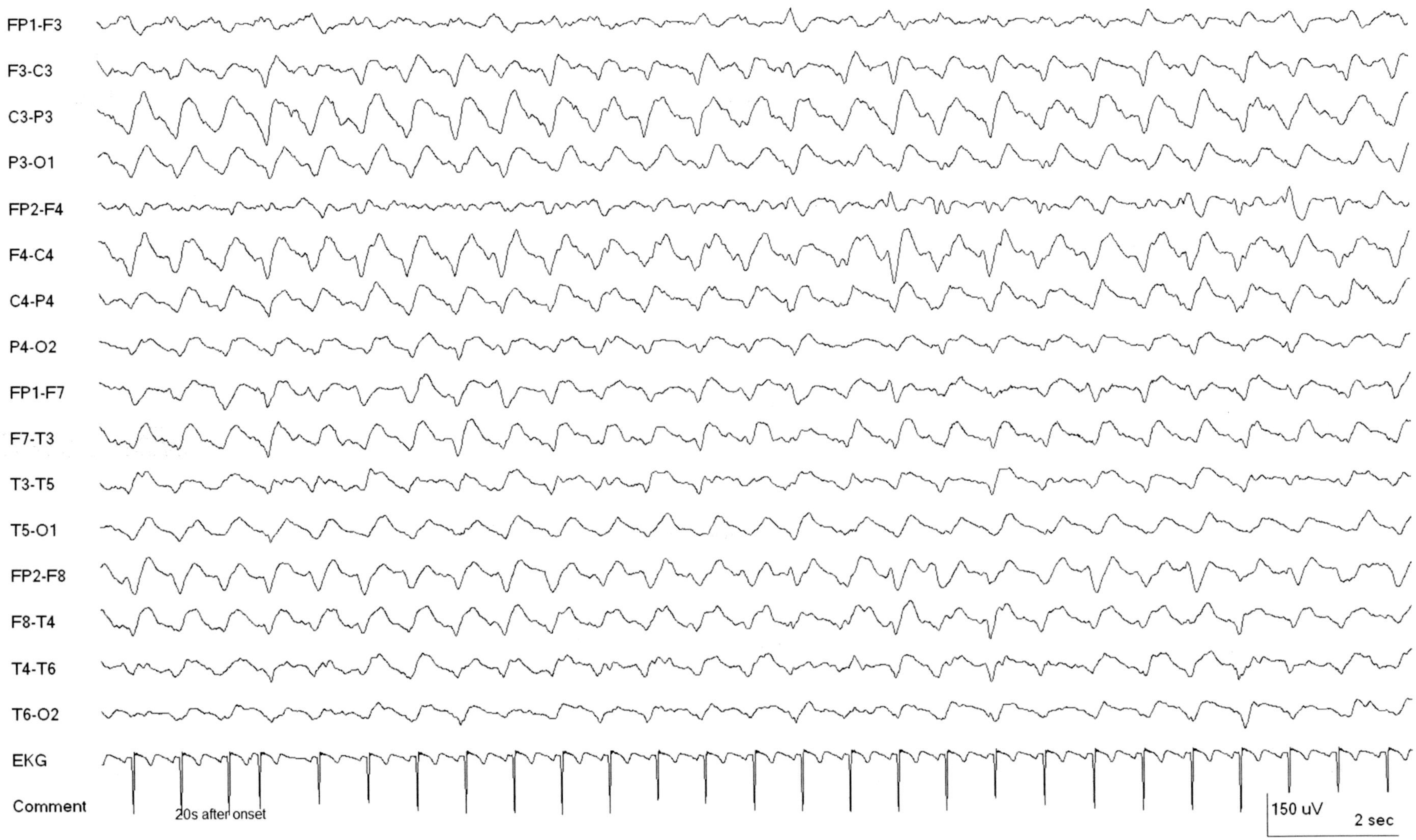

Figure 4.17 (*Continued*) (b) Twenty seconds after onset, the pattern is similar but slightly slower and slightly different in morphology.

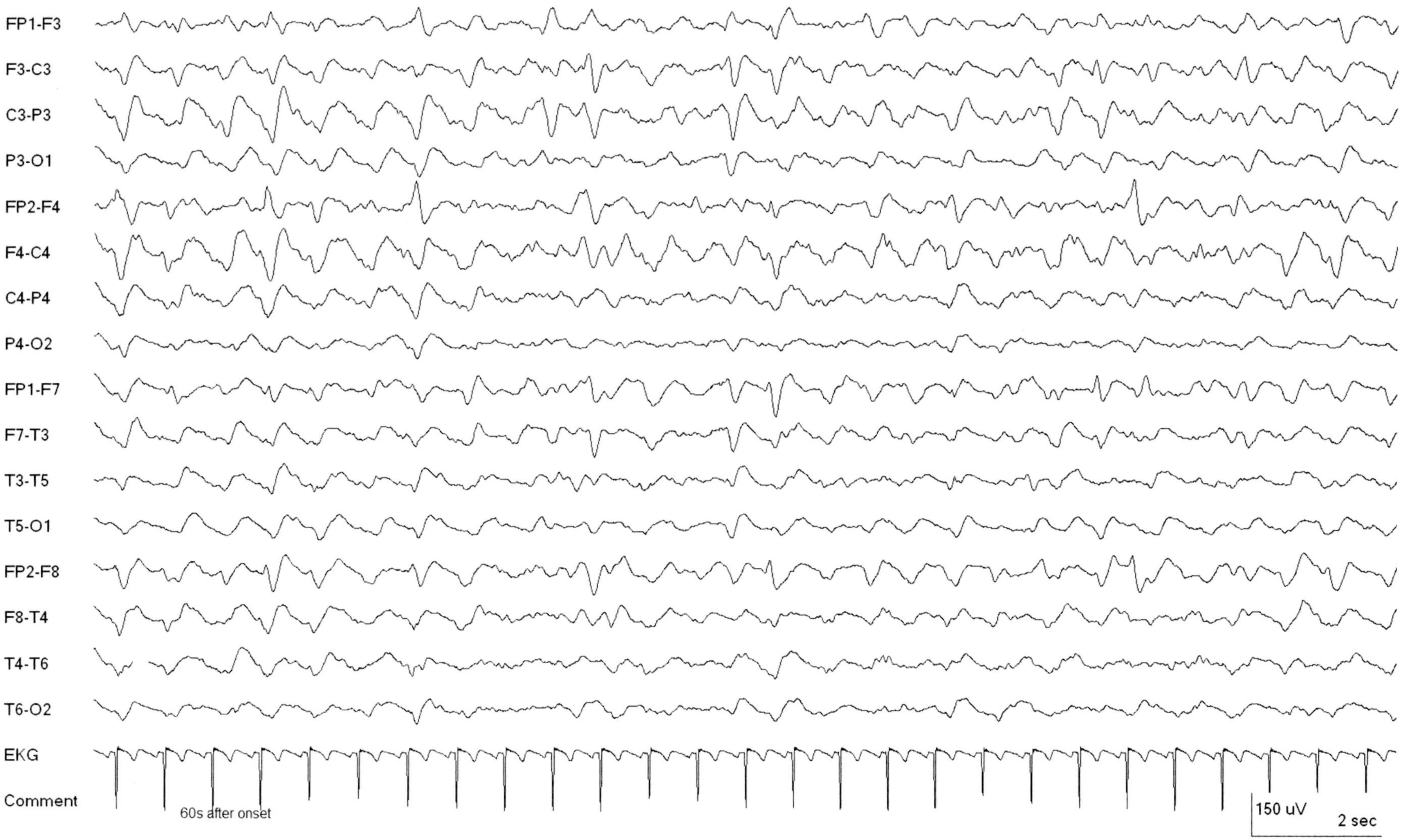

Figure 4.17 (*Continued*) (c) Sixty seconds after onset the pattern is becoming lower amplitude and less regular.

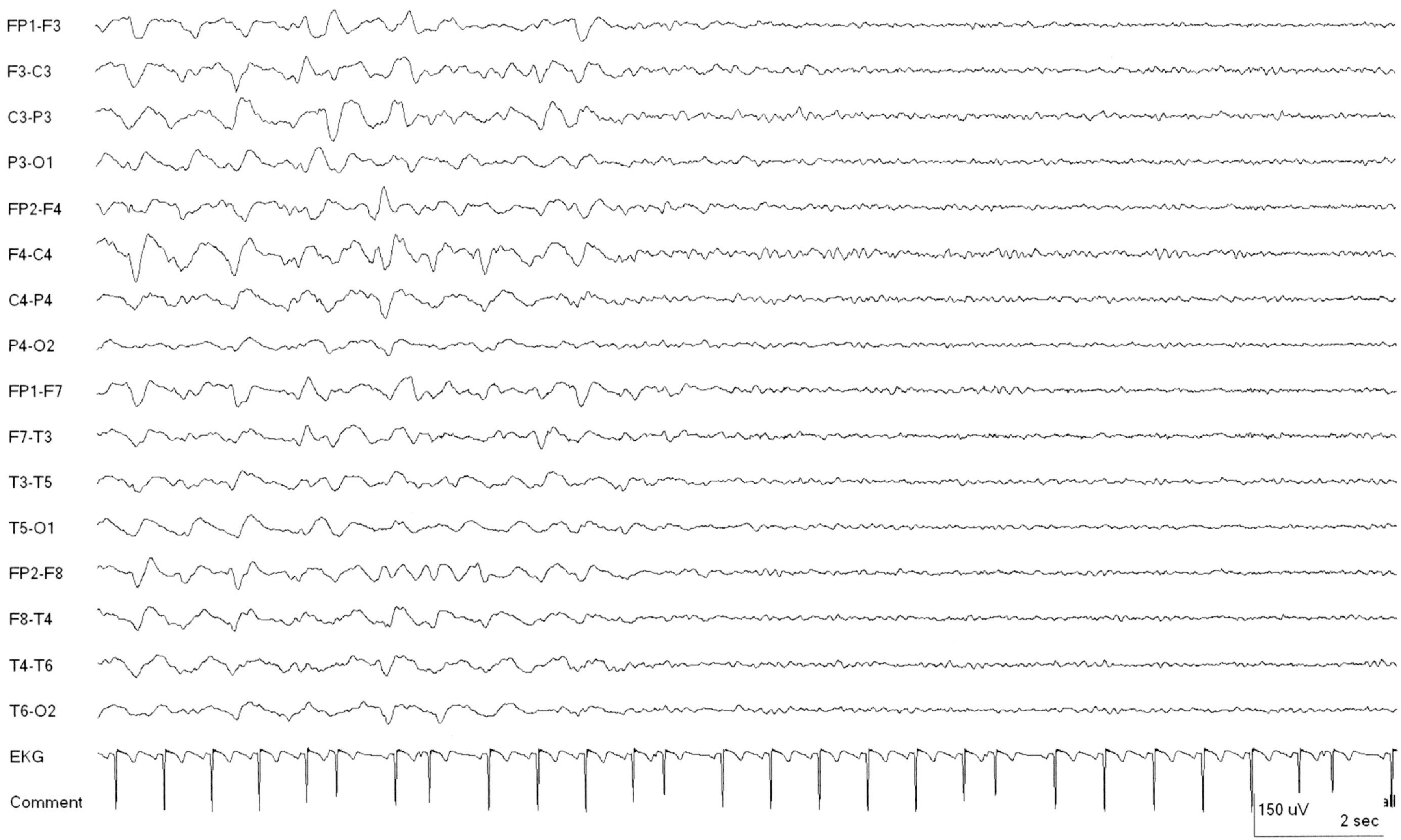

Figure 4.17 (*Continued*) (d) Eighty-three seconds after onset the discharge ceases. There was no clinical accompaniment. This is another example of SIRPIDs. It is unclear if this represents stimulus-induced seizure activity or not, but in the absence of a clear metabolic problem, with probable subtle evolution and with a history of recent seizures it probably is seizure activity.

ACNS proposal name: SI-GRDA+ or SI-GPDs+, evolving.

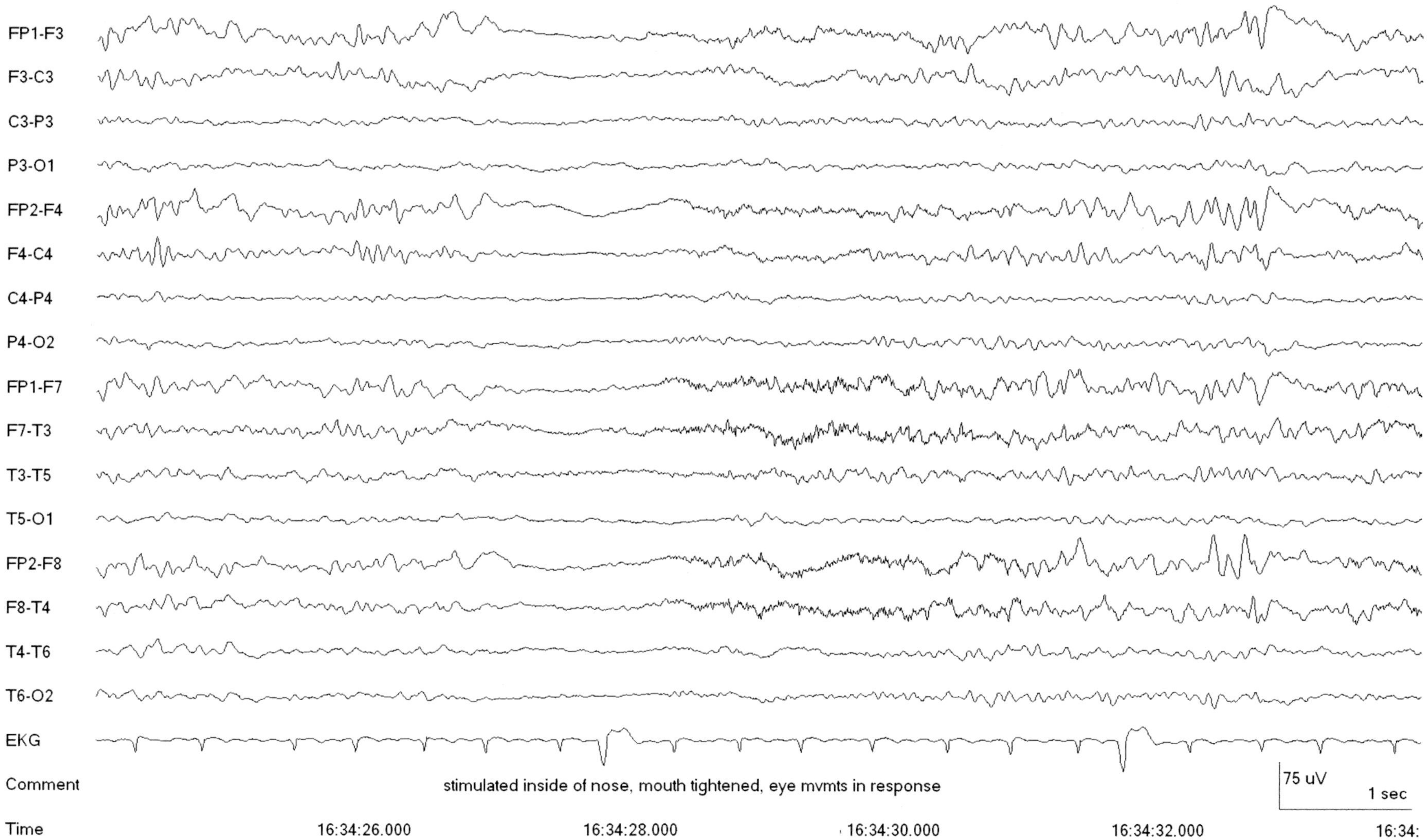

Figure 4.18 SIRPIDs with clinical correlate. (a) In this 73-year-old comatose woman with bilateral watershed infarcts, stimulation by the EEG technician (nostril tickle, labeled) in the middle of this segment results in diffuse attenuation, followed by nondescript continuous low-amplitude alpha and beta activity. This turns out to be the subtle onset of a subsequent evolving electrographic followed by clinical seizure.

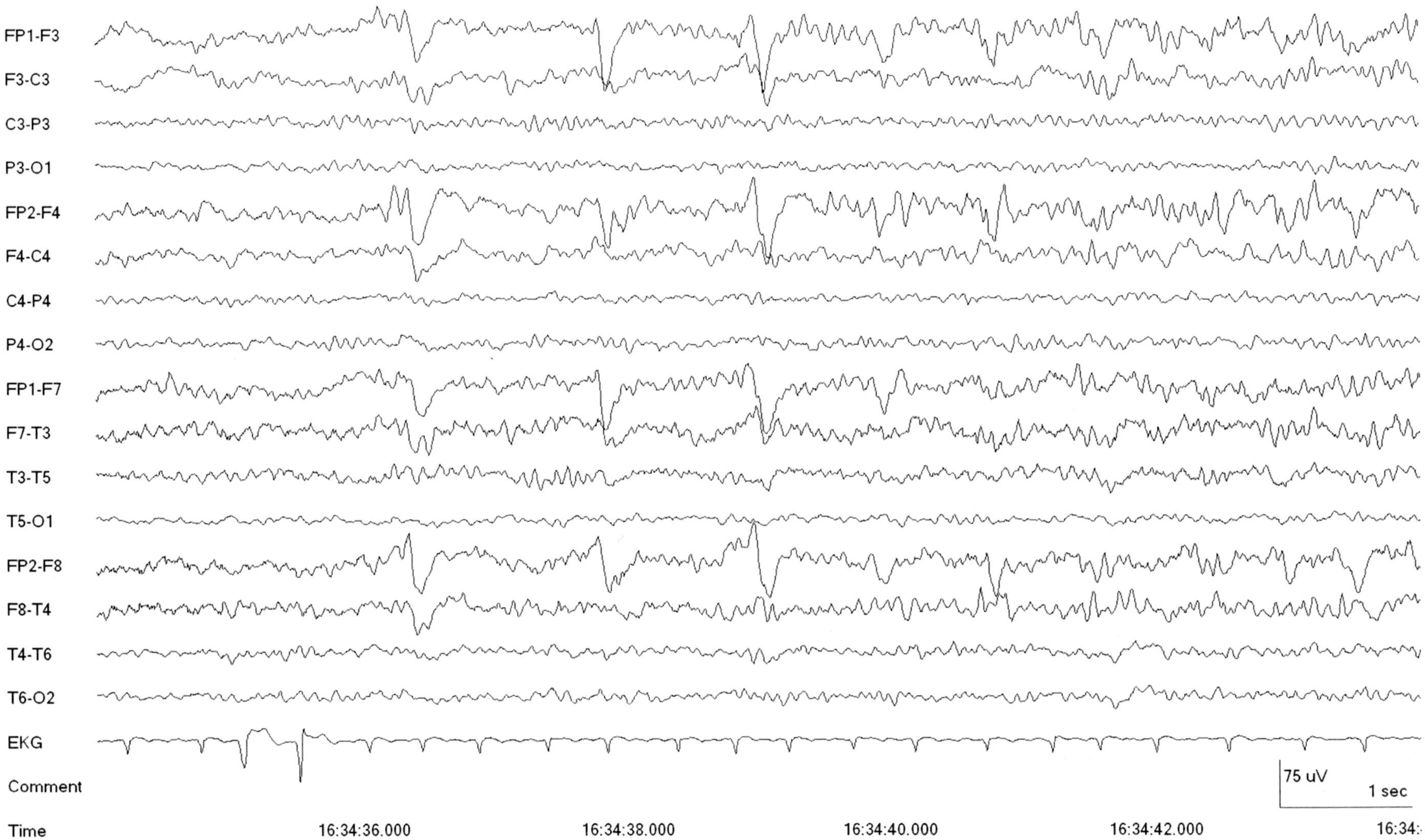

Figure 4.18 (*Continued*) (b) The next 10 s show diffuse fast activity becoming slightly higher in amplitude.

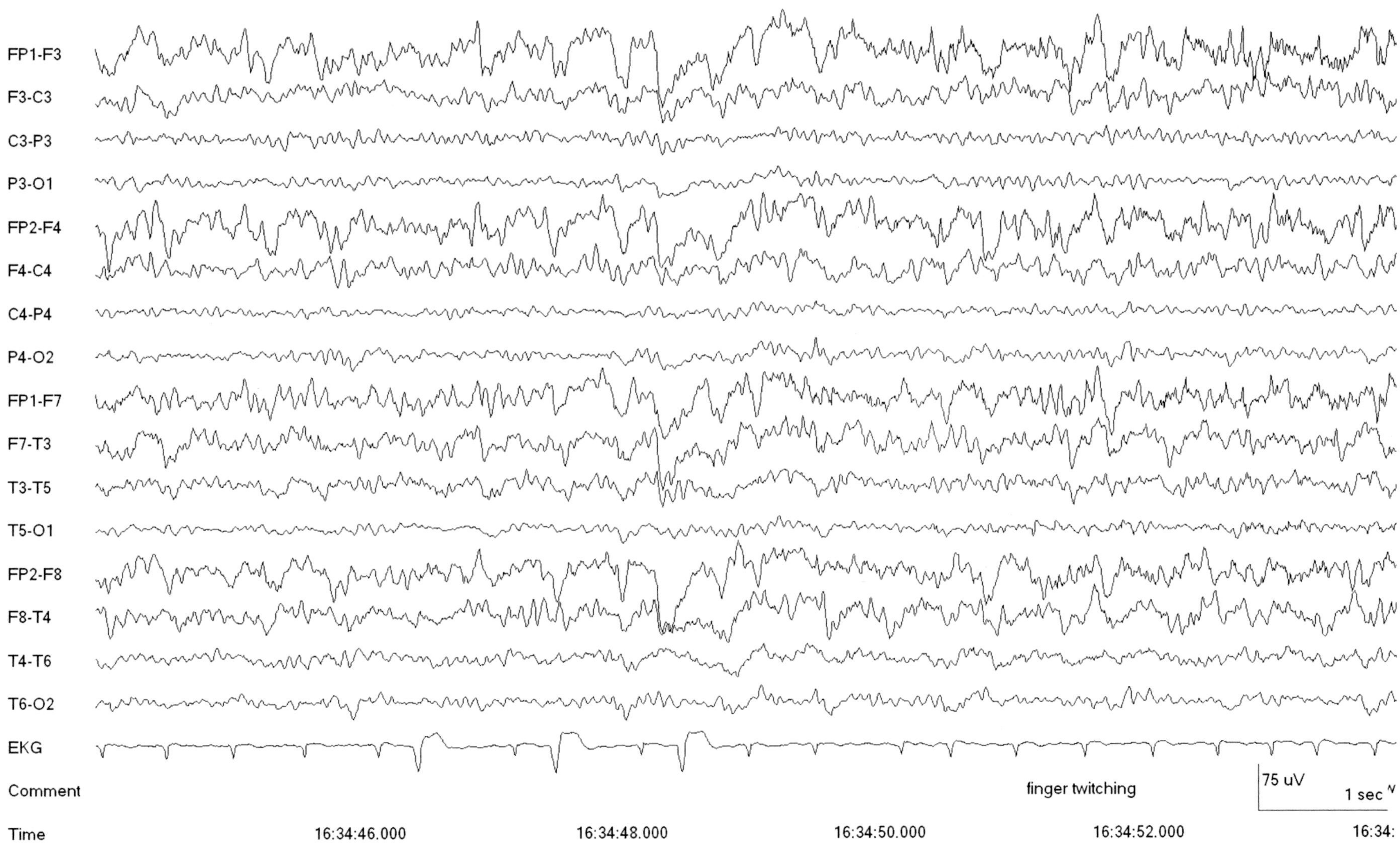

Figure 4.18 (*Continued*) (c) During the subsequent 10 s, this fast activity continues to become more prominent, and now semirhythmic superimposed delta is seen bilaterally, maximal anteriorly. Her eyes opened wide, then left-hand finger twitching became visible near the end of this segment, as seen on video and noted by the technician.

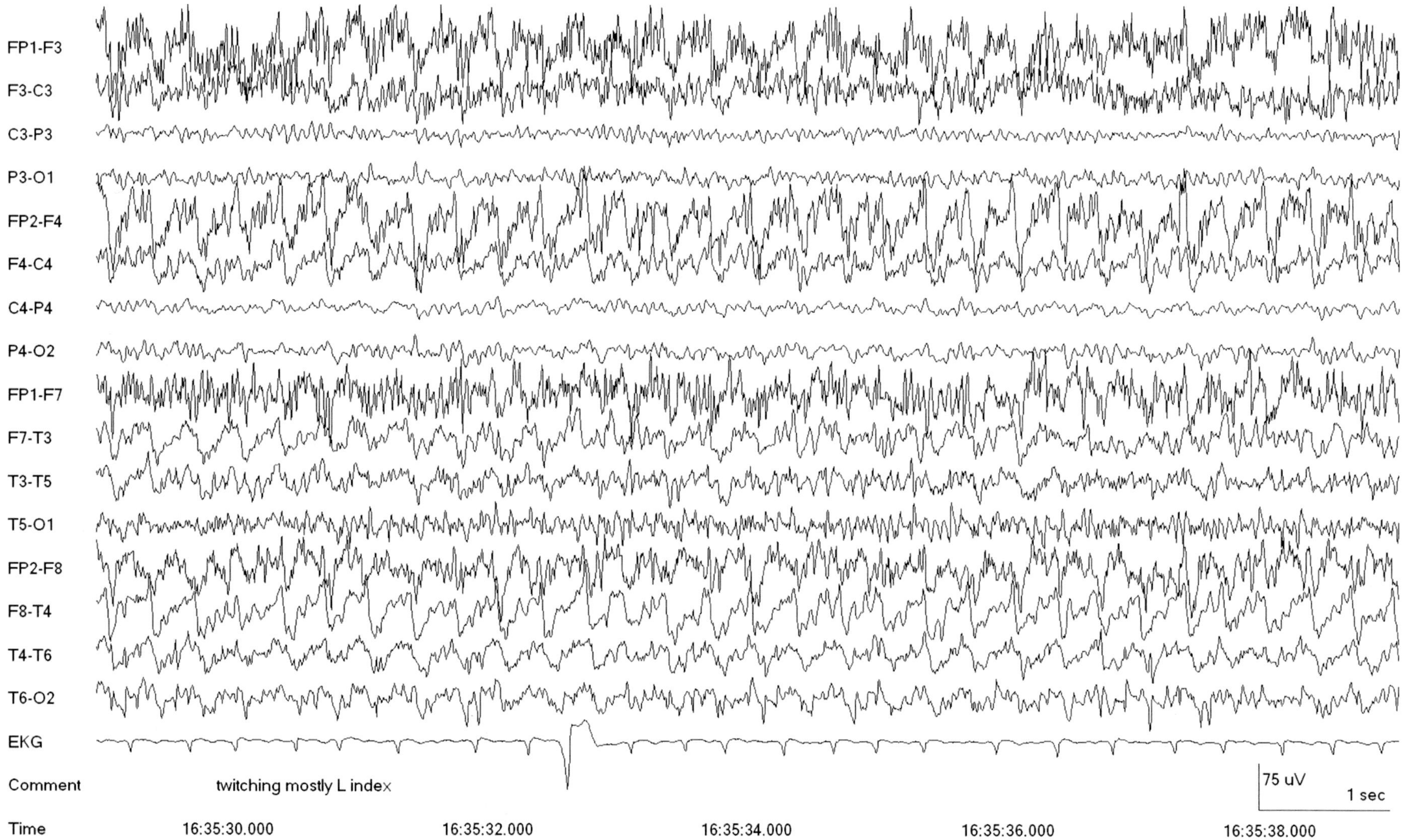

Figure 4.18 (*Continued*) (d) By 10 s later, the pattern has clearly become ictal with higher amplitude and rhythmic sharply contoured 3 Hz activity (maximal on the right) with superimposed fast activity. Left-hand twitching continued. Thus, this is a clinical and electrographic seizure induced by stimulation (SIRPIDs with clinical correlate). This clinical and electrographic pattern recurred each time the patient was stimulated that day.

ACNS term: not applicable; would still be termed a seizure (stimulus-induced).

5 EEG in cerebrovascular disease

5.1 Ischemia

As cerebral blood flow decreases, the EEG changes in the following manner. First, there is subtle loss of faster frequencies (beta and alpha, sometimes including sleep spindles). Then, as flow drops further, slowing appears – first excess theta, then excess delta. All of this occurs while ischemia is at a reversible stage and standard anatomical imaging, including MRI with diffusion weighted imaging, remains normal. As flow continues to decline, there is suppression of all frequencies, which corresponds with irreversible neuronal death (infarction). Thus, EEG can detect ischemia when standard imaging cannot, although perfusion imaging can also detect this. This ability of EEG to detect ischemia early with a procedure that can be done continuously is the basis for continuous EEG monitoring in patients at high risk for ischemia, such as those with subarachnoid hemorrhage (see Chapter 7).

5.2 Hemorrhage

Intracerebral hemorrhage tends to produce nonspecific focal slowing in the EEG. Recently, EEG has begun to be used to monitor patients with ischemic stroke receiving tissue plasminogen activator (TPA) to detect hemorrhagic transformation as soon as it occurs. With intraventricular and subarachnoid hemorrhage, diffuse slowing and frontal intermittent rhythmic delta activity (FIRDA) are commonly seen, and may correlate with raised intracranial pressure. Subdural and epidural hemorrhages tend to produce focal slowing and attenuation of normal faster frequencies. The attenuation is from the underlying cortical dysfunction as well as the extra distance between the brain and the electrodes; this can also occur with extracranial soft tissue swelling. All intracranial hemorrhages can be associated with epileptiform discharges, periodic lateralized epileptiform discharges (PLEDs) or seizures, especially, but not only, when the bleed affects the cortex.

After neurosurgical procedures, there is sometimes a confusing combination of attenuation of faster frequencies from underlying injury and extra-axial fluid, and accentuation of the same activity from the skull defect.

Figure list

Figure 5.1 Unilateral attenuation from infarct.

Figure 5.2 Attenuation, PLEDs and SIRPIDs from infarct.

Figure 5.3 Unilateral attenuation from infarct.

Figure 5.4 PLEDs vs. asymmetric triphasic waves after stroke.

Figure 5.5 Seizure and PLEDs mimicking stroke.

Figure 5.6 Slowing and attenuation from infarct.

Atlas of EEG in Critical Care Lawrence J. Hirsch and Richard P. Brenner

Figure 5.7 Slowing and spindle asymmetry from stroke.

Figure 5.8 Spindle coma from posterior fossa hemorrhage.

Figure 5.9 PLEDs from intracerebral hemorrhage.

Figure 5.10 FIRDA from intraventricular hemorrhage.

Figure 5.11 Slowing and breach from intracerebral hemorrhage and hemicraniectomy.

Figure 5.12 Slowing and breach from subdural hematomas and hemicraniectomy.

Figure 5.13 Focal seizure from subdural hematoma.

Figure 5.14 SIRPIDs and GPEDs from subarachnoid hemorrhage.

Figure 5.15 Asymmetry after subdural hematoma evacuation.

Figure 5.16 Asymmetry after traumatic brain injury.

Figure 5.17 Breach after subdural hematoma evacuation.

Figure 5.18 Focal slowing after subarachnoid hemorrhage.

Suggested reading

Bazil, C.W., Herman, S.T. and Pedley, T.A. (2003) Focal electroencephalographic abnormalities In: Ebersole, J.S. and Pedley, T.A. (eds), *Current Practice of Clinical Electroencephalography*, pp. 303–347. Lippincott, Williams and Wilkins, Philadelphia.

Claassen, J., Hirsch, L.J., Frontera, J.A. *et al.* (2006) Prognostic significance of continuous EEG monitoring in patients with poor-grade subarachnoid hemorrhage. *Neurocritical Care* **4**(2), 103–112.

Claassen, J., Jetté, N., Chum, F. *et al.* (2007) Electrographic seizures and periodic discharges after intracerebral hemorrhage. *Neurology* **69**(13), 1356–1365.

Cobb, W.A., Guiloff, R.J. and Cast, J. (1979) Breach rhythm: The EEG related to skull defects. *Electroencephalography and Clinical Neurophysiology*; **47**, 251–271.

de Vos, C.C., van Maarseveen, S.M., Brouwers, P.J. *et al.* (2008) Continuous EEG monitoring during thrombolysis in acute hemispheric stroke patients using the brain symmetry index. *Journal of Clinical Neurophysiology* **25**(2), 77–82.

Finnigan, S.P., Rose, S.E., Walsh, M. *et al.* (2004) Correlation of quantitative EEG in acute ischemic stroke with 30-day NIHSS score: comparison with diffusion and perfusion MRI. *Stroke*. **35**(4), 899–903.

Finnigan, S.P., Walsh, M., Rose, S.E. *et al.* (2007) Quantitative EEG indices of sub-acute ischaemic stroke correlate with clinical outcomes. *Clinical Neurophysiology* **118**(11), 2525–2532.

Fountain, N.B. (2007) Is it time for routine EEG monitoring after intracerebral hemorrhage? *Neurology* **69**(13), 1312–1313.

Hansotia, P., Gottschalk, P., Green, P. *et al.* (1981) Spindle coma: Incidence, clinicopathologic correlates, and prognostic value. *Neurology* **31**, 83–87.

Jordan, K.G. (2004) Emergency EEG and continuous EEG monitoring in acute ischemic stroke. *Journal of Clinical Neurophysiology* **21**(5), 341–352.

Kaplan, P.W., Genoud, D., Ho, T.W. *et al.* (2000) Clinical correlates and prognosis in early spindle coma. *Journal of Clinical Neurophysiology* **111**, 584–590.

Nuwer, M.R., Jordan, S.E. and Ahn, S.S. (1987) Evaluation of stroke using EEG frequency analysis and topographic mapping. *Neurology* **37**(7), 1153–1159.

Passero, S., Rocchi, R., Rossi, S. *et al.* (2002) Seizures after spontaneous supratentorial intracerebral hemorrhage. *Epilepsia* **43**(10), 1175–1180.

van Putten, M.J. and Tavy, D.L. (2004) Continuous quantitative EEG monitoring in hemispheric stroke patients using the brain symmetry index. *Stroke* **35**(11), 2489–2492.

Vespa, P.M., O'Phelan, K., Shah, M. *et al.* (2003) Acute seizures after intracerebral hemorrhage: a factor in progressive midline shift and outcome. *Neurology* **60**(9), 1441–1446.

Wood, J.H., Polyzoidis, K.S., Epstein, C.M. *et al.* (1984) Quantitative EEG alterations after isovolemic-hemodilutional augmentation of cerebral perfusion in stroke patients. *Neurology* **34**(6), 764–768.

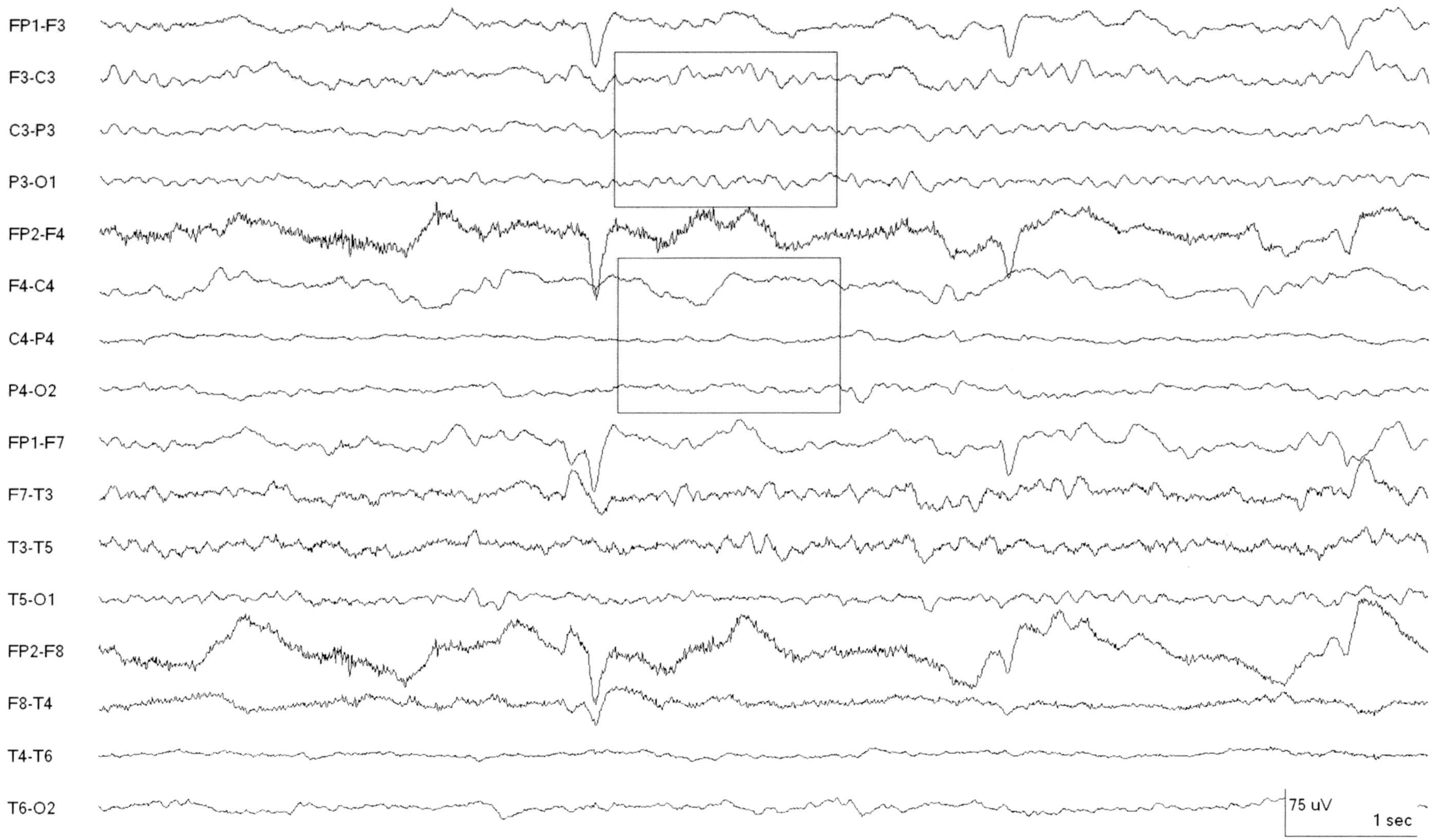

Figure 5.1 Unilateral attenuation from stroke. The EEG in this 42-year-old man with a history of a right MCA/ACA stroke and status post (s/p) 'strokectomy' shows prominent hemispheric differences. Background activity is markedly suppressed over the right hemisphere. The boxes highlight homologous electrodes with faster (alpha frequency) activity on the left that is absent on the right. This attenuation of faster activity signifies either cortical dysfunction (such as from an infarct or resection, as in this case) or an extra-axial collection on the right.

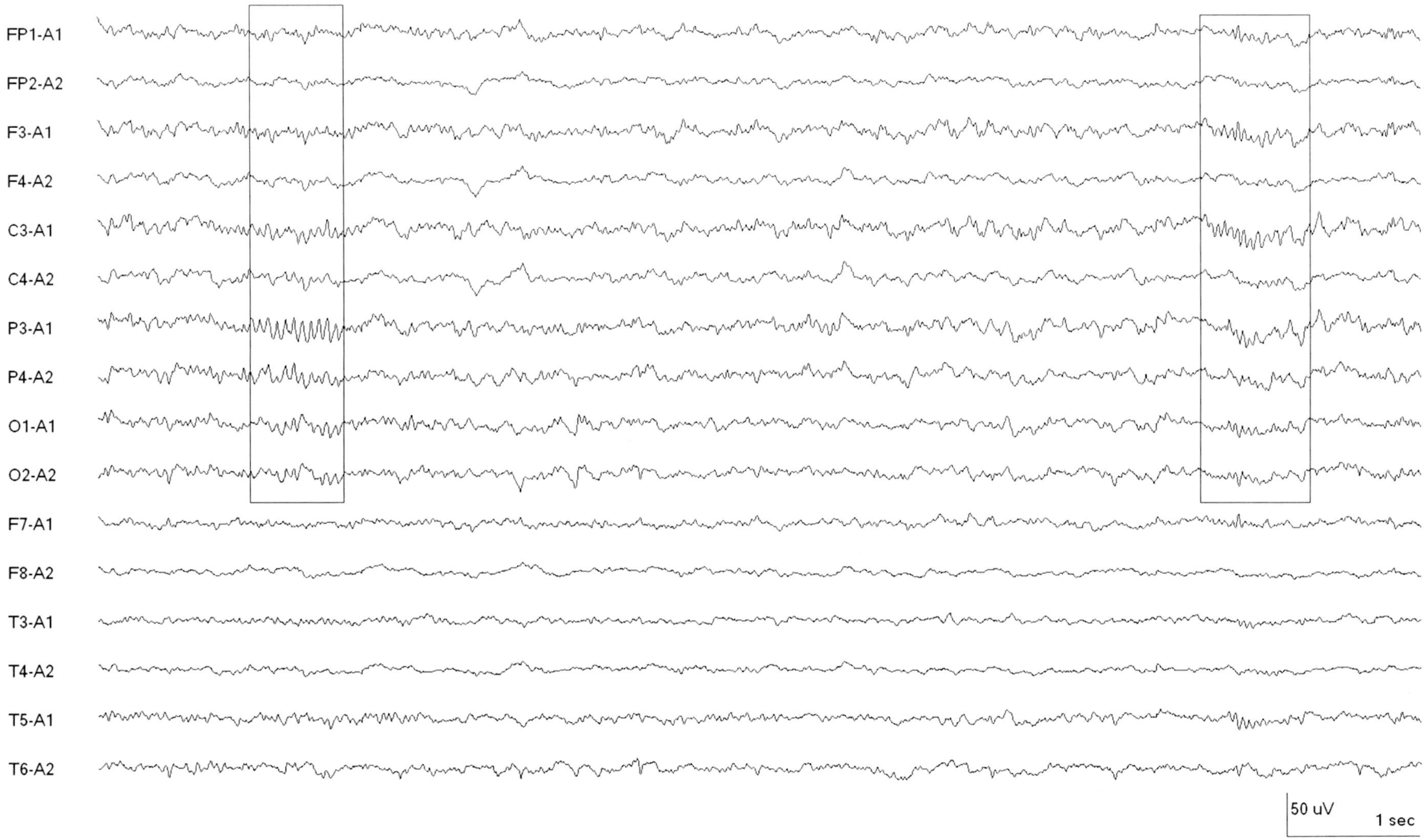

Figure 5.2 Unilateral attenuation, PLEDs and SIRPIDs from stroke. (a) The EEG in this 57-year-old woman s/p right 'strokectomy' shows an asymmetry of beta activity (decreased on the right; compare Fp2-A2 and F4-A2 to Fp1-A1 and F3-A1) and spindles (also decreased on the right; compare C4-A2 and P4-A2 to C3-A1 and P3-A1 in the boxes during sleep. The decreased fast activity suggests cortical dysfunction or an extra-axial collection on the right. The decrease in spindles on the right suggests the same or other involvement of thalamocortical pathways on the right.

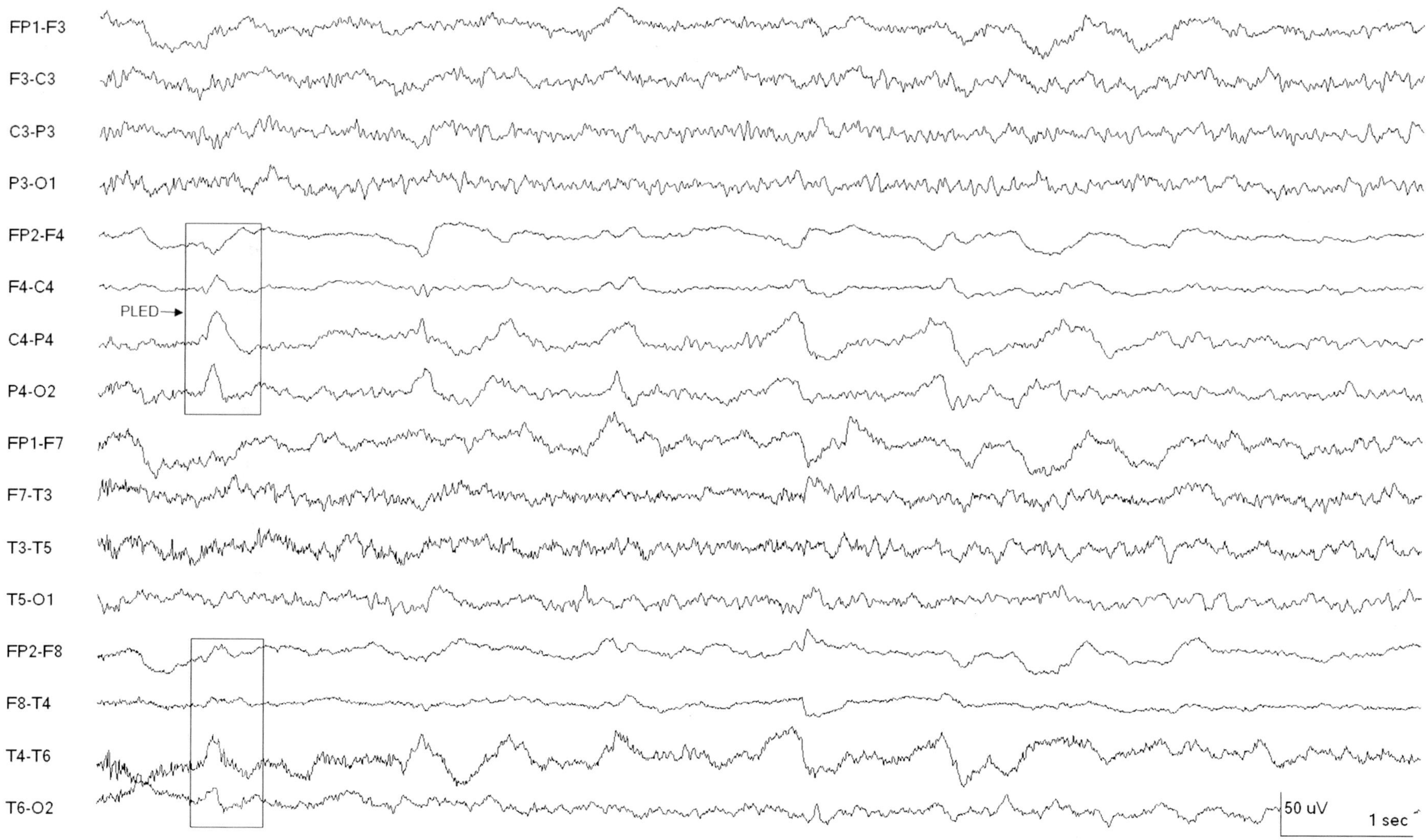

Figure 5.2 (*Continued*) (b) PLEDs are present on the right following stimulation (focal SIRPIDs, see Chapter 4); the first of the periodic discharges is shown in the box. Faster frequencies are better developed on the left, even more obvious after stimulation

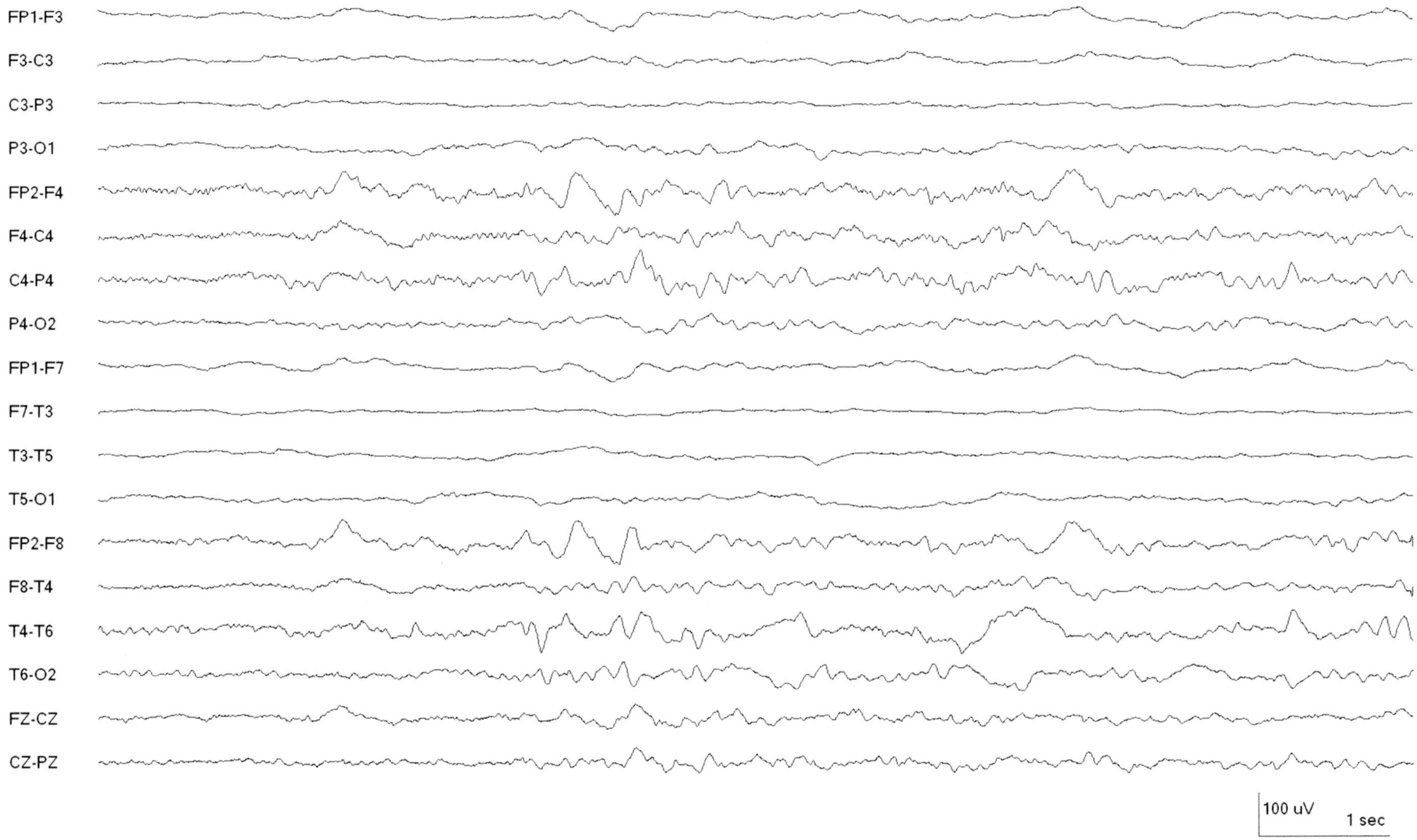

Figure 5.3 Unilateral attenuation from stroke. The EEG in this 31-year-old man with a massive left hemispheric infarct secondary to a carotid dissection shows marked suppression over the left hemisphere.

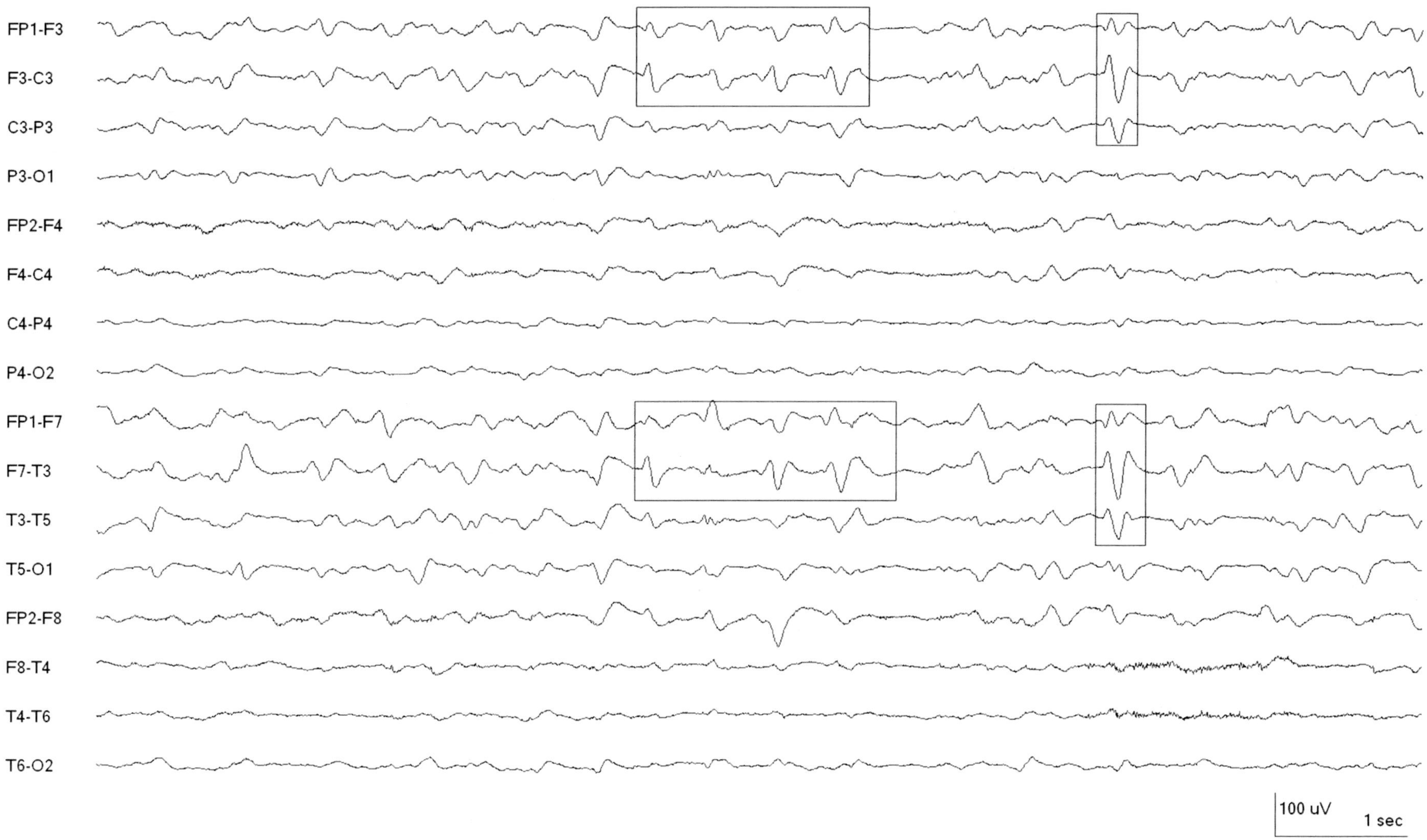

Figure 5.4 Asymmetric triphasic waves vs. PLEDs. (a) Bipolar. Asymmetric (left >> right) triphasic periodic discharges are present in this 75-year-old man with a right hemisphere stroke, left hemiparesis and acute renal failure.

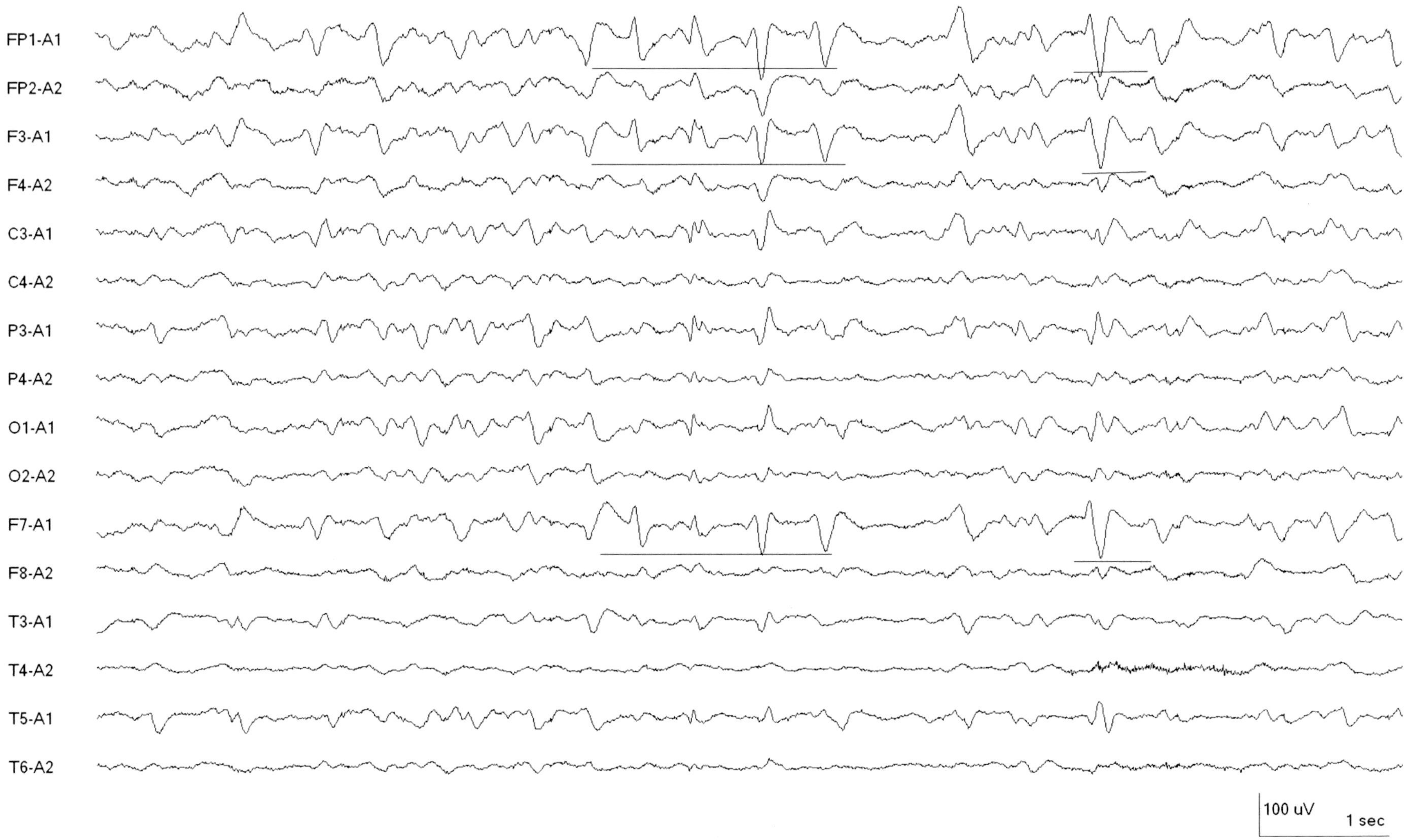

Figure 5.4 (*Continued*) (b) Referential. A reformatted referential montage to ipsilateral ears in the same patient. If this patient's infarct had been on the left with a right hemiparesis (not the case here), these would most likely represent PLEDs and suggest a high risk of seizures. But given that the patient's infarct was on the right, these are most likely triphasic waves related to renal failure that are generalized but attenuated on the right due to the infarct.

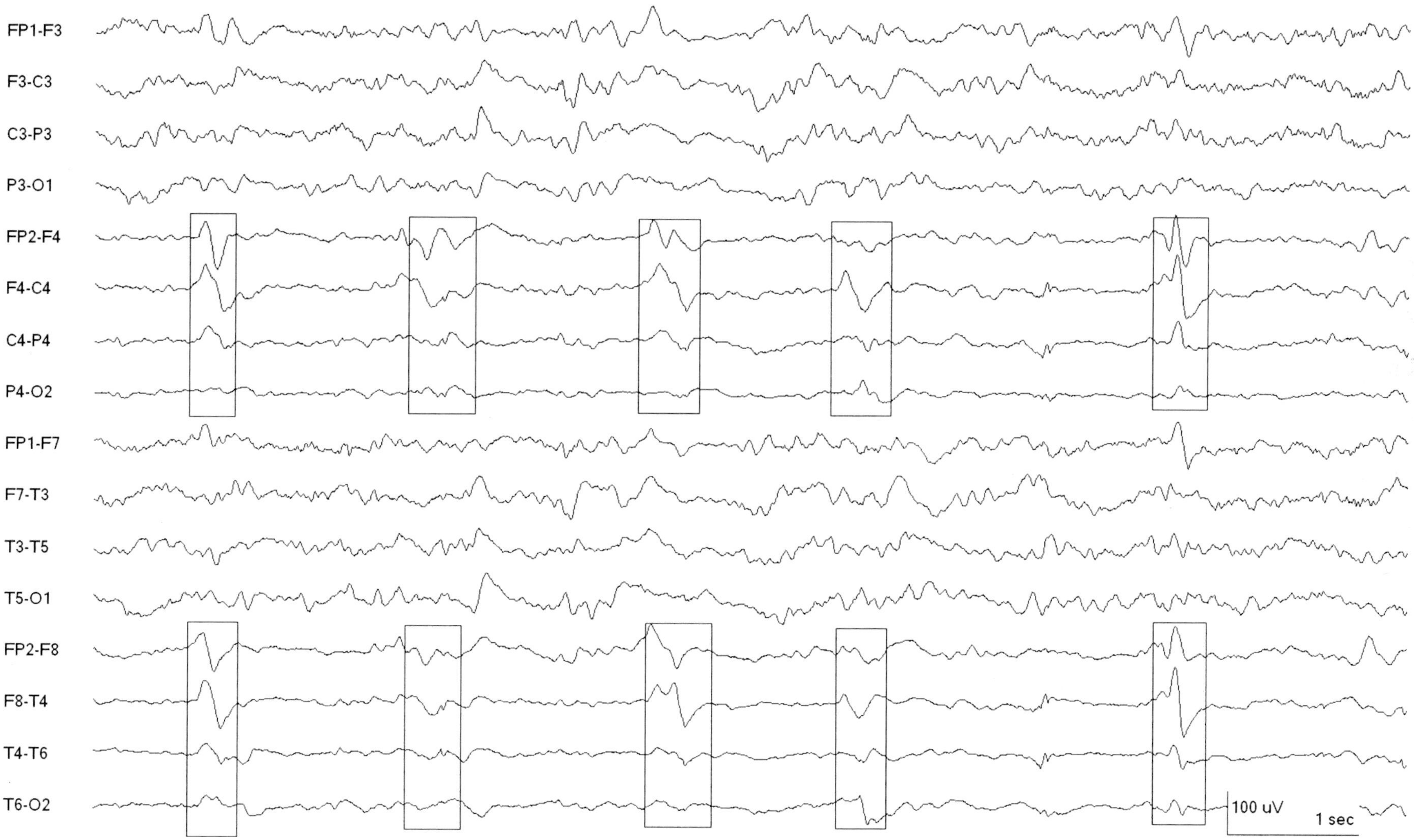

Figure 5.5 Seizure with PLEDs mimicking stroke. This 56-year-old woman with a history of epilepsy since childhood was found unresponsive and not moving her left side. She was felt to have a probable stroke. EEG shows right-sided PLEDs (boxes) and attenuation of background activity on the right between PLEDs. Imaging showed no stroke, but did show left hemisphere calcification. This is an example of a postictal state (or perhaps even ictal if intracranial recordings were available) mimicking an infarct, not an unusual occurrence.

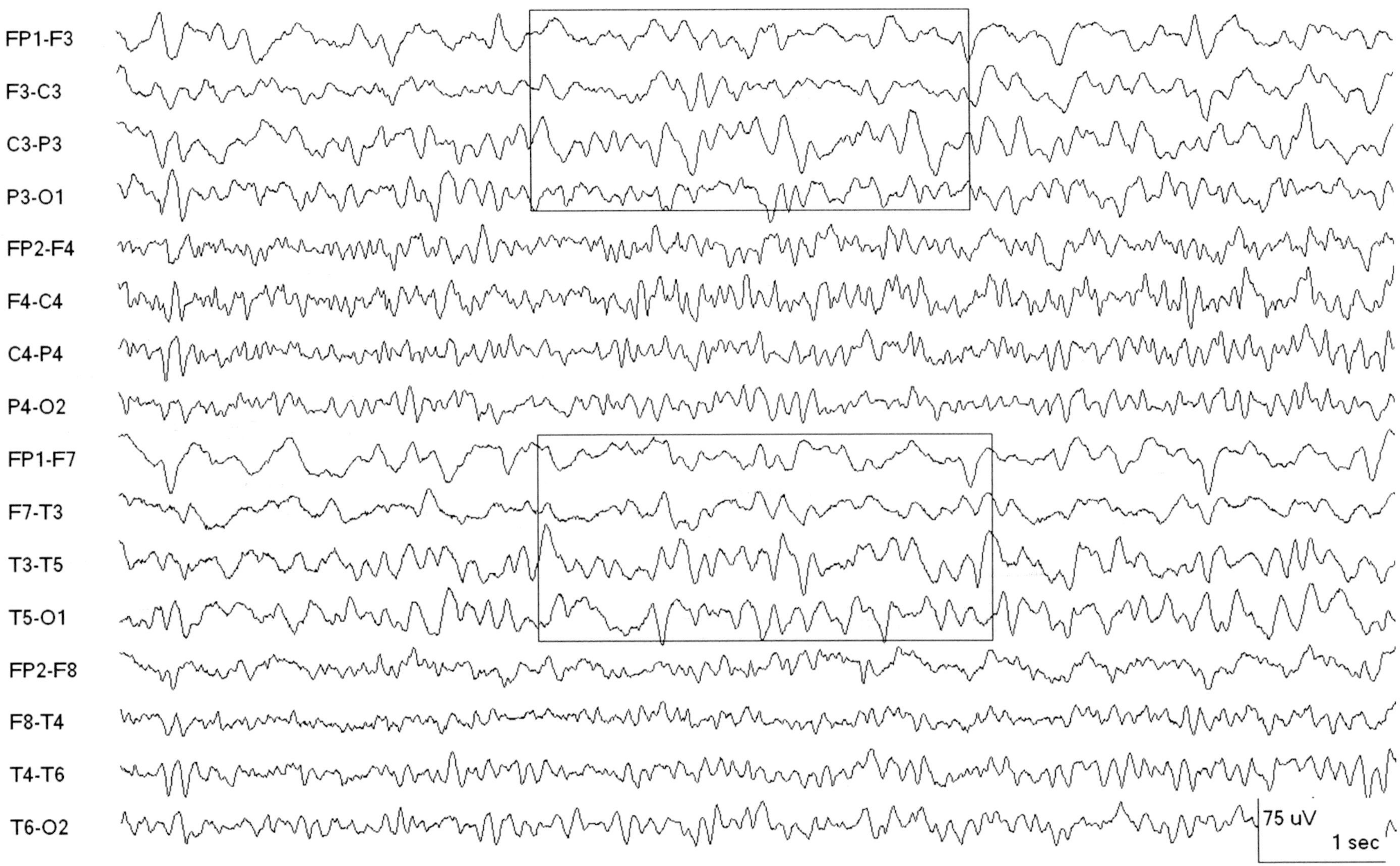

Figure 5.6 Slowing and attenuation from stroke. (a) A longitudinal bipolar montage in this 54-year-old woman with a stroke and acute onset of aphasia and a right hemiparesis shows prominent slowing and attenuation of faster frequencies over the left hemisphere (box). This suggests both cortical (attenuation) and subcortical (slowing) dysfunction.

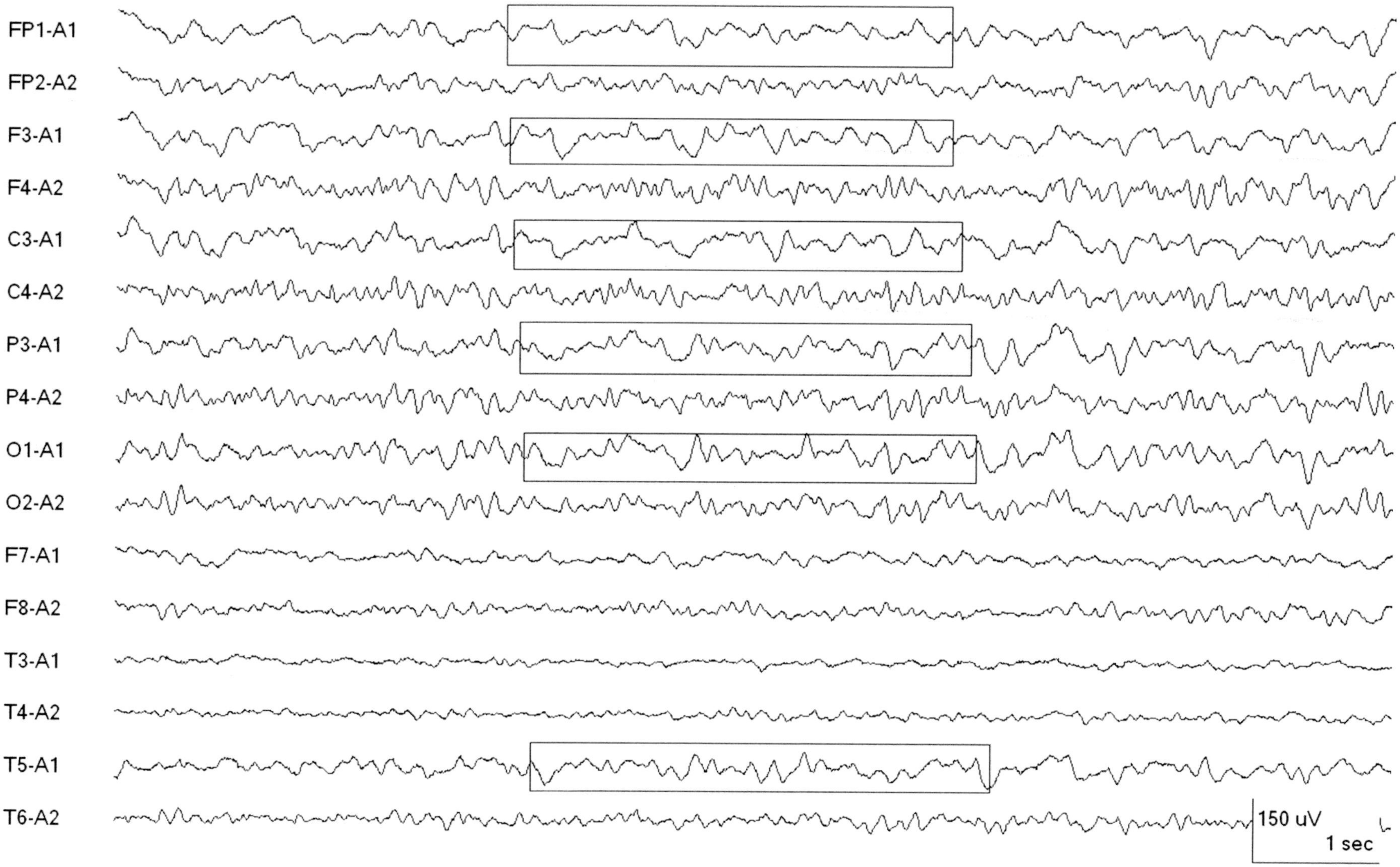

Figure 5.6 (*Continued*) (b) A reformatted epoch utilizing ipsilateral ears as the reference. The left-sided attenuation and slowing are highlighted in the boxes.

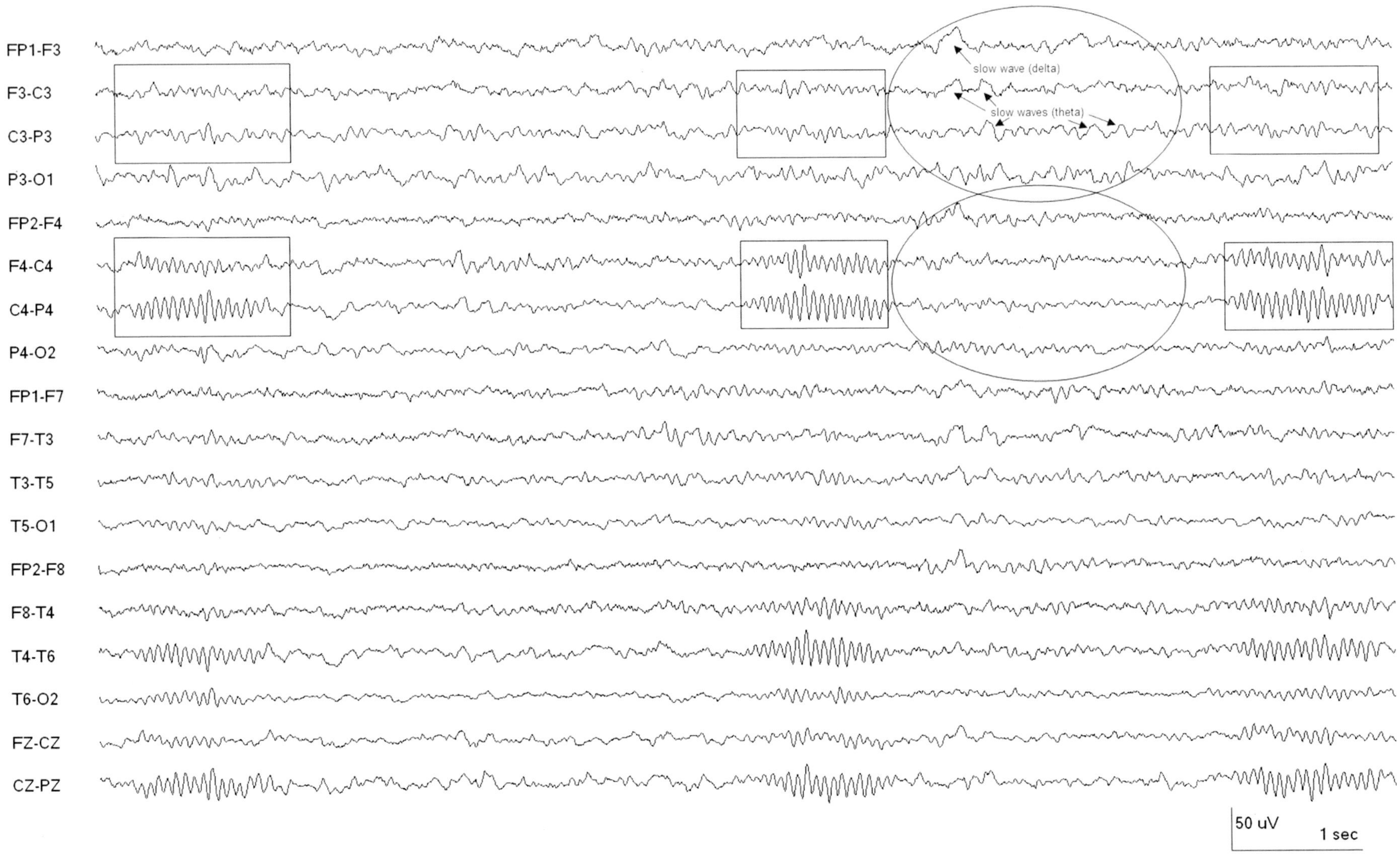

Figure 5.7 Slowing and spindle asymmetry from stroke. An EEG taken during sleep in a 68-year-old woman with an acute left hemispheric stroke shows a prominent asymmetry of sleep spindles being decreased on the left (compare homologous channels during spindles, in boxes), suggesting dysfunction in the thalamocortical pathways involved with spindles. In addition, slower frequencies are present throughout the left hemisphere, maximal in the parasagittal region (compare homologous channels in ellipses), suggesting subcortical white matter dysfunction. Several left-sided slow waves are marked with arrows and labeled.

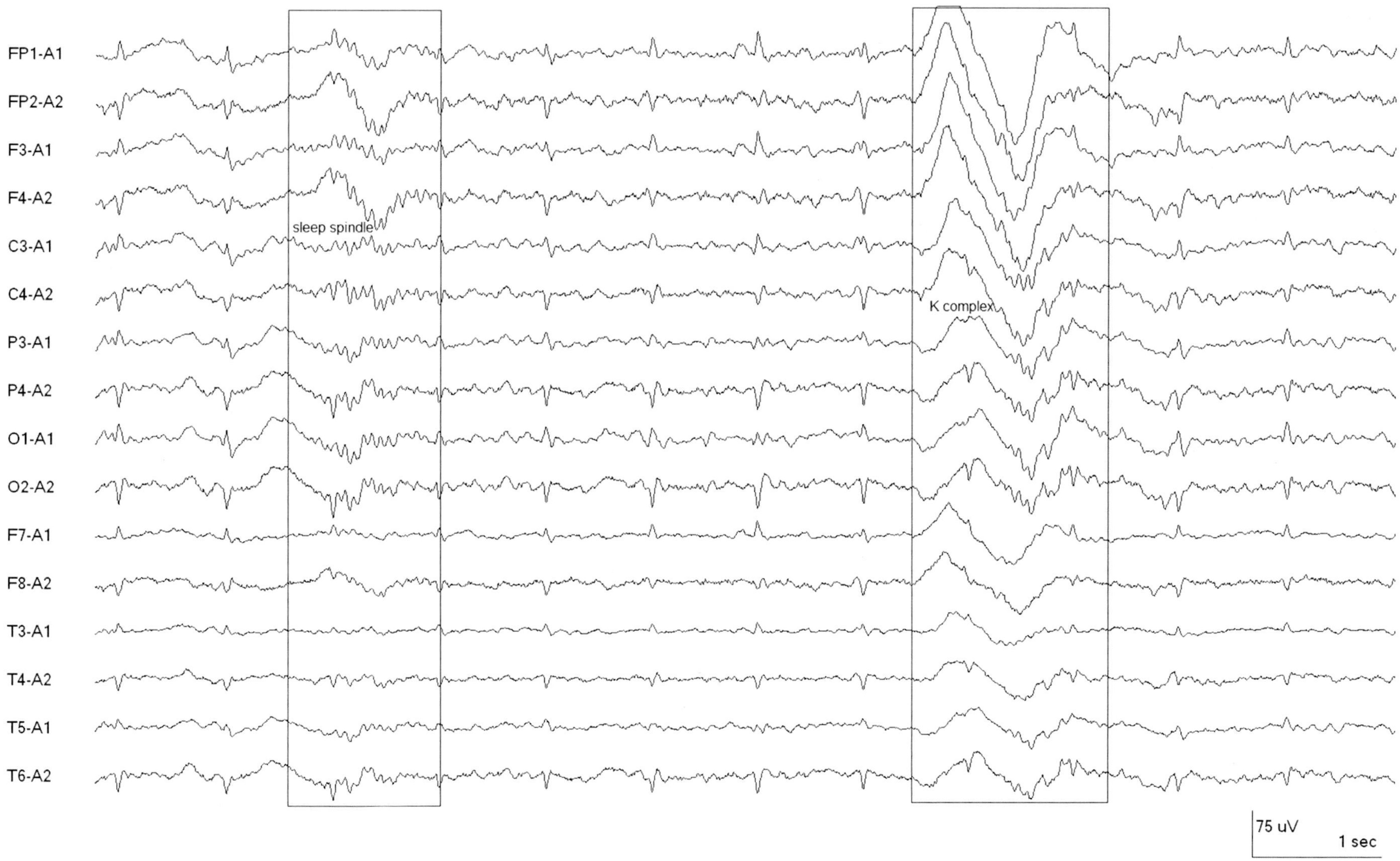

Figure 5.8 Spindle coma from posterior fossa hemorrhage. A spindle-coma pattern is seen in this 35-year-old comatose woman with a left cerebellar hemorrhage. Although this could represent normal sleep, this patient could not be awoken.

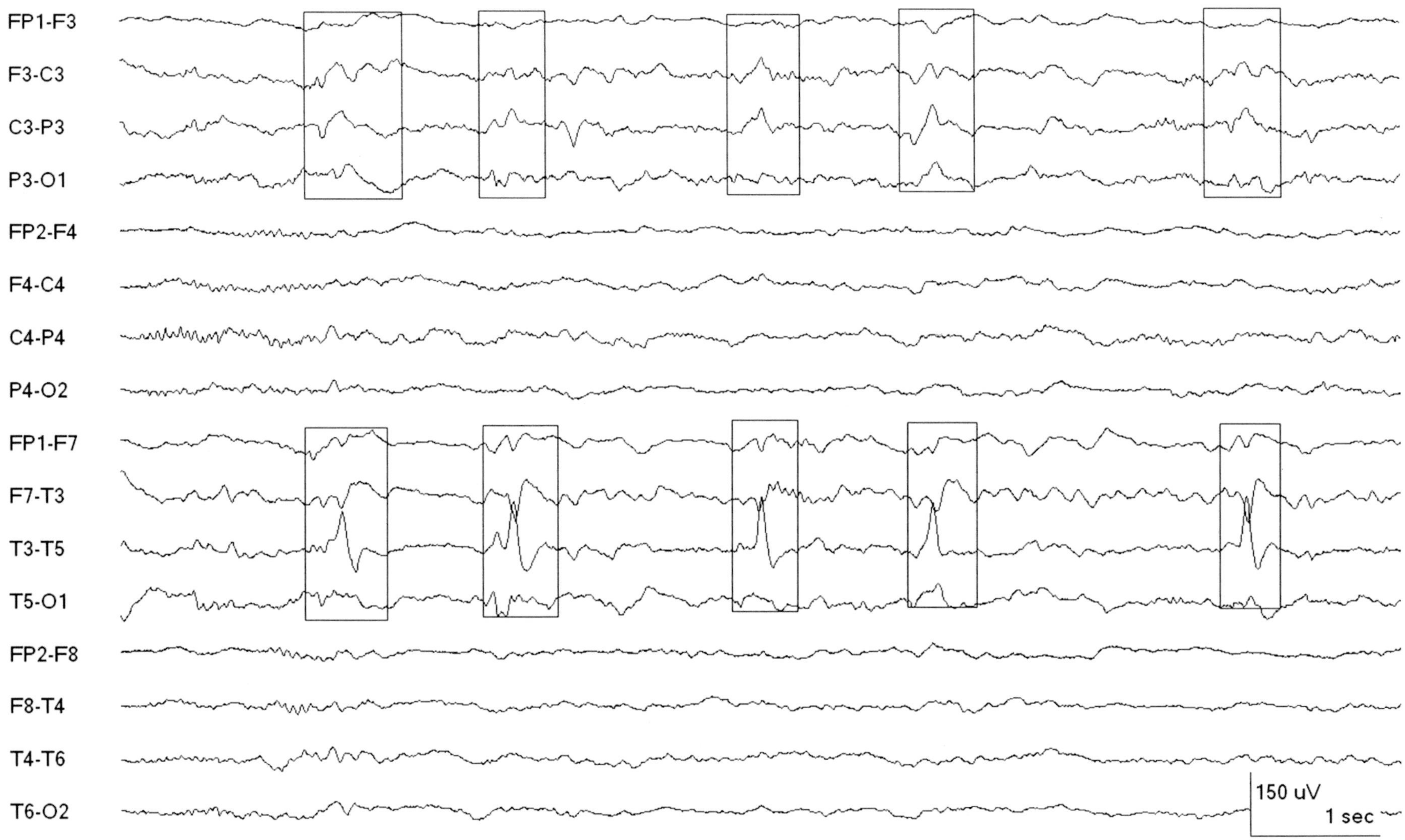

Figure 5.9 PLEDs from intracerebral hemorrhage. Left-sided PLEDs (boxes), maximal in the temporal region, in an 83-year-old woman with a left intracerebral hemorrhage.

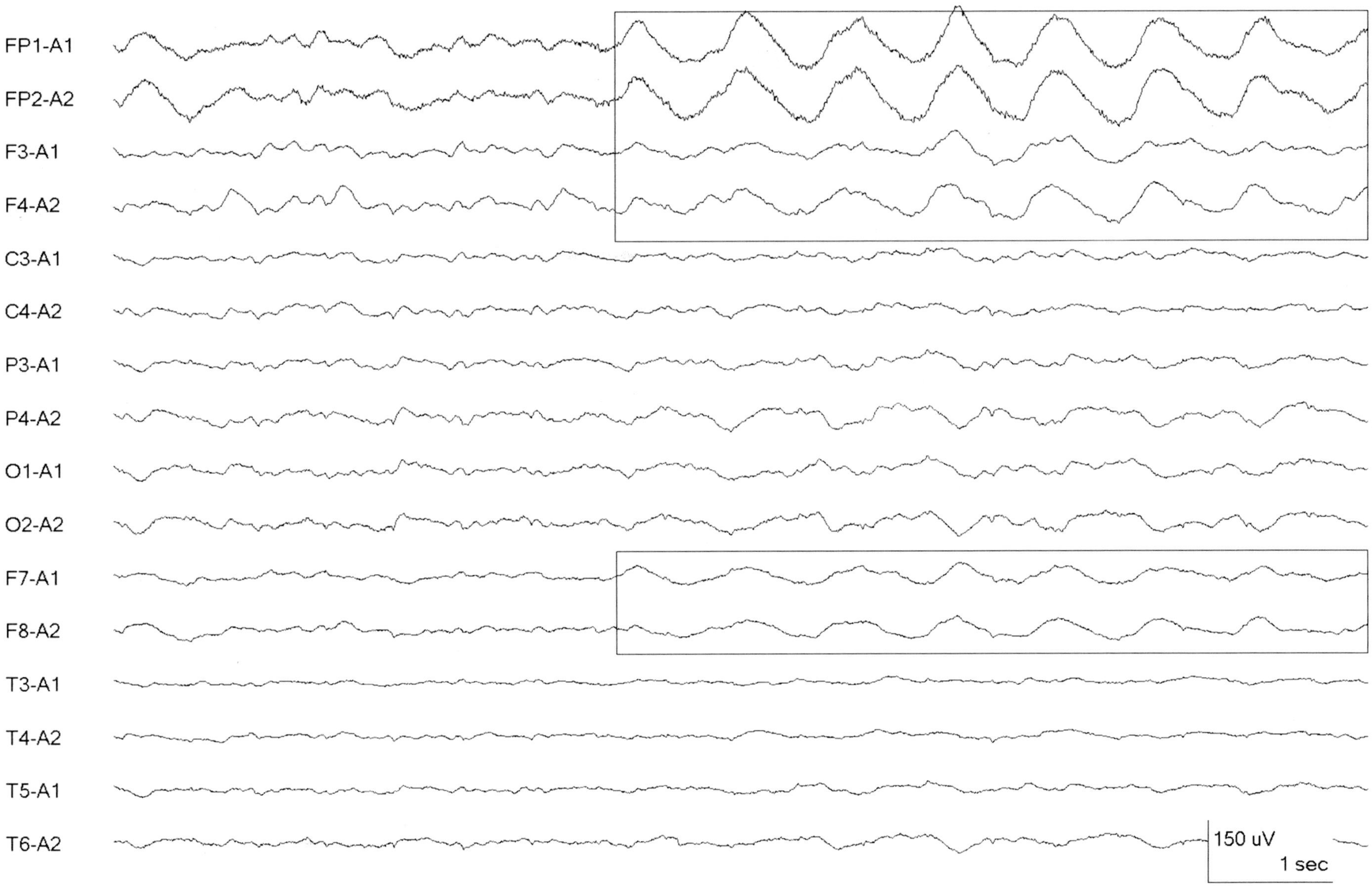

Figure 5.10 Frontal intermittent rhythmic delta activity (FIRDA). FIRDA (boxes) is seen in this 19-year-old woman with an intraventricular hemorrhage. Although FIRDA is most commonly a non-specific indicator of diffuse dysfunction, typically toxic/metabolic, it can also be seen with increased intraventricular pressure or disturbances of deep midline structures.

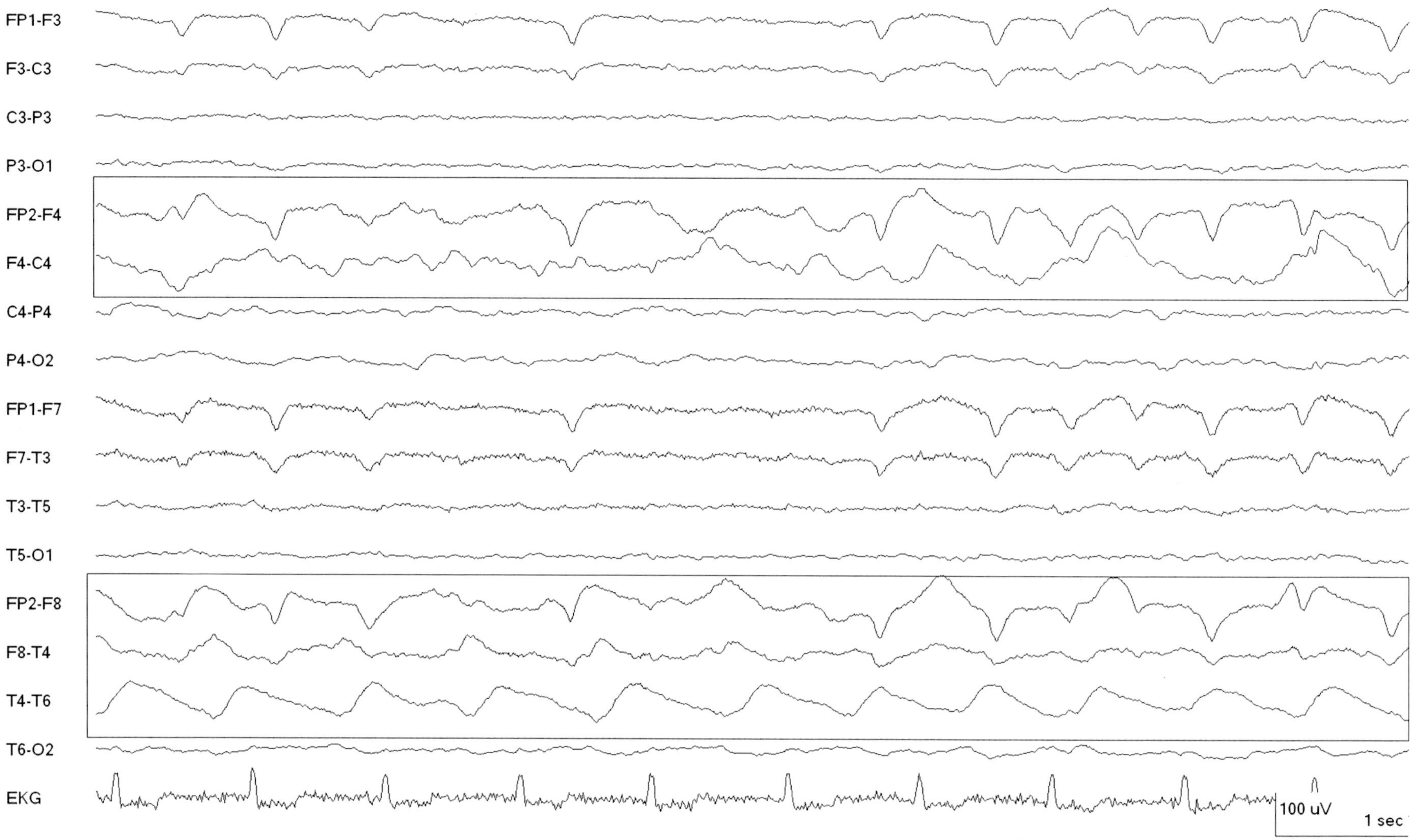

Figure 5.11 Hemicraniectomy. This 56-year-old man with a right-sided intracerebral hemorrhage was alert throughout the recording. The patient had a craniectomy for decompression. Slow delta activity (~1 Hz), somewhat rhythmic, is prominent over the right fronto-temporal region (boxes). This type of high amplitude, rhythmic or semirhythmic 1 Hz activity, sometimes sharply contoured, is common in patients after hemicraniectomy.

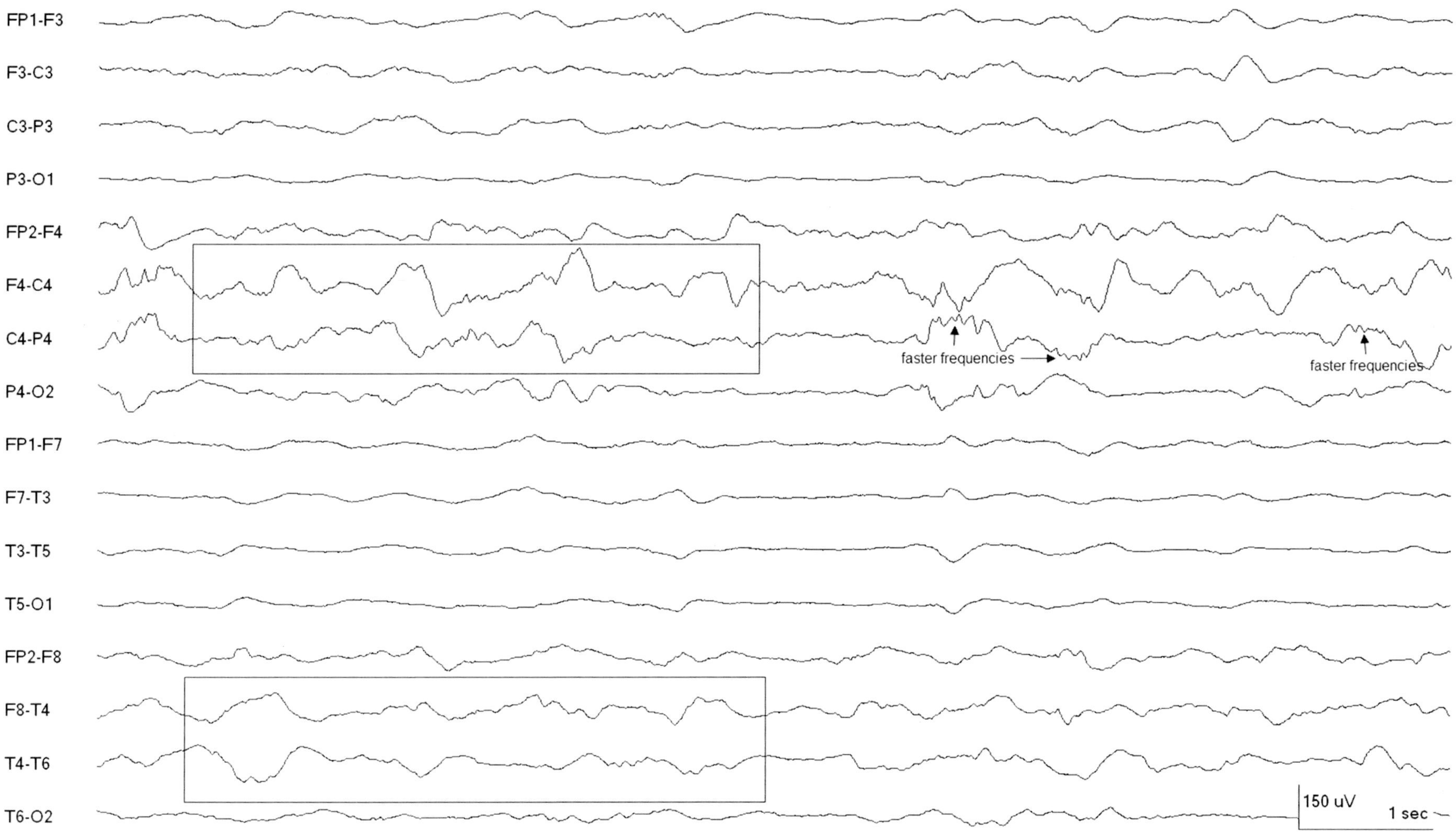

Figure 5.12 Bilateral subdural hematomas and hemicraniectomy. The EEG in this 32-year-old woman s/p right-sided craniectomy shows marked hemispheric differences. High-voltage diffuse slowing is present over the right hemisphere (boxes) and lower voltage slowing on the left. Faster frequencies are also more prominent on the right (labeled), suggesting either a breach effect with sparing of some degree of cortical function on the right, or an abnormality on the other side (cortical or extraaxial). In fact, this patient had both a skull defect on the right *and* a subdural hematoma on the left.

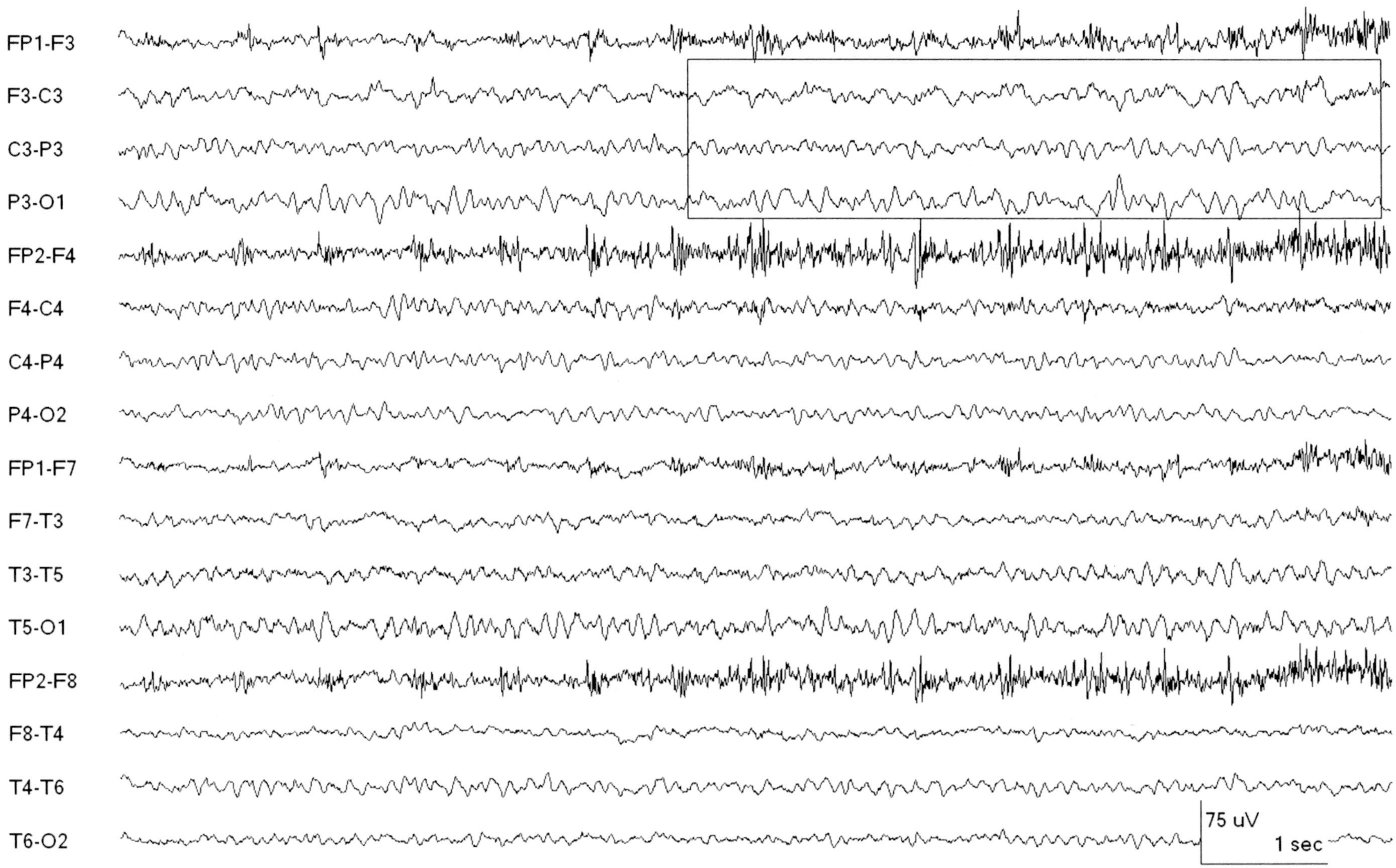

Figure 5.13 Focal seizure from subdural hematoma. (a) This 82-year-old man with a left-sided subdural hematoma developed new onset of twitching of the right thumb. This sample shows subtle rhythmic activity beginning in the left central parietal region near the end of the sample (box).

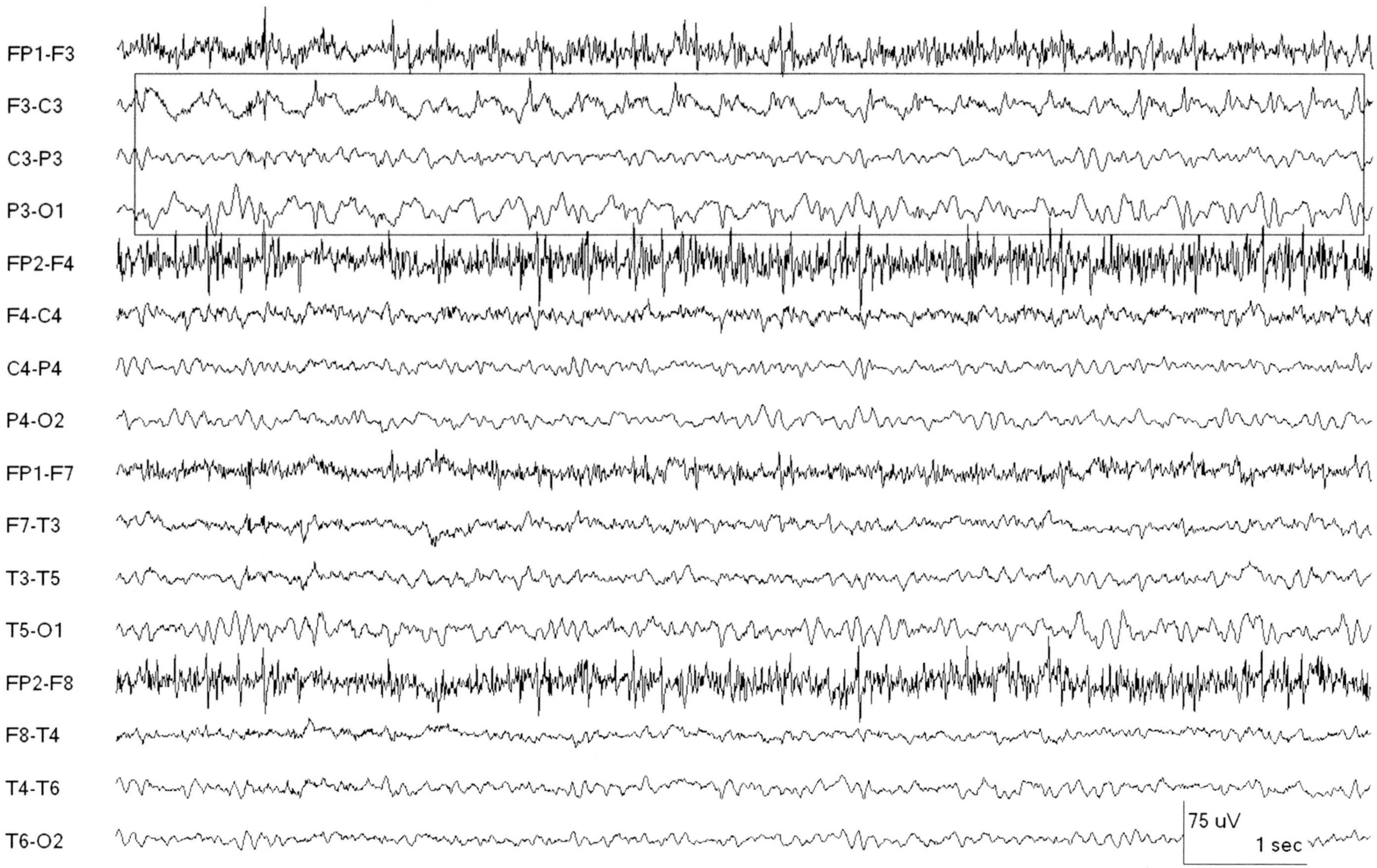

Figure 5.13 (*Continued*) (b) The left parasagittal rhythmic delta activity (box) is now more prominent, evolving and associated with superimposed spikes. Fp1 and Fp2 show prominent muscle artifact.

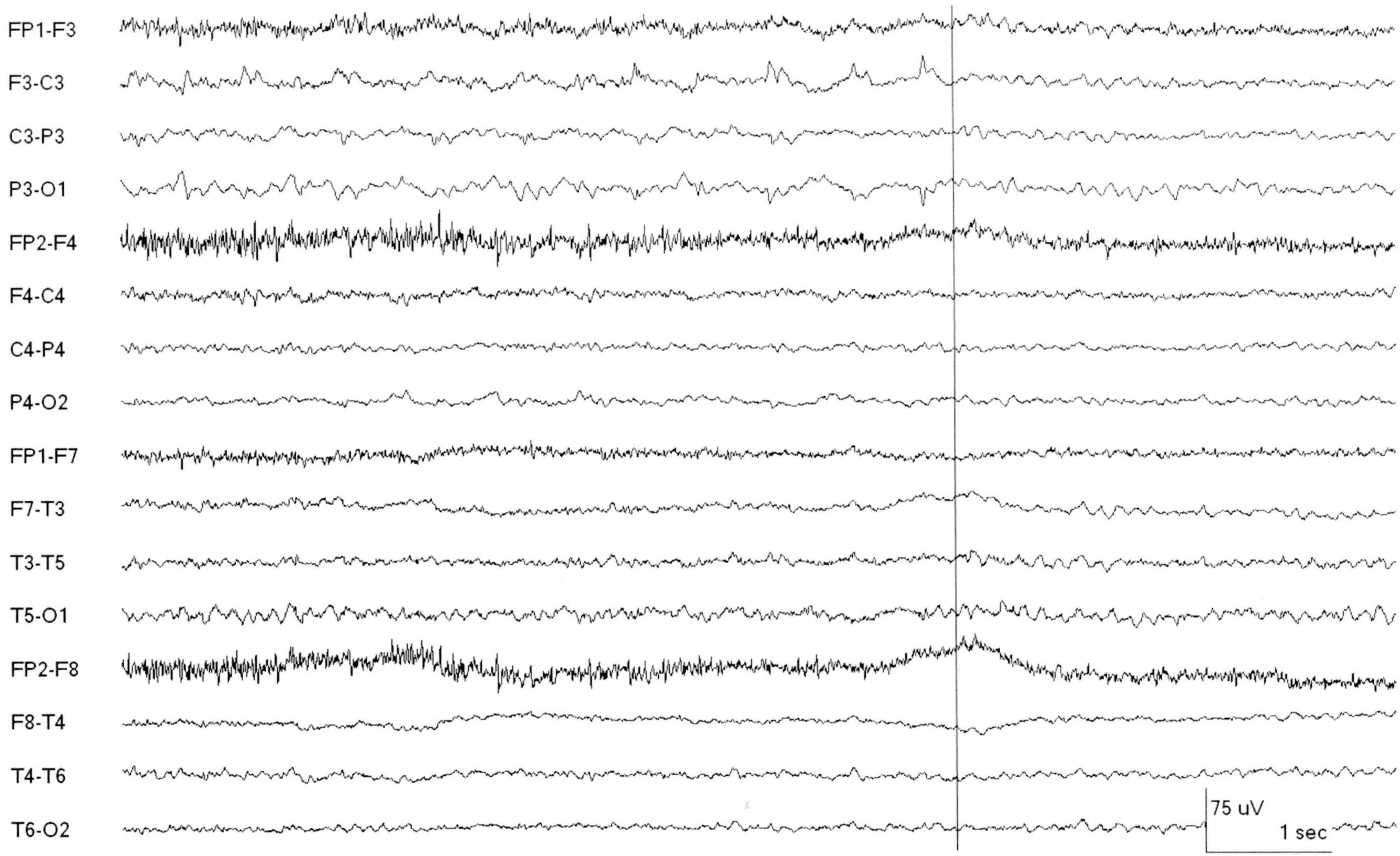

Figure 5.13 (*Continued*) (c) The discharge ends (vertical line). This is a focal seizure.

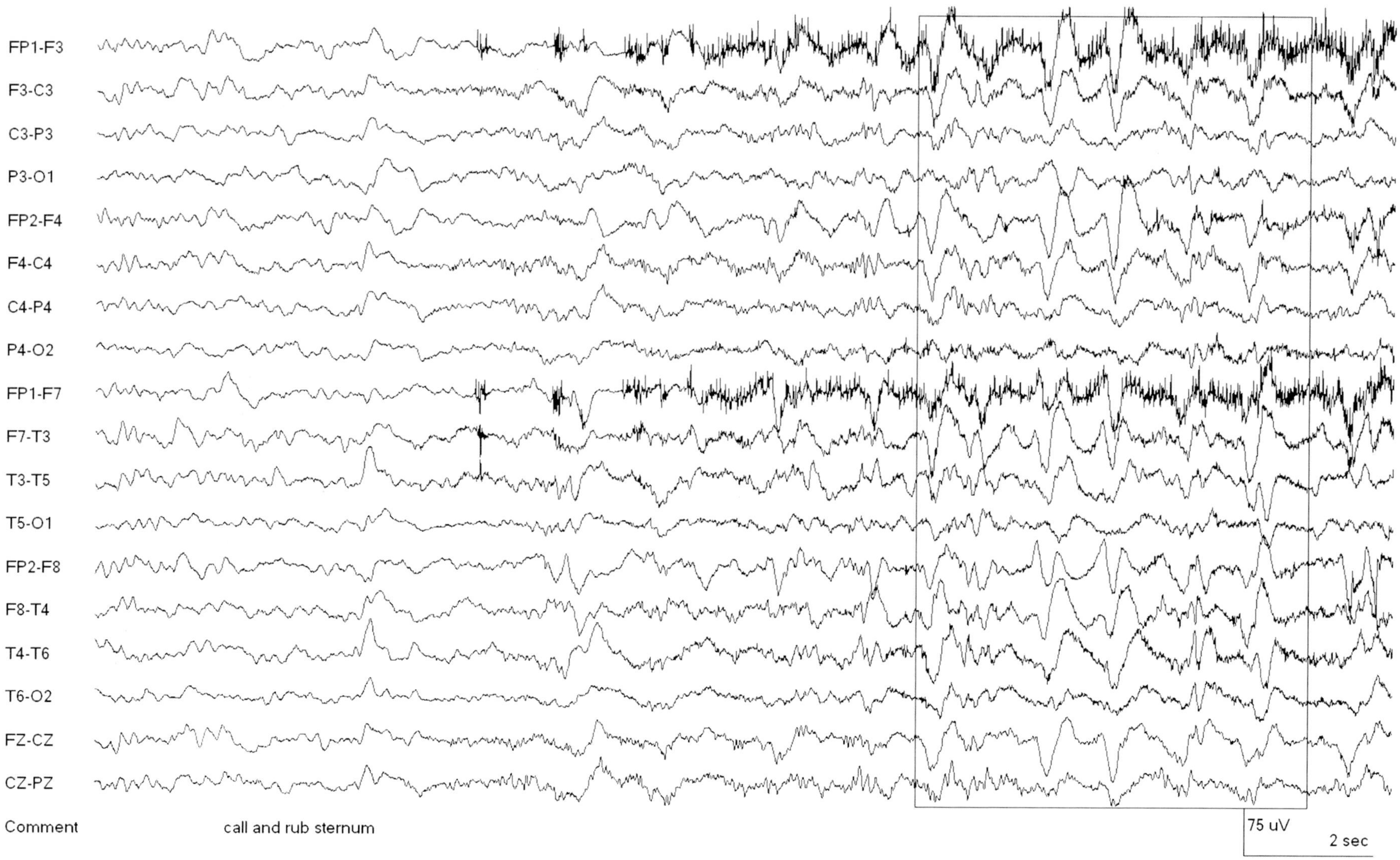

Figure 5.14 Subarachnoid hemorrhage and SIRPIDs. The EEG in this 71-year-old woman with a subarachnoid hemorrhage demonstrates SIRPIDs that consist of generalized periodic discharges (box) induced by sternal rub. Note that this epoch represents 20 s, rather than 10 s. See Chapter 4 for further examples of SIRPIDs.

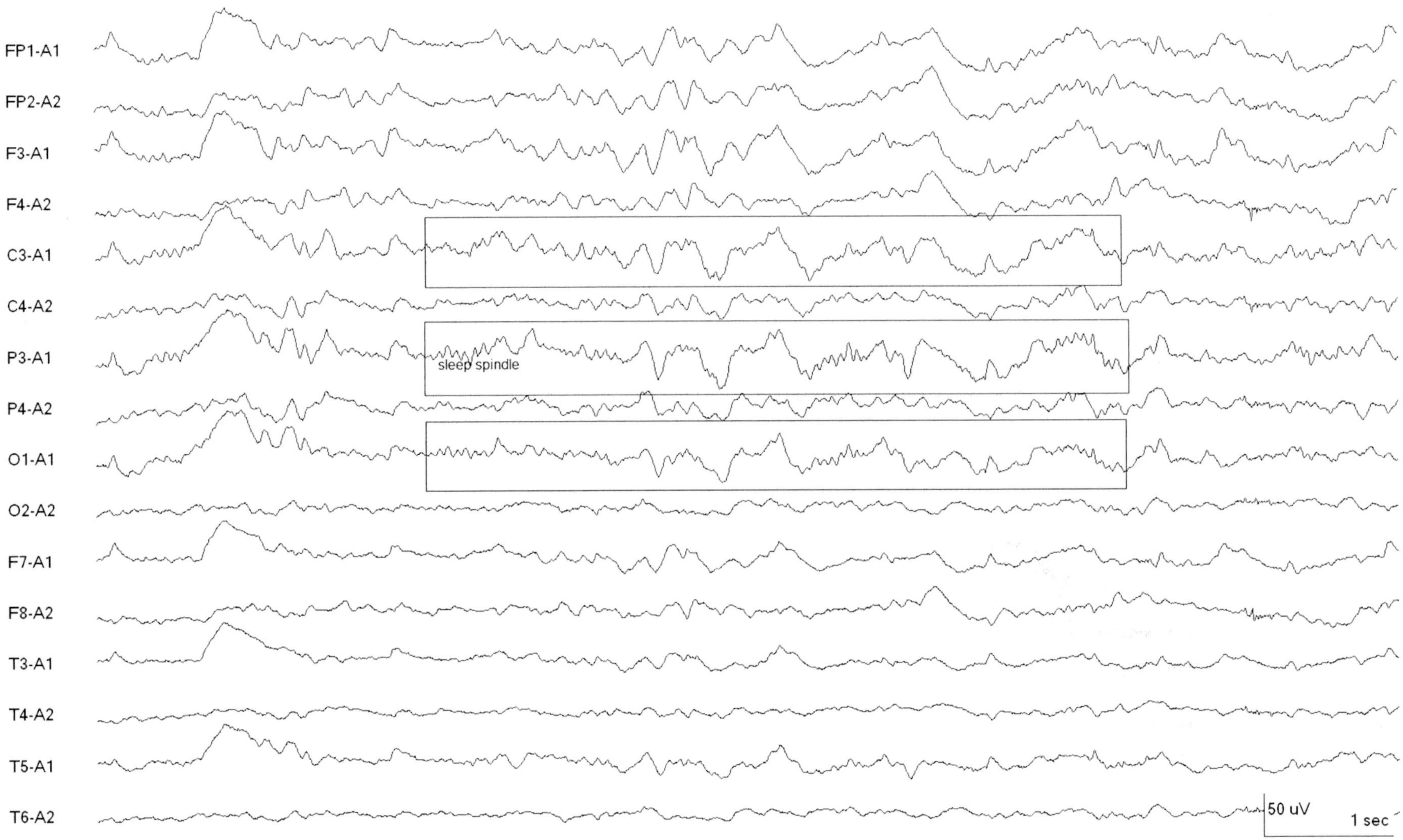

Figure 5.15 Asymmetry after subdural hematoma evacuation. The EEG in this 85-year-old man shows hemispheric differences with both faster activity (including sleep spindles, labeled) and slow activity being of higher voltage over the left hemisphere (boxes). The patient had suffered a fall and is 2 days s/p evacuation of a chronic right-sided subdural hematoma. Normal sleep activity is seen, higher voltage over the healthier left hemisphere (despite the skull defect on the right).

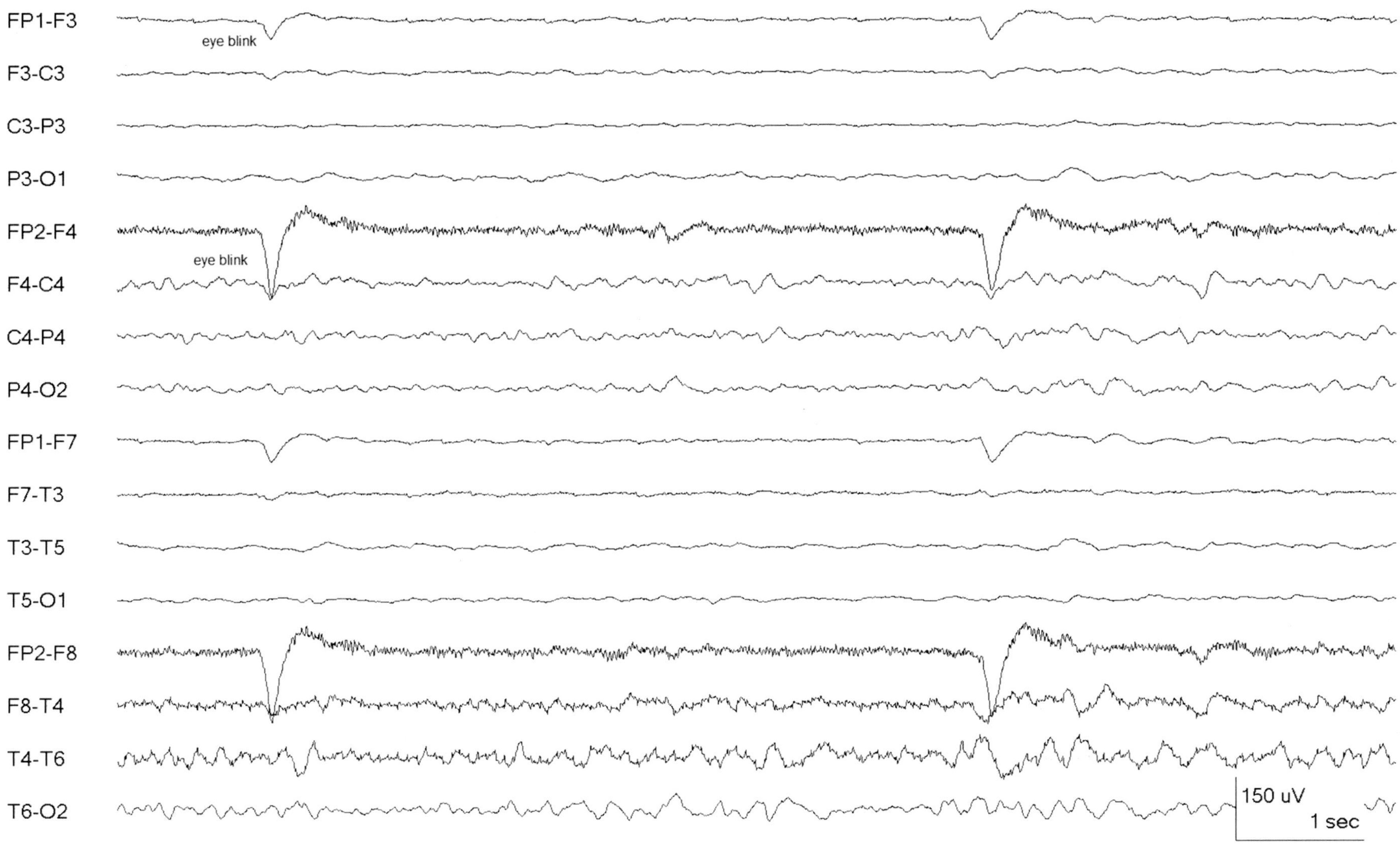

Figure 5.16 Traumatic brain injury. The EEG in this 25-year-old comatose woman involved in a motor vehicle accident shows marked hemispheric differences with activity suppressed over the left side. Faster frequencies are better developed over the right hemisphere and eye blinks are asymmetric, being decreased on the left. This patient had a left-sided subdural hematoma as well as a left hemispheric infarct. The asymmetric blinks suggest possible decreased (but not absent) upgaze on the left.

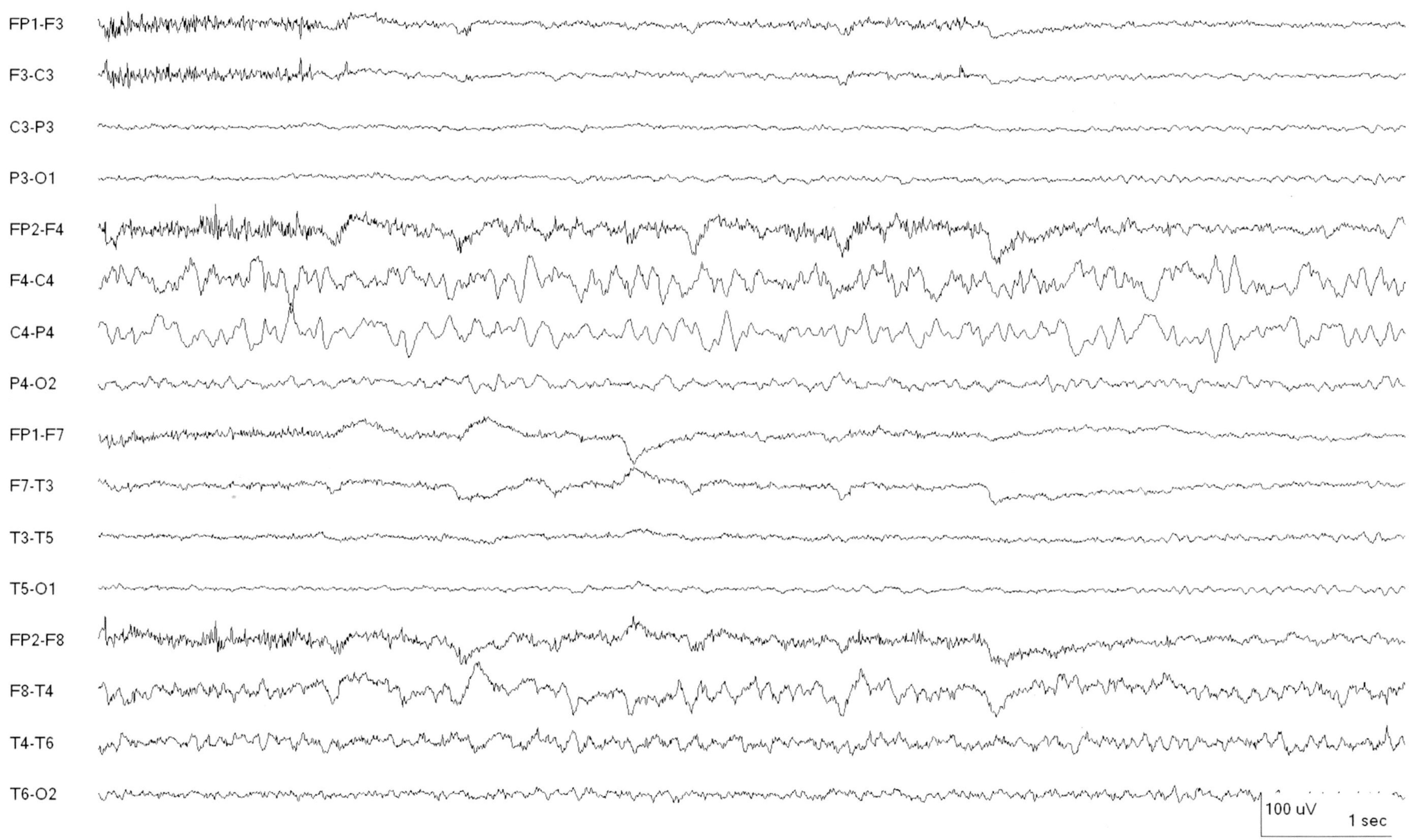

Figure 5.17 Breach effect after subdural hematoma evacuation. The EEG in this 52-year-old man s/p evacuation of a right subdural hematoma shows marked hemispheric differences. Background activity including faster frequencies are of higher voltage over the right side. The patient had a right craniectomy. This is a prominent example of the effects of a skull defect. The higher voltage slowing on the right suggests underlying dysfunction in addition to the craniectomy.

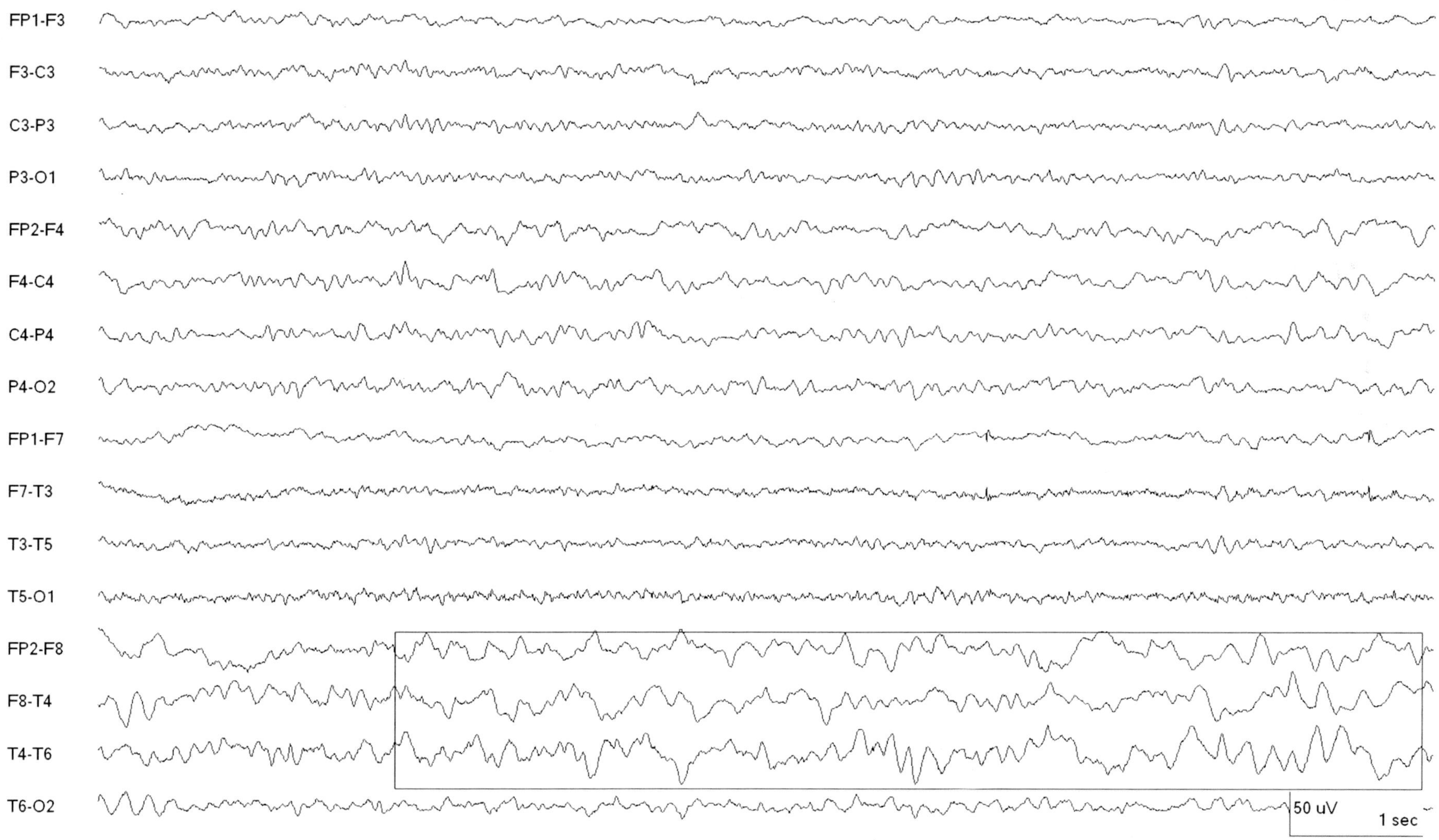

Figure 5.18 Focal slowing after subarachnoid hemorrhage. (a) The EEG in this 40-year-old woman with a history of a subarachnoid hemorrhage s/p right MCA aneurysm coiling, shows prominent right-sided focal slowing maximal in the temporal region (box).

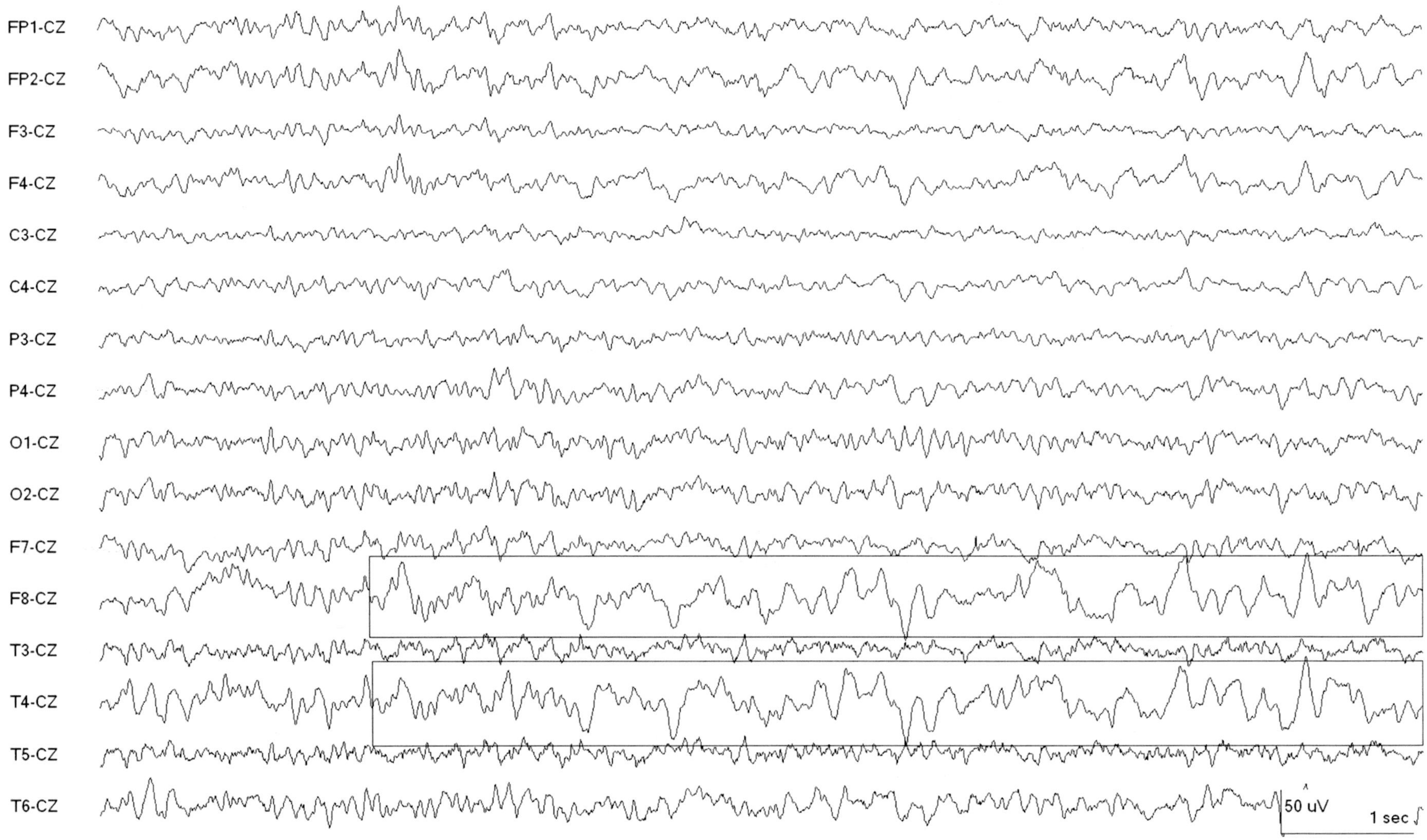

Figure 5.18 (*Continued*) (b) The midline vertex electrode Cz is often a very good reference to demonstrate temporal slowing. The slowing is maximal in the F8 and T4 electrodes (boxes) with lesser involvement of the Fp2 and F4 electrodes.

6 Artifacts that can mimic seizures or other physiologic patterns

A major problem in obtaining high-quality recordings is the proper identification and elimination, when possible, of artifacts. EEGs performed in the intensive care unit (ICU) are often contaminated by artifacts arising from monitoring equipment, life-support systems and personnel. From the viewpoint of an electroencephalographer or technologist, an artifact may be defined as any recorded signal not originating in the brain. Artifacts are not always undesirable and physiological artifacts frequently provide clinically useful information, such as eye movements, including nystagmus, muscle artifact, tremors, body movements, respiration artifact and electrocardiogram (EKG).

Artifacts do need to be properly identified. Sherlockian deduction and reasoning are helpful in interpreting EEGs; however, there are many artifacts that may appear identical to cerebral discharges. The ideal time to answer the question as to whether the activity being recorded is cerebral or artifact is during the recording, although this is often not possible with prolonged monitoring. The use of additional electrodes, the monitoring of the EKG, movements (e.g. body, tongue and eye), respiration and the temporary disconnection of other equipment may be needed to identify the noncerebral origin of such activity. Failure to properly identify artifacts may have serious consequences. For example, misinterpretation of artifact as spikes or seizures may lead to misdiagnosis and inappropriate treatment.

Artifacts may be divided into two groups: physiological and nonphysiological. At times, there is an overlap between these two categories. Physiological artifacts originate in the body but outside the brain. They include:

(1) ocular – eye movement, eyelid flutter, nystagmus, electroretinogram (ERG)

(2) muscle

(3) sweat

(4) tongue and mouth – glossokinetic potential (GKP), sobbing, chewing, dissimilar metals, palatal myoclonus

(5) vascular – EKG, pulse, cardioballistic artifact, pacemaker

(6) movement – tremor, respiration, facial, extremities

(7) skull defect.

The eyeballs and eyelids are factors in the production of eye movement artifact. The former acts as a dipole with the cornea being positive with respect to the retina. With eye closure, the eyeball rotates upward and the Fp1 and Fp2 electrodes become surface positive. The reverse is true

Atlas of EEG in Critical Care Lawrence J. Hirsch and Richard P. Brenner

with downward eye movement as seen with eye opening. Vertical eye movements are always maximal in the Fp1 and Fp2 electrodes and, therefore, the voltage gradient of this potential often indicates its source. If the activity is not greatest in Fp1 and Fp2, it cannot be a vertical eye movement. The converse, however, is not always true; some cerebral potentials may be maximal in the Fp1 and Fp2 electrodes. In order to resolve this difficulty, the simplest solution is to place additional electrodes below the eyes. Vertical eye movements will be out of phase when comparing superior (Fp1 and Fp2) and inferior orbital (left and right, LIO and RIO) electrodes referred to ipsilateral ear, while frontal slowing of cerebral origin will be in phase. There are some artifacts, such as a GKP, which can be mistaken for frontal slowing. This potential will be in phase between the superior and inferior orbital electrodes, and of higher voltage in inferior orbital electrodes, which are closer to the tongue. Further monitoring of this potential is discussed later in this chapter. Lateral eye movements are maximal in the F7 and F8 electrodes and are of opposite polarity. Additional electrodes placed at the outer canthus of the eyes and referred to the ipsilateral ear may help further delineate this activity since these electrodes (left and right, LOC and ROC) are closer to the source.

An ERG – electrical signals generated in the retina – can be seen in normal individuals if the Fp1 and Fp2 electrodes are used during photic stimulation. However, this artifact is most often seen in patients with cerebral death. In part this is due to the increased sensitivities employed in such recordings as well as the absence of cerebral potentials. It does not invalidate the diagnosis of electrocerebral inactivity or cerebral death if other criteria are met. Eyelid flutter is also maximal in the Fp1 and Fp2 electrodes and often not well detected with infraorbital electrodes. At times, rapid eyelid flutter or nystagmus can give rise to confusion if not properly identified. In patients with a prosthetic eye or third nerve palsy, unilateral eye movement artifact may be mistaken for focal frontal delta activity.

Muscle artifact is common in routine EEG recordings. Getting the patient more relaxed, if possible, is the best way to reduce this artifact. Occasionally the artifact can be unilateral, persist in sleep and, if severe, can obscure underlying cerebral potentials. Shivering artifact during therapeutic hypothermia is becoming a common source of continuous prominent muscle artifact even when shivering is not obvious on clinical observation. The use of high-frequency filter (HFF) to reduce this activity can lead to difficulties in interpretation. For example, prominent muscle artifact may appear as beta activity when a HFF of 15 Hz is employed or muscle spikes may be misinterpreted as epileptiform at this filter setting. The same is true of isolated muscle spikes seen with eye movements, particularly in the anterior temporal electrodes (F7 and F8). Occasionally paralytics are recommended to allow interpretation of the underlying EEG.

Artifacts from tongue and mouth movements may be misinterpreted. The tongue acts as a dipole with the tip being surface negative and the base positive. Tongue movements in some patients result in a prominent burst of slow waves, which may have a widespread distribution but are usually maximal anteriorly. If the technologist is aware of this, the artifact can easily be reproduced by having the awake patient say 'Tom Thumb' or 'lilt'. If that is not effective, performing vertical and/or lateral tongue movements may reproduce the pattern. This type of artifact can resemble a 'projected' rhythm or frontal intermittent rhythmic delta activity (FIRDA). Unfortunately, a GKP artifact can occur in patients who are confused and lethargic, and who may also have anterior frontal slowing that is cerebral. To help resolve this, additional electrodes can be placed above and below the mouth, and slightly off-center in opposite directions on either side. A bipolar derivation from these perioral electrodes (above the mouth on one side and below the mouth on the other) displays this artifact clearly.

Perspiration or sweat artifact is a long-duration potential that usually involves several electrodes. Although the use of a short time constant (i.e. a higher low-frequency filter setting) eliminates this artifact, it also affects slow-frequency cerebral activity. This is therefore not recommended, but rather one should try to decrease the sweating by cooling the head, applying alcohol or an antiperspirant to the area and having adequate air conditioning.

An EKG artifact is usually recognized by its regular and stereotyped appearance. It is best seen on montages employing the ipsilateral ear as a reference and is less noticeable in bipolar montages or in referential recordings using Cz as a reference. Occasionally, irregular beats may be mistaken for cerebral potentials or the coincidental coupling of an EKG artifact and a slow wave may give rise to the appearance of a 'spike and wave complex'. Cardiac activity is best monitored by placing two additional electrodes on the chest and recording between them (to record cardiac potentials only, not a combination of cerebral and cardiac). Ear electrodes should not be used because they may record temporal spikes as well as the EKG. Occasionally EKG complexes may be mistaken for lambda waves.

A pulse artifact can be mistaken for focal delta activity. This artifact is due to the movement of the electrode due to pulsation, is timelocked to the QRS complex and usually occurs approximately 200 ms after the R wave. A similar but more widespread artifact is seen in cerebral death recordings, which is due to movement of electrodes, electrode wires or the head from the recoil effect of the beating heart (cardioballistic artifact). A pacemaker artifact is cardiac related and results in 'spikes' that will be intermittent or regular, depending on the type of pacemaker.

There are a wide variety of movement artifacts affecting the EEG. These include head tremors, such as seen in patients with Parkinson's disease, and body movements. The tremor can often be monitored with additional electrodes. Muscle and movement artifacts are often prominent in patients having psychogenic nonepileptic seizures. Rhythmic activity in occipital regions due to head movement can be eliminated by raising the patient's head from the bed. Facial movement, such as during a focal motor seizure, hemifacial spasm, facial myokymia or facial synkinesias, can result in muscle artifact.

A skull defect, such as a craniectomy, results in an increase in the voltage and sharpness of underlying cerebral activity known as a breach rhythm. Faster frequencies are accentuated more than slower activity.

Nonphysiological artifacts include:

(1) electrodes – disc, wire, connection, jackbox, placement

(2) external sources – 60 Hz, electrostatic, ICU equipment

(3) instrumentation – amplifier, settings, cables

(4) patient care – chest percussion, cleaning patient, suctioning

An electrode pop is a common occurrence in any recording and appears in all channels of the montage in which that electrode is present, but not in others. An electrode artifact can occur intermittently or occasionally be regular. Findings limited to a single electrode should be viewed with suspicion. The use of an additional electrode placed next to the one in question can indicate whether the discharge is cerebral or artifact, if simple measures such as filling or replacing the electrode, etc. have not eliminated it. Electrodes with high impedance, usually due to poor electrical contact with the scalp, are more prone to show artifact and unequal resistances frequently result in 60 Hz artifact. The electrode problem may be with the disc itself, but can also involve the wire, its connections or the jackbox. Occasionally, one can get a ground electrode recording artifact without 60 Hz interference. The type of artifact seen depends on the location of the ground electrode. In addition to low and equal impedances, accurate placement of electrodes is crucial to good recording technique and a spurious asymmetry may result from inaccurate placement.

Of the external sources of artifacts, 60 Hz is the most common. Although often encountered routinely in the laboratory, it can become a difficult problem in the ICU. Here, judicious disconnection of various equipment is often required to eliminate the artifact. A 60 Hz artifact is not necessarily bad since it often indicates electrode problems. Furthermore, the indiscriminate use of a 60 Hz 'notch' filter makes recognition of electrode artifact more difficult. Artifacts may result from electrostatic interference. This often occurs with movement of persons in the vicinity of the patient and is most common in the ICU. Another artifact, which is rare, is due to an intravenous drip and is also probably electrostatic in origin. There are a variety of instrumentation artifacts, including those due to an amplifier, settings (filters, sensitivity) and cables.

During prolonged EEG monitoring when a technologist is not present throughout the recording, there are many other artifacts. The most troublesome are those that cause rhythmic artifact that can mimic seizures, such as patting and chest percussion by respiratory therapists. Recording video is very helpful for the quick and accurate identification of these artifacts (see also Chapter 7).

Thus, there are multiple causes of artifact, both of a physiological and nonphysiological nature, and these need to be recognized by both the technologist and the electroencephalographer. They may not always be able to be eliminated, but they must be properly identified and proven, when in doubt, at the time of the recording.

Figure list

Figure 6.1 Facial twitching mimicking PLEDs.

Figure 6.2 Muscle artifact.

Figure 6.3 Filtered muscle mimicking brain activity.

Figure 6.4 Shivering artifact.

Figure 6.5 Muscle artifact vs. cerebral activity.

Figure 6.6 Sweat artifact.

Figure 6.7 Chewing artifact.

Figure 6.8 Breach rhythm.

Figure 6.9 Electrode artifact.

Figure 6.10 Breach rhythm.

Figure 6.11 Muscle artifact mimicking brain activity.

Figure 6.12 Snore artifact.

Figure 6.13 Breach rhythm.

Figure 6.14 Dialysis artifact.

Figure 6.15 Generalized spike-wave vs. EKG artifact.

Figure 6.16 Pulse and electrode artifacts.

Figure 6.17 Ocular bobbing artifact.

Figure 6.18 Cardioballistic artifact.

Figure 6.19 Vertical nystagmus artifact.

Figure 6.20 Respirator artifact.

Suggested reading

Cobb, W.A., Guiloff, R.J. and Cast, J. (1979) Breach rhythm: The EEG related to skull defects. *Electroencephalography and Clinical Neurophysiology* **47**, 251–271.

Klass, D.W. (1995) The continuing challenge of artifacts in the EEG. *American Journal of EEG Technology* **35**, 239–269.

Reilly, E.L. (2005) EEG recording and operation of the apparatus. In: Niedermeyer, E., Lopes de Silva, F. (eds), *Electroencephalography: Basic principles, clinical applications and related fields*, pp. 167–192. Lippincott, Williams and Wilkins, Philadelphia.

Tyner, F.S., Knott, J.R. and Mayer, W.B. Jr. (1983) Artifacts. In: *Fundamentals of EEG Technology*, Volume 1, pp. 280–311. Raven Press, New York.

Westmoreland, B.F., Espinosa, R.E. and Klass, D.W. (1973) Significant prosopoglossopharyyngeal movements affecting the electroencephalogram. *American Journal of EEG Technology* **13**, 59–70.

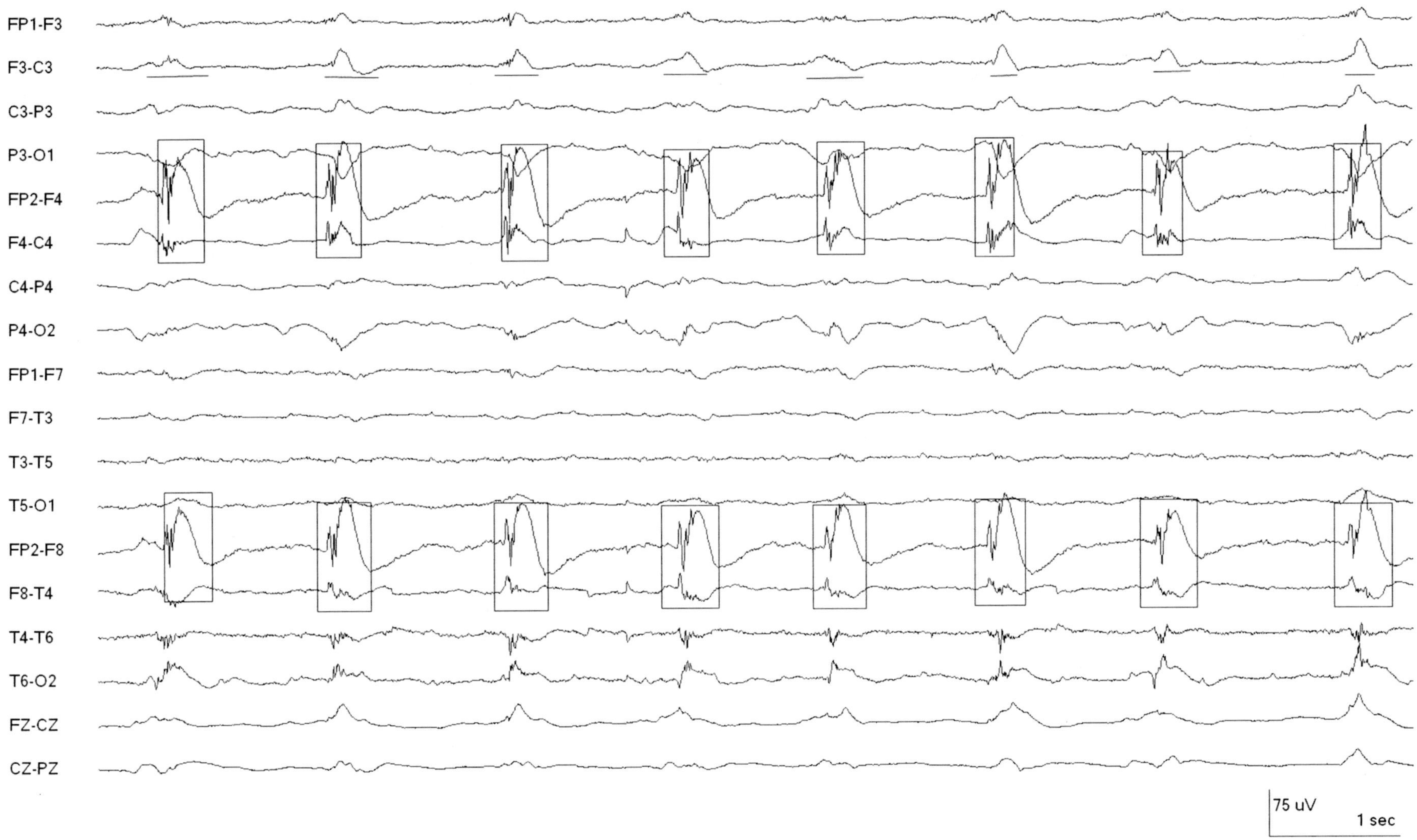

Figure 6.1 Facial-twitching artifact mimicking periodic lateralized epileptiform discharges (PLEDs). (a) The EEG in this 39-year-old woman shows periodic spike-wave- or polyspike-wave-like potentials over the right hemisphere (boxes). Lower voltage periodic slow waves (blunt PLEDs) are present on the left (underlined).

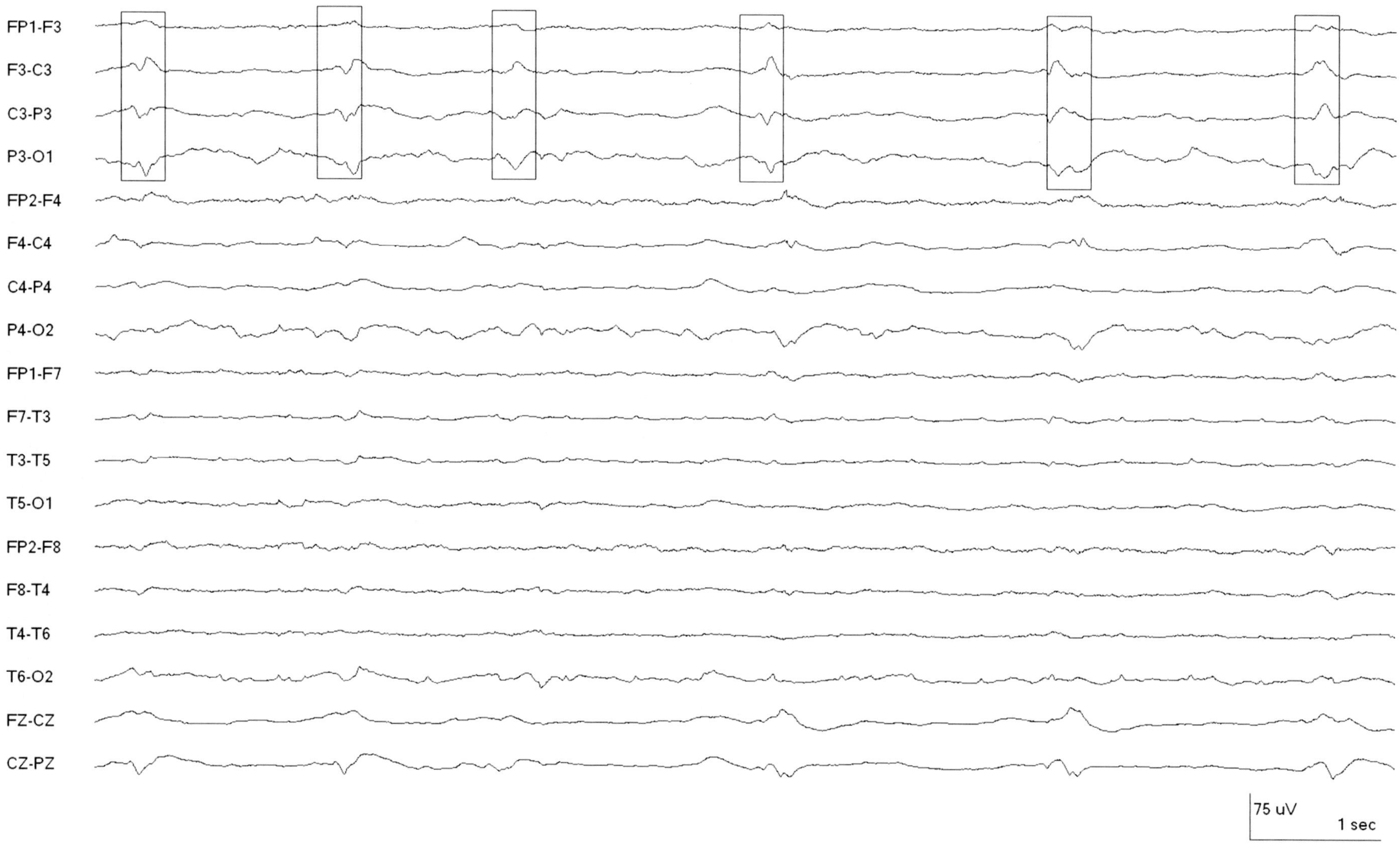

Figure 6.1 (*Continued*) (b) Following the administration of vecuronium the right-sided 'spikes' are no longer present. They were due to muscle artifact associated with twitching movements on the right side of the face. The movements were associated with the low-voltage PLEDs present over the left hemisphere (now in boxes), maximal in the parasagittal region. Thus, the left PLEDs were real (and ictal in this case), but the right 'PLEDs' were artifact.

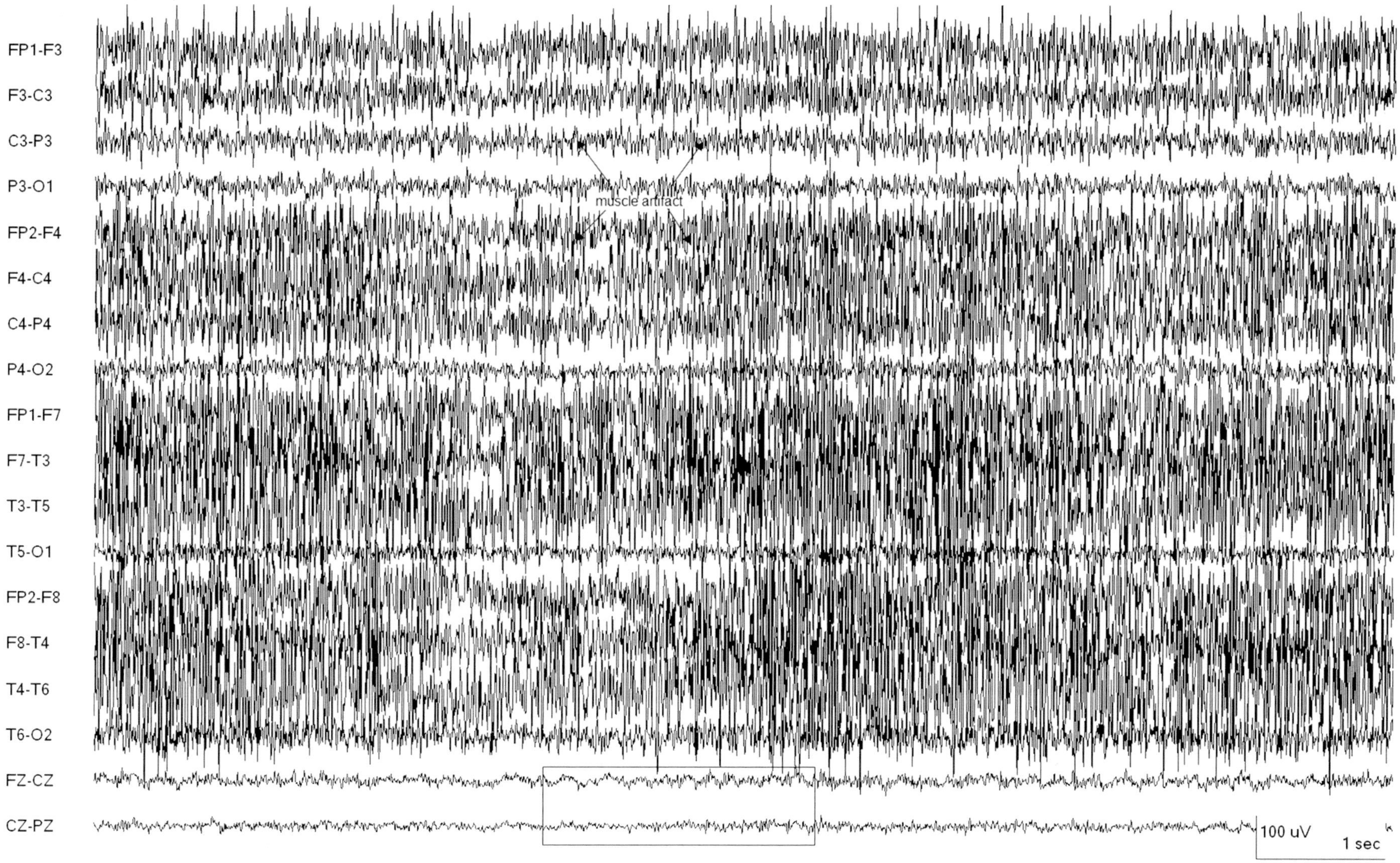

Figure 6.2 Widespread muscle artifact. (a) The EEG in this 25-year-old woman status post (s/p) cardiac arrest shows muscle artifact in a widespread distribution. Note the relative sparing of this activity in the midline derivations.

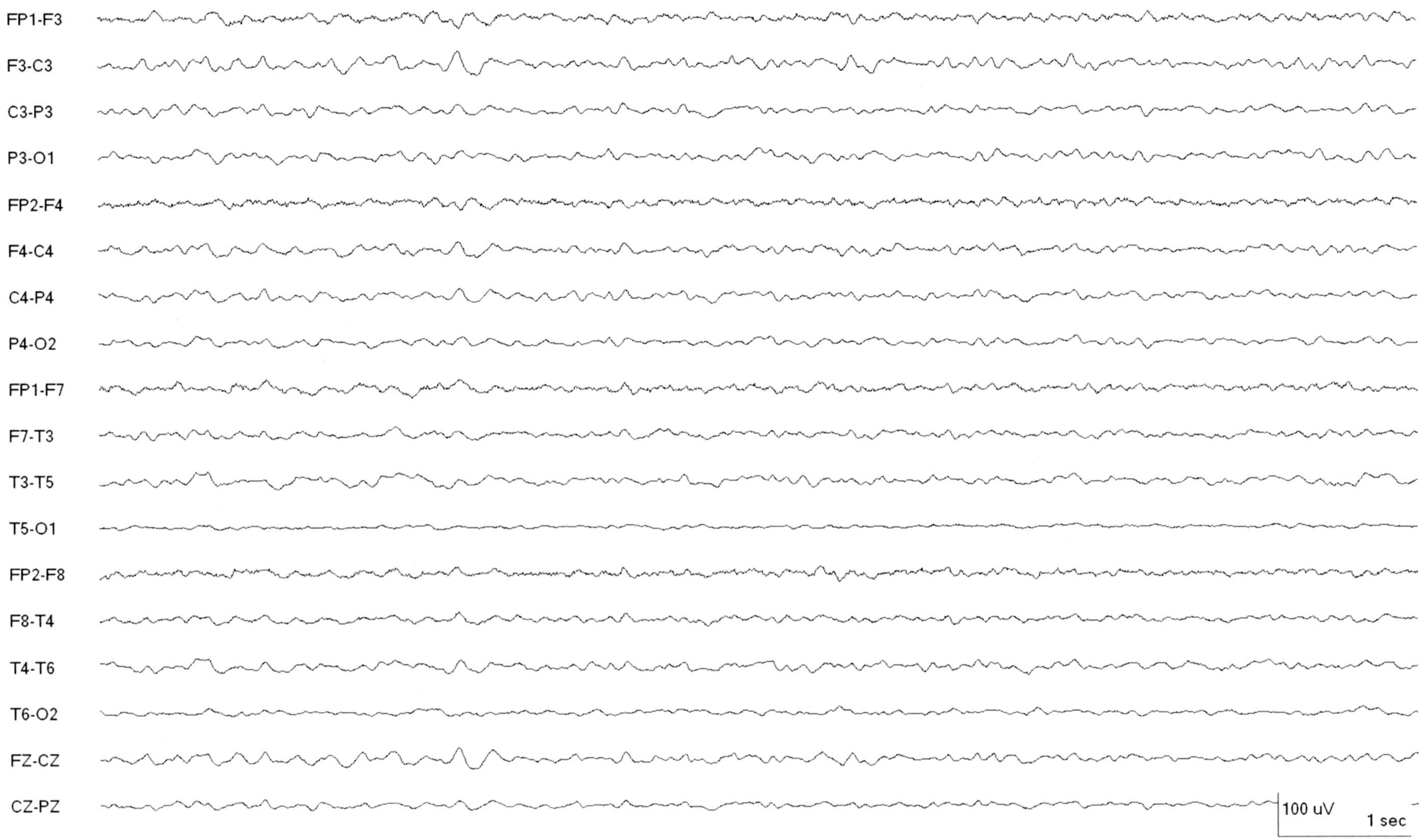

Figure 6.2 (*Continued*) (b) Following the administration of vecuronium, muscle artifact disappears. Background EEG can now be seen predominantly in the theta and alpha range in a widespread distribution.

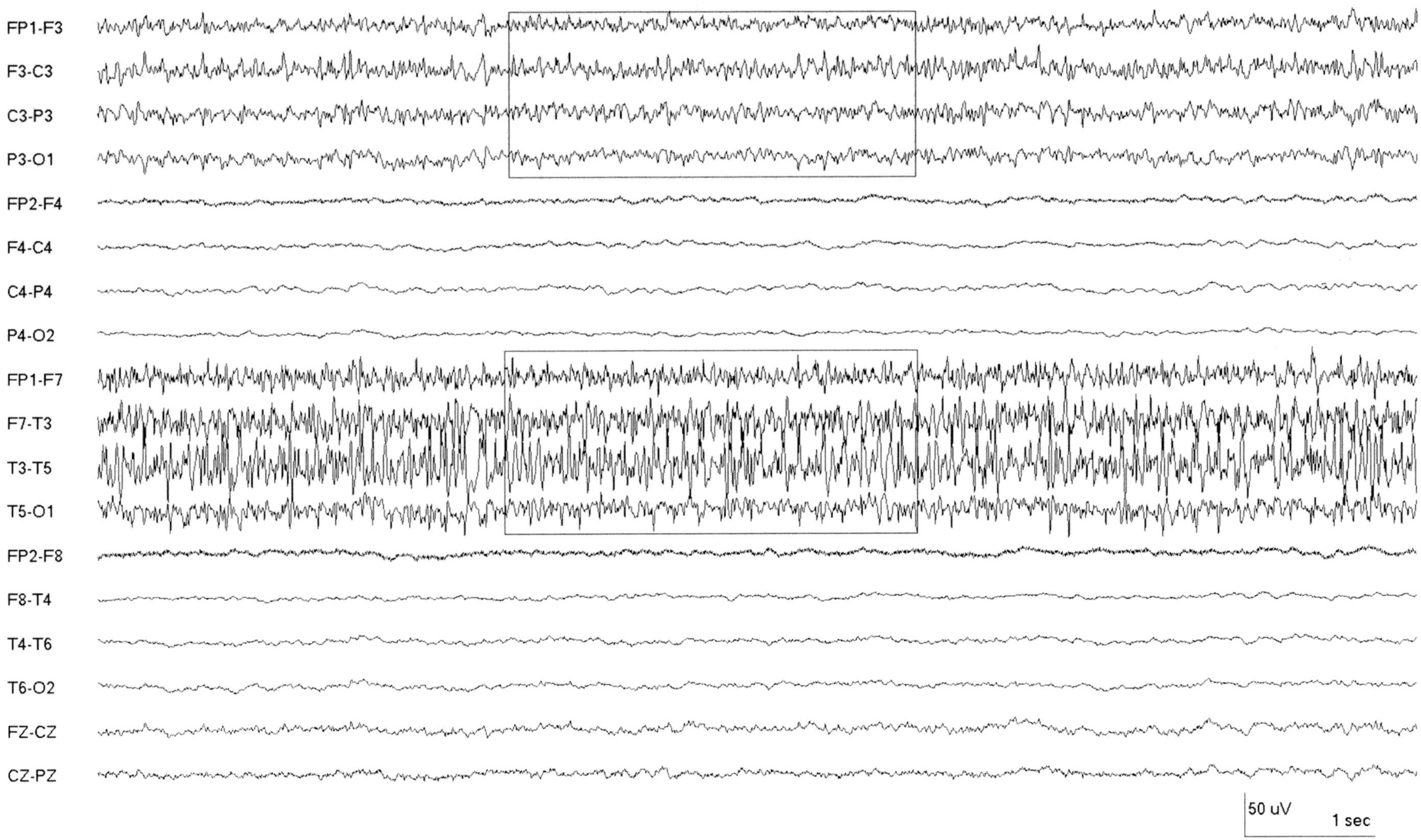

Figure 6.3 Filtered muscle mimicking brain activity. (a) Faster frequency activity is present on the left (boxes) in this 79-year-old man. The high-frequency filter (HFF) is set at a low setting of 15 Hz.

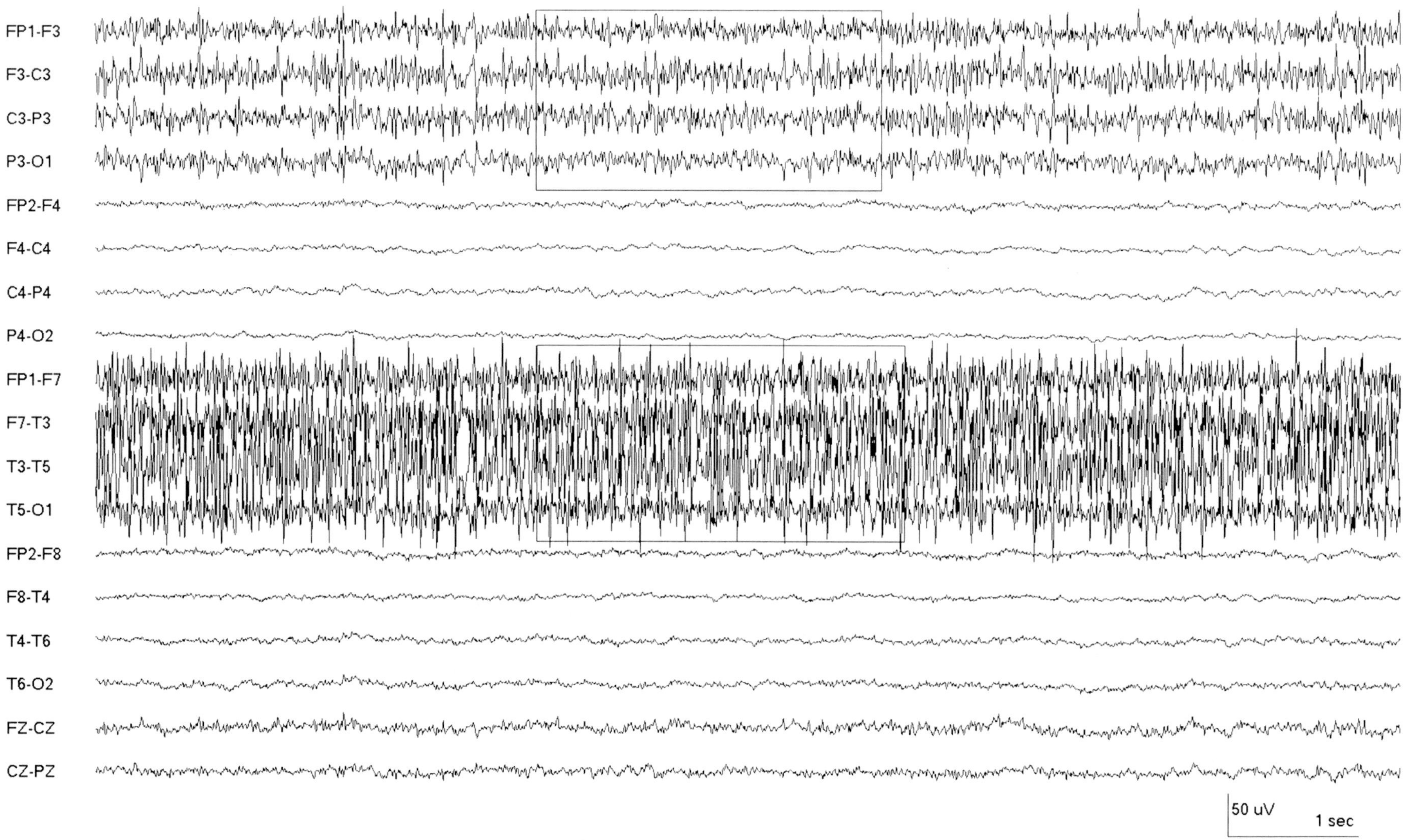

Figure 6.3 (*Continued*) (b) The HFF, also known as a low-pass filter, is now set at a more standard 70 Hz. The fast activity on the left is due to unilateral muscle artifact. The 15 Hz filter decreases muscle artifact, which is in the faster frequency range. With the 15 Hz filter, muscle artifact can be mistaken for cerebral beta activity or even epileptiform discharges. Filters do not distinguish between artifact or cerebral activity and inappropriate use of filters can often lead to misinterpretation.

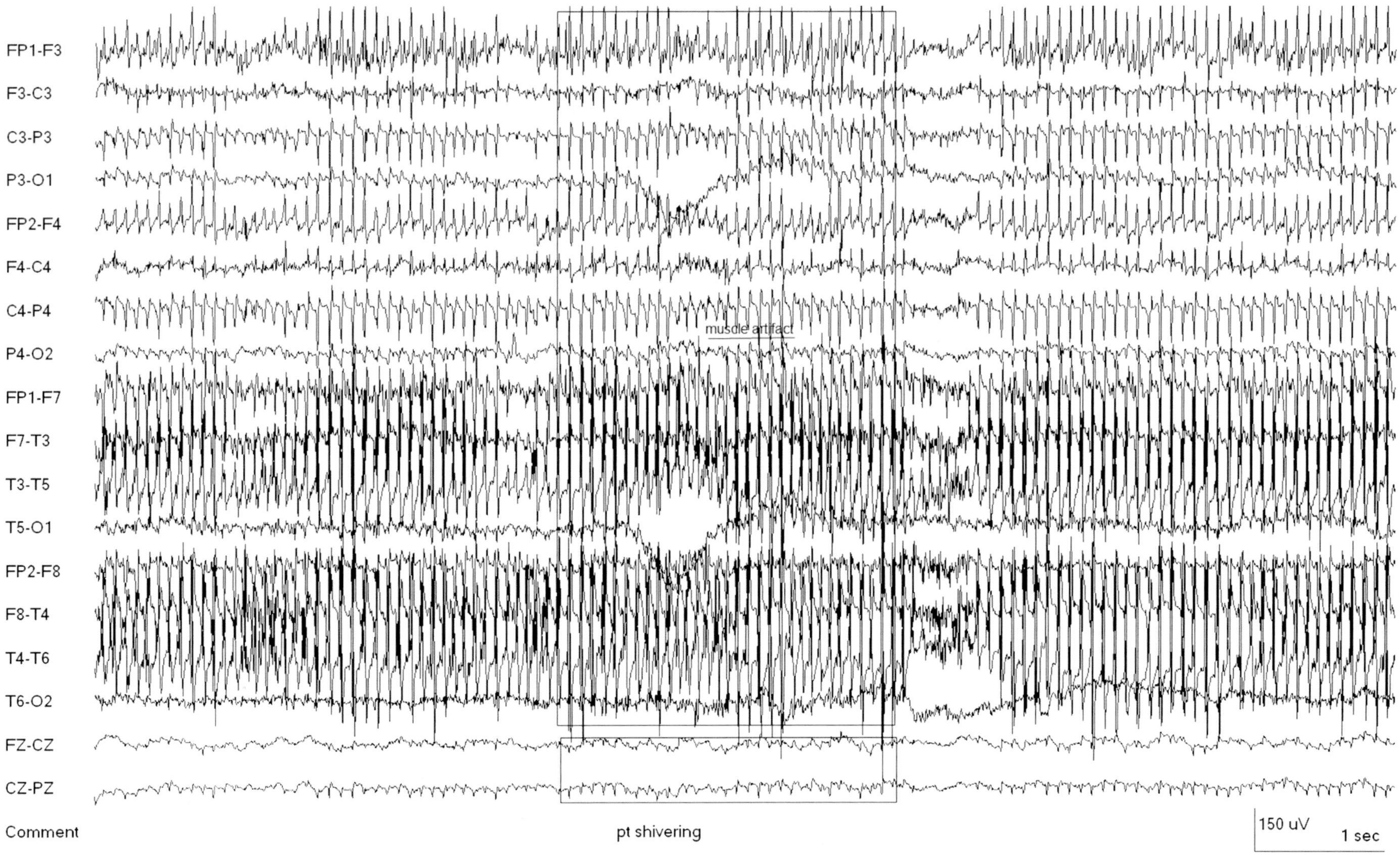

Figure 6.4 Muscle artifact from shivering. The EEG in this 61-year-old man demonstrates repetitive muscle spikes due to shivering. This activity is not well represented in the midline derivations (bottom two channels) as is typical of muscle artifact.

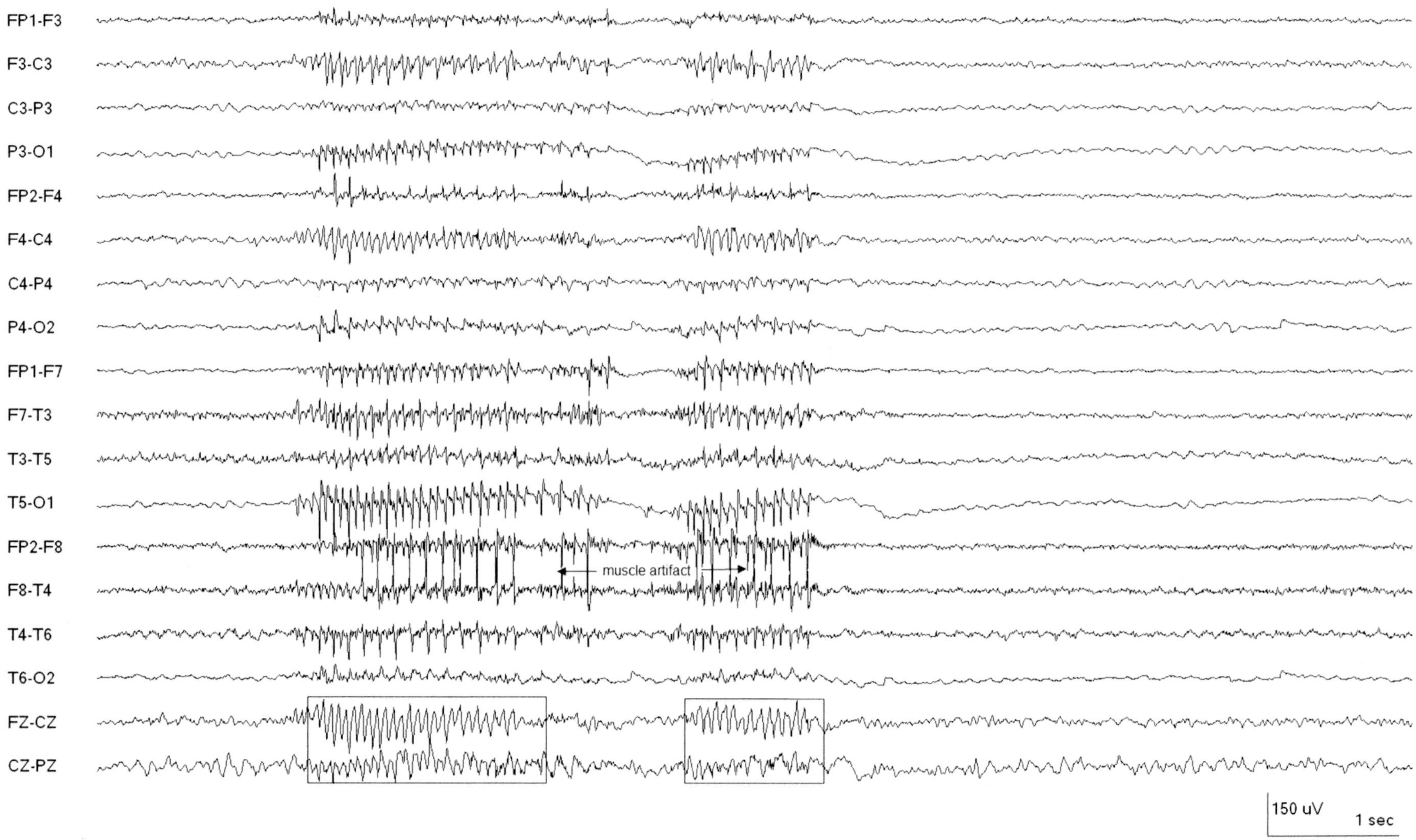

Figure 6.5 Muscle artifact vs. cerebral activity. The EEG in this 60-year-old man, being evaluated for a confusional state, shows muscle artifact, mostly marked in the right temporal region. However, there is also fast activity best-represented in the midline derivations (boxes), strongly suggesting that there is a cerebral discharge as well. In fact, he was having tonic seizures (a rare seizure type at this age).

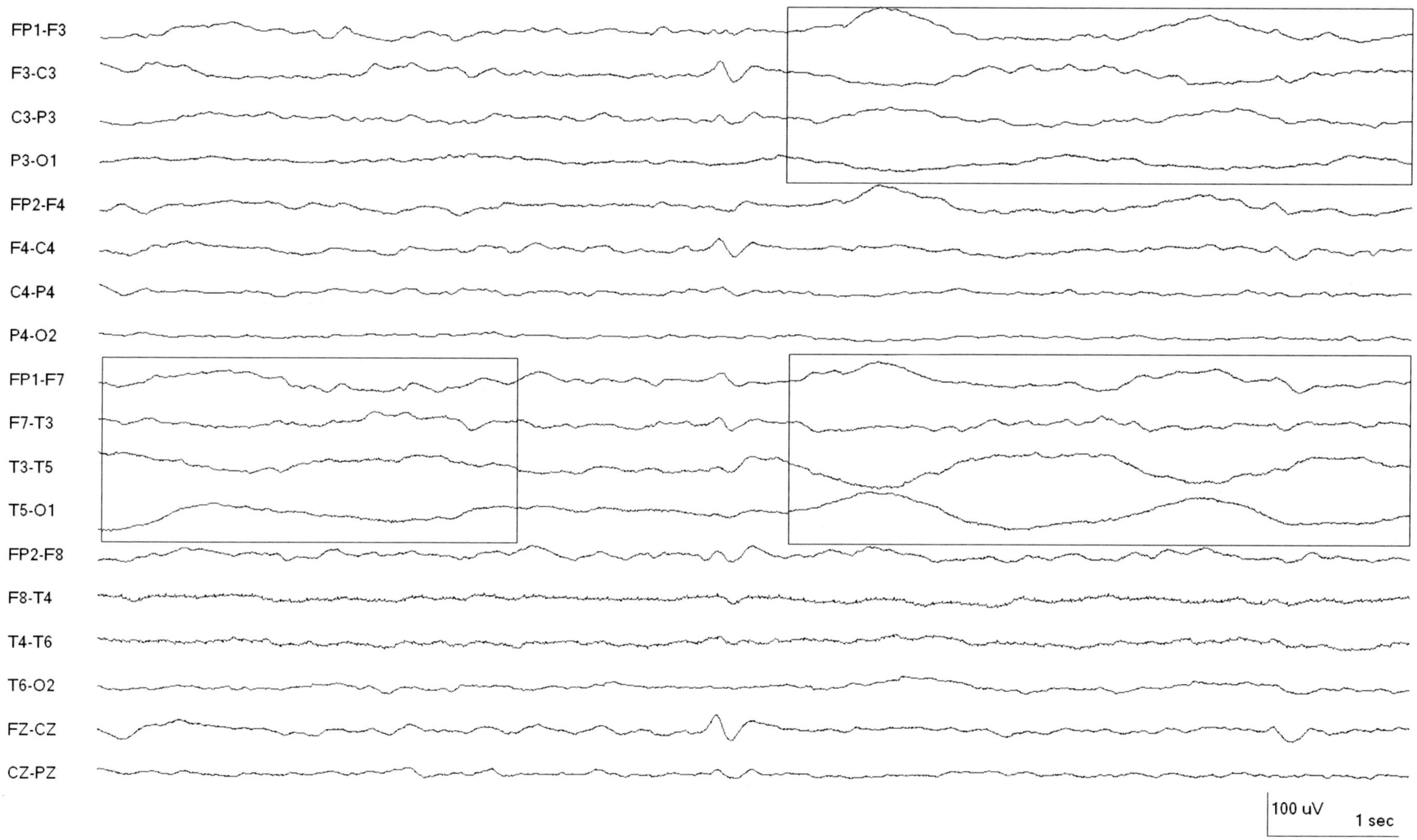

Figure 6.6 Sweat artifact. The EEG in this 66-year-old female with possible metastatic carcinoma shows prominent slowing, particularly over the left hemisphere (boxes). This represents sweat artifact. Sweat artifact usually involves several electrodes and consists of very slow and irregular delta activity. Delta slower than 1 Hz such as this is often either sweat artifact or slow-roving horizontal eye movements seen during drowsiness.

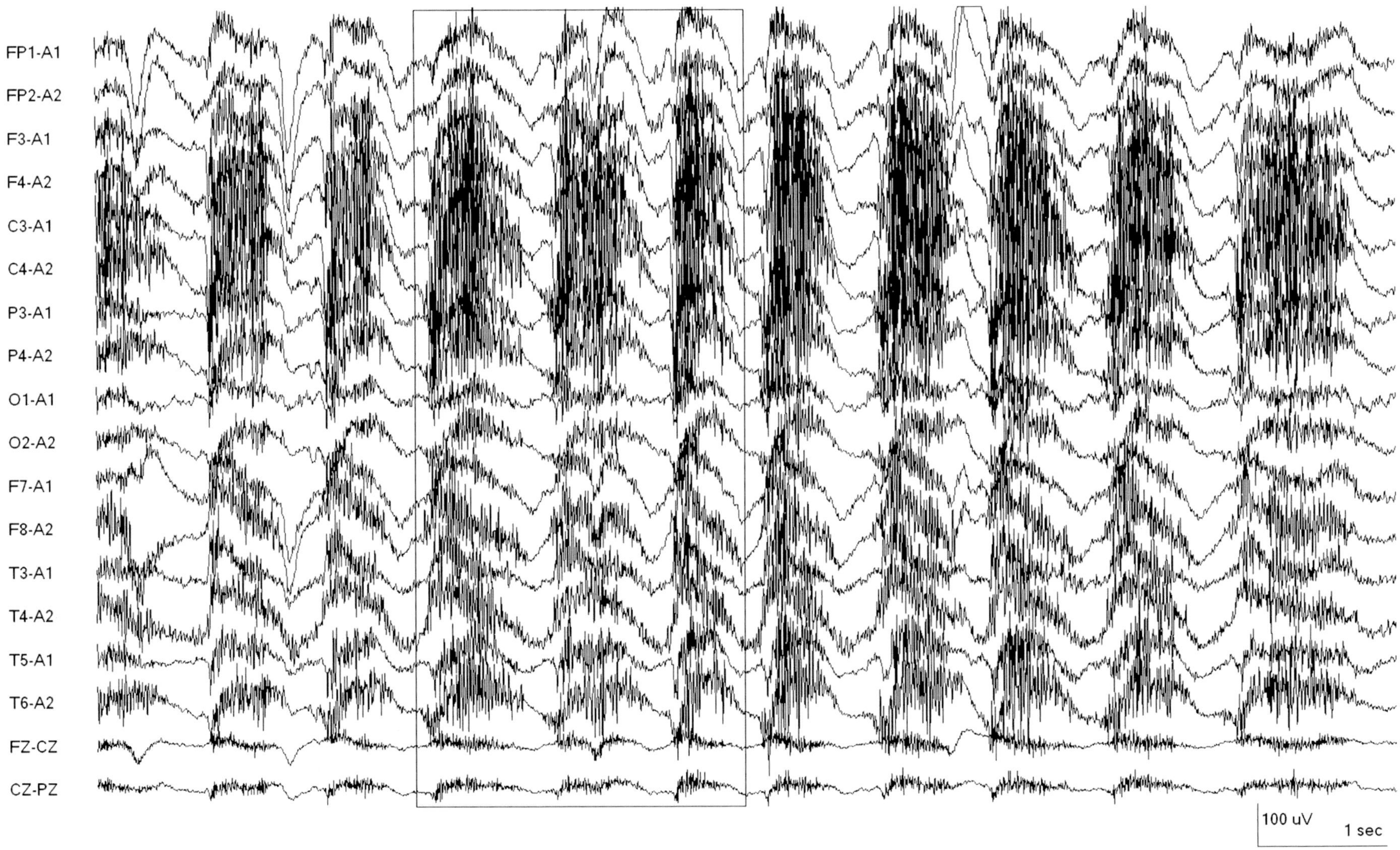

Figure 6.7 Chewing artifact. The EEG in this 41-year-old woman demonstrates repetitive muscle artifact that was due to chewing movements. Note the relative sparing of the midline derivations (bottom two channels).

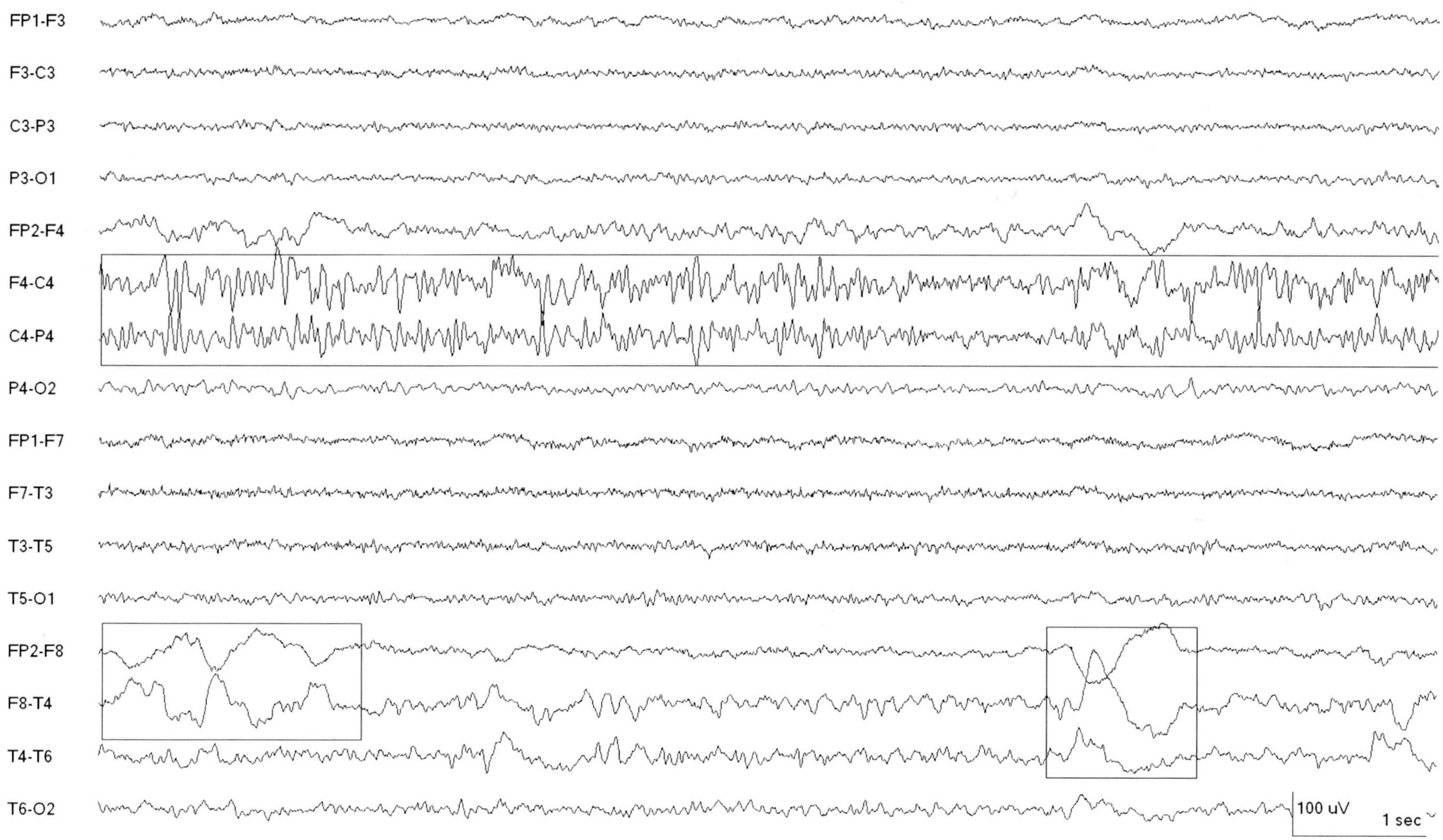

Figure 6.8 Breach rhythm. The EEG in this 36-year-old woman demonstrates high-voltage beta activity, particularly in the right central region (long box). Activity is also of higher voltage and slower over the right side, particularly in the frontal temporal area. The patient had a right-sided craniotomy. This is a breach rhythm (enhanced fast activity due to a skull defect, most marked at C4) as well as underlying dysfunction as manifest by the focal slowing (two smaller boxes).

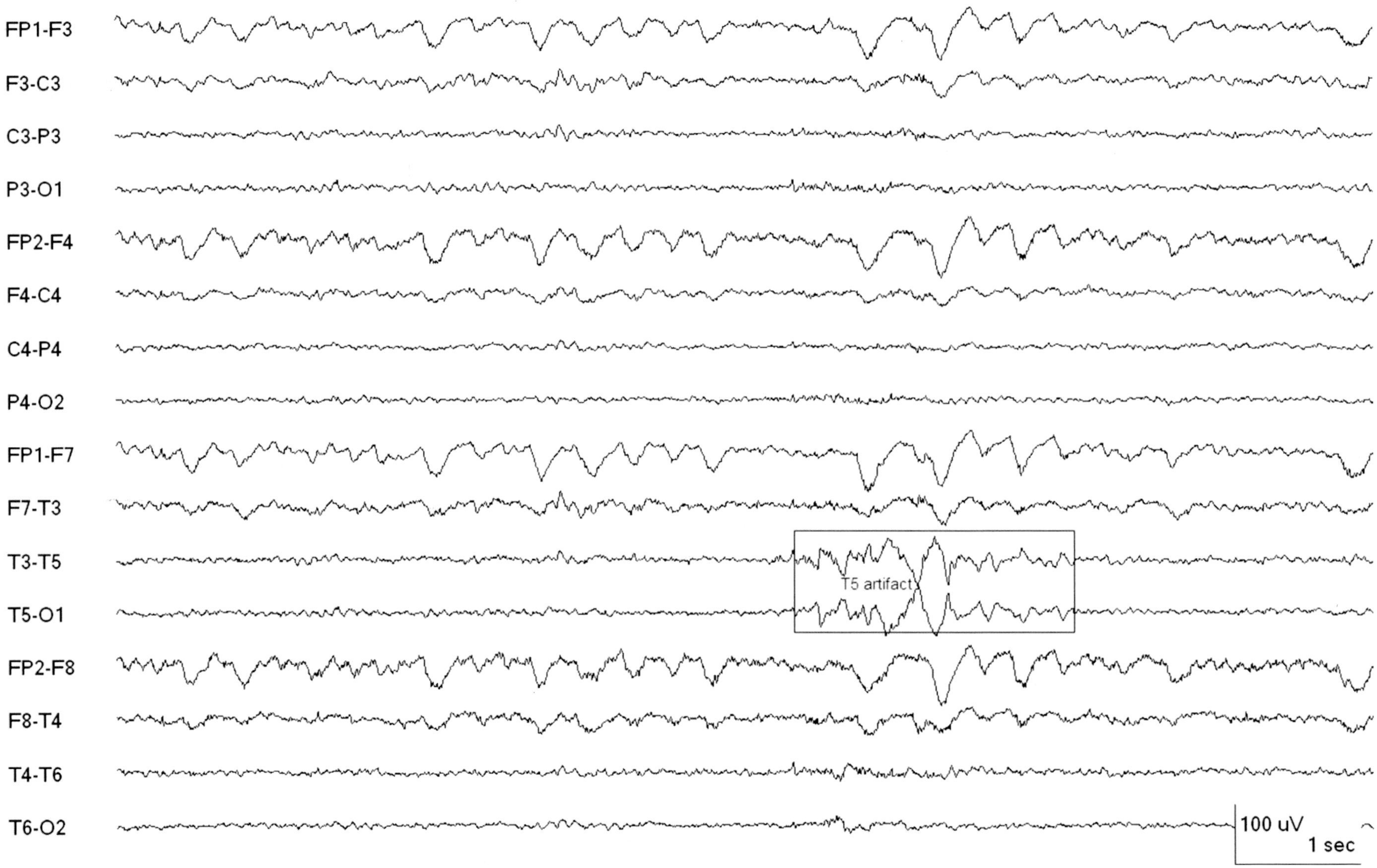

Figure 6.9 Electrode artifact. (a) Longitudinal bipolar. Eye blink or eye flutter artifact is prominent in Fp1 and Fp2 in this 24-year-old man. In addition, in the seventh second, a sharp wave admixed with slow waves is present in the T3-T5 and T5-01 derivations (box). This has a mirror image appearance, suggesting a T5 electrode artifact.

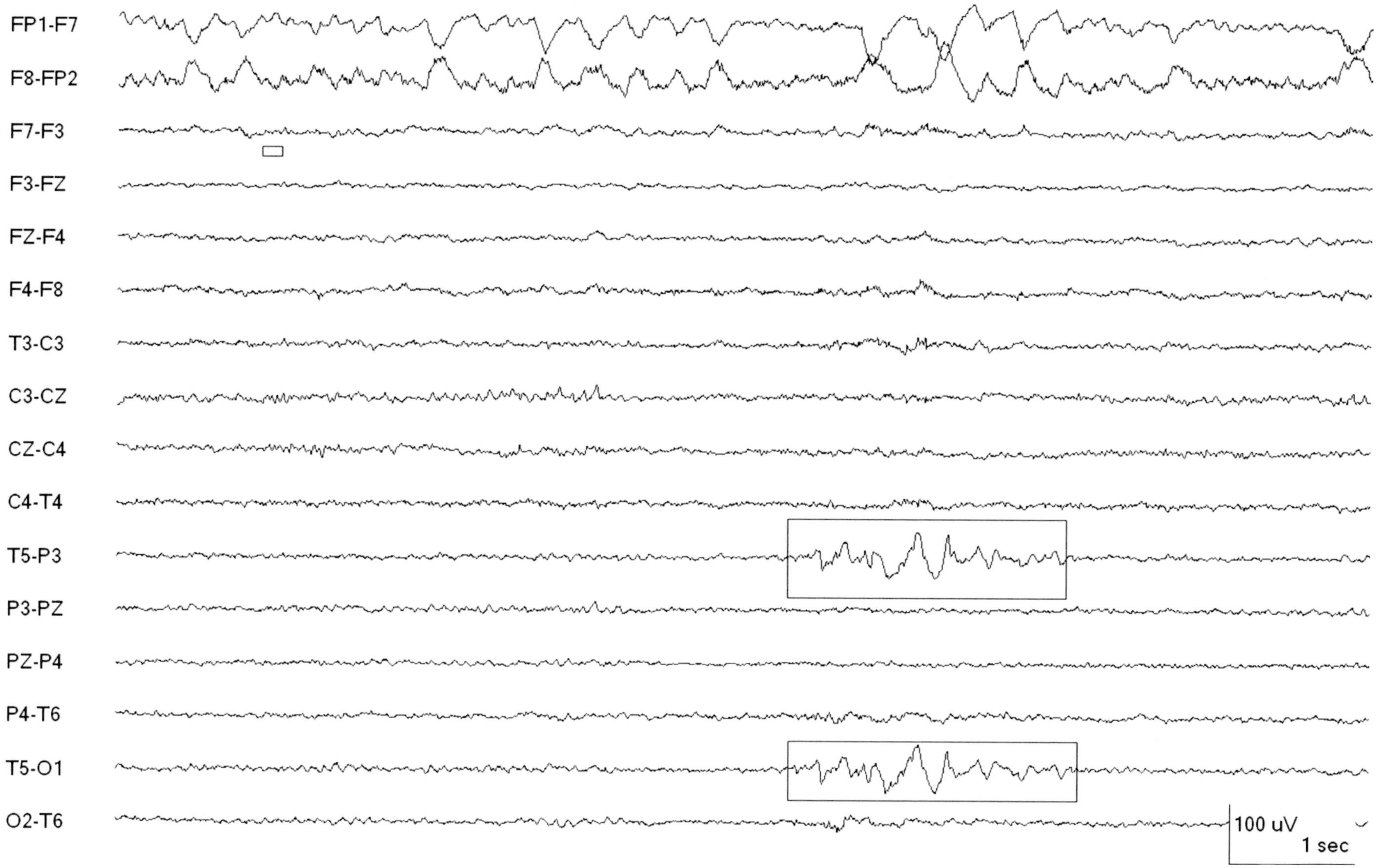

Figure 6.9 (*Continued*) (b) Transverse bipolar. This is a reformatted montage of the same epoch. Notice that the artifact (boxes) appears in all channels that have electrode T5, and only those channels.

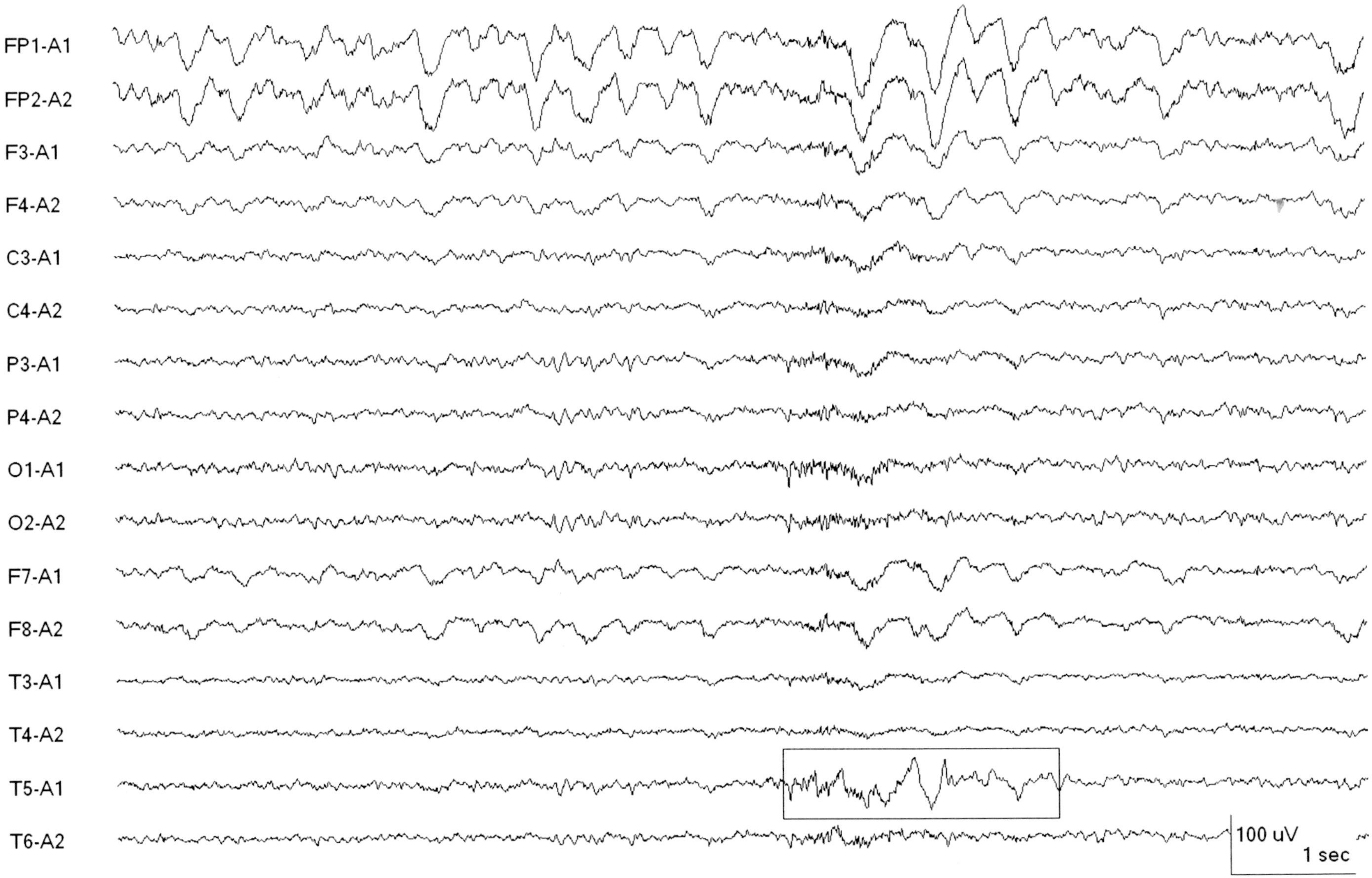

Figure 6.9 (*Continued*) (c) Referential. This is a referential montage of the same epoch. Notice that the artifact is present only in the channel that contains electrode T5 (box).

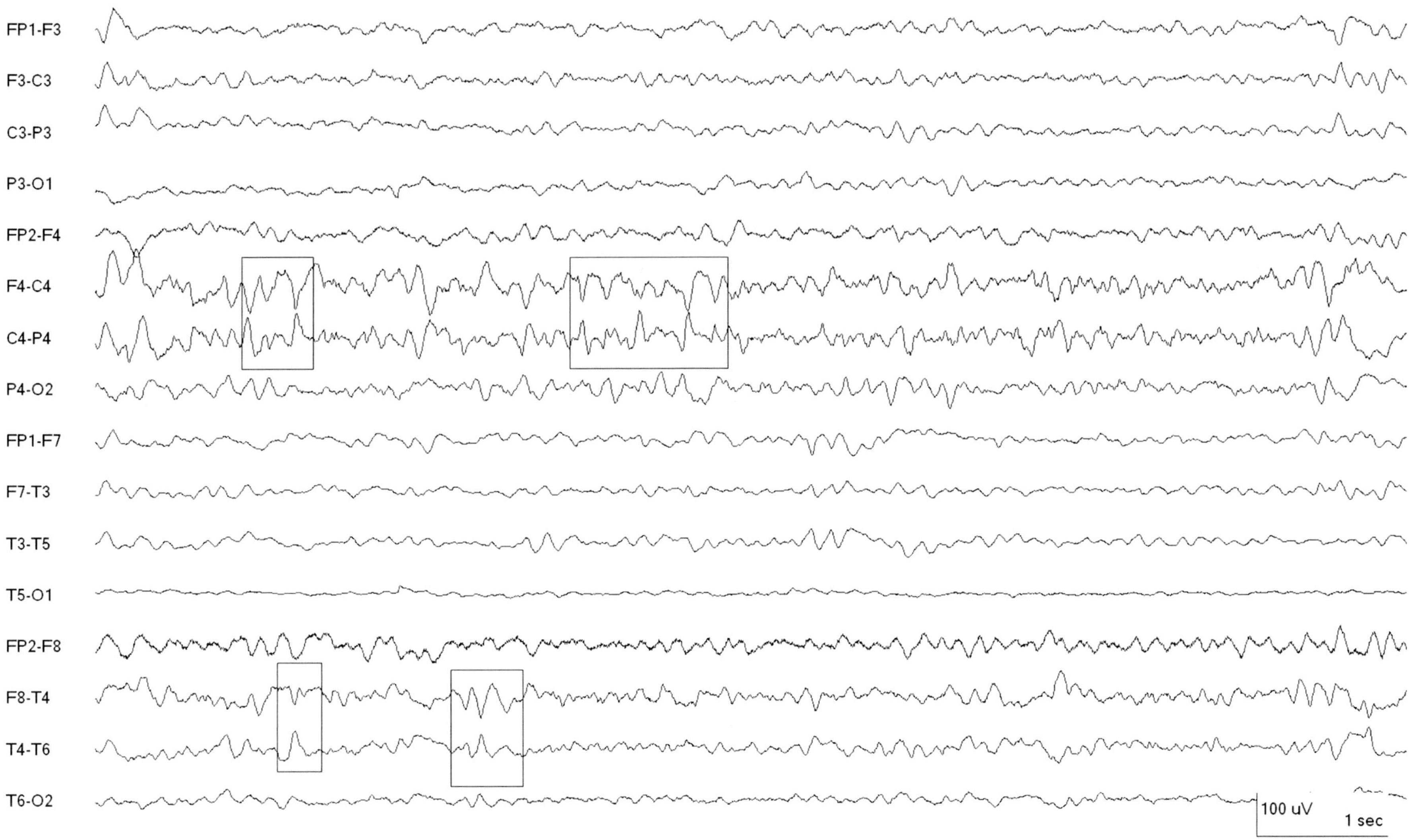

Figure 6.10 Breach effect. The EEG in this 80-year-old woman s/p right craniectomy for evacuation of a right subdural hematoma shows higher voltage activity over the right hemisphere. There are a several sharply contoured waves present in the central and mid-temporal regions (boxes); however, this degree of sharpness in an area of a clear skull defect could be simply due to the skull defect (breach effect) and not indicative of epileptogenic potential.

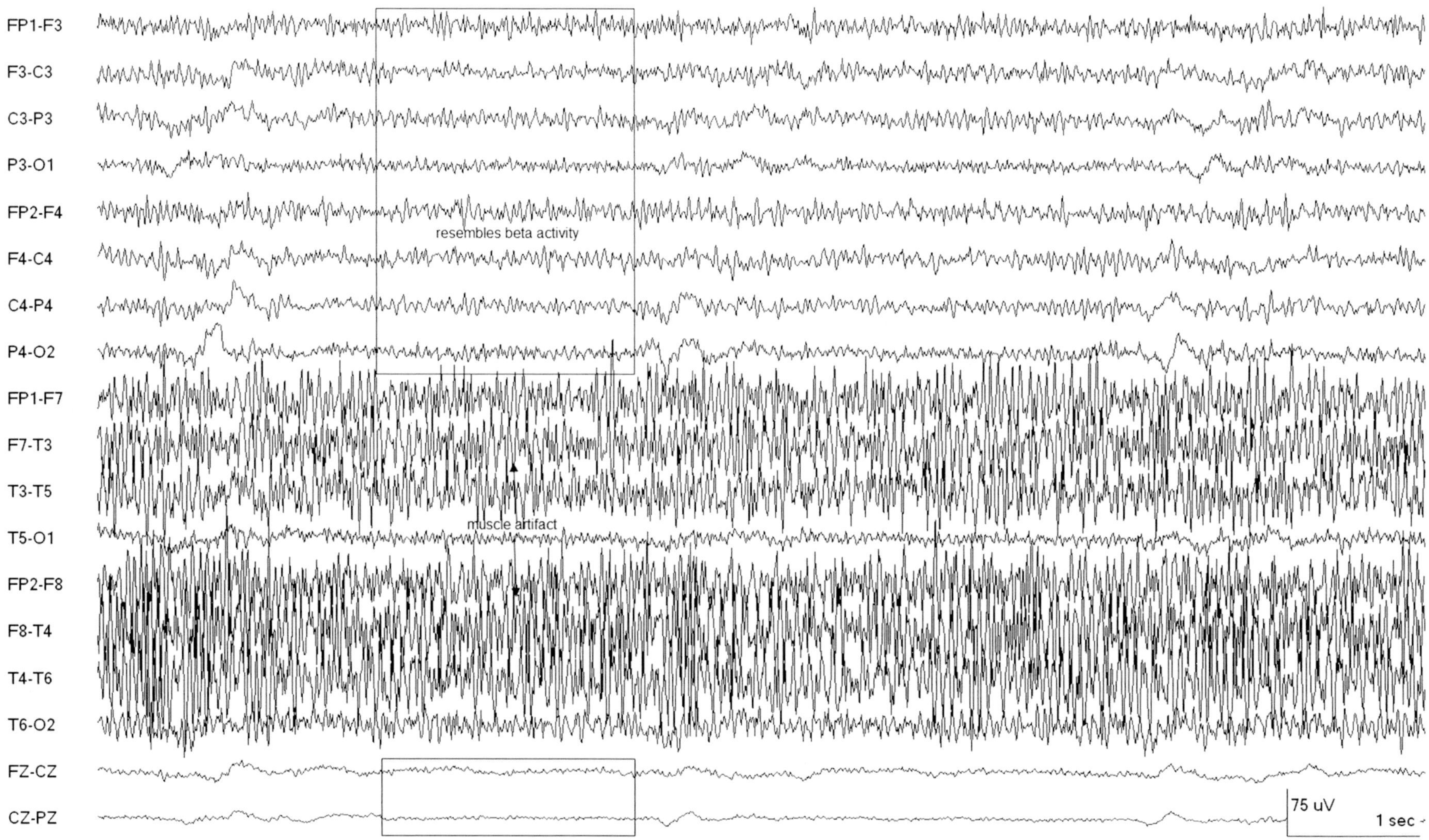

Figure 6.11 Muscle artifact mimicking cerebral activity. (a) The EEG in this 77-year-old woman s/p revision of a right frontal craniotomy shows muscle artifact that is prominent in the temporal areas. There appears to be beta activity (the high-frequency filter was 70 Hz) in the parasagittal regions. However, this activity is not well seen in the midline derivations (Fz-Cz and Cz-Pz), suggesting that it is more likely to be muscle artifact rather than beta activity.

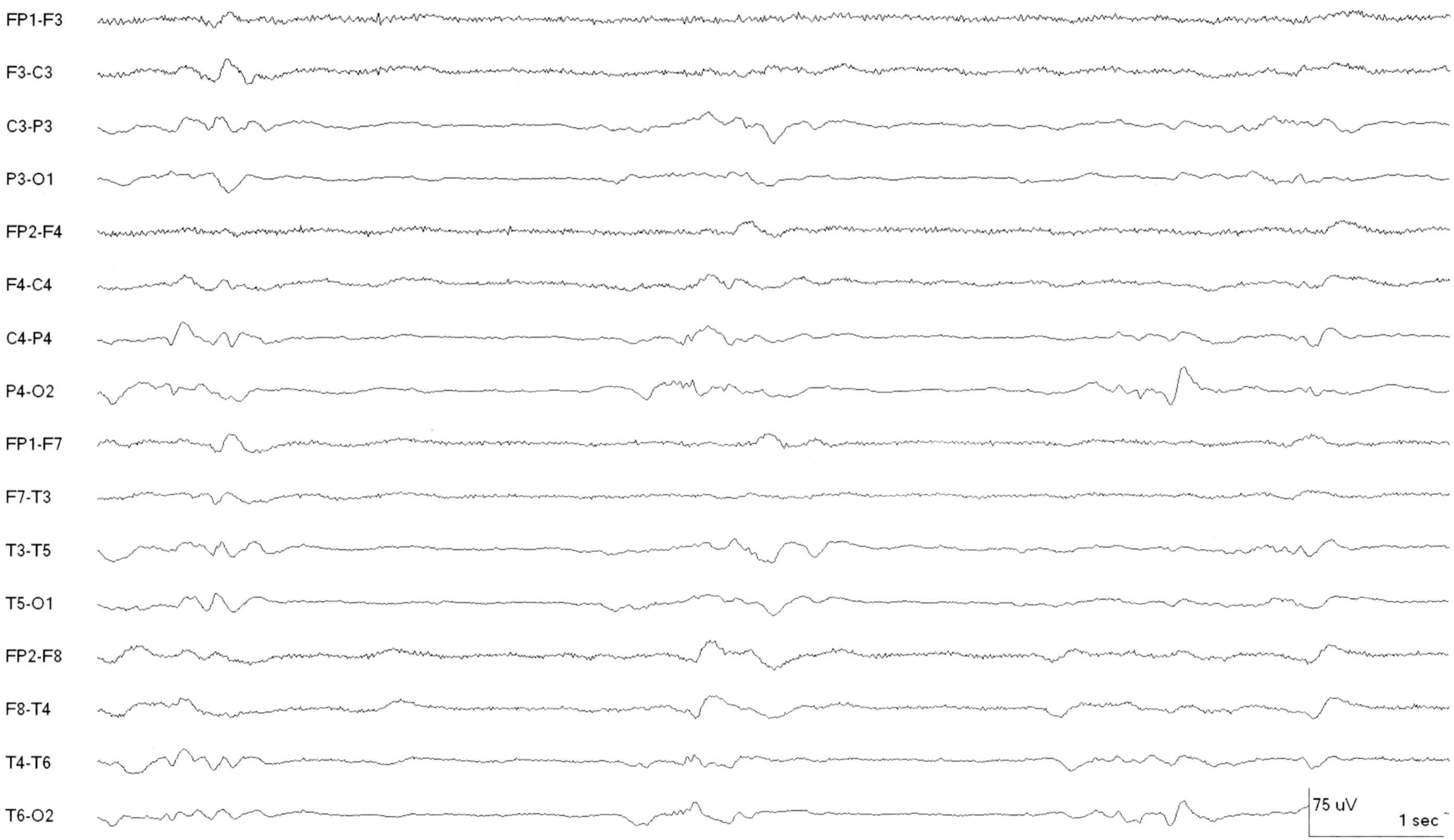

Figure 6.11 (*Continued*) (b) Following the administration of vecuronium, a burst-suppression pattern, previously largely obscured by muscle artifact, is now much more apparent.

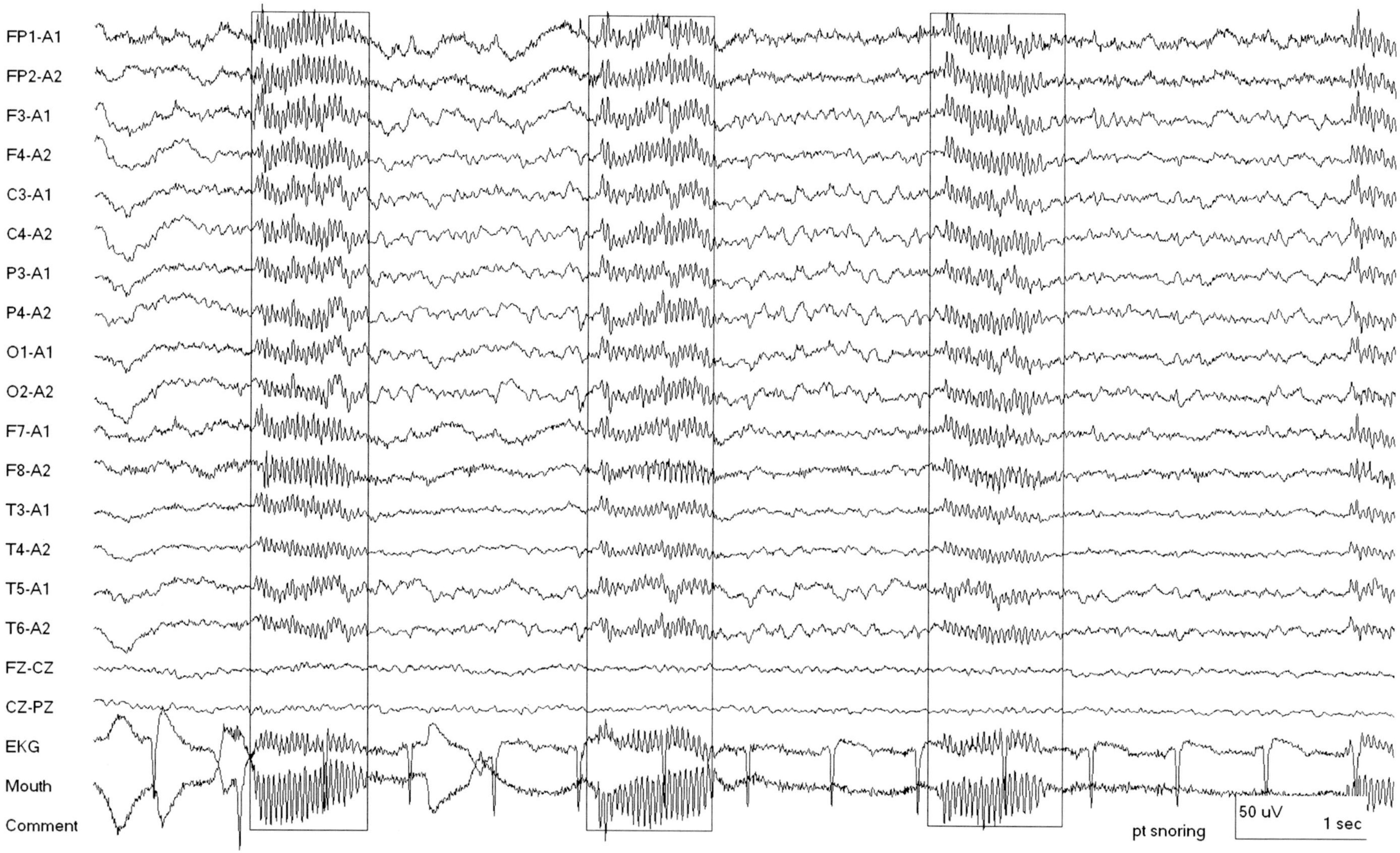

Figure 6.12 Snore artifact. The EEG in this 72-year-old man shows groups of fast activity (approximately 25 Hz), present in a widespread distribution. The discharges, however, are not present in the midline electrodes, which usually are relatively free of artifact, but are present near the mouth and in the EKG electrodes. This is an artifact and was due to snoring.

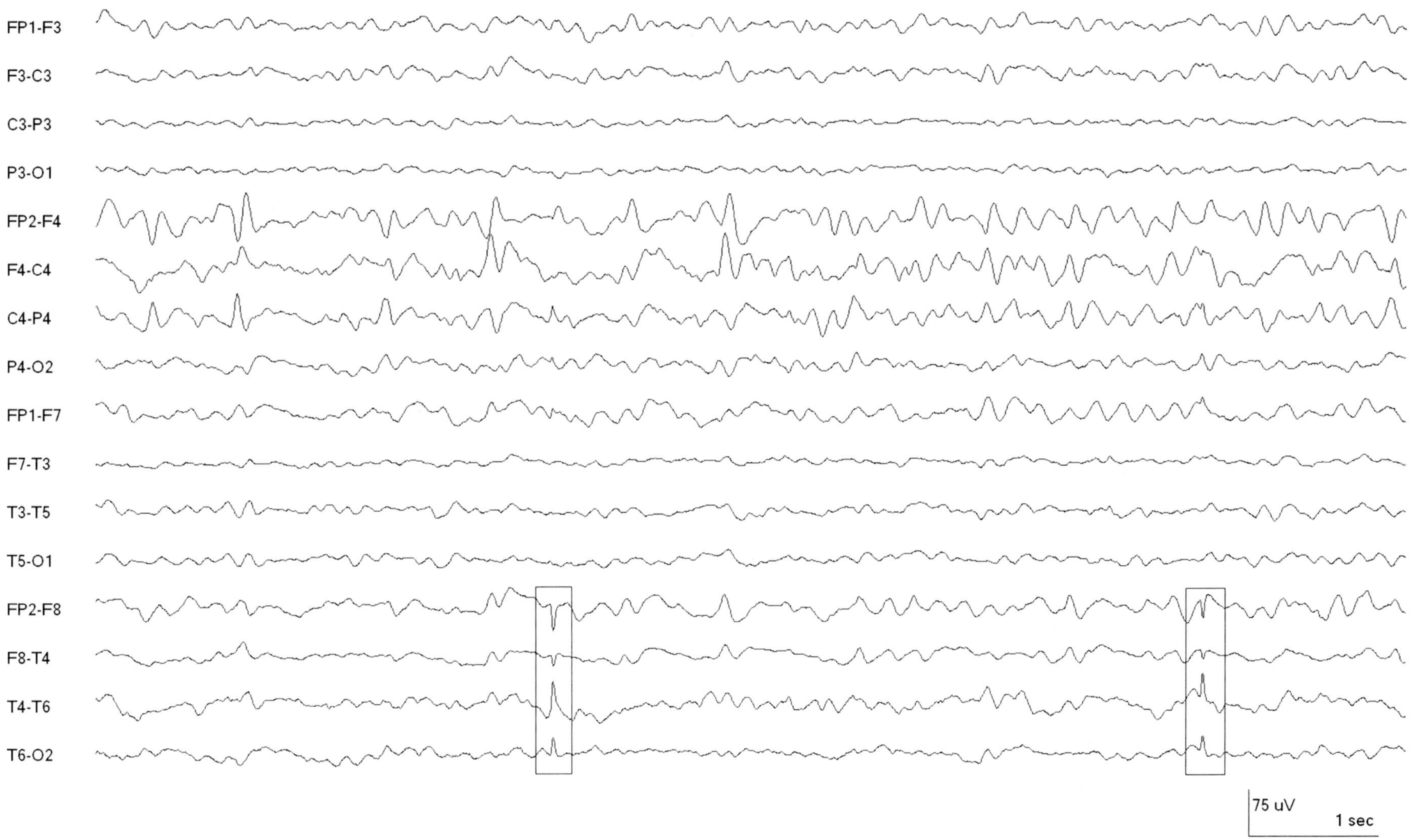

Figure 6.13 Asymmetry with skull defect (breach). The EEG in this 73-year-old man shows prominent hemispheric differences. Background activity is of higher voltage and slower over the right hemisphere. These are right anterior to mid-temporal spikes (boxes) and slowing over the frontal regions. The patient suffered a head injury and developed a right subdural hematoma, which was evacuated. Thus, part of the changes (increased amplitude of faster frequencies on the right) was due to a skull defect. However, the EEG does show bilateral abnormalities (slowing) and right-sided epileptiform discharges.

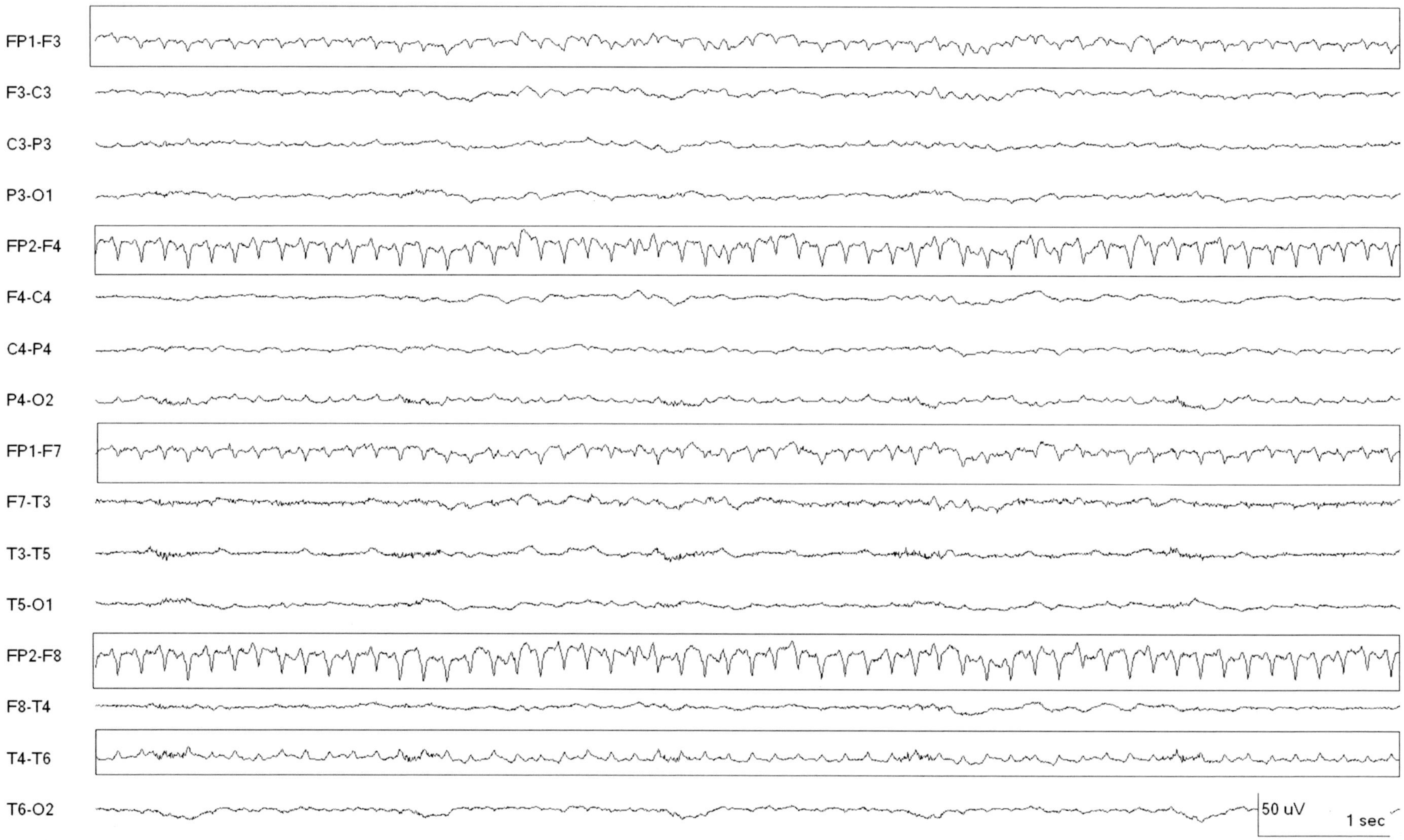

Figure 6.14 Dialysis artifact. The EEG in this 92-year-old man with mental status changes and renal failure shows rhythmic artifact (boxes), predominantly involving the anterior head regions (electrodes Fp1 and Fp2), more marked on the right. The discharges are also present in the T4-T6 derivation, which provides evidence that this could not represent eye movement artifact. The patient was being dialyzed utilizing slow continuous ultra filtration (SCUF) that resulted in this artifact.

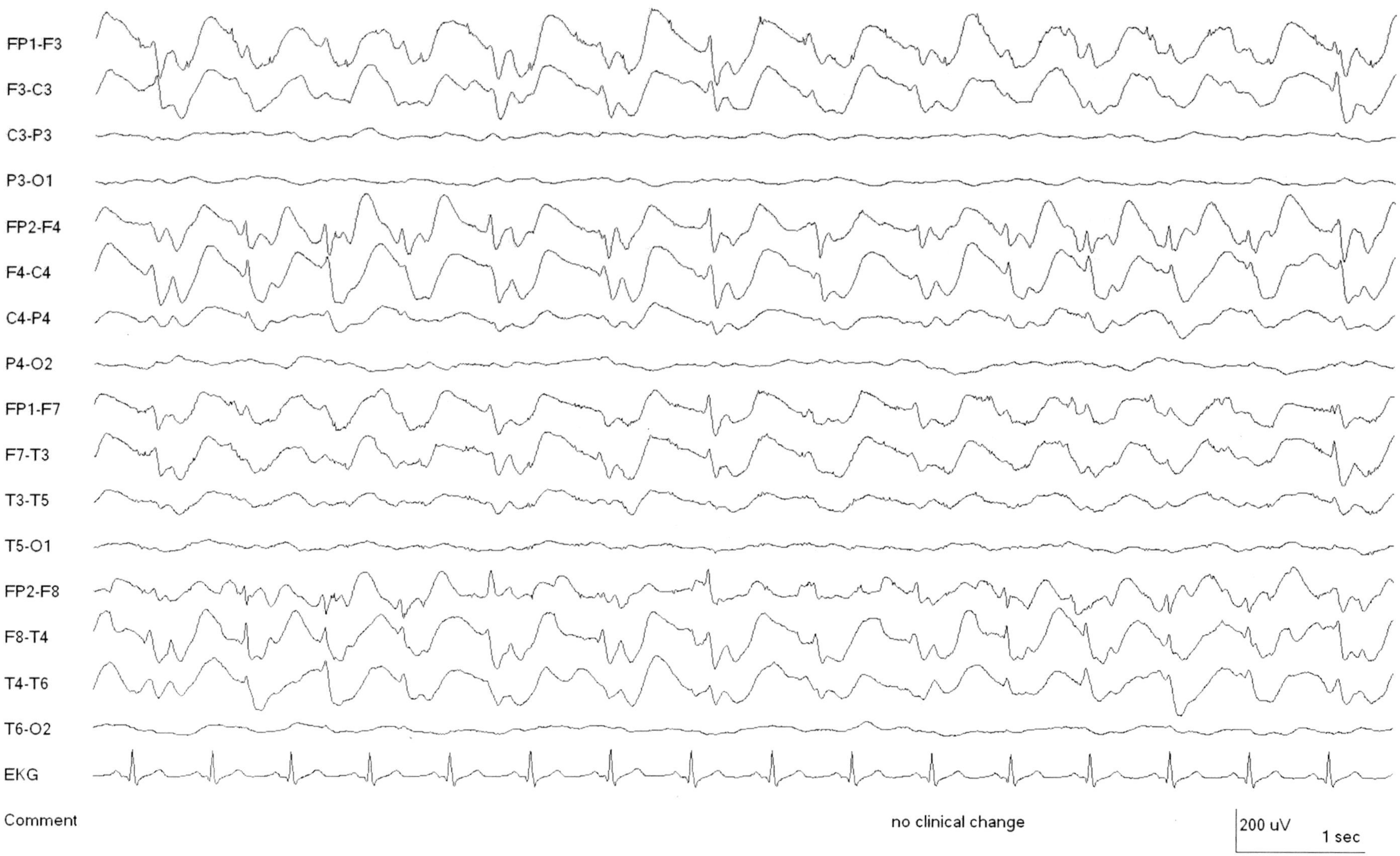

Figure 6.15 Generalized spike-wave vs. EKG artifact. Rhythmic spike and wave activity is present in a widespread distribution, maximal anteriorly, in this 21-year-old woman. Although this rhythmic activity is regular and has a rate of approximately that of the EKG, it does not represent EKG artifact (monitored in the bottom channel). The patient was in generalized nonconvulsive status epilepticus.

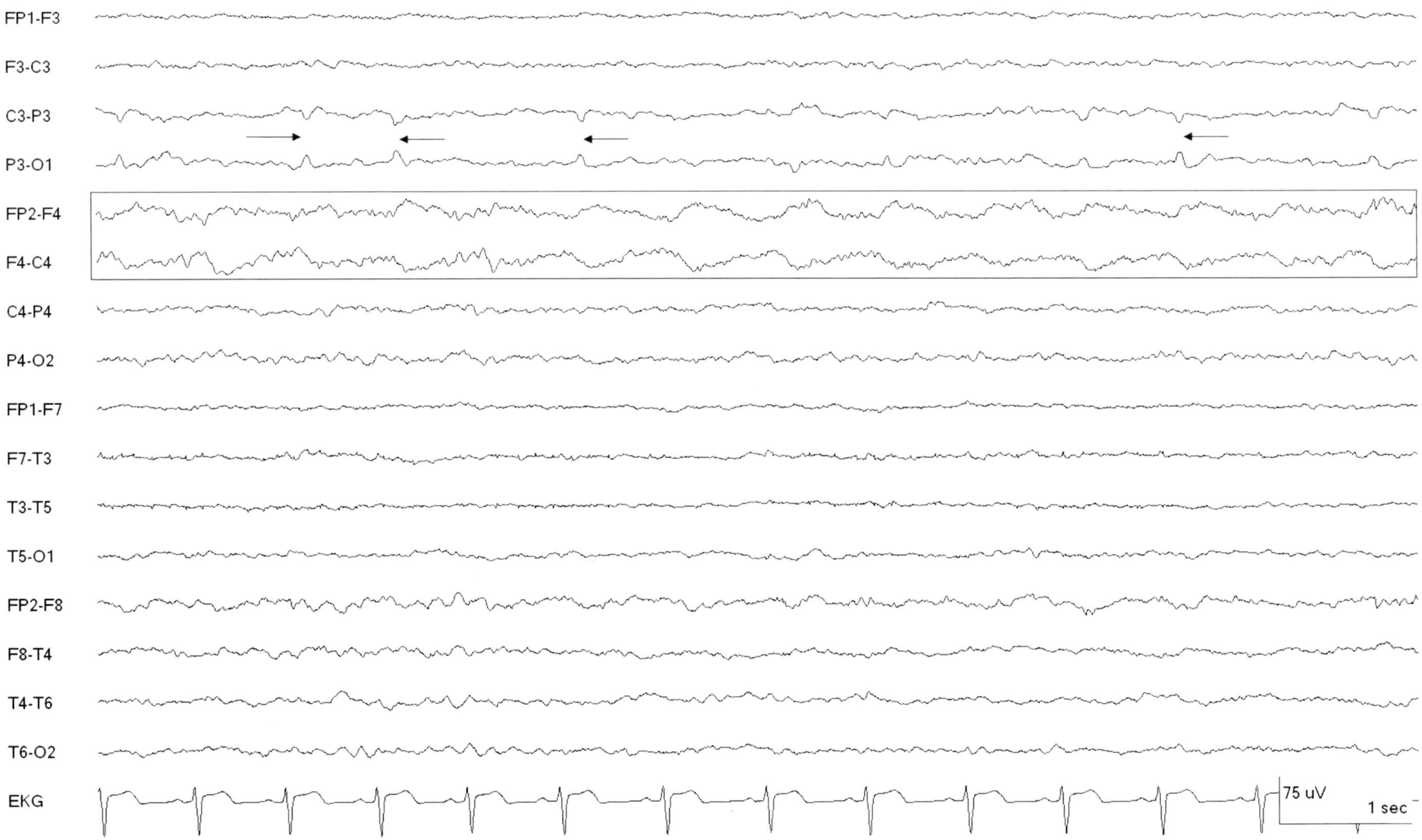

Figure 6.16 Pulse artifact and electrode artifact. Rhythmic slowing is present in the F4 electrode (box) and has a mirror image appearance in derivations FP2-F4 and F4-C4. In addition, intermittent, repetitive, low-voltage sharp potentials are present in electrode P3 (arrows). The slowing at F4 is due to a pulse artifact. The slow wave follows the QRS complex by approximately 200 ms. The sharp activity in the P3 electrode was due to a P3 electrode artifact.

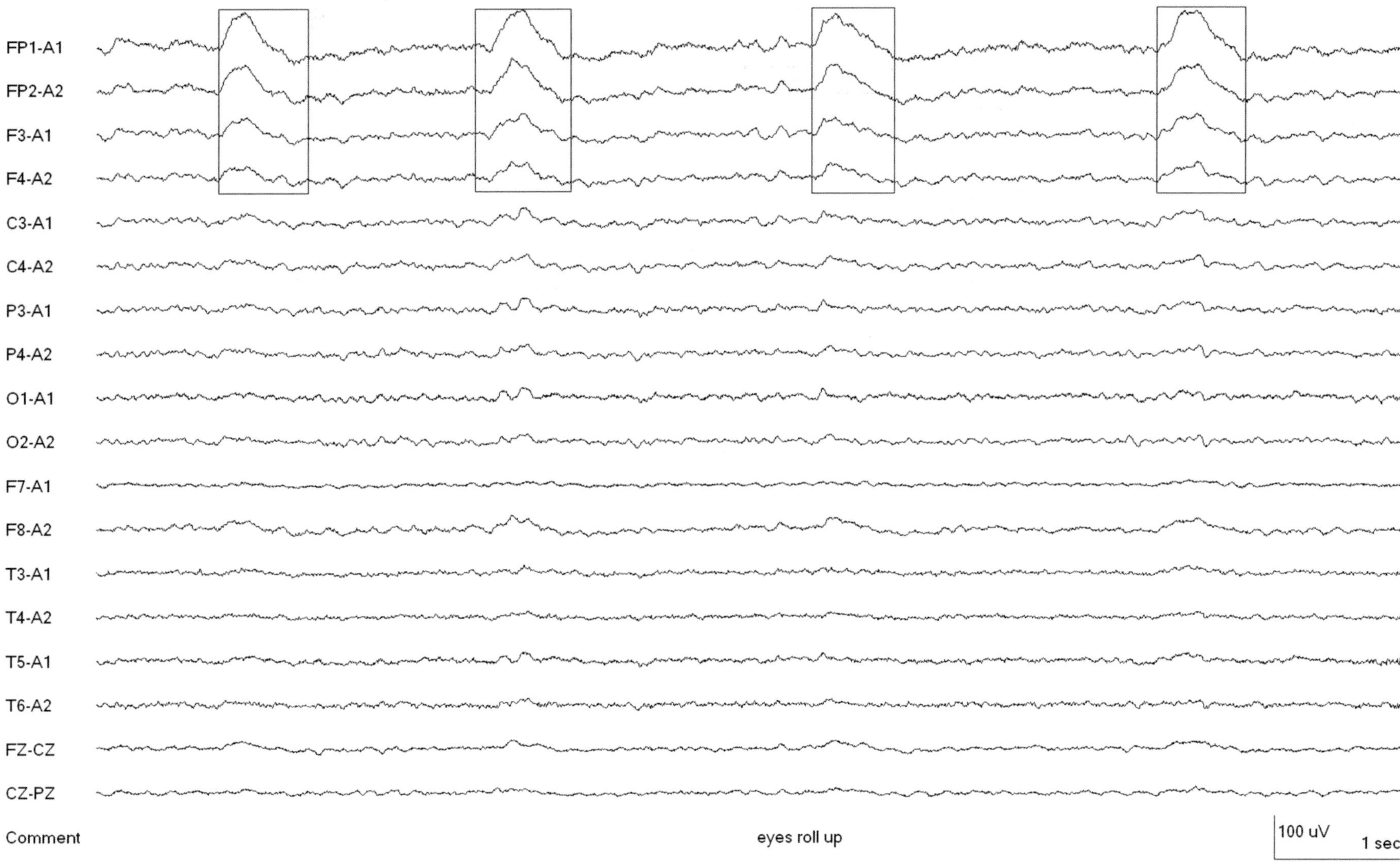

Figure 6.17 Ocular bobbing. The EEG shows repetitive slow waves present in the frontal regions, maximal at electrodes Fp1 and Fp2 (boxes). The ascending portion of the waveform in the Fp1 and Fp2 electrodes is more rapid than its descending portion, that is it has a steeper slope. This is because the upward deflection is due to the fact that the eyes are quickly moving down and then coming up more slowly. Examination revealed ocular bobbing corresponding with the bifrontal slow waves in this 75-year-old man with a brainstem stroke.

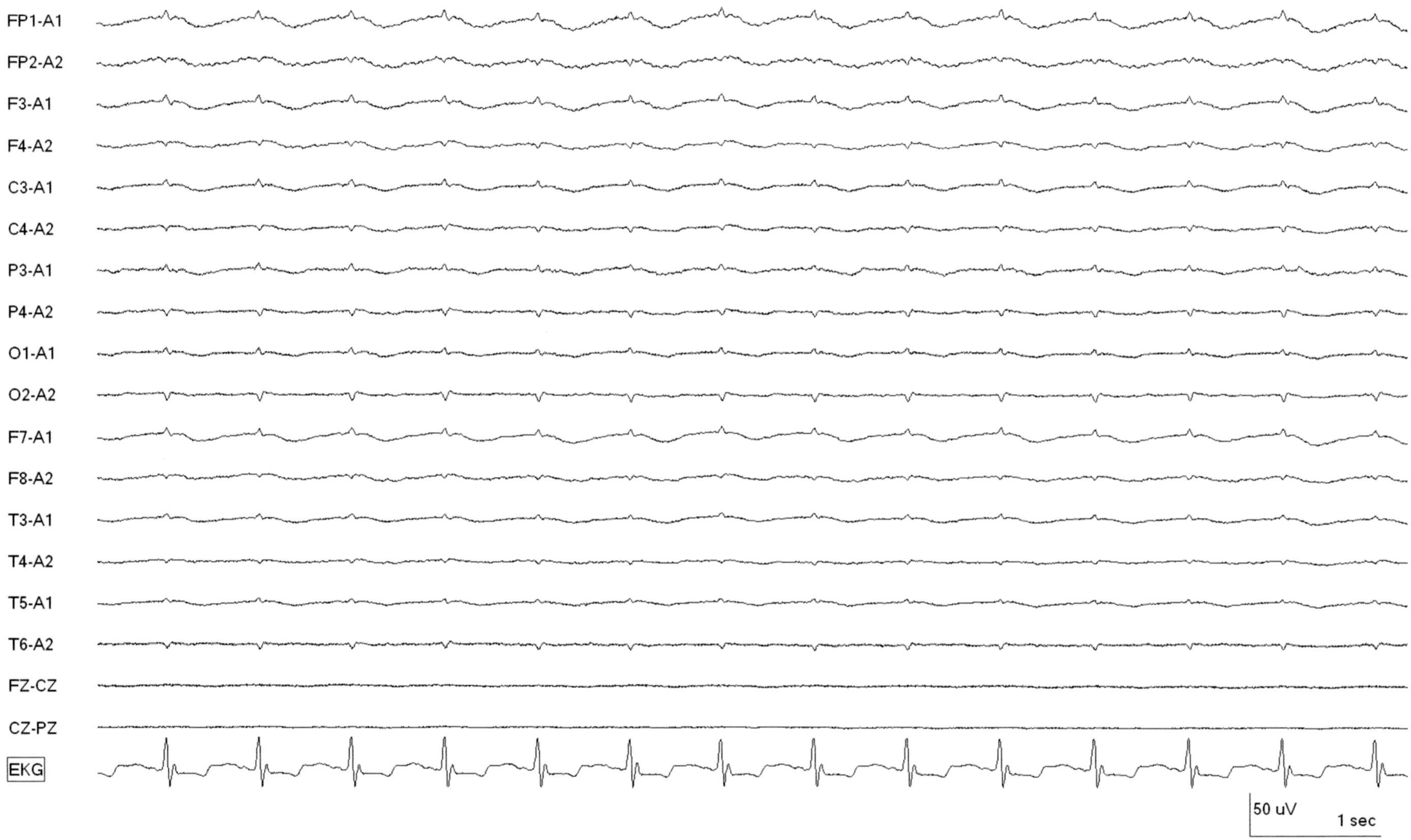

Figure 6.18 Cardioballistic artifact. Rhythmic delta activity is present in a widespread distribution. This represents a cardioballistic artifact (head movement with each pulse) in a 62-year-old man being evaluated for brain death. The slow waves have a fixed relationship to the QRS complex.

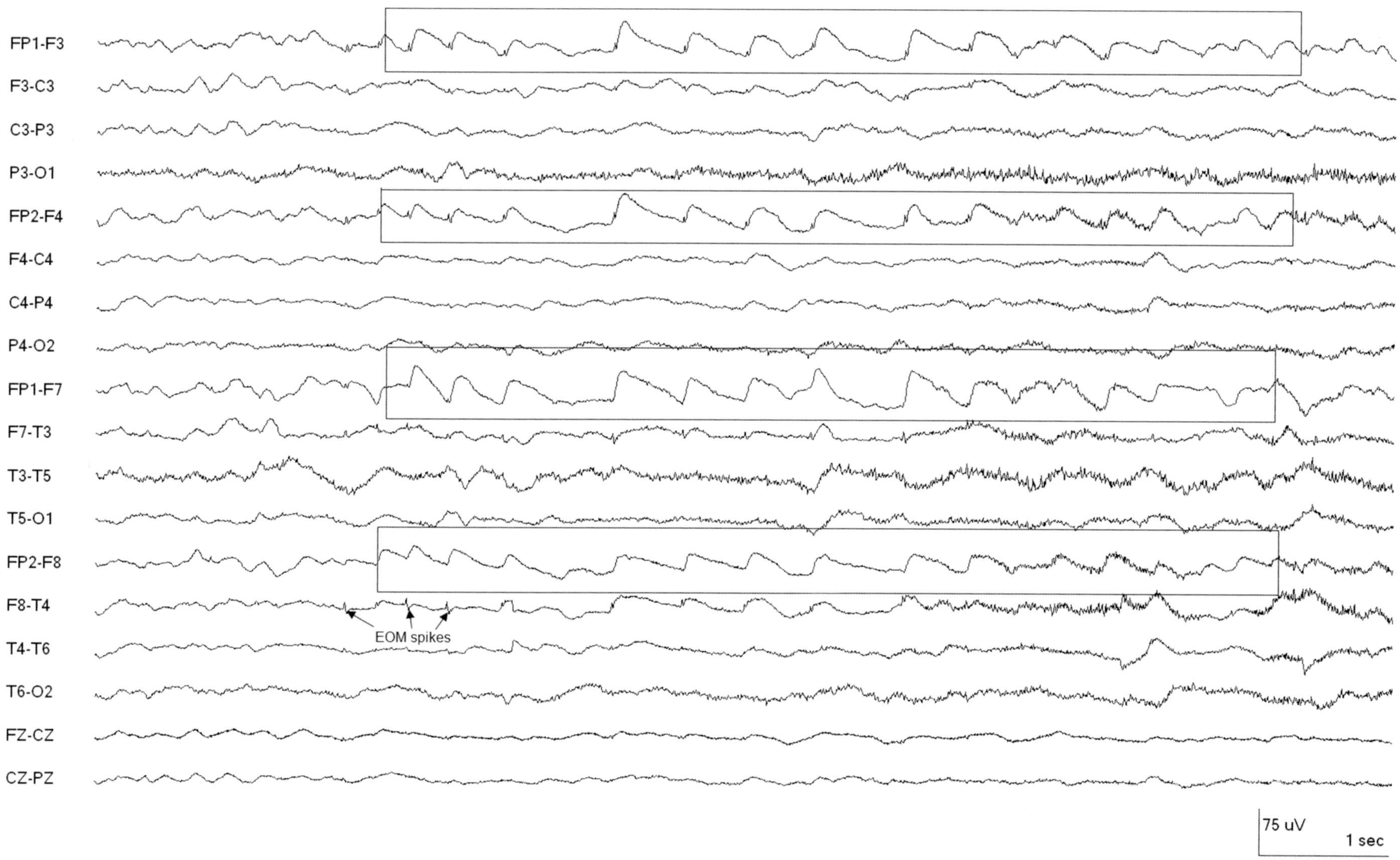

Figure 6.19 Vertical nystagmus. The prominent feature in this 65-year-old man with an intracerebral hemorrhage is the slowing in the frontal electrodes (boxes). This activity has a very steep field and is consistent with vertical eye movement, although rarely cerebral activity may have a similar field. In this case, the eye movements have a quick phase, at which time electrodes Fp1 and Fp2 become surface negative, indicating a downward eye deflection (the positive cornea moving away from Fp1 and Fp2). Following this, there is a slower return. In addition, small extraocular muscle spikes (arrows) can be seen at the start of most of these discharges, particularly in F8-T4. These movements represent downbeat nystagmus.

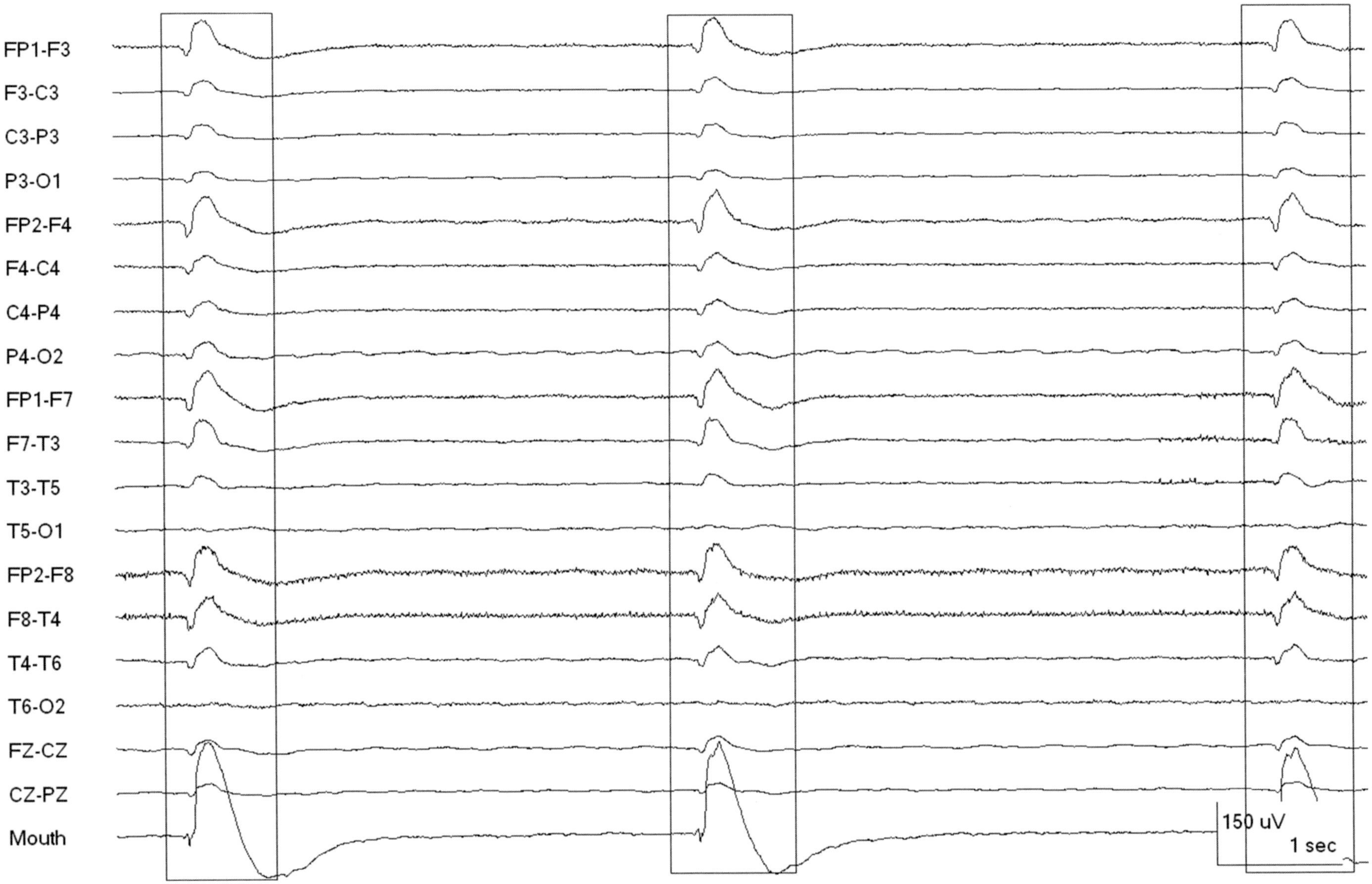

Figure 6.20 Respirator artifact. The EEG in this 84-year-old woman shows regular repetitive bursts of slow waves (boxes). This activity does not represent widely spaced periodic discharges or a burst-suppression pattern, but was due to respirator artifact, as demonstrated in the electrodes placed about the mouth.

7 Prolonged EEG monitoring and quantitative EEG techniques for detecting seizures and ischemia

Due to technical advances and increased awareness of the high prevalence of nonconvulsive seizures (see Chapter 3, Introduction), prolonged EEG recording in the critically ill is rapidly increasing in use. It is clear that the majority of seizures in the intensive care unit (ICU) are nonconvulsive and can only be recognized with EEG. It is also clear that it is quite labor-intensive to review these studies. Quantitative EEG (QEEG) techniques have helped speed this up. Although many are intimidated by these techniques, they are actually quite simple in principle and easy to learn. As software programs have improved, QEEG has become more and more useful. Not only can seizures be detected, but also other acute brain events, such as ischemia, hydrocephalus, hemorrhage and so on. Several existing software programs enable alarms to be set and, theoretically, allow true real-time monitoring once the infrastructure has been put in place and someone is available to respond to alarms and interpret the study (currently a rare scenario). In the not too distant future, this type of real-time monitoring or 'neurotelemetry' will be available in many centers, akin to cardiac telemetry today. This chapter describes many of the QEEG techniques that can aid in review of prolonged EEGs.

After covering the basics of QEEG, this chapter includes examples of intracranial EEG recordings in the ICU via subdural strips or intraparenchymal 'depth' electrodes. These electrodes can detect seizure activity that is otherwise not visible on the scalp, can provide artifact-free recordings for real-time monitoring, can help clarify equivocal patterns seen on the scalp and can detect peri-injury depolarization (PIDs). Peri-injury depolarizations are related to cortical spreading depression and seem to be very common in acute brain injury, including ischemia, trauma and hemorrhages. Similar to seizures, they seem to contribute to secondary neuronal injury and are potentially treatable or preventable. Finally, examples of the use of EEG as part of multimodality monitoring with a variety of invasive monitoring techniques are shown. This type of multimodal monitoring is now part of standard care in many neurological/neurosurgical ICUs.

Figure List

Figures 7.1–7.10 Quantitative EEG (QEEG) basics

Figure 7.1 Introduction to spectral arrays/spectrograms: multiple seizures.

Figure 7.2 Spectrogram basics: muscle artifact and state changes.

Figure 7.3 Spectrogram basics: muscle artifact and effect of paralytic.

Figure 7.4 Spectrogram basics: state changes and alpha rhythm.

Figure 7.5 Spectrogram basics: mechanical artifact–bed oscillator.

Atlas of EEG in Critical Care Lawrence J. Hirsch and Richard P. Brenner

Figure 7.6 QEEG basics: unilateral ischemia and basics of symmetry measures.

Figure 7.7 QEEG basics: normal study with state changes, including basics of amplitude-integrated EEG (aEEG).

Figure 7.8 QEEG basics: asymmetry, breach, rhythmic run detector, and aEEG 'false positives'.

Figure 7.9 QEEG basics: pentobarbital bolus and mechanical artifact with harmonics.

Figure 7.10 QEEG basics: multiple seizures and identical-appearing false positives on amplitude-integrated EEG.

Figures 7.11–7.17 Basics of seizure detection

Figure 7.11 Bilateral independent seizures.

Figure 7.12 Multiple seizures arising from complete suppression.

Figure 7.13 Nonconvulsive status epilepticus culminating with convulsion.

Figure 7.14 Nonconvulsive status epilepticus.

Figure 7.15 Nonconvulsive status epilepticus with gradual onset and offset.

Figure 7.16 Breach and highly focal nonconvulsive seizure, sometimes with spread.

Figure 7.17 Evolving nonconvulsive seizures and rhythmic run detector.

Figures 7.18–7.21 Cyclic seizures and PLEDs

Figure 7.18 Cyclic nonconvulsive seizures.

Figure 7.19 Cyclic nonconvulsive seizures.

Figure 7.20 Cyclic 'ping-pong' seizures.

Figure 7.21 Cyclic PLEDs

Figures 7.22–7.25 Other QEEG techniques and uses in patients with seizures

Figure 7.22 Pentobarbital coma, suppression-burst, depth electrode and QEEG alarms.

Figure 7.23 Glucose load effect in glucose transporter deficiency.

Figure 7.24 Envelope trend analysis for neonatal seizure recognition.

Figure 7.25 Envelope (amplitude) trending: multiple seizures in an adult.

Figures 7.26–7.31 Detecting other (non-seizure) events

Figure 7.26 Multimodality monitoring for vasospasm after subarachnoid hemorrhage (SAH); alpha-delta ratio.

Figure 7.27 CO_2 retention, acidosis and resolution of nonconvulsive seizures.

Figure 7.28 Hydrocephalus and multiple QEEG alarms.

Figure 7.29 Detecting delayed cerebral ischemia after subarachnoid hemorrhage, including setting alarms and use of depth electrode.

Figure 7.30 Brain symmetry index during carotid clamping.

Figure 7.31 Brain symmetry index and seizures.

Figures 7.32–7.35 Long-term trends

Figure 7.32 Long-term trends: wearing off of pentobarbital.

Figure 7.33 Long-term trends: worsening of nonconvulsive status epilepticus (NCSE); ictal-interictal continuum.

Figure 7.34 Long-term trends: gradual resolution of nonconvulsive status epilepticus (NCSE), ictal-interictal continuum and bilateral independent PLEDs (BIPLEDs).

Figure 7.35 Long-term trends: patient death.

Figures 7.36–7.46 ICU artifacts

Figure 7.36 Ventilator artifact.

Figure 7.37 Chest percussion artifact.

Figure 7.38 Chest percussion artifact.

Figure 7.39 Chest percussion artifact.

Figure 7.40 Chewing (glossokinetic) artifact.

Figure 7.41 'Pseudoalpha' artifact.

Figure 7.42 'Virtual'or disconnected patient.

Figure 7.43 'Virtual' or disconnected patient.

Figure 7.44 Wearing off of paralytic; shivering artifact.

Figure 7.45 Drug-induced beta and asymmetry.

Figure 7.46 Artifact mimicking seizures on amplitude-integrated EEG (aEEG).

Figures 7.47–7.48 Spreading depression/peri-injury depolarizations

Figure 7.47 Electrocorticogram (ECoG) of cortical spreading depression of Leão (CSD) in the human brain.

Figure 7.48 Electrocorticogram (ECoG) of periinjury depolarisations (PIDs) in the human brain.

Figures 7.49–7.54 Multimodality monitoring and intracranial EEG in the ICU

Figure 7.49 Multimodality monitoring of hemorrhagic transformation of a large infarct, including with depth electrode.

Figure 7.50 Multimodality monitoring of seizures on intracranial EEG after meperidine bolus.

Figure 7.51 Seizures and periodic discharges on intracranial EEG only.

Figure 7.52 Cyclic seizures on intracranial EEG only.

Figure 7.53 Multimodality monitoring after traumatic brain injury, including depth electrode.

Figure 7.54 Ictal-appearing SIRPIDs on intracranial EEG only.

Suggested Reading

Abend, N.S., Dlugos, D. and Herman, S. (2008) Neonatal seizure detection using multichannel display of envelope trend. *Epilepsia* **49**(2), 349–352.

Claassen, J., Hirsch, L.J., Kreiter, K. *et al.* (2004) Quantitative continuous EEG for detecting delayed cerebral ischemia in subarachnoid hemorrhage. *Journal of Clinical Neurophysiology* **115**, 2699–2710.

Claassen, J., Mayer, S.A., Kowalski, R.G. *et al.* (2004) Detection of electrographic seizures with continuous EEG monitoring in critically ill patients. *Neurology* **62**(10), 1743–1748.

Claassen, J., Hirsch, L.J., Frontera, J.A. *et al.* (2006) Prognostic significance of continuous EEG monitoring in patients with poor grade subarachnoid hemorrhage. *Neurocritical Care* **4**(2), 103–112.

Claassen, J., Jette, N., Chum, F. *et al.* (2007) Electrographic seizures and periodic discharges after intracerebral hemorrhage. *Neurology* **69**(13), 1356–1365.

DeLorenzo, R.J., Waterhouse, E.J., Towne, A.R. *et al.* (1998) Persistent nonconvulsive status epilepticus after the control of convulsive status epilepticus. *Epilepsia* **39**(8), 833–840.

de Vos, C.C., van Maarseveen, S.M., Brouwers, P.J. *et al.* (2008) Continuous EEG monitoring during thrombolysis in acute hemispheric stroke patients using the brain symmetry index. *Journal of Clinical Neurophysiology* **25**(2), 77–82.

Dohmen, C., Sakowitz, O.W., Fabricius, M. *et al.* (2008) Co-Operative Study of Brain Injury Depolarisations (COSBID). Spreading depolarizations occur in human ischemic stroke with high incidence. *Annals of Neurology* **63**(6), 720–728.

Dreier, J.P., Woitzik, J., Fabricius, M. *et al.* (2006) Delayed ischaemic neurological deficits after subarachnoid haemorrhage are associated with clusters of spreading depolarizations. *Brain* **129**(Pt 12), 3224–3237.

Fabricius, M., Fuhr, S., Bhatia, R. *et al.* (2006) Cortical spreading depression and peri-infarct depolarization in acutely injured human cerebral cortex. *Brain* **129**(Pt 3), 778–790.

Fabricius, M., Fuhr, S., Willumsen, L. *et al.* (2008) Association of seizures with cortical spreading depression and peri-infarct depolarisations in the acutely injured human brain. *Journal of Clinical Neurophysiology*. **119**(9), 1973–1984.

Friedman, D.E., Schevon, C., Emerson, R.G. *et al.* (2008) Cyclic electrographic seizures in critically ill patients. *Epilepsia* **49**(2), 281–287.

Friedman, D. and Hirsch, L.J. EEG monitoring in the ICU – indications and interpretation. *Anesthesia and Analgesia*.

Hirsch, L.J. (2004) Brain monitoring: the next frontier of ICU monitoring. *Journal of Clinical Neurophysiology* **21**, 305–306.

Hirsch, L.J., Claassen, J., Mayer, S.A. *et al.* (2004) Stimulus-induced rhythmic, periodic, or ictal discharges (SIRPIDs): a common EEG phenomenon in the critically ill. *Epilepsia* **45**, 109–123.

Hirsch, L.J., Brenner, R.P., Drislane, F.W. *et al.* (2005) The ACNS Subcommittee on Research Terminology for Continuous EEG Monitoring: Proposed standardized terminology for rhythmic and periodic EEG patterns encountered in critically ill patients. *Journal of Clinical Neurophysiology* **22**, 128–135.

Hirsch, L.J., Pang, T., Claassen, J. *et al.* (2008) Focal motor seizures induced by alerting stimuli in critically ill patients. *Epilepsia* **49**, 968–973.

Jette, N., Claassen, J., Emerson, R.G. *et al.* (2006) Frequency and predictors of nonconvulsive seizures during continuous electroencephalographic monitoring in critically ill children. *Archives of Neurology* **63**(12), 1750–1755.

Jirsch, J. and Hirsch, L.J. (2007) Nonconvulsive seizures: developing a rational approach to the diagnosis and management in the critically ill population. *Journal of Clinical Neurophysiology*. **118**(8), 1660–1670.

Jordan, K.G. (1993) Continuous EEG and evoked potential monitoring in the neuroscience intensive care unit. *Journal of Clinical Neurophysiology* **10**(4), 445–475.

Jordan, K.G. (1995) Neurophysiologic monitoring in the neuroscience intensive care unit. *Neurology Clinic* **13**(3), 579–626.

Jordan, K.G. (2004) Emergency EEG and continuous EEG monitoring in acute ischemic stroke. *Journal of Clinical Neurophysiology*. **21**(5), 341–352.

Leão, A.A.P. (1944) Spreading depression of activity in the cerebral cortex. *Journal of Neurophysiology* **7**(6), 359–390 .

Oddo, M., Carrera, E., Claassen, J. *et al.* (2009) Continuous electroencephalography in the medical intensive care unit. *Critical Care Medicine* **37**(6), 2051–2056.

Pandian, J.D., Cascino, G.D., So, E.L. *et al.* (2004) Digital video-electroencephalographic monitoring in the neurological-neurosurgical intensive care unit: clinical features and outcome. *Archives of Neurology* **61**(7), 1090–1094.

Privitera,, M., Hoffman,, M., Moore, J.L. *et al.* (1994) EEG detection of nontonic-clonic status epilepticus in patients with altered consciousness. *Epilepsy Research* **18**(2), 155–166.

Scheuer, M.L. and Wilson, S.B. (2004) Data analysis for continuous EEG monitoring in the ICU: Seeing the forest and the trees. *Journal of Clinical Neurophysiology*. **21**(5), 353–378.

Shah, D.K., Mackay, M.T., Lavery, S. *et al.* (2008) Accuracy of bedside electroencephalographic monitoring in comparison with simultaneous continuous conventional electroencephalography for seizure detection in term infants. *Pediatrics* **121**(6), 1146–1154.

Shellhaas, R.A., Soaita, A.I. and Clancy, R.R. (2007) Sensitivity of amplitude-integrated electroencephalography for neonatal seizure detection. *Pediatrics* **120**(4), 770–777.

Strong, A.J., Anderson, P.J., Watts, H.R. *et al.* (2007) Peri-infarct depolarizations lead to loss of perfusion in ischaemic gyrencephalic cerebral cortex. *Brain* **130**(Pt 4), 995–1008.

Toet, M.C., Van Der Meij, W., de Vries, L.S. I. *et al.* (2002) Comparison between simultaneously recorded amplitude integrated electroencephalogram (cerebral function monitor) and standard electroencephalogram in neonates. *Pediatrics* **109**(5), 772–779.

Towne, A.R., Waterhouse, E.J., Boggs, J.G. *et al.* (2000) Prevalence of nonconvulsive status epilepticus in comatose patients. *Neurology* **54**(2), 340–345.

van Putten,, M.J. (2006) Extended BSI for continuous EEG monitoring in carotid endarterectomy. *Journal of Clinical Neurophysiology* **117**(12), 2661–2666.

van Putten, M.J. (2007) The revised brain symmetry index. *Journal of Clinical Neurophysiology*. **118**(11), 2362–2367.

van Putten, M.J. and Tavy, D.L. (2004) Continuous quantitative EEG monitoring in hemispheric stroke patients using the brain symmetry index. *Stroke* **35**(11), 2489–2492.

Vespa, P. (2005) Continuous EEG monitoring for the detection of seizures in traumatic brain injury, infarction, and intracerebral hemorrhage: 'to detect and protect'. *Journal of Clinical Neurophysiology* **22**(2), 99–106.

Vespa, P. (2006) Continuous electroencephalography for subarachnoid hemorrhage has come of age. *Neurocritical Care* **4**(2), 99–100.

Vespa, P.M., Nuwer, M.R., Juhász, C. *et al.* (1997) Early detection of vasospasm after acute subarachnoid hemorrhage using continuous EEG ICU monitoring. *Electroencephalography and Clinical Neurophysiology*. **103**(6), 607–615.

Vespa, P.M., Nuwer, M.R., Nenov, V. *et al.* (1999) Increased incidence and impact of nonconvulsive and convulsive seizures after traumatic brain injury as detected by continuous electroencephalographic monitoring. *Journal of Neurosurgery* **91**(5), 750–760.

Vespa, P.M., O'Phelan, K., Shah, M. *et al.* (2003) Acute seizures after intracerebral hemorrhage: a factor in progressive midline shift and outcome. *Neurology* **60**(9), 1441–1446.

Vespa, P.M., Miller, C., McArthur, D. *et al.* (2007) Nonconvulsive electrographic seizures after traumatic brain injury result in a delayed, prolonged increase in intracranial pressure and metabolic crisis. *Critical Care Medicine* **35**(12), 2830–2836.

Waziri, A., Claassen, J., Stuart, R.M. *et al.* (2009) Intracortical EEG in acute brain injury. *Annals of Neurology* in press.

Wittman, J.J. Jr. and Hirsch, L.J. (2005) Continuous electroencephalogram monitoring in the critically ill. *Neurocritical Care*. **2**(3), 330–341.

Young, G.B., Jordan, K.G. and Doig, G.S. (1996) An assessment of nonconvulsive seizures in the intensive care unit using continuous EEG monitoring: an investigation of variables associated with mortality. *Neurology* **47**(1), 83–89.

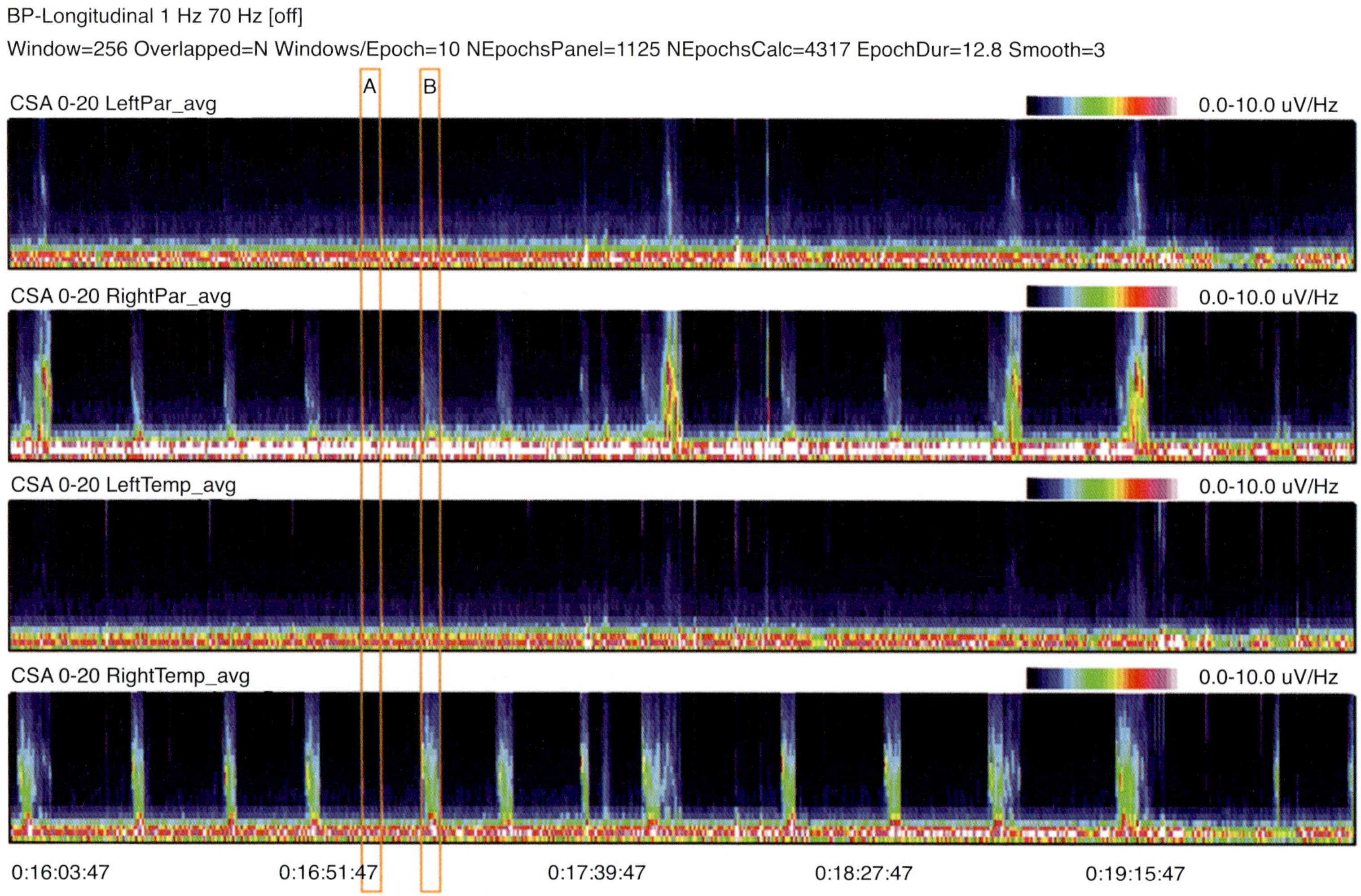

Figure 7.1 Introduction to spectral arrays/spectrograms: multiple seizures. **Main:** Four hours of EEG in a young woman with a leukodystrophy and intractable nonconvulsive seizures. This quantitative EEG (QEEG) sample shows time along the *x*-axis (4 h shown), frequency on the *y*-axis (0–20 Hz) and power in the *z*-axis, with power shown on a color scale where the highest power is white, followed by lavender, pink and red (see color scales in the upper right of each panel). Power is simply a calculation of the total 'amount' (based on amplitude) of a given frequency. To make these types of calculations, the EEG undergoes fast fourier transformation (FFT), a mathematical technique that breaks up the EEG signal into its components based on frequency. There are four panels (rows) shown in this example, representing different electrode chains (left parasagittal, right parasagittal, left temporal and right temporal); this is essentially the QEEG montage. Most power is near the bottom in the delta range for most of the tracing. There are intermittent bursts of power in higher frequencies on the right, usually maximal in the temporal region; one example is shown in (b). These represent seizures, although review of the raw EEG at that point is necessary to confirm this. QEEG should never be interpreted without reviewing portions of the original waveforms as well. This three-dimensional type of display is called a *density spectral array*, although it is commonly referred to by its two-dimensional counterpart term, *compressed spectral array* (CSA). It is also known as a *'spectrogram'*. **(a)** EEG at A: baseline, showing diffuse delta activity. **(b)** EEG at B: right temporal seizure (box).

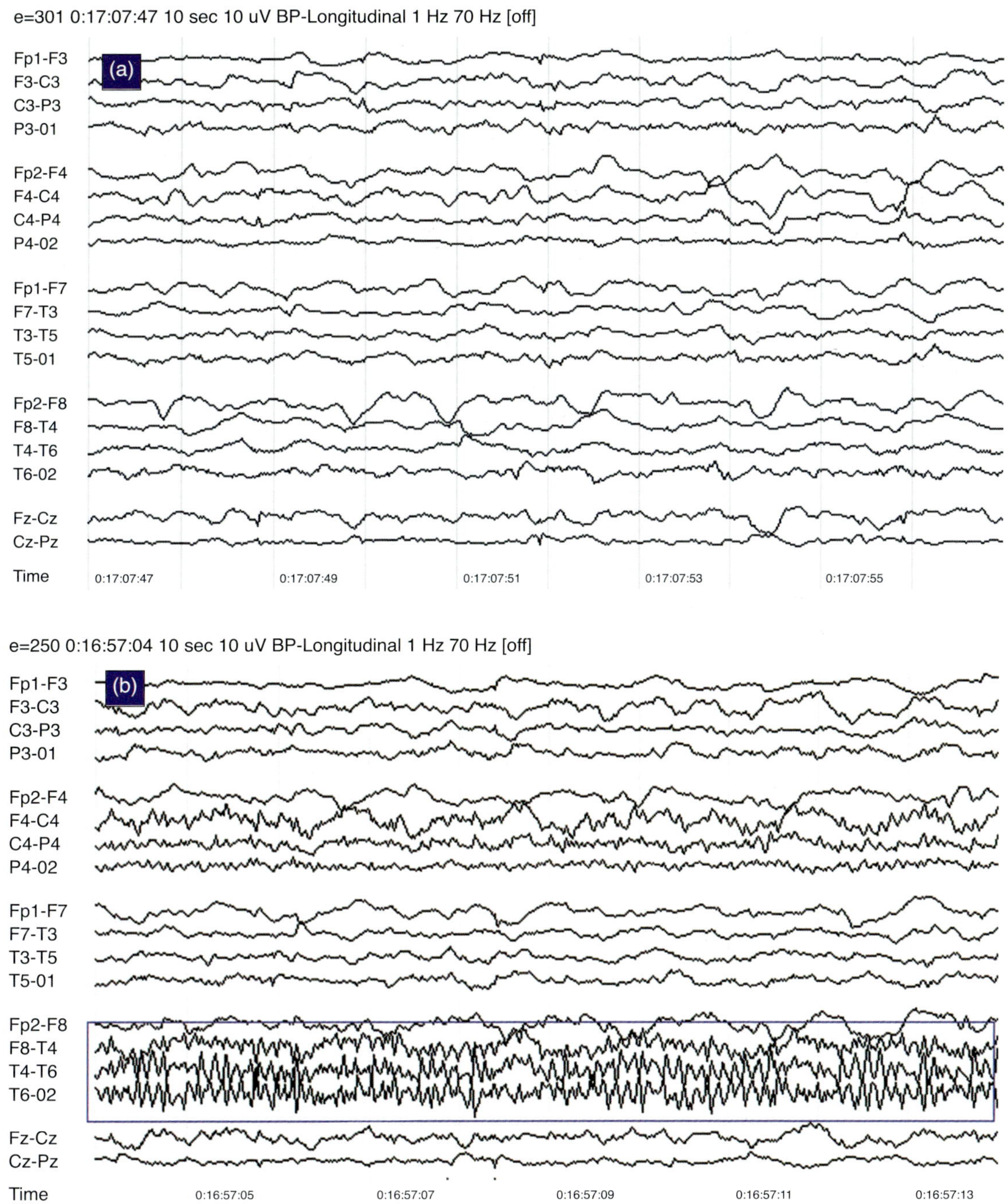
e=301 0:17:07:47 10 sec 10 uV BP-Longitudinal 1 Hz 70 Hz [off]
(a)
Fp1-F3
F3-C3
C3-P3
P3-01
Fp2-F4
F4-C4
C4-P4
P4-02
Fp1-F7
F7-T3
T3-T5
T5-01
Fp2-F8
F8-T4
T4-T6
T6-02
Fz-Cz
Cz-Pz
Time
0:17:07:47
0:17:07:49
0:17:07:51
0:17:07:53
0:17:07:55
e=250 0:16:57:04 10 sec 10 uV BP-Longitudinal 1 Hz 70 Hz [off]
(b)
Fp1-F3
F3-C3
C3-P3
P3-01
Fp2-F4
F4-C4
C4-P4
P4-02
Fp1-F7
F7-T3
T3-T5
T5-01
Fp2-F8
F8-T4
T4-T6
T6-02
Fz-Cz
Cz-Pz
Time
0:16:57:05
0:16:57:07
0:16:57:09
0:16:57:11
0:16:57:13

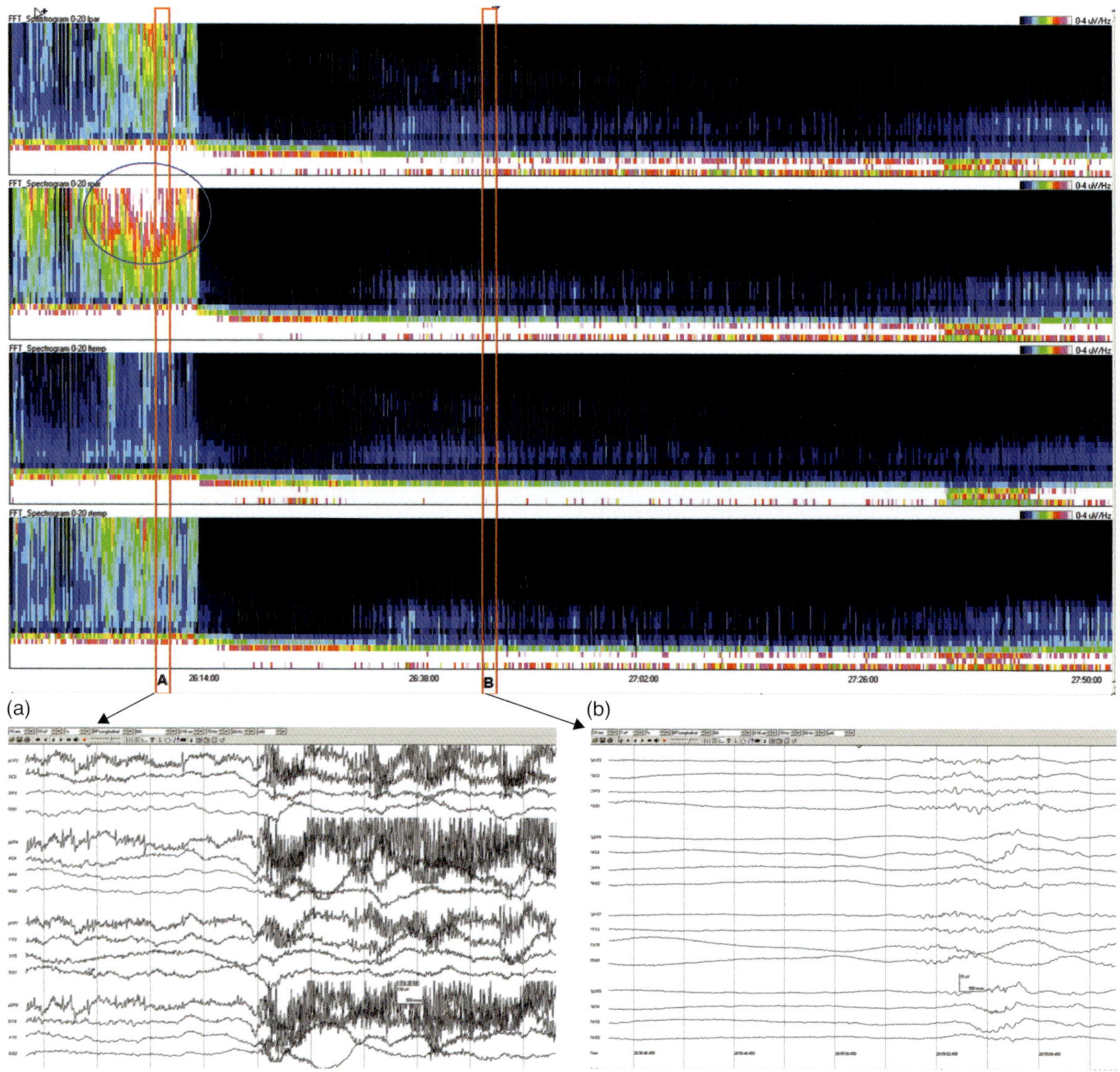

Figure 7.2 Spectrogram basics: muscle artifact and state changes. **Main:** Two hours of EEG showing an initial period with prominent muscle artifact, maximal in the right parasagittal region (circle). Muscle artifact on a spectrogram tends to appear as if it is coming down from the top of the tracing, as in this example, since it is usually composed primarily of frequencies greater than those being displayed (>20 Hz in this example). A sample of EEG during this time period is shown in A. There is then a period with no muscle artifact and with most power in the lower frequencies, corresponding to sleep. **(a)** EEG at A: awake recording with prominent muscle artifact, maximal in the right parasagittal region as seen on the spectrogram. **(b)** EEG at B: sleep recording with no muscle artifact.

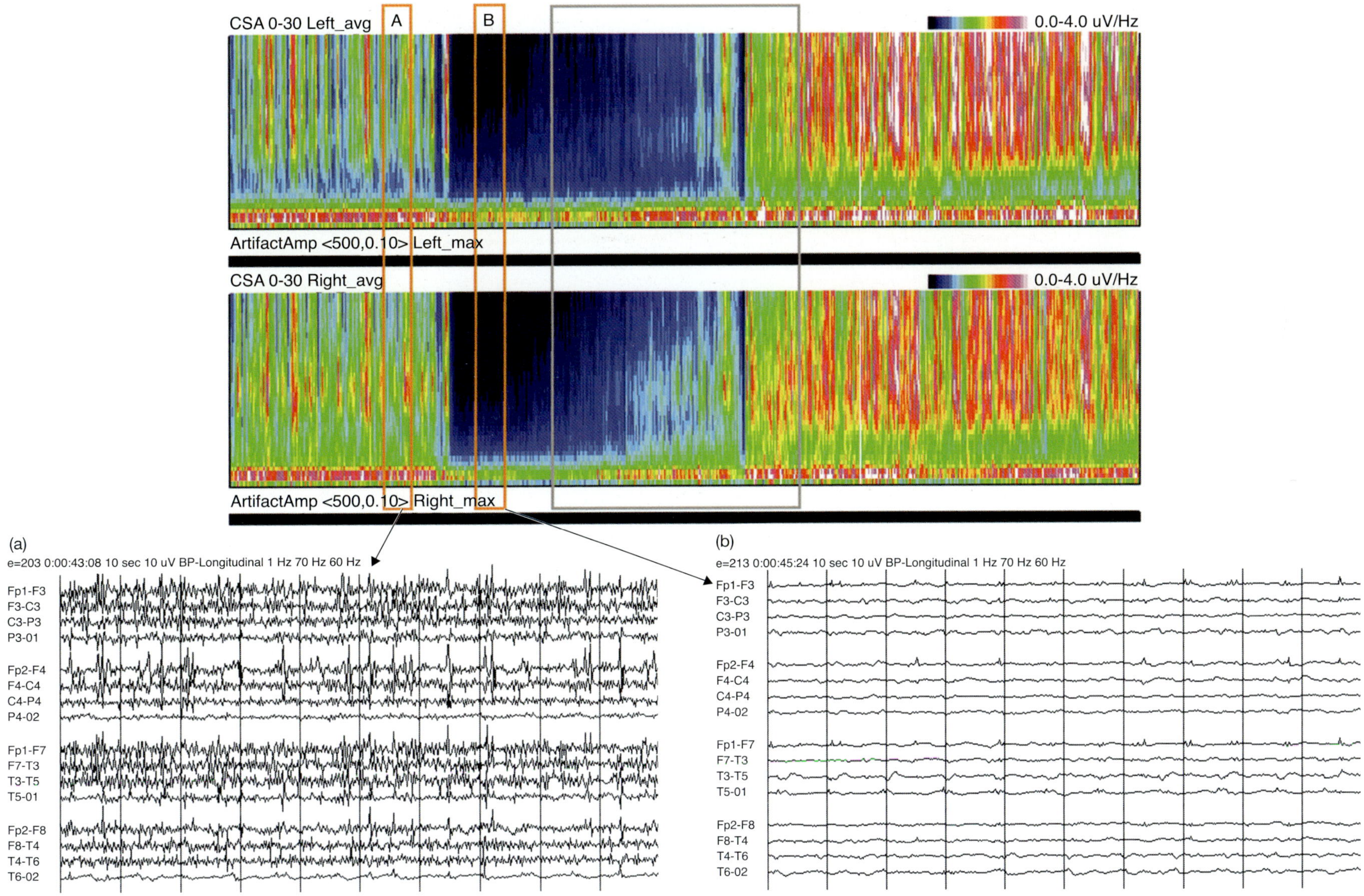

Figure 7.3 Spectrogram basics: muscle artifact and effect of paralytic. **Main:** Four hours of EEG. There is prominent muscle artifact (A), followed by administration of a paralytic. One can then appreciate that the background EEG is composed only of slow frequencies (B). Gradual wearing off of the paralytic can then be appreciated (gray box), with gradual re-appearance of the muscle artifact. This slow change over an hour or more is easier to appreciate on a compressed QEEG tracing such as a spectrogram than on the raw EEG. Note that the muscle artifact appears to come down from the top of the tracing as usual. **(a)** EEG at A: prominent muscle artifact. **(b)** EEG at B: no muscle artifact. Diffuse attenuation and slowing can now be appreciated.

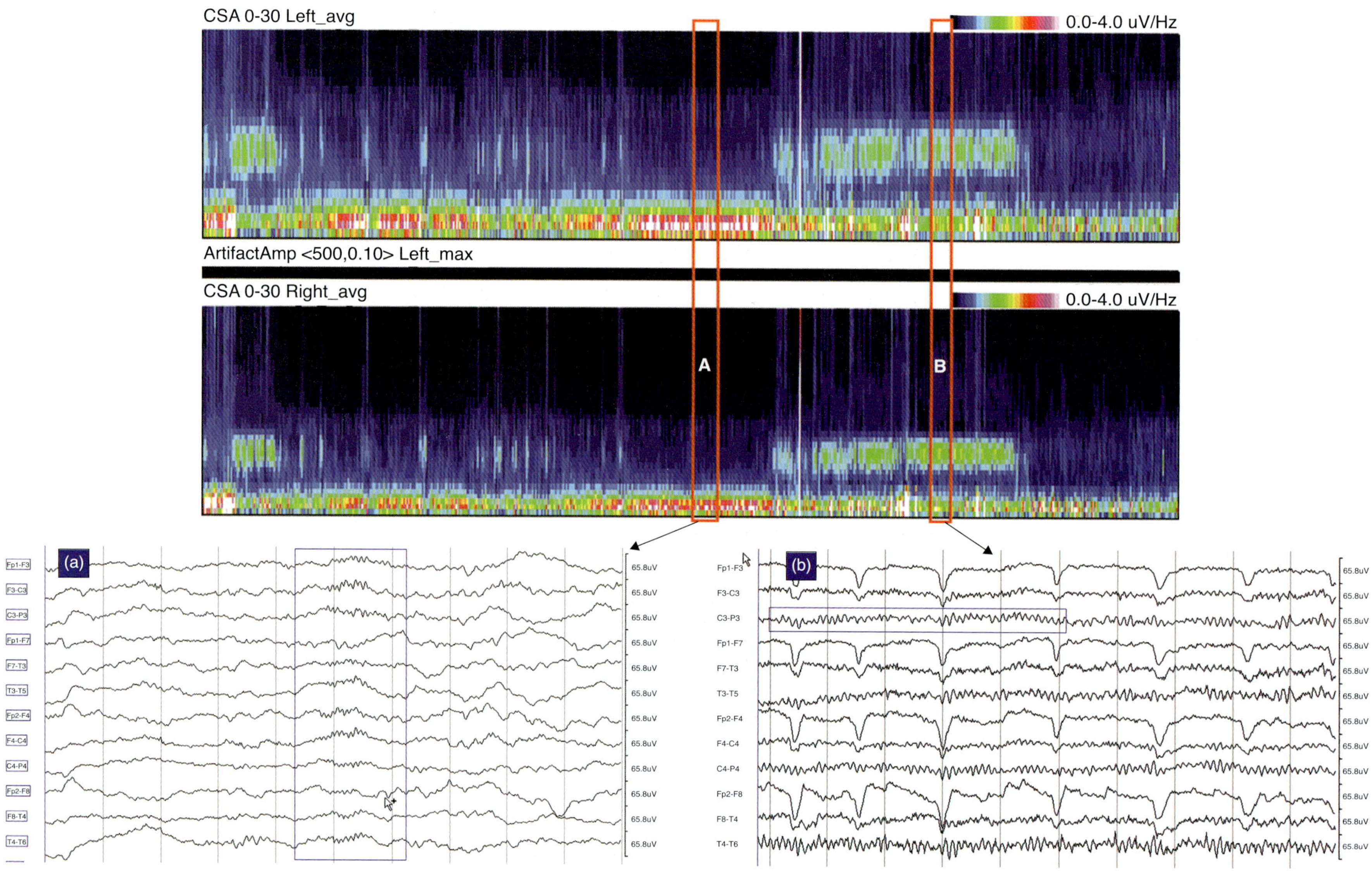

Figure 7.4 Spectrogram basics: state changes and alpha rhythm. **Main:** Four hours of normal EEG. While the patient is asleep (A), most power is in the delta frequency. While awake (B), there is less delta (the white and red are no longer seen at the bottom of the tracings), and there is a prominent horizontal green band at ~10 Hz. The 10 Hz activity is due to the alpha rhythm (see raw EEG). **(a)** EEG at A: normal stage II sleep with a spindle shown in the box. **(b)** EEG at B: normal awake EEG with a 9.5–10 Hz alpha rhythm (box).

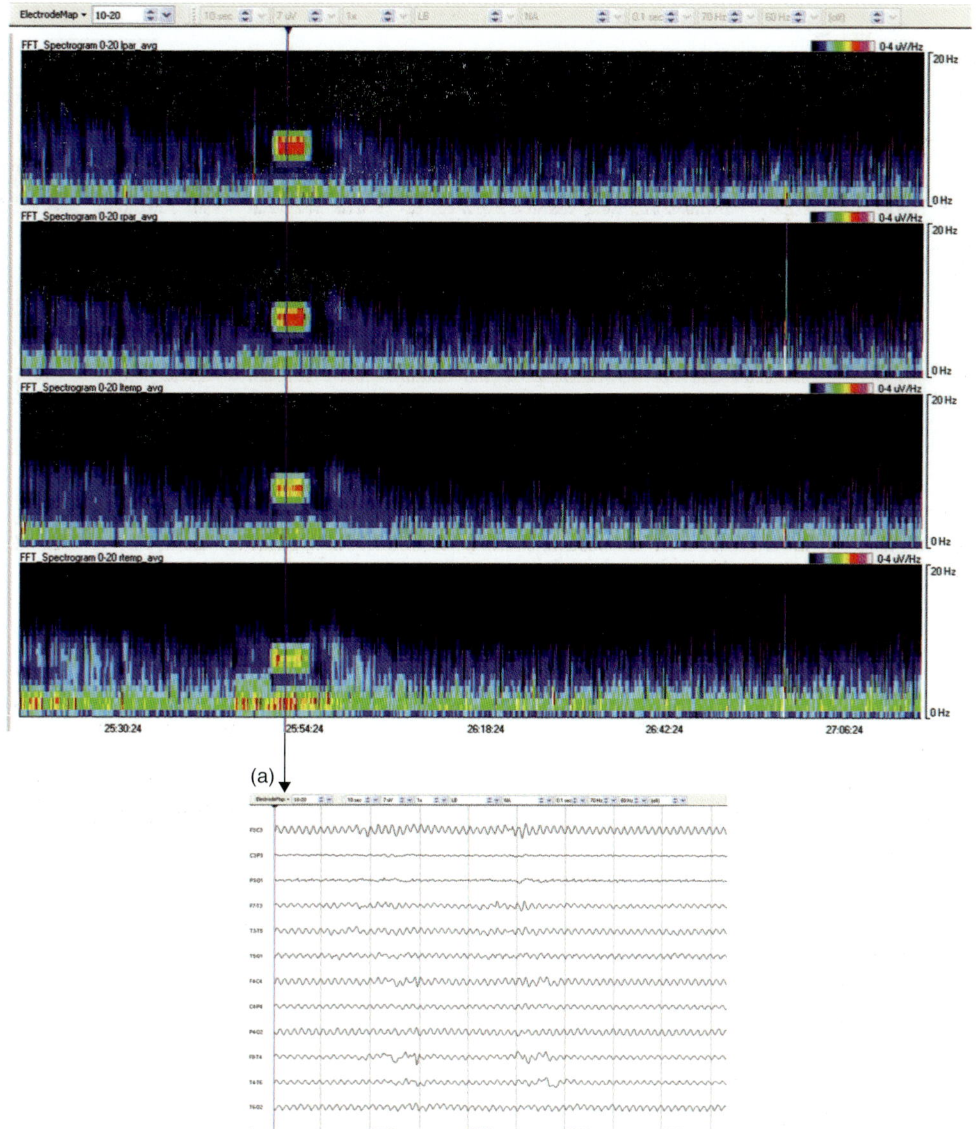

Figure 7.5 Spectrogram basics: mechanical artifact–bed oscillator. **Main:** Spectrogram showing 3 h of QEEG with diffuse slow activity (most activity delta with some theta). There is then a period lasting several minutes with sudden appearance of activity between 5 and 10 Hz, remaining constant, then stopping suddenly (cursor line is during this activity). This causes a square shape on the spectrogram. Raw EEG at that time shows widespread 7 Hz activity. This was caused by a vibrating bed. Sharp edges on a spectrogram and constant frequency activity with little change as seen in this example should raise suspicion of mechanical artifact. **(a)** EEG at line.

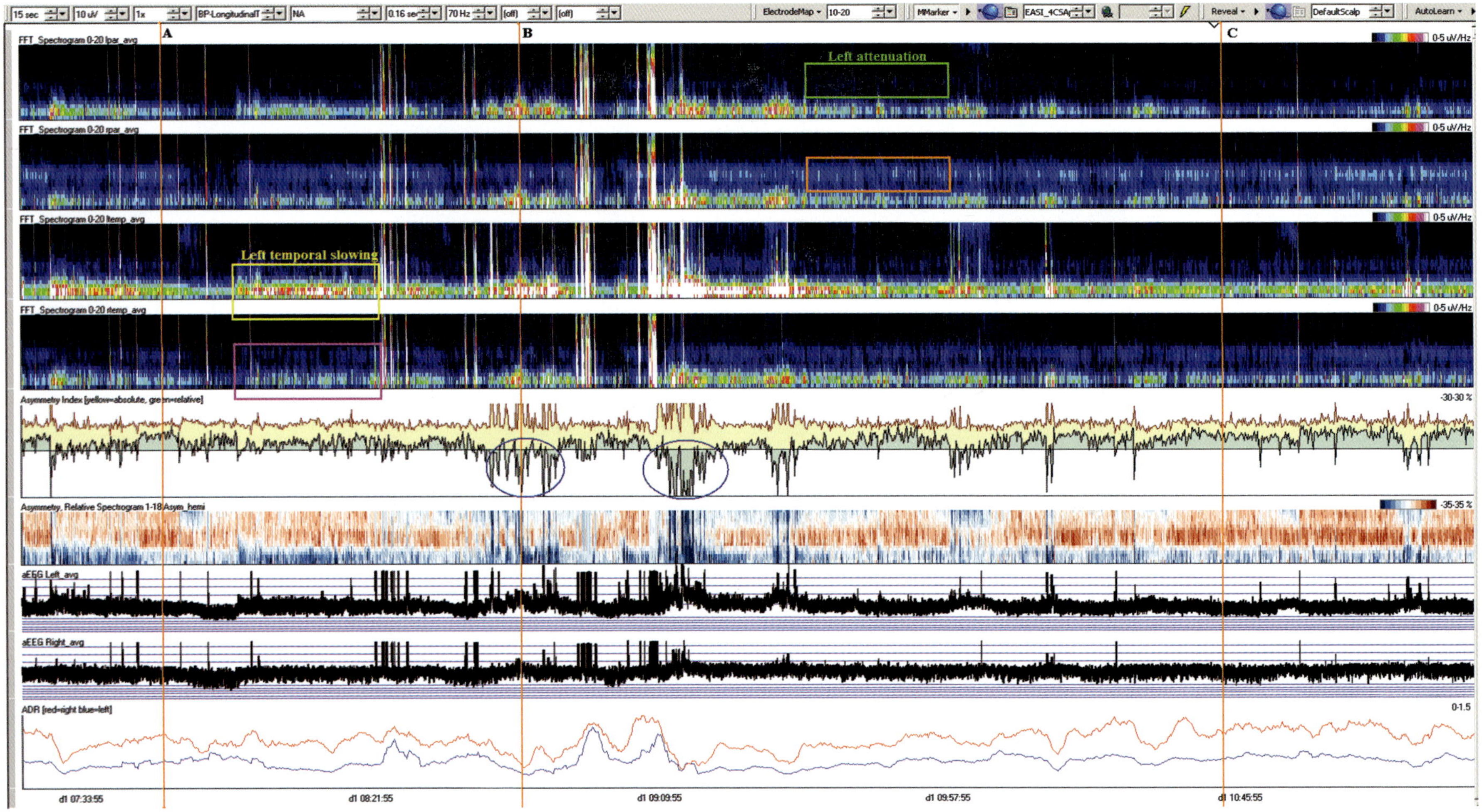

Figure 7.6 Quantitative EEG (QEEG) basics: Unilateral ischemia and basics of symmetry measures. **Main:** Four hours of QEEG in a middle-aged man with right hemiparesis after a left carotid endarterectomy. At the time of this study, postoperative CT and MRI had been unremarkable, but hemiparesis and neglect were marked and persistent, and EEG showed findings typical of cortical dysfunction from ischemia. No seizures occurred, clinically or on EEG. Repeat MRI days later showed widespread laminar necrosis. *Ischemia on spectrograms*: The first four panels (rows) show spectrograms from 0 to 20 Hz in the parasagittal and temporal regions. Left temporal slowing can be seen as higher delta power (yellow box, compared to pink box in right temporal region). Left hemisphere attenuation (decreased power) of faster frequencies, mainly affecting alpha frequencies, can be seen in the left parasagittal region (green box, compared to orange box on right). These findings can be seen on the raw EEG in C below. These are the classic findings with ischemia: loss of faster frequencies and increased slowing. *Ischemia on asymmetry measures*: The fifth and sixth panels measure symmetry. The asymmetry index shows total absolute asymmetry in yellow; this is calculated by comparing asymmetry at each pair of homologous electrodes and summing their absolute values to give a total asymmetry score; this can only be positive and upward on this display. This measure goes up with asymmetry in any frequency

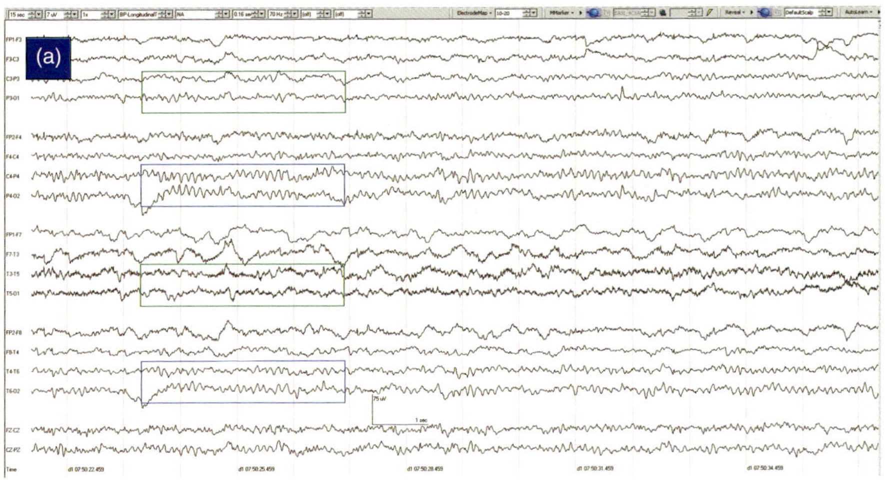

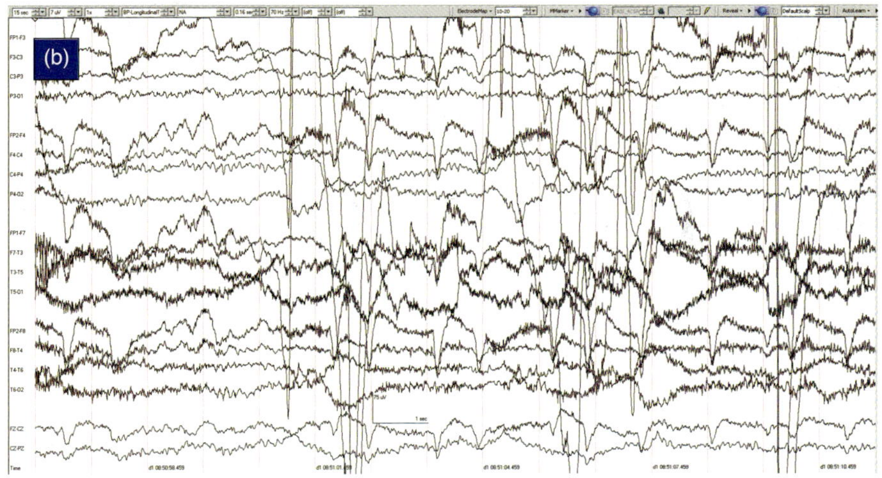

Figure 7.6 (*Continued*) or direction. The green relative asymmetry tracing is the same, but shows laterality: downgoing indicates more power on the left and upgoing on the right. Note in this case the green tracing is usually upgoing, suggesting more power on the right overall, although variable. The sixth panel in red and blue is an asymmetry spectrogram. It shows asymmetry at each frequency from 1 to 18 Hz averaged over the entire hemisphere. Red means more power on the right in that frequency. In this case the asymmetry spectrogram is much more useful than the total asymmetry measures in the fifth panel. It shows that higher frequencies (>∼6 Hz) are greater on the right (red) and slower frequencies (<∼4 Hz) are greater on the left (blue). This is the typical pattern with ischemia, although it is also seen with other processes that cause both increased slowing and attenuation of faster frequencies on one side. *Ischemia on alpha/delta ratio*: Since alpha frequencies decrease and delta increases with ischemia, the alpha/delta ratio is used to magnify this difference when looking for ischemia. The bottom panel shows the alpha/delta ratio (ADR) on each side (red = right). Note that the ADR is persistently higher on the right, suggesting ischemia on the left. The aEEG traces are amplitude-integrated EEG, which will be described in Figure 7.7c. **(a)** EEG at A: note the attenuation of faster frequencies in the left hemisphere, including the alpha rhythm (8 Hz and fairly well developed on the right, blue boxes; nearly absent on the left, green box). There is also continuous left temporal slowing. **(b)** EEG at B: this is at the point where there appears to be a switch in the

(continues on next page)

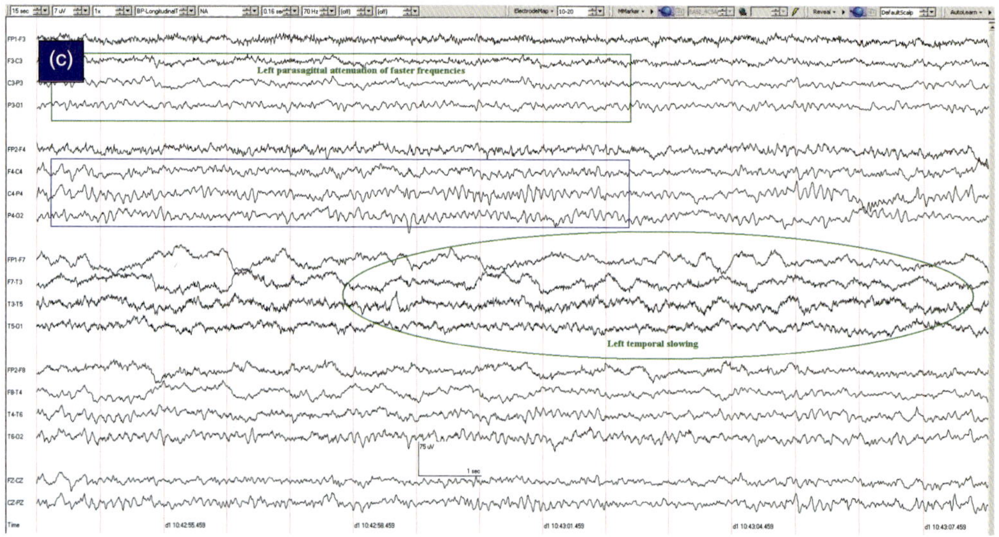

Figure 7.6 (*Continued*) direction of overall asymmetry, with the green relative symmetry trace going downward. Review of the raw EEG shows that this is due to movement artifact, most prominent in the left temporal region. This artifactual asymmetry can also be recognized by turning on artifact rejection, shown below in (d). **(c)** EEG at C: the raw EEG at a relatively random point shows the asymmetries already mentioned (labeled).

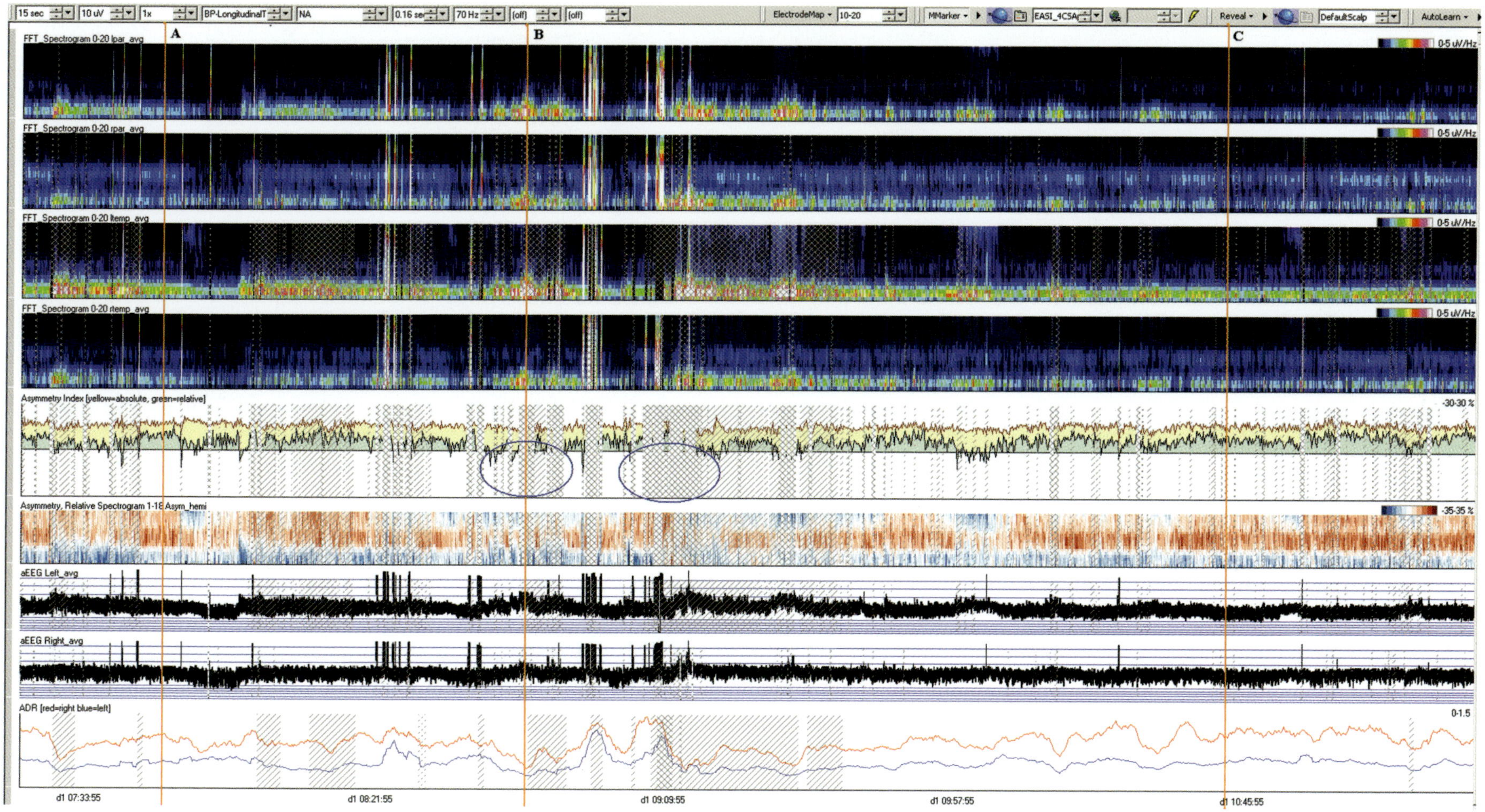

Figure 7.6 (*Continued*) QEEG with artifact rejection: the same QEEG is shown after applying artifact rejection. Software detects probable artifacts on each channel. If a channel has an artifact, it is removed from the QEEG calculation, but calculations continue on the other channels. If too many channels have to be removed, the artifact rejection display shows this with single-hatching (if two or more channels, but <25% of the total, have to be removed from the calculation), double hatching (if 25–50% of channels have to be removed) or blanking-out of the display completely if >50% of channels are removed. Note the areas in the blue circles on both versions of the QEEG: It is now clear that the apparent change in asymmetry on the green relative asymmetry tracing was all artifactual, as it is now simply blanked out since it was not a reliable calculation. Artifact rejection like this is crucial for allowing setting of alarms, as they can continue to function effectively even if a few electrodes are not functioning. This is also one reason to apply more electrodes than necessary: in order to allow continued monitoring when some of them get dislodged.

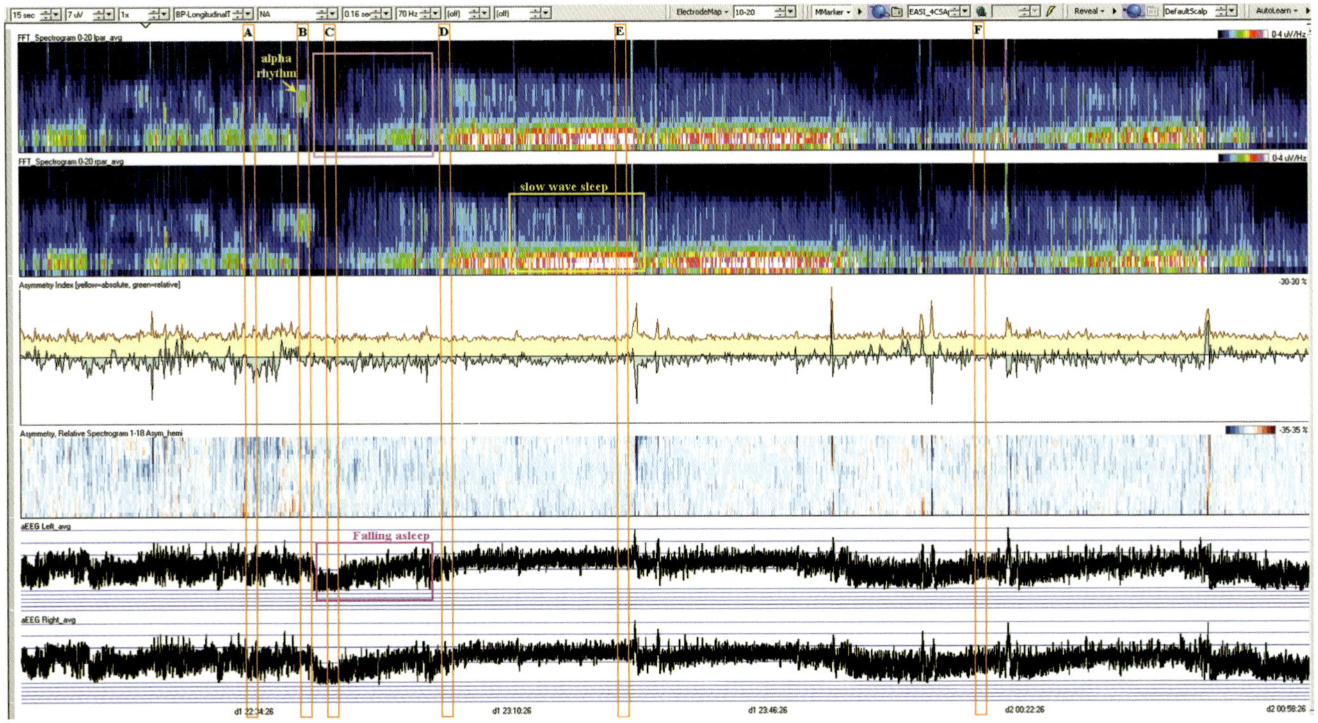

Figure 7.7 QEEG basics: normal study with state changes, including basics of amplitude-integrated EEG (aEEG). **Main:** Three hours of QEEG in a normal middle-aged man. Patient is awake at first (A and B), becomes drowsy (C), then falls asleep (magenta boxes), progressing from stage II (D) to slow-wave sleep (E and yellow box). **(a)** EEG at A: normal awake recording with eyes open. **(b)** EEG at B: eyes closed, with prominent alpha rhythm. Note the band appearing on the spectrogram around 9 Hz due to this activity (labeled 'alpha rhythm' on QEEG). Also note the lack of any delta power at this time to distinguish this pattern on the QEEG from sleep. **(c)** EEG at C: typical drowsy EEG pattern. Note that after this, there is gradual increase in power at slower frequencies (mainly delta) seen on the spectrogram as he falls asleep (upper magenta box). A sudden drop (between B and C), followed by gradual increase in amplitude can also be appreciated on the *amplitude-integrated EEG* (aEEG). With aEEG, there is a minimum amplitude and maximum amplitude for each data point (i.e. each short EEG epoch), connected by a vertical line. Thus, the tracing is a band with width. The horizontal scale lines show the absolute value of the amplitudes: the bottom portion is a linear scale from 0 to 10 uV, and the upper portion is a logarithmic scale for higher voltages. A very thick band that reaches the bottom of the tracing suggests suppression-burst (parts with very low amplitude and parts with high amplitude in each epoch). In the current example, the amplitudes (both minimum and maximum) drop as his alpha rhythm attenuates and drowsiness ensues (C). The amplitudes then gradually increase as the patient falls further asleep (lower magenta box). aEEG can be applied to a single channel (as is commonly done with neonatal EEG monitoring, sometimes via a bedside device known as a 'cerebral function monitor') or to a group of channels; in this setup shown, all channels in one hemisphere are averaged into one aEEG trace. The above description is an oversimplification of aEEG. The raw EEG signal undergoes filtering and mathematical modification prior to amplitude calculations in order to enhance the power of faster frequencies, which are normally lower amplitude than slower frequencies (see Scheuer and Wilson, 2004 for technical details of this and many other QEEG techniques). **(d)** EEG at D: normal stage II sleep with spindles (labeled) and K complexes. **(e)** EEG at E: slow wave sleep, consisting of mostly moderate-to-high voltage delta. **(f)** EEG at F: back to stage II sleep.

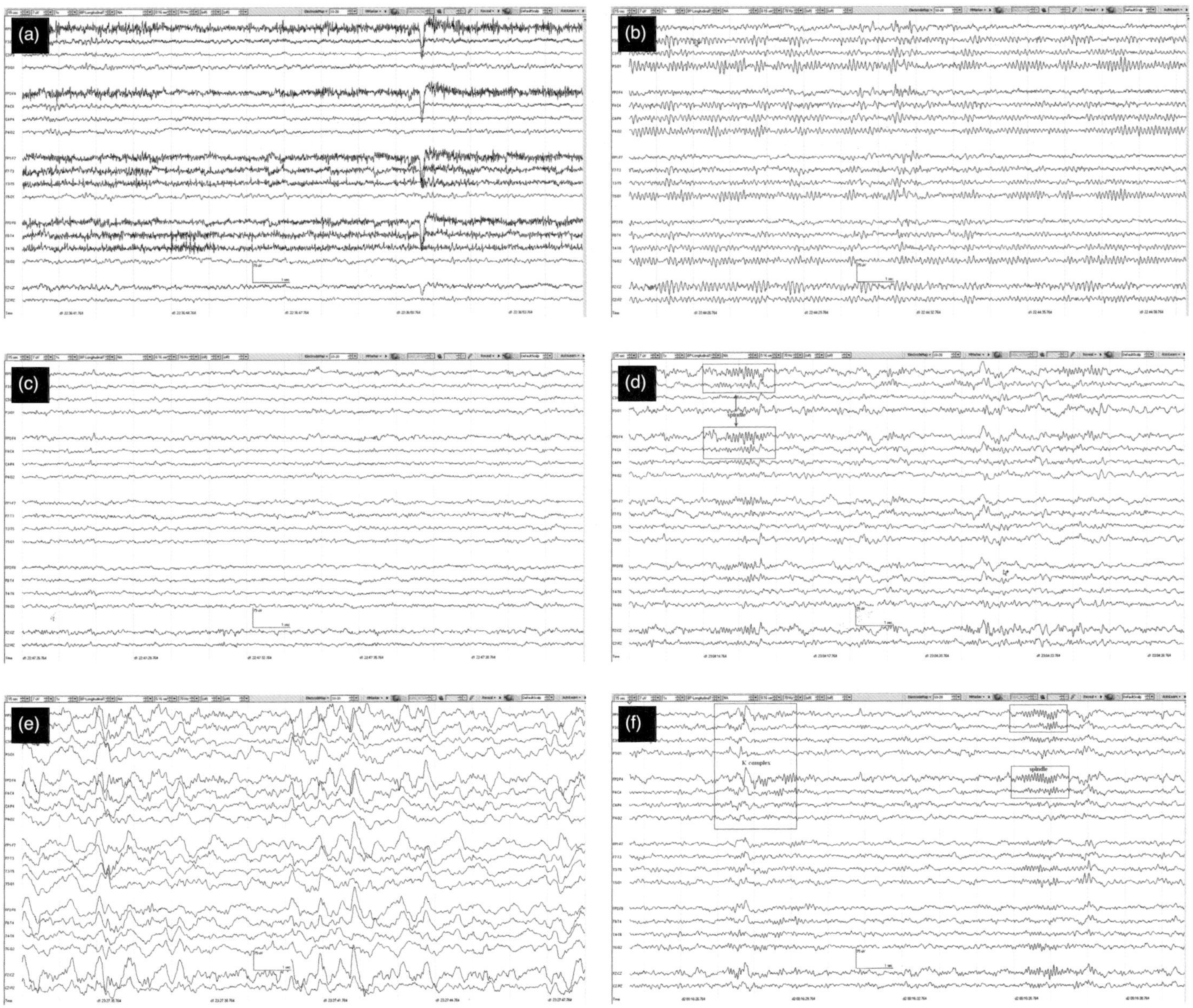
(a)
(b)
(c)
(d)
spindle
(e)
(f)
K complex
spindle

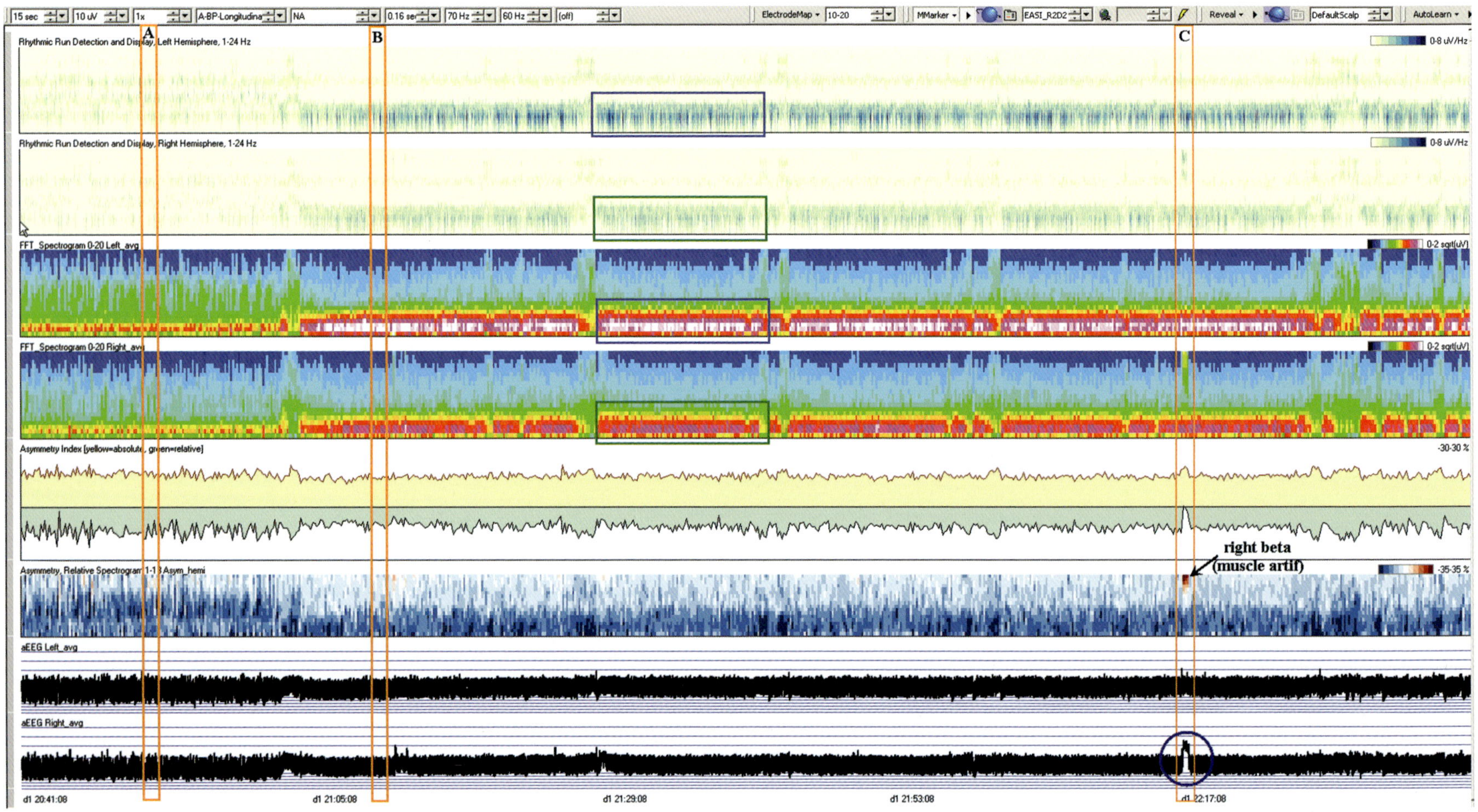

Figure 7.7 QEEG basics: asymmetry, breach, rhythmic run detector and aEEG 'false positives'. **Main:** Two to three hours of QEEG in a 70-year-old man with a left hemisphere mass, s/p biopsy and evacuation of a left-sided subdural hematoma. The spectrograms (panels 3 and 4) show a persistent asymmetry, initially with greater power in all frequencies (A) on the left, later with this difference only notable on the spectrogram in the delta frequency (B) with faster frequencies roughly symmetric. This asymmetry is also well appreciated with the green relative asymmetry index tracing (fifth panel), always below zero and downgoing (meaning greater power on the left). The asymmetry spectrogram (sixth panel) adds additional information, again initially showing much greater power on the left (darker blue) in all frequencies (e.g. at A), then only showing dark blue in the lower frequencies with less asymmetry at higher frequencies for most of this page (including at B). Increase in all frequencies on one side is suggestive of a skull defect as in this case: increase in slower frequencies is due to the underlying brain dysfunction (i.e. focal slowing), whereas the increase in faster frequencies is due to the skull defect (breach effect). At C, there is a sudden, brief elevation of amplitude seen in the aEEG trace on the right (blue circle), typical for a seizure. However, one can tell that this is likely due to muscle artifact (or accompanied by muscle artifact) via the asymmetry spectrogram, which shows a burst of red (more power on right) at the highest frequencies (arrow labeled 'right beta').

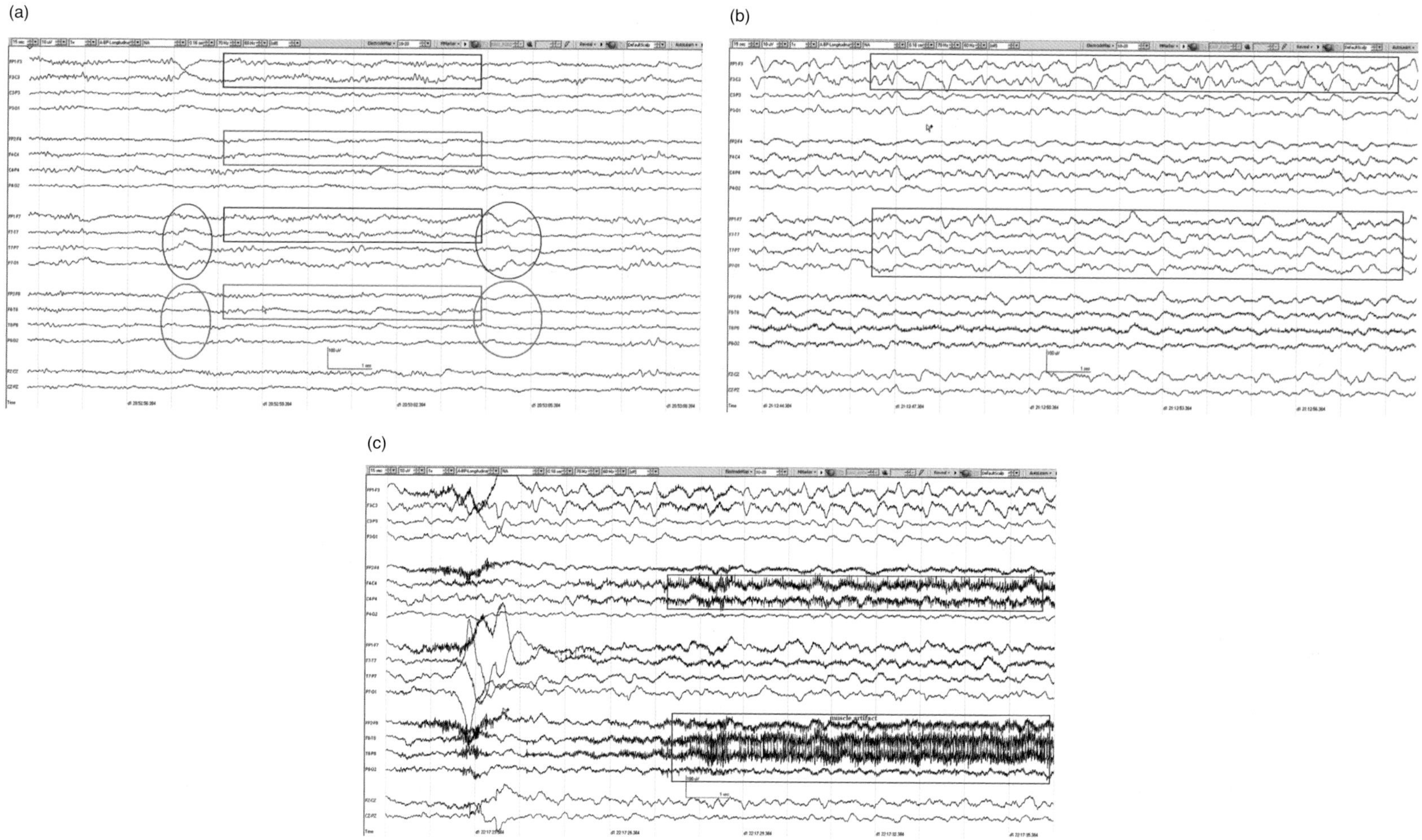

Figure 7.8 (*Continued*) The spectrogram also shows high-frequency activity on the right at this point, seemingly coming down from the top of the tracing and suggesting artifact. Review of the raw EEG confirms that the change is due to muscle artifact and is a 'false positive' change on aEEG that is not due to seizure. This pattern, which looks identical to a seizure on an aEEG trace, is common, and is one reason it is crucial to never diagnose seizures on an aEEG trace alone (or any single QEEG measure) without reviewing the raw EEG (shown in part c). The top two panels are *rhythmic run detectors*, a measure of rhythmicity in which the tracing becomes darker when there is rhythmic or periodic activity, and shows a dark band at the frequency of the rhythmic pattern. This allows detection of evolution at times as well (via a diagonal line as the dominant rhythmic frequency gradually changes). There is an obvious asymmetry in rhythmicity here as well as power, with much higher rhythmicity on the left, especially at lower frequencies (delta; boxes). The left side has fairly rhythmic delta for much of the recording, including at B and C, due to rhythmic delta on that side (see parts b and c). **(a)** EEG at A: there is more slowing on the left (circles), as well as more prominent faster frequencies on the same side (squares). **(b)** EEG at B: semirhythmic delta on the left, maximal at F3. **(c)** EEG at C: left frontal rhythmic delta continues, still now sharply contoured, maximal at F3. Then prominent right-sided muscle artifact is seen (blue boxes, labeled), leading to the aEEG amplitude change.

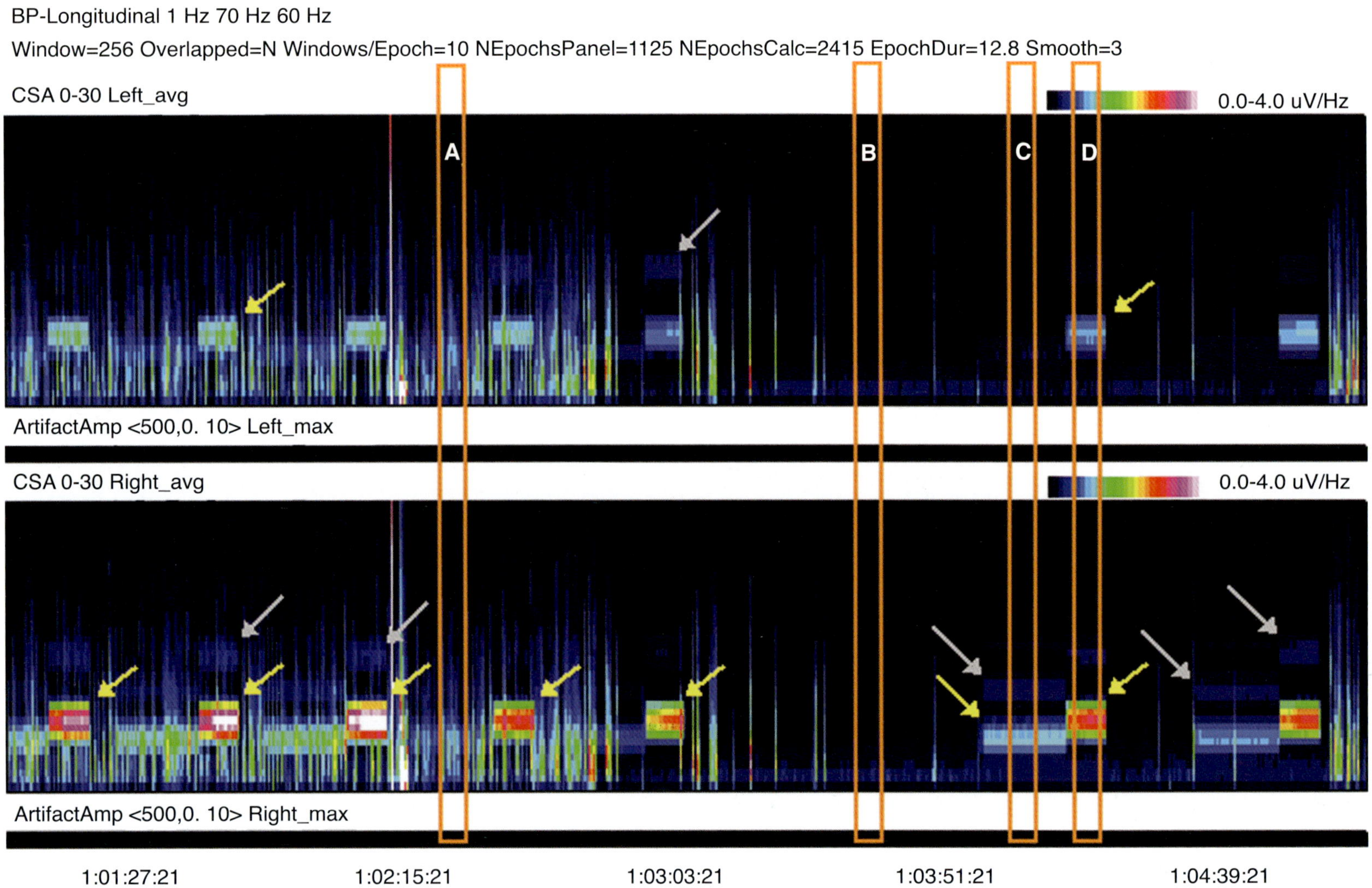

Figure 7.9 QEEG basics: Pentobarbital bolus and mechanical artifact with harmonics. **Main:** Four hours of QEEG in a young man with refractory status epilepticus being treated with pentobarbital coma. At point A, suppression-burst is seen. An additional pentobarbital bolus is given between A and B, and the rest of the EEG shows suppression only (including at B). Yellow arrows highlight mechanical artifact due to bed vibration (automatic chest percussion), initially at ~5 Hz (C), then switching to ~7 Hz (D). Note the square or rectangular shape of this artifact on the spectrograms. Also note the similar but fainter artifact at a harmonic of the main artifact (10 Hz, then 14 Hz; gray arrows). **(a)** EEG at A: ~5 Hz rhythmic artifact from the oscillating bed, plus two short bursts of cerebral activity on a background of suppression (suppression-burst). **(b)** EEG at B: complete suppression with the bed oscillator off. There is also bifrontal artifact, likely from a machine rather than EKG as it is at exactly 1 per second and unvarying in shape and frequency. An EKG channel would easily resolve this. **(c)** EEG at C: ~5 Hz rhythmic artifact is back, with complete background suppression. **(d)** EEG at D: ~7 Hz rhythmic artifact as the bed oscillator changes frequency.

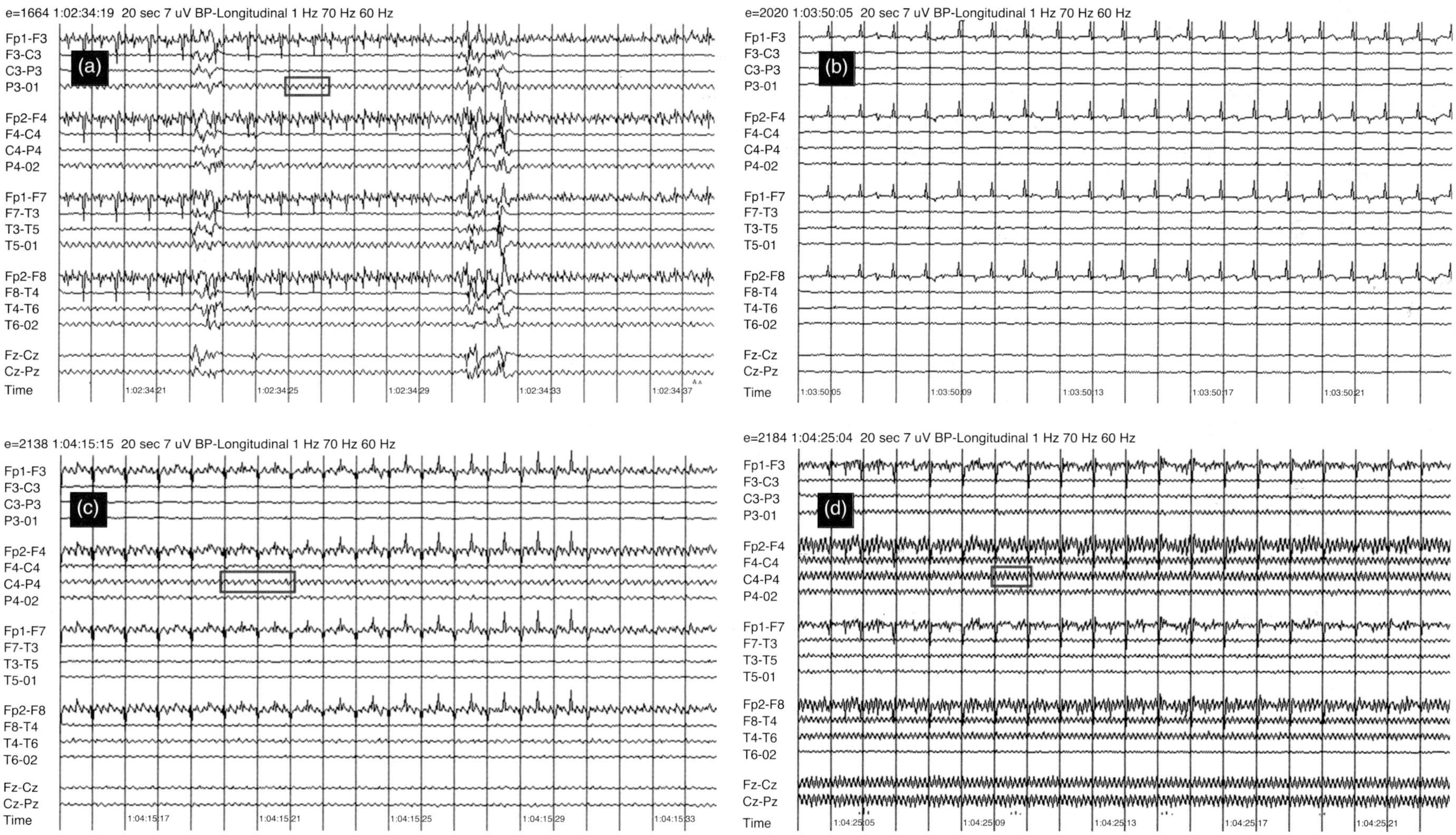
e=1664 1:02:34:19 20 sec 7 uV BP-Longitudinal 1 Hz 70 Hz 60 Hz
(a)
Fp1-F3
F3-C3
C3-P3
P3-01
Fp2-F4
F4-C4
C4-P4
P4-02
Fp1-F7
F7-T3
T3-T5
T5-01
Fp2-F8
F8-T4
T4-T6
T6-02
Fz-Cz
Cz-Pz
Time
1:02:34:21
1:02:34:25
1:02:34:29
1:02:34:33
1:02:34:37
e=2020 1:03:50:05 20 sec 7 uV BP-Longitudinal 1 Hz 70 Hz 60 Hz
(b)
1:03:50:05
1:03:50:09
1:03:50:13
1:03:50:17
1:03:50:21
e=2138 1:04:15:15 20 sec 7 uV BP-Longitudinal 1 Hz 70 Hz 60 Hz
(c)
1:04:15:17
1:04:15:21
1:04:15:25
1:04:15:29
1:04:15:33
e=2184 1:04:25:04 20 sec 7 uV BP-Longitudinal 1 Hz 70 Hz 60 Hz
(d)
1:04:25:05
1:04:25:09
1:04:25:13
1:04:25:17
1:04:25:21

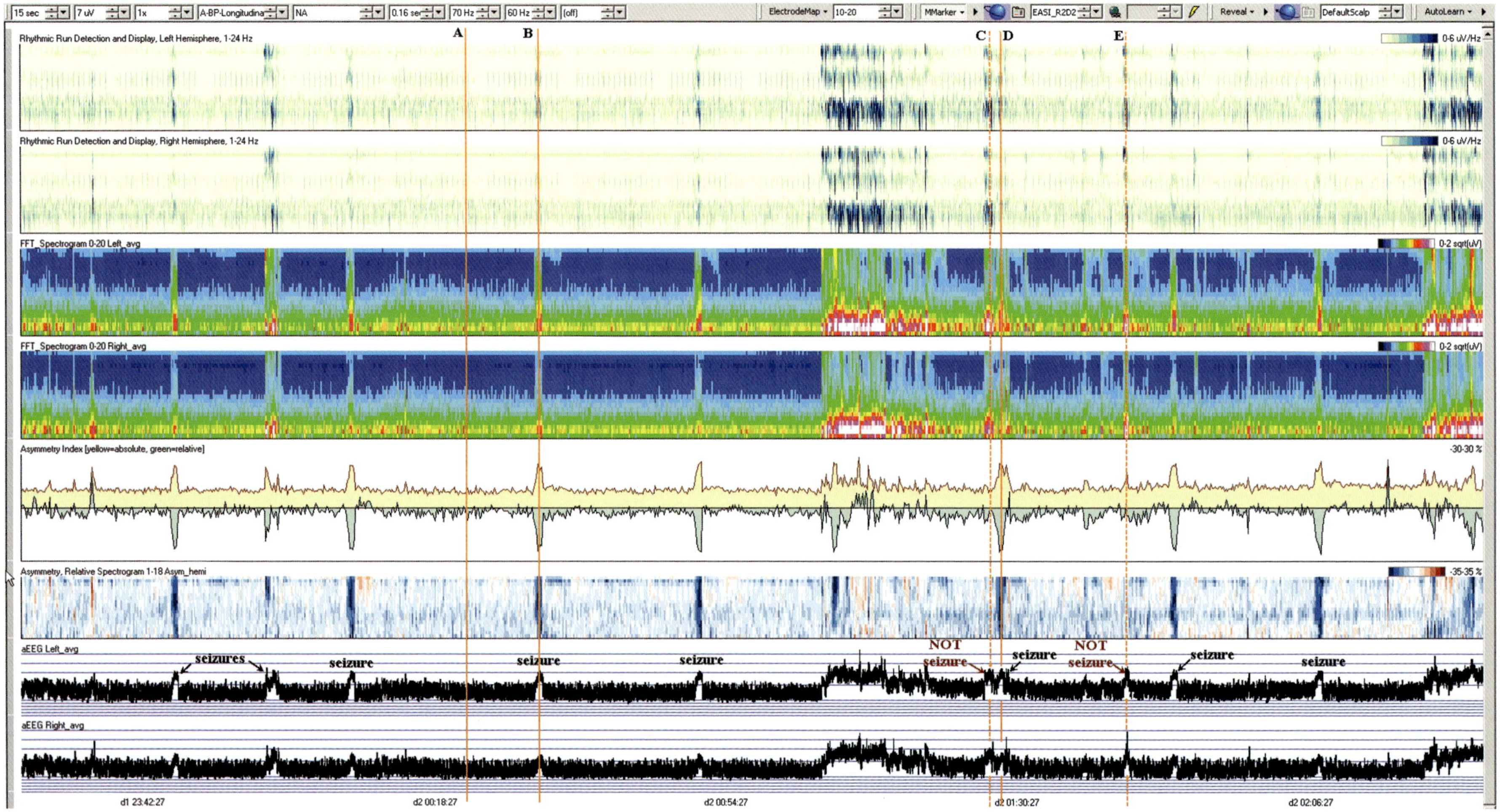

Figure 7.10 QEEG basics: Multiple seizures and identical-appearing false positives on amplitude-integrated EEG. **Main:** Three to four hours of QEEG from a man in his 60s with a left hemisphere brain tumor, presenting with worsening memory and language. Multiple nonconvulsive seizures were recorded (labeled), maximal on the left as evident on the aEEG (higher amplitudes on left) and the relative asymmetry index, going sharply downward (more power on left) with each seizure. The standard spectrogram and the asymmetry spectrogram both demonstrate involvement of all frequencies, and the rhythmic run detector shows a burst of rhythmicity with most of them. Note the two episodes labeled 'not seizure' (and with dashed lines) in which the aEEG tracing jumps up in a manner almost identical to the prior and subsequent seizures. However, these are due to muscle artifact. Note that the two asymmetry panels do not show the typical seizure pattern with these artifactual increases in amplitude. This example shows the benefit of using multiple QEEG measures simultaneously, and again stresses the importance of not relying on one measure alone without reviewing the raw EEG. **(a)** EEG at A: interictal baseline. **(b)** EEG at B: left hemisphere seizure, maximal in the temporal chain and composed of mixed frequencies. **(c)** EEG at C: blinking, movement and muscle artifact only. No seizure. **(d)** EEG at D: another left-sided seizure. **(e)** EEG at E: muscle artifact and a couple blinks. No seizure.

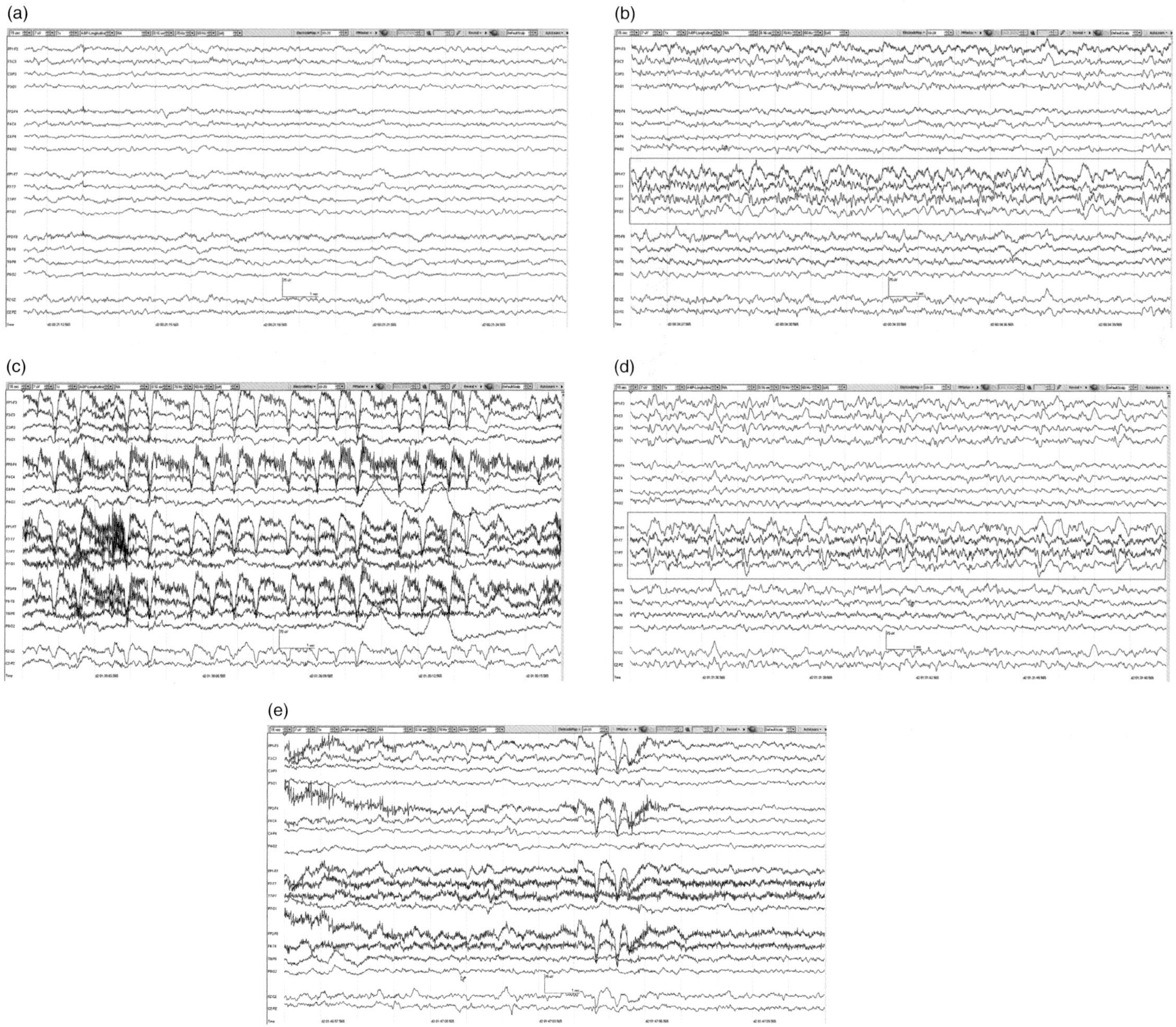

Figure 7.10 (*Continued*)

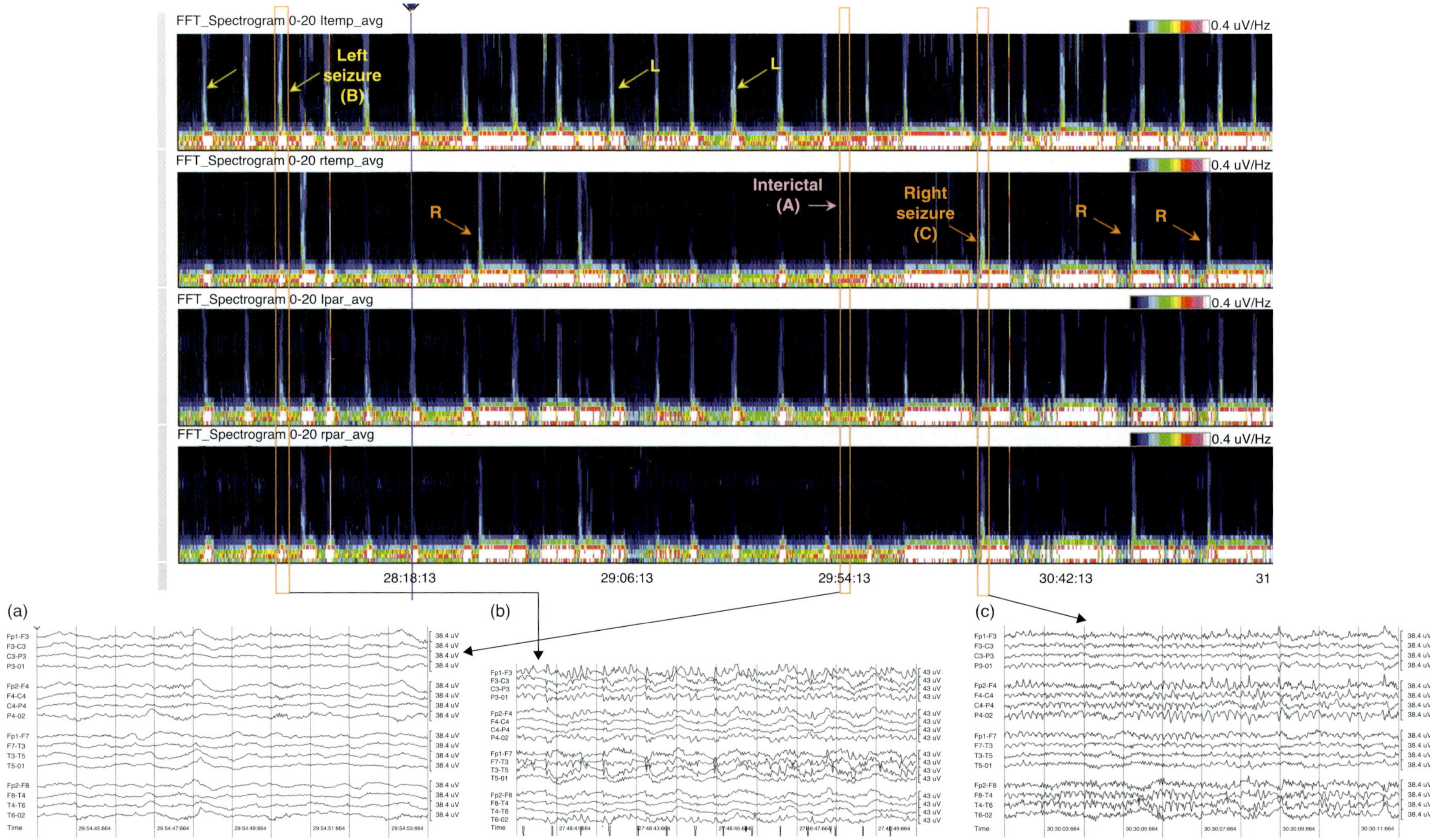

Figure 7.11 Bilateral independent seizures. **Main:** Four hours of QEEG in a middle-aged woman with confusion, initially found to be in nonconvulsive status epilepticus (NCSE), now treated. The top two spectrograms are the temporal chains and the bottom two are parasagittal; all depict 0–20 Hz. Interictally, (A), all power is in the delta range. There are intermittent bursts of power into the theta and alpha ranges, more often on the left (B; and a few labeled with L), and each representing a seizure. Some of the bursts are on the right (C, and a few labeled with R). **(a)** EEG at A: interictal background (asleep). **(b)** EEG at B: left-sided seizure, with most activity in the theta–alpha range. **(c)** EEG at C: right-sided seizure, with most activity in the theta range.

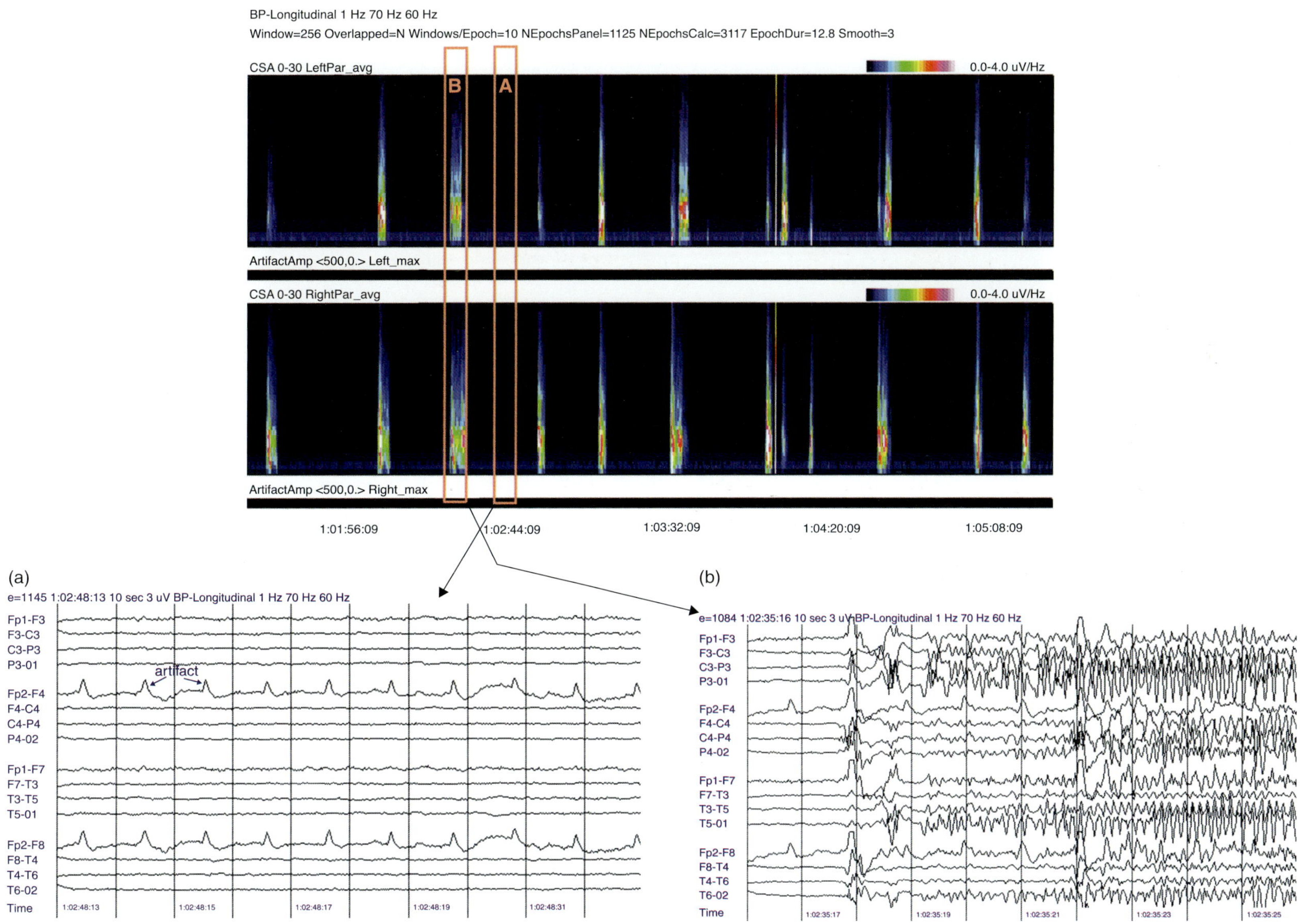

Figure 7.12 Multiple seizures arising from complete suppression. **Main:** Six hours of QEEG in a 12-year-old boy with refractory status epilepticus being treated with pentobarbital coma. The background was completely suppressed (A) with no bursts, yet well-developed seizures still occurred about twice per hour (B). This example demonstrates the limitations of intermittent short EEGs for monitoring barbiturate-induced coma. **(a)** EEG at A: interictal, showing complete suppression and Fp2 artifact. Sensitivity 3 uV/mm (high gain). **(b)** EEG at B: start of a seizure, beginning maximally on the left, but rapidly becoming bilateral.

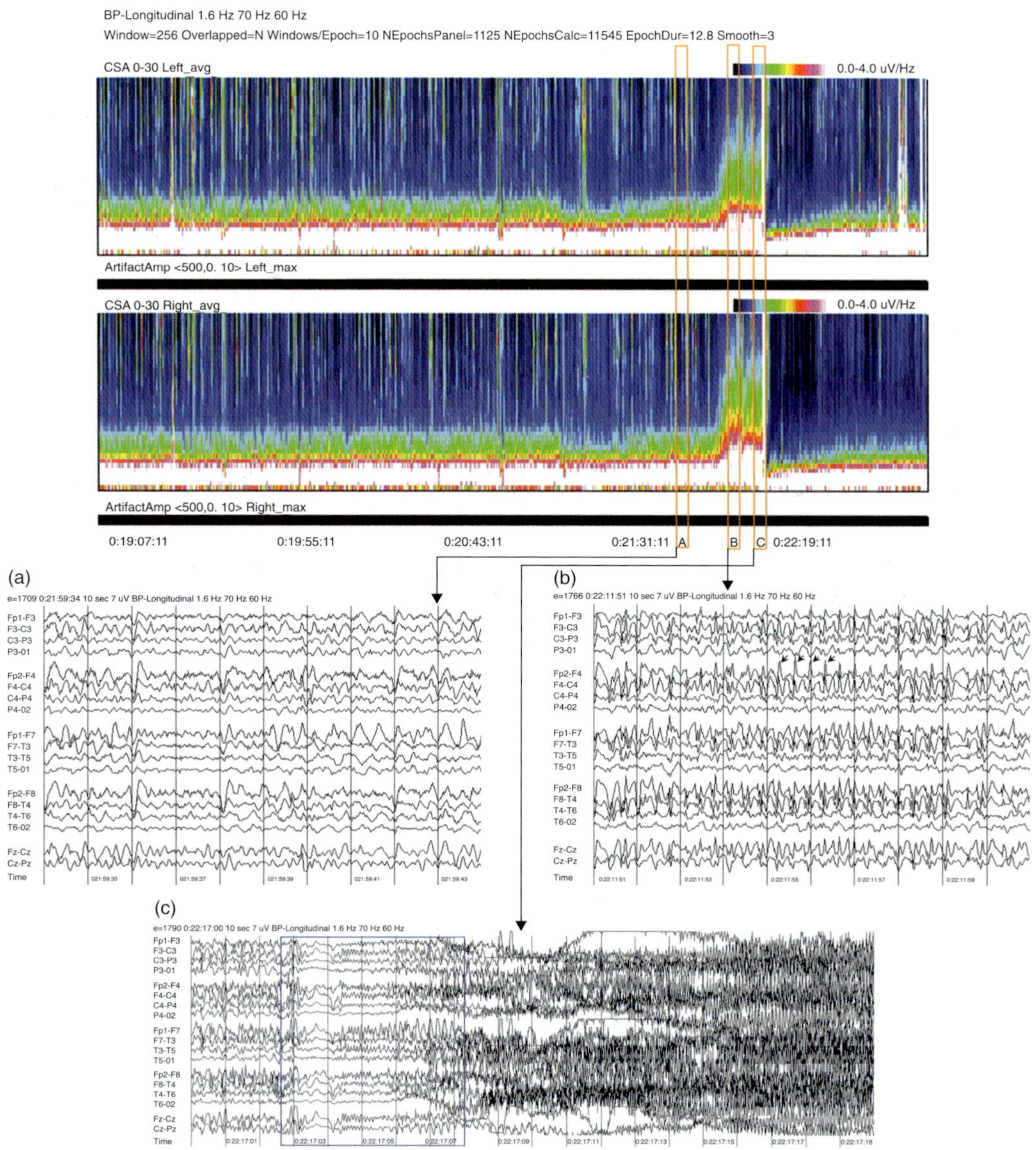

Figure 7.13 Nonconvulsive status epilepticus culminating with convulsion. **Main:** Spectrogram showing 4 h of EEG in a middle-aged man with primary generalized epilepsy and seizures since age 9, now admitted with intermittent confusion. Baseline EEG (A) shows diffuse slowing. He then develops nonconvulsive status epilepticus for 15–20 min (B), which continues until he develops a generalized tonic-clonic seizure (C). **(a)** EEG at A: diffuse slowing with no definite ictal activity. **(b)** EEG at B: nonconvulsive status epilepticus (NCSE), with irregular, ~3 Hz generalized spike-wave. Arrows highlight a few of the spikes. **(c)** EEG at C: transition from NCSE (first few seconds) into a typical primary generalized tonic-clonic seizure.

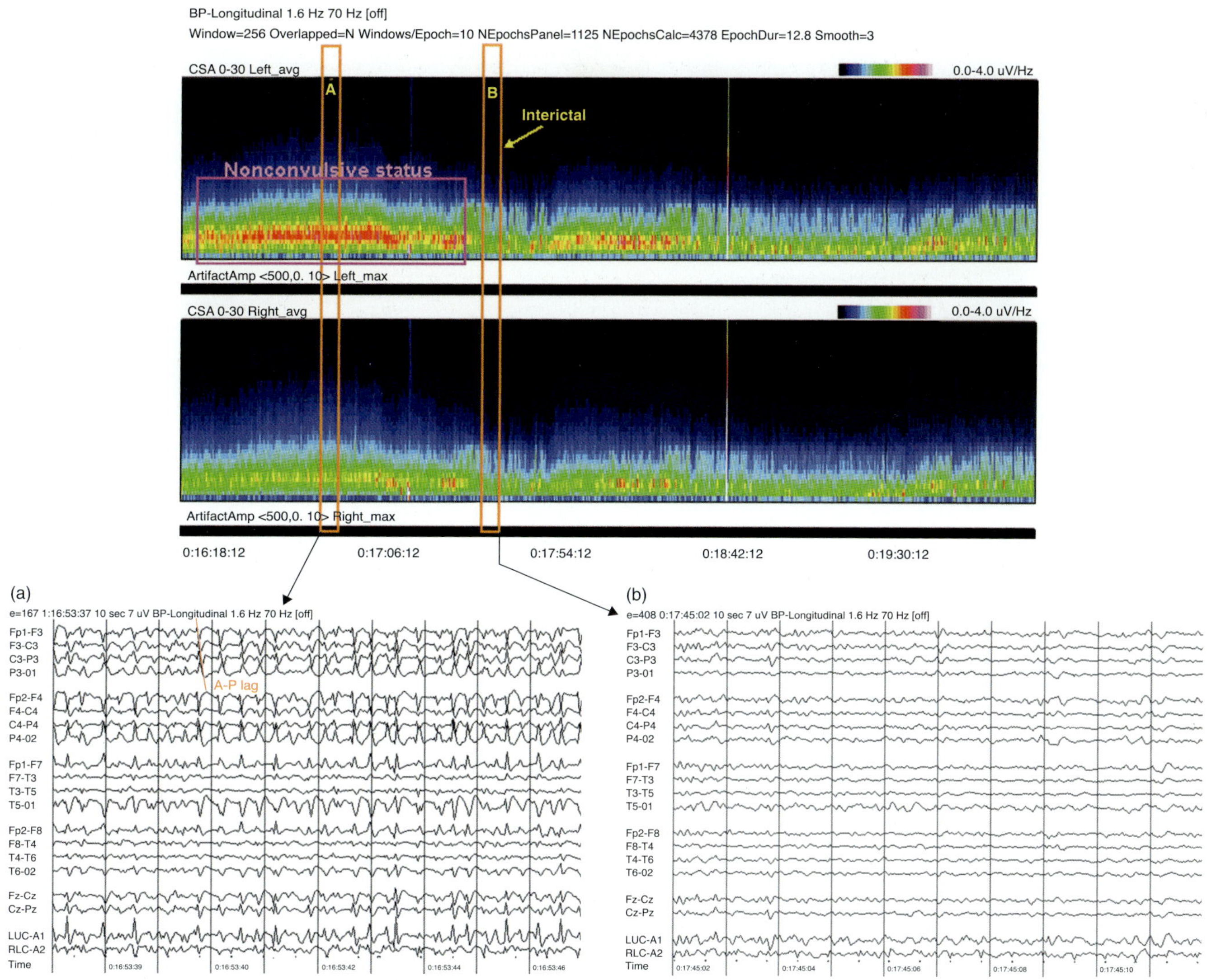

Figure 7.14 Nonconvulsive status epilepticus. **Main:** Spectrogram showing 4 h of EEG in a middle-aged woman with meningoencephalitis. The patient was in nonconvulsive status epilepticus for the first 90 min or so (purple box and A), bilateral but more obvious on the left. This then resolved by point B, then resumed but less prominently after this. Quantitative EEG such as this helps for recognition of long-term trends and for assessing the effects of interventions. **(a)** EEG at A: nonconvulsive status epilepticus, with bilateral, irregular ~3 Hz spike and wave activity. (Also note the so-called 'anterior-posterior lag', in which a single discharge seems to occur later posteriorly than anteriorly. This lag has been described with triphasic waves seen in metabolic encephalopathy and it has been suggested that this feature suggests a metabolic process. However, it occurs commonly with definite nonconvulsive status epilepticus as well, such as in this example.) **(b)** EEG at B: interictal EEG.

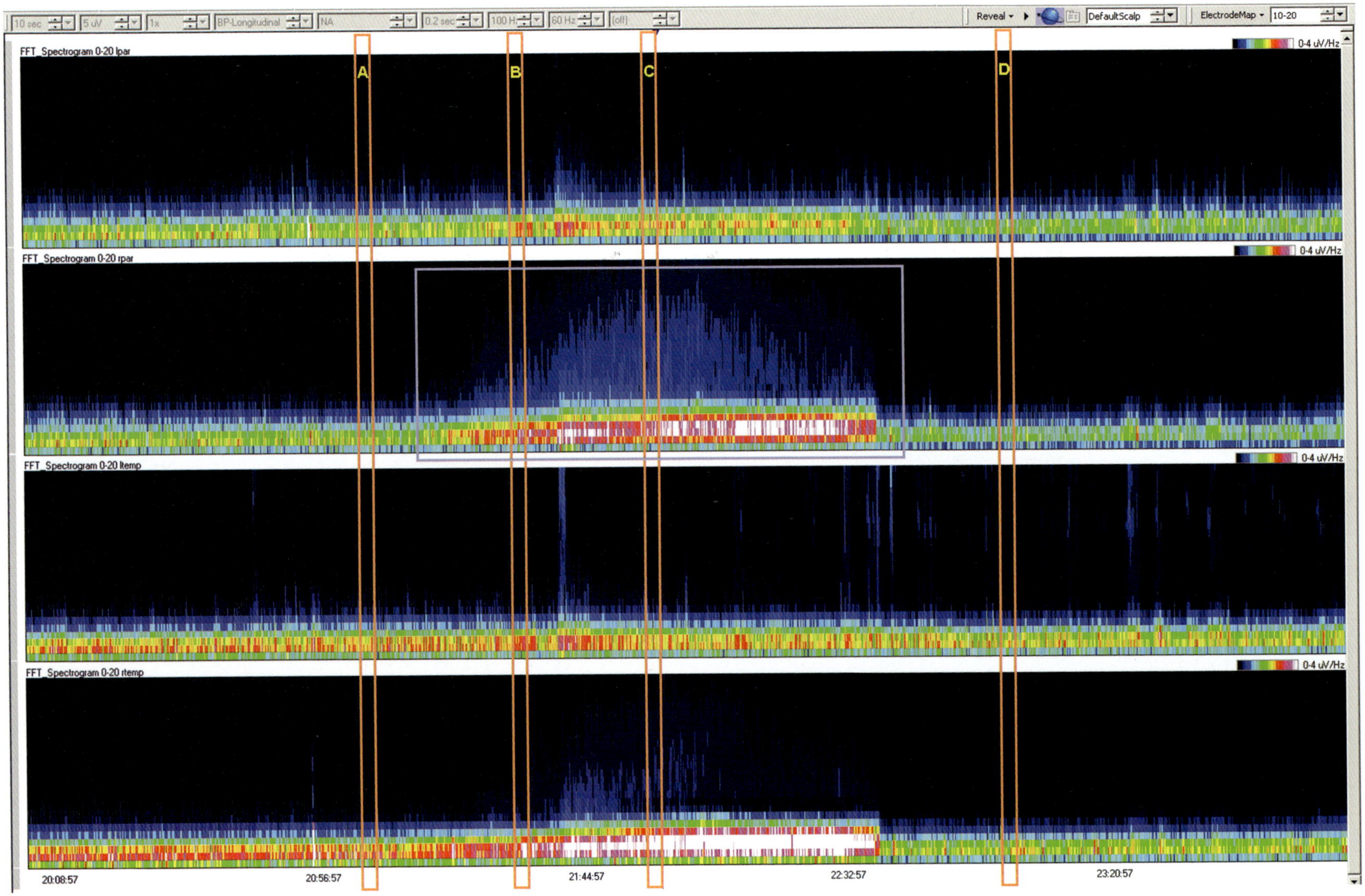

Figure 7.15 Nonconvulsive status epilepticus with gradual onset and offset. **Main:** Spectrogram showing 4 h of QEEG in a 72-year-old woman s/p subarachnoid hemorrhage complicated by vasospasm. It is easy to appreciate a gradual onset and offset over about an hour of a pattern on the right, maximal in the parasagittal region, which corresponded to a gradually evolving focal seizure. **(a)** EEG at A: baseline EEG, with marked diffuse slowing and some artifact. **(b)** EEG at B: early portion of focal nonconvulsive status epilepticus (NCSE) with semirhythmic slow delta on the right, maximal anteriorly, and superimposed faster activity (beta). **(c)** EEG at C: focal NCSE, well developed. There is now a more prominent right hemisphere rhythmic delta at 1.5–2 Hz with superimposed sharp beta. **(d)** EEG at D: back to nonictal baseline.

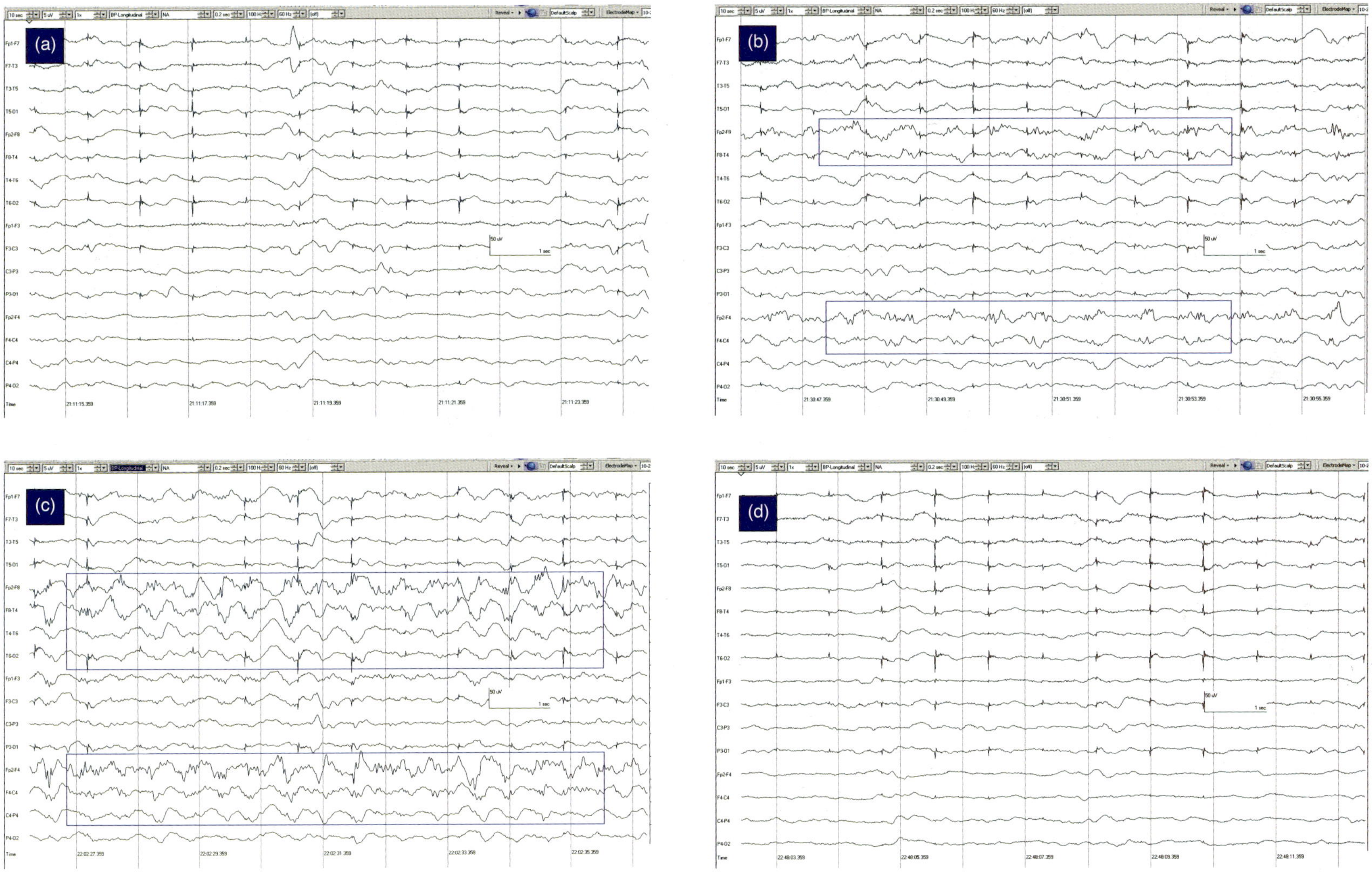
(a)
(b)
(c)
(d)

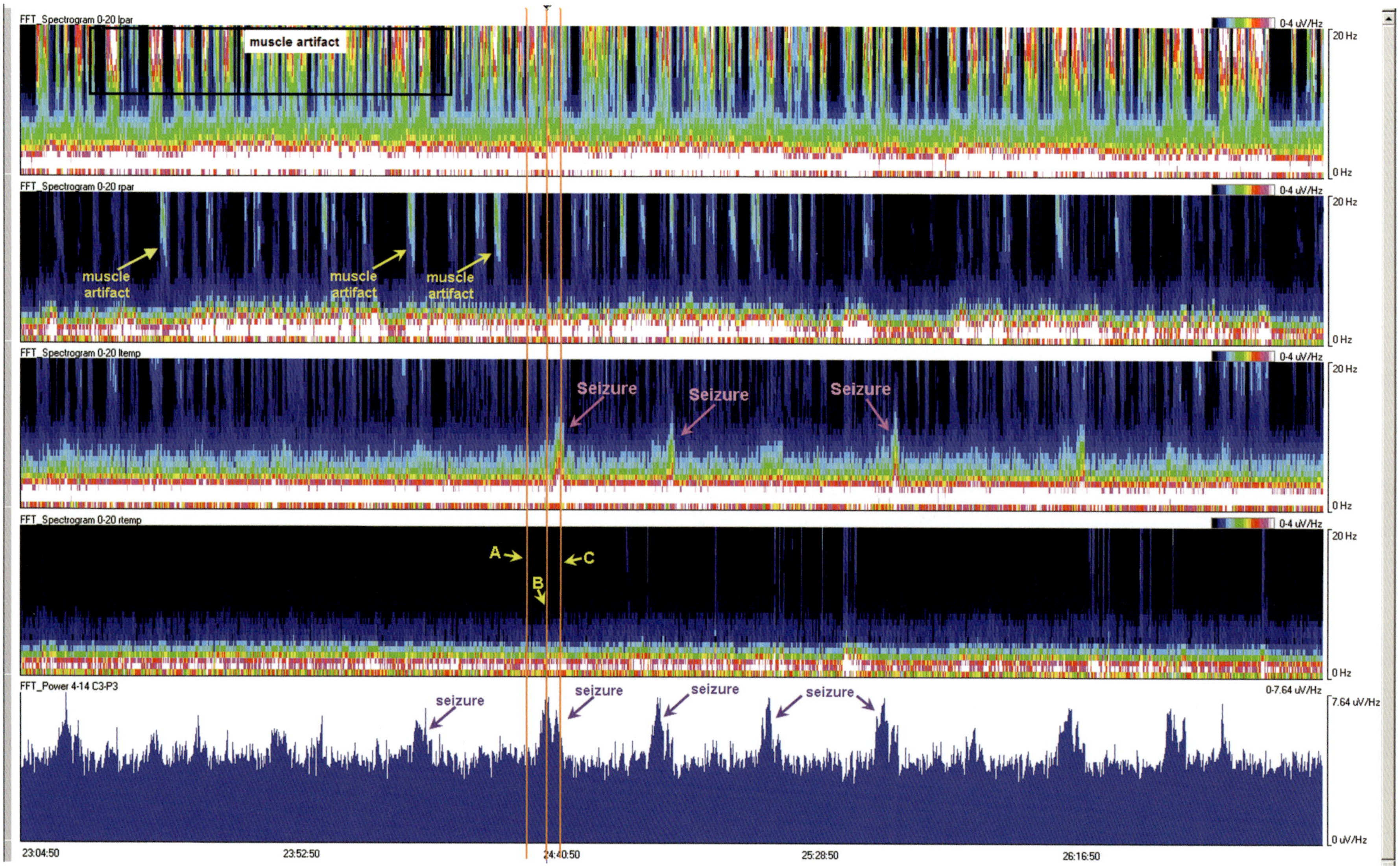

Figure 7.16 Breach and highly focal nonconvulsive seizure, sometimes with spread. **Main:** Four hours of QEEG in a man in his 70s s/p resection of a tumor in the left parietal region. The background shows more power in all frequencies on the left throughout the recording, including delta; this is typical with a skull defect (causing increased faster frequencies) over an area of abnormality (causing increased slowing) as in this case. Also note the muscle artifact (coming down from the top of the spectrograms and labeled). This patient was having frequent focal nonconvulsive seizures from P3 (left parietal; B) that remained very focal most of the time and were hard to recognize on the standard spectrogram.

(a)

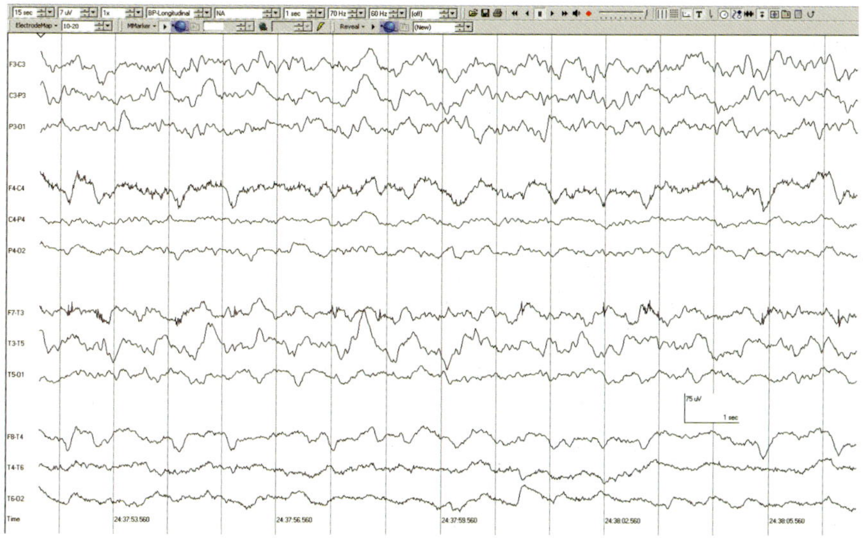

(b)

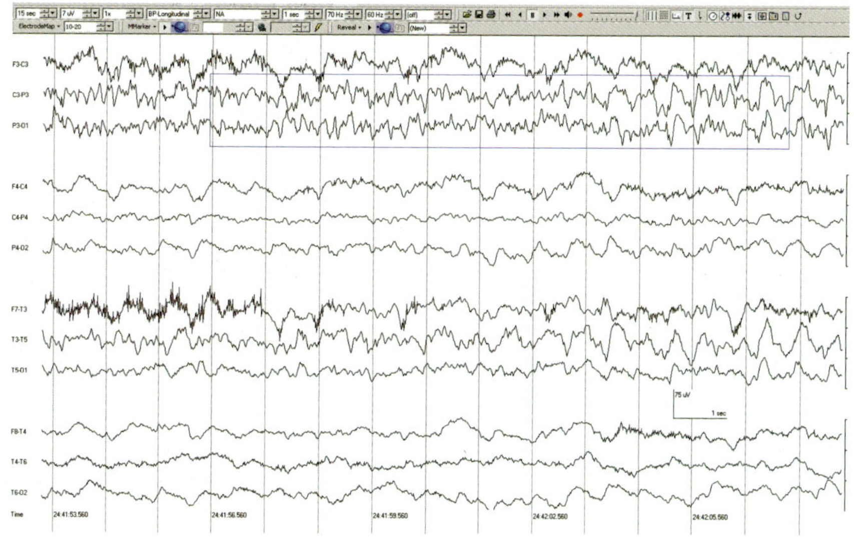

(c)

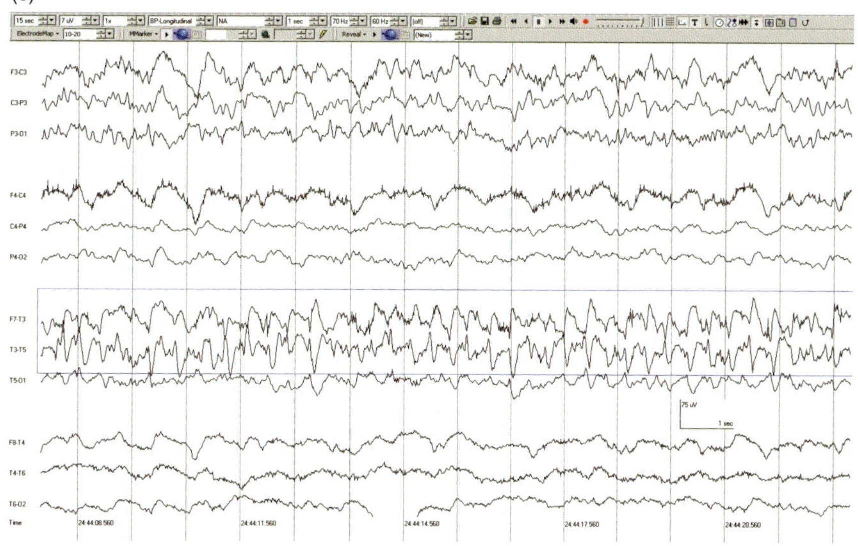

Figure 7.16 (*Continued*) Thus, an additional panel was added (bottom) showing total power from 4 to 14 Hz at C3-P3, the most relevant channel and frequencies. This tracing showed each seizure rather clearly. Some of the seizures spread to the left temporal lobe and were well visualized on the spectrogram on the temporal panel (C, and purple 'seizure' labels). Interictal EEG is shown in A, left parietal seizure in B and spread to left temporal lobe in C. **(a)** EEG at A: baseline, with prominent slowing and breach effect on the left. **(b)** EEG at B: evolving ictal pattern predominantly at C3 (box). Note that this portion was readily identifiable on the last panel (C3–P3 4–14 Hz total power), but is not visible on the standard spectrograms. **(c)** EEG at C: ictal pattern has now spread to the left temporal region (box), when it becomes obvious on the left temporal spectrogram as well.

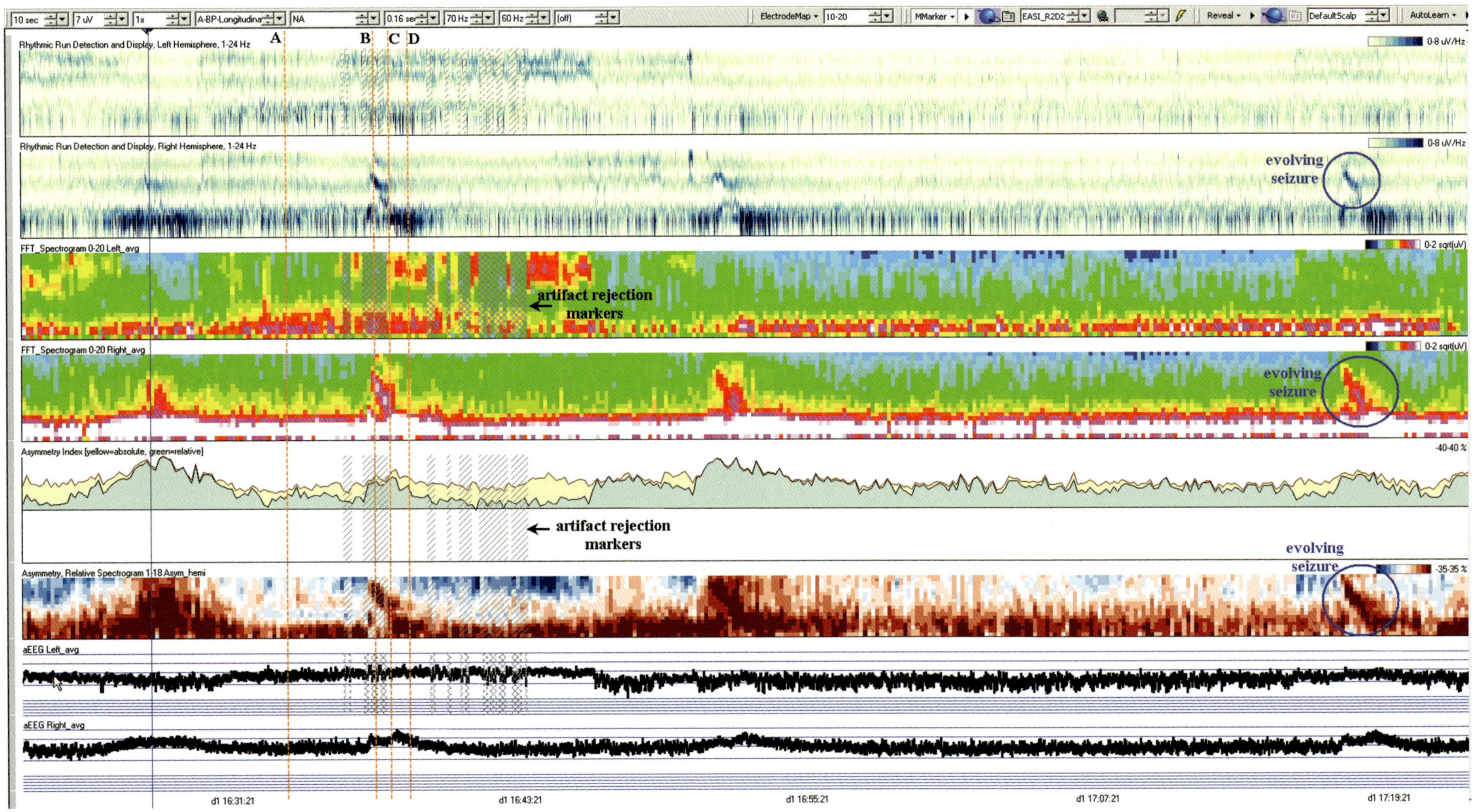

Figure 7.17 Evolving nonconvulsive seizures and rhythmic run detector. **Main:** Two hours of QEEG in a 58-year-old man with remote subarachnoid hemorrhage admitted with a generalized convulsion followed by confusion. The spectrograms (third and fourth panels) show greater delta on the right throughout, which results in the green relative asymmetry index remaining positive and upgoing (more power on right; fifth panel), and dark red at lower frequencies on the asymmetry spectrogram (sixth panel). A few right-sided seizures are seen with clear evolution visible on the QEEG (blue circles and B–D). The top two panels show rhythmicity at 1–24 Hz (essentially a rhythmicity spectrogram; see Figure 7.8). The seizures appear as rhythmicity

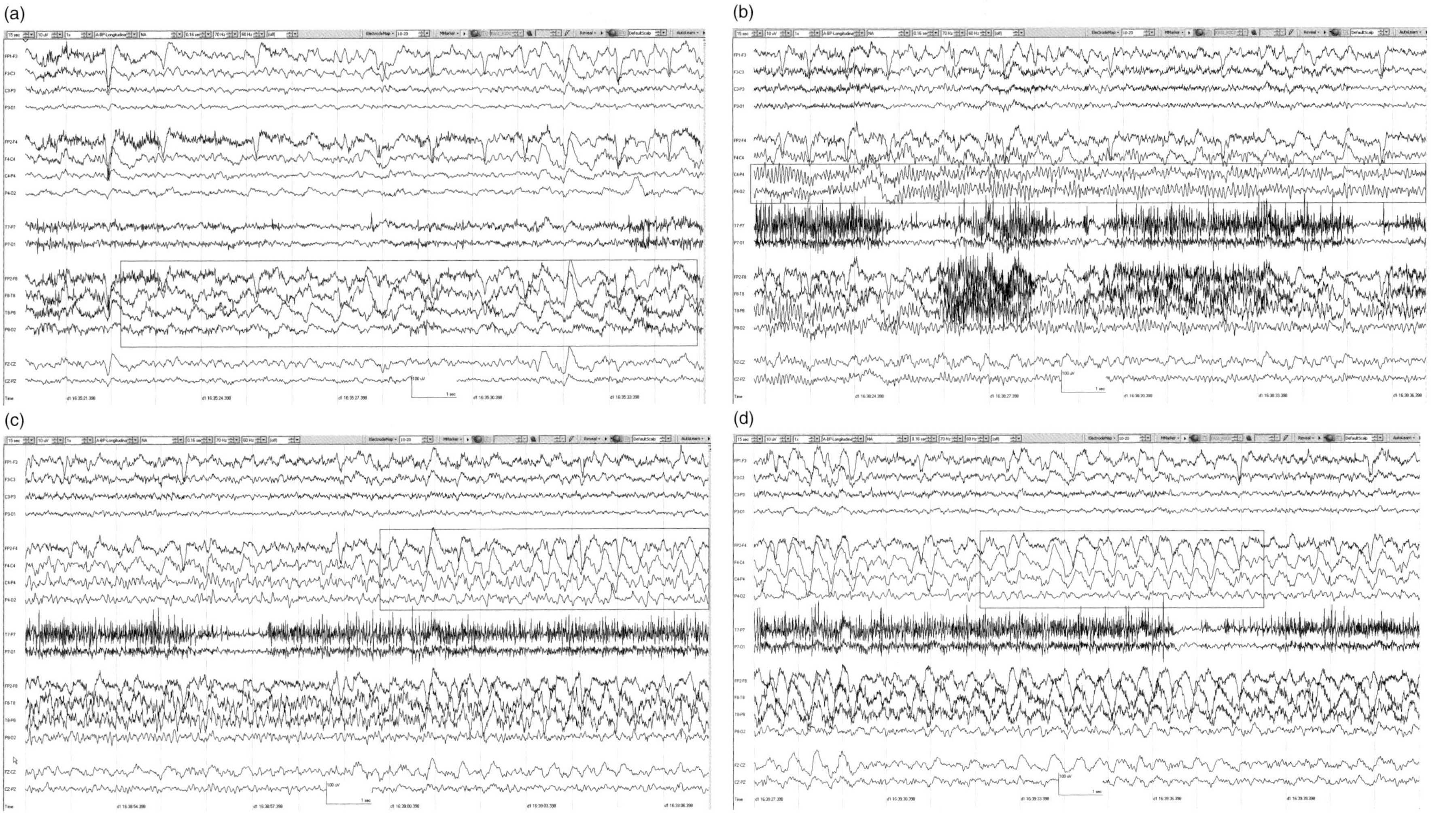

Figure 7.17 (*Continued*) on the right, initially above 12 Hz (B), then gradually decreasing in frequency (C), resulting in a diagonal line (circled). Rhythmicity eventually settles into the delta frequency (D). The same diagonal evolution can be seen on the standard spectrogram and the asymmetry spectrogram (in red as the seizures are on the right) (circles). Overall amplitude gradually increases on the right during the seizures, as can be seen on the amplitude-integrated EEG tracing on the bottom panel. Note the stereotyped QEEG findings from seizure to seizure. **(a)** EEG at A: interictal, with delta range slowing in the right temporal region. **(b)** EEG at B: early ictal, with rhythmic 12–13 Hz activity maximal in the right parieto-temporal region (P4–P8). **(c)** EEG at C: middle ictal, as the ictal pattern transitions to slower frequencies, now widespread in the right hemisphere. **(d)** EEG at D: late ictal, with rhythmic delta in the right hemisphere, mainly ~2 Hz.

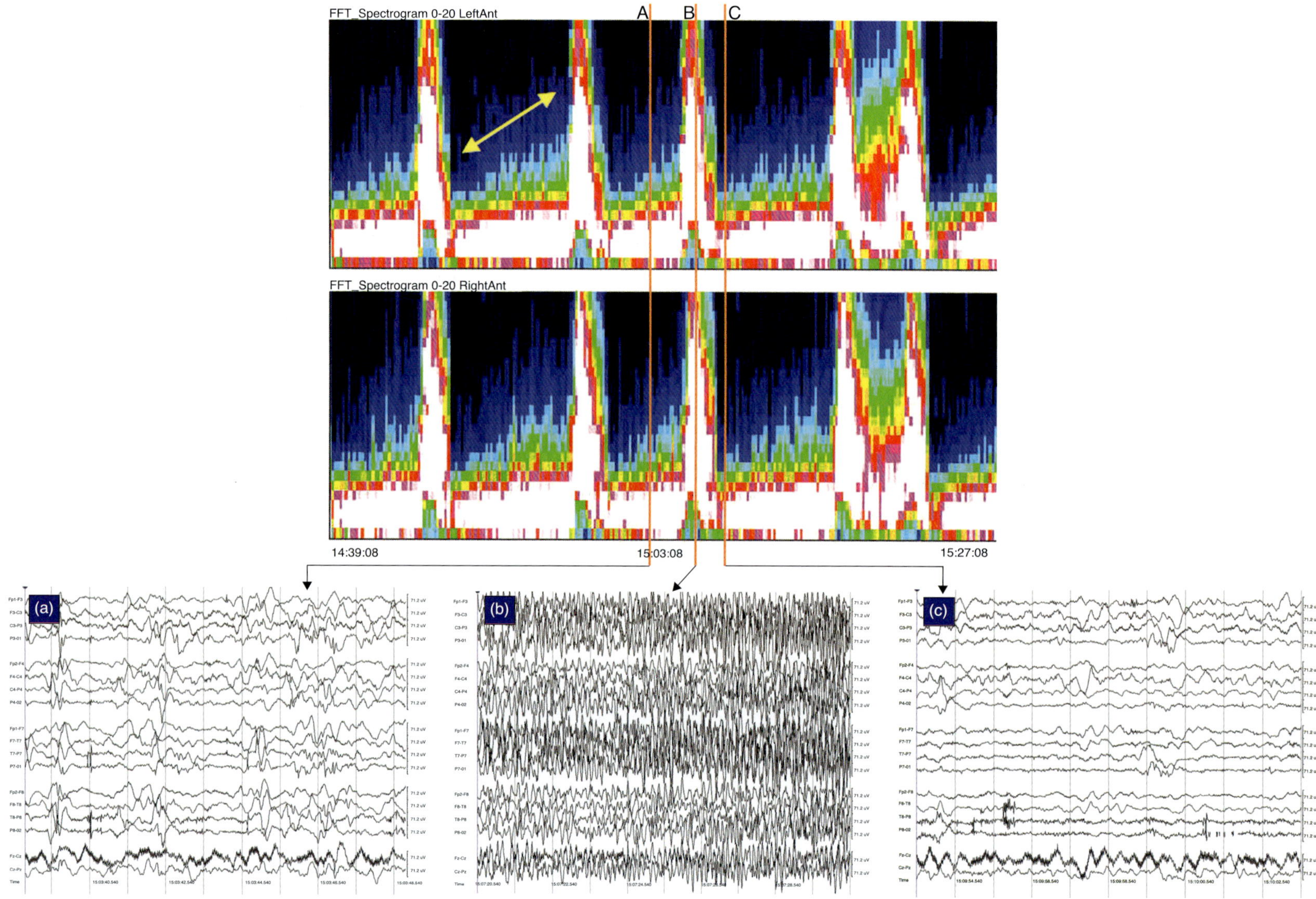

Figure 7.18 Cyclic nonconvulsive seizures. **Main:** One-hour spectrogram in a 2-year-old with a progressive encephalopathy of unknown etiology. Nonconvulsive seizures were occurring every ~15 min, with a fairly stable cyclical pattern consisting of a gradual buildup of amplitude at low frequencies, then gradually higher frequencies (arrow and A), culminating with a well-developed high-amplitude bilateral seizure (B), followed by postictal attenuation (C). Postictal attenuation then gradually transitioned into the same pattern of gradually increasing power (arrow) until the next seizure occurred. This pattern is easy to recognize on QEEG such as this, but difficult on review of raw EEG. **(a)** EEG at A: middle of period of gradually increasing power diffusely. **(b)** EEG at B: fully developed, high amplitude, bilateral seizure activity. **(c)** EEG at C: postictal, with relative attenuation diffusely.

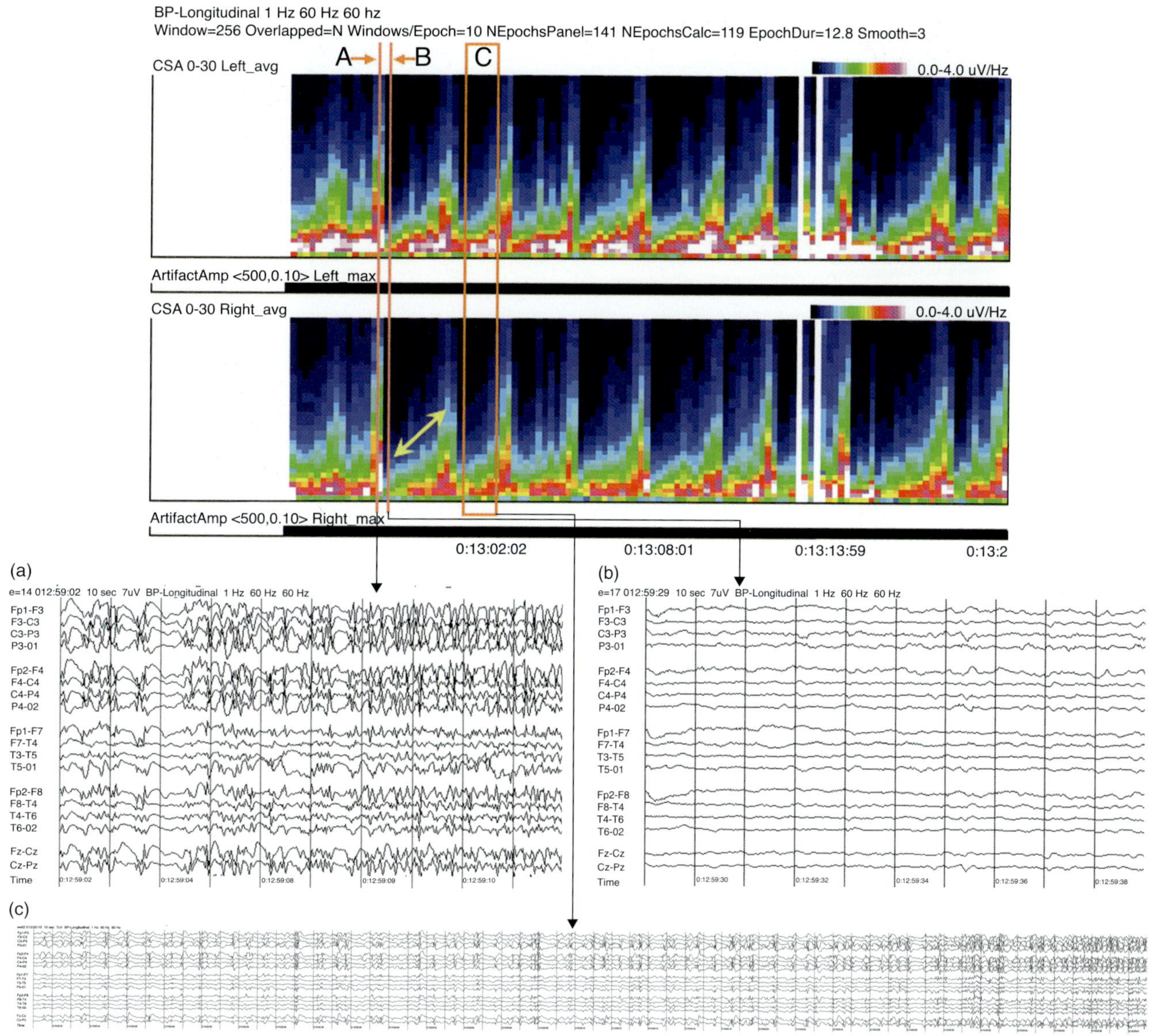

Figure 7.19 Cyclic nonconvulsive seizures. **Main:** ~30 min of QEEG in a middle-aged woman with encephalitis, seizures and s/p 10 min cardiac arrest. Brief nonconvulsive seizures were occurring every ~3 min in a very stable pattern of seizure (A), postictal attenuation (B), then gradual buildup of epileptiform activity (yellow arrow and C) until another seizure occurs. **(a)** EEG at A: definite electrographic seizure, maximal in bilateral parasagittal chains. **(b)** EEG at B: postictal, with marked diffuse attenuation. **(c)** One minute of raw EEG at C: gradual build-up of epileptiform activity between seizures.

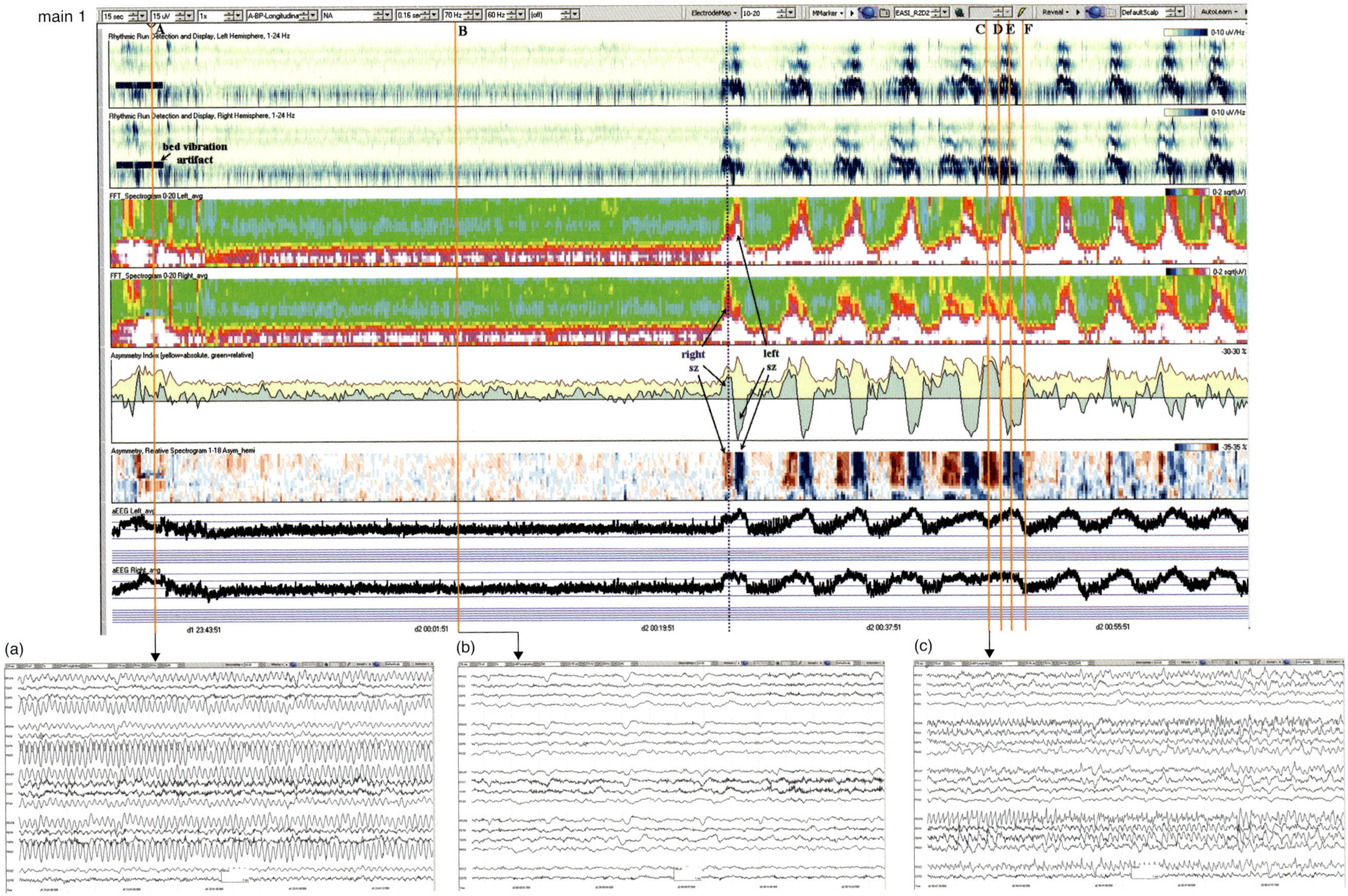

Figure 7.20 Cyclic 'ping-pong' seizures. **Main 1:** Two hours of QEEG in a 7-year-old boy with refractory nonconvulsive seizures from probable viral encephalitis. Near the beginning, there is classic mechanical artifact (perfect rectangular shape at 5 Hz in the spectrogram at (A) from an oscillating bed. There is then a nondescript period (including B), followed by the onset of cyclic seizures in the second half of this sample. The QEEG shows that each seizure starts on the right (dotted line labeled 'right sz' and C) as seen on the regular spectrogram (burst on right precedes left), the green relative asymmetry index (upward first), the asymmetry spectrogram (burst of red first), then spreads to the left (labeled 'left sz' and E) with the green asymmetry index switching to downwards (more power on left) and the asymmetry spectrogram switches to blue. **(a)** EEG at A: rhythmic 5 Hz artifact from a

(d)

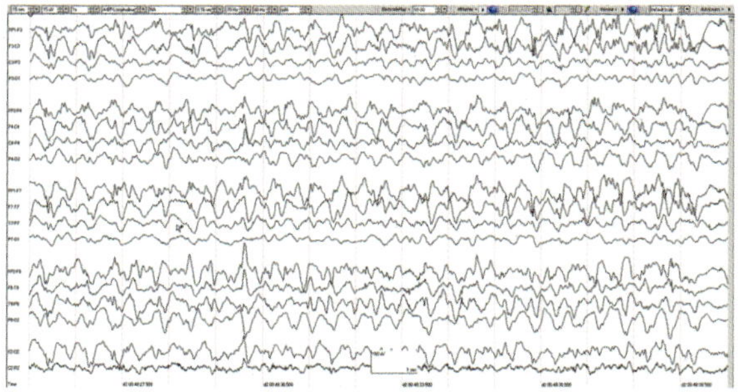

(e)

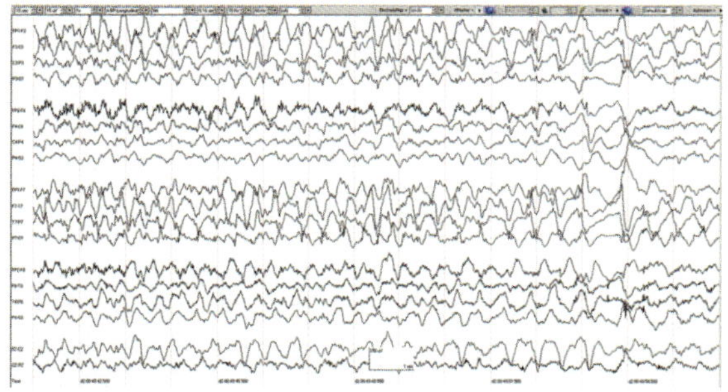

(f)

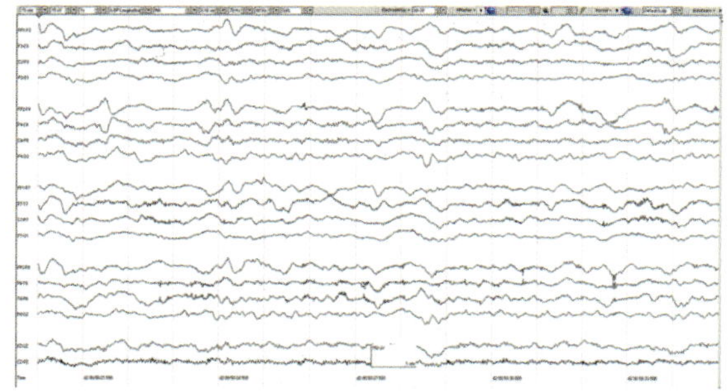

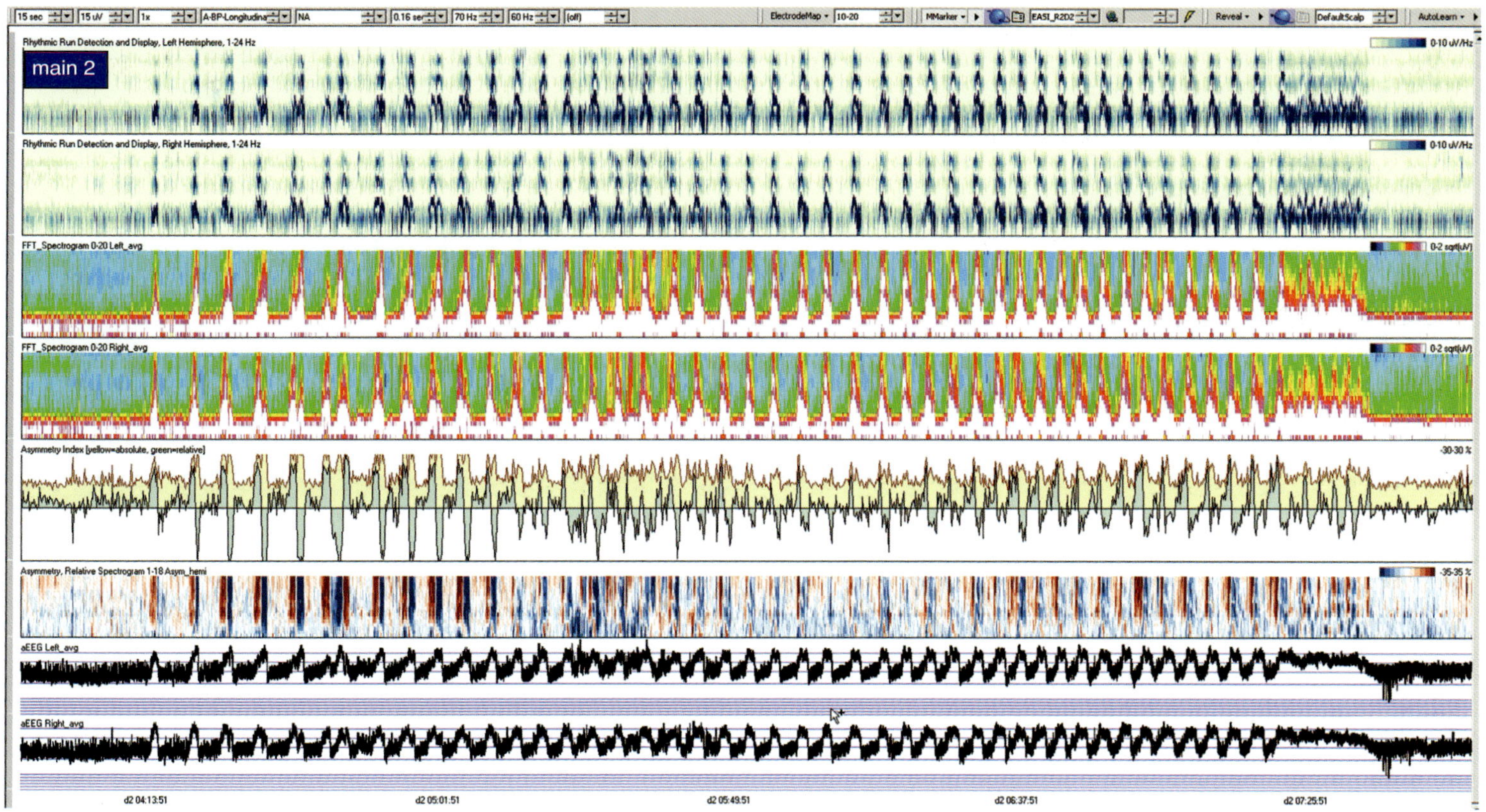

Figure 7.20 (*Continued*) vibrating bed. **(b)** EEG at B: baseline EEG. **(c)** EEG at C: right side seizure. **(d)** EEG at D: evolving seizure, now bilateral and symmetric; hence the asymmetry measures show no asymmetry at this point. **(e)** EEG at E: evolving seizure, now maximal on the left. **(f)** EEG at F: postictal EEG. **Main 2:** Four hours of QEEG beginning 3 h later. There is a stable pattern of seizures alternating from side to side. This is a form of cyclic seizures which we refer to as 'ping-pong' seizures.

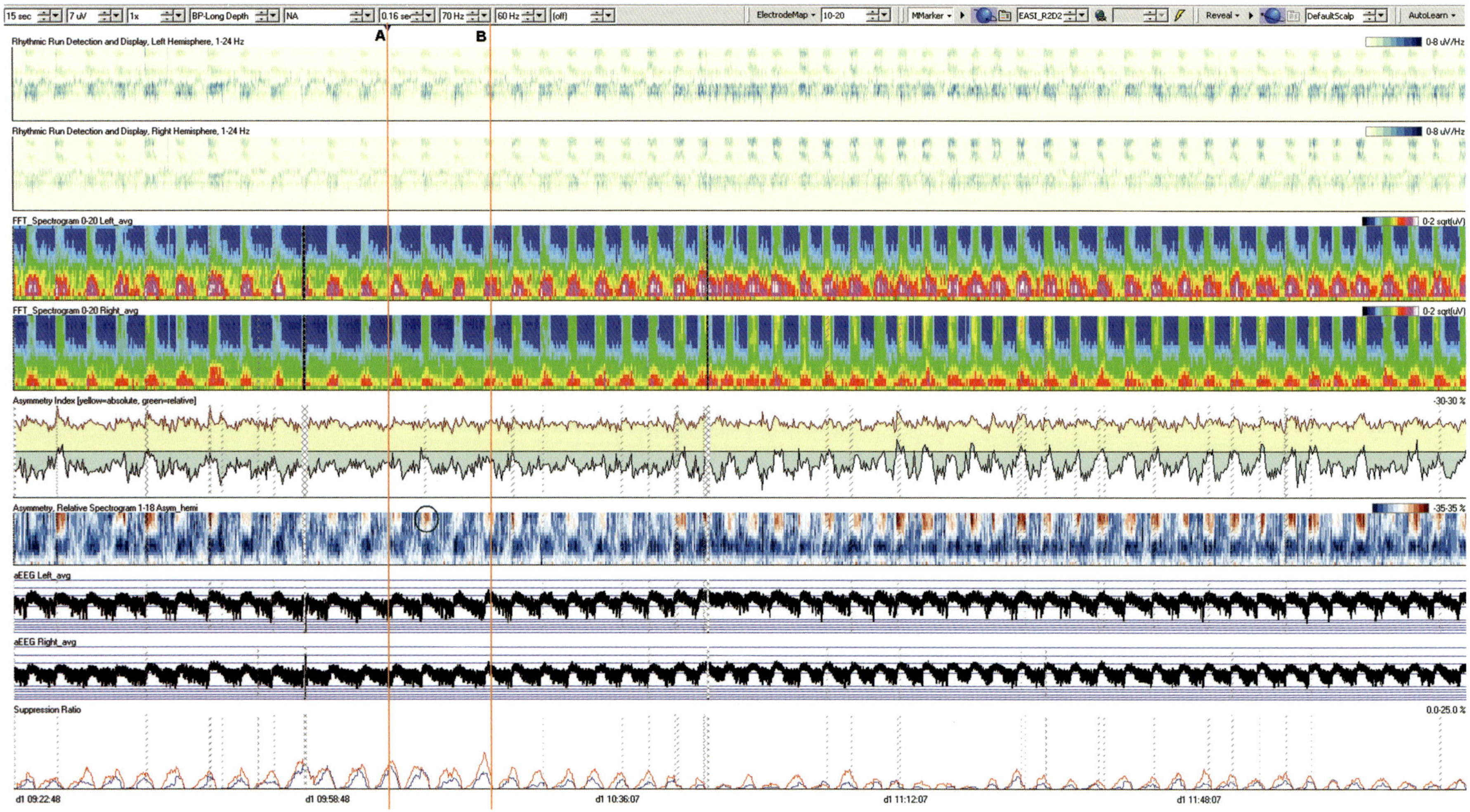

Figure 7.21 Cyclic PLEDs. **Main:** Three hours of QEEG in an elderly man with a large right frontal intracerebral hemorrhage with ventricular extension. A cyclic pattern is evident. In this case, there are left-sided PLEDs (periodic lateralized epileptiform discharges; from the opposite side of the hemorrhage) coming and going every ~3 min. At the same time, muscle artifact appears on the right, best appreciated on the asymmetry spectrogram (appearing in red at high frequencies; circle). There was no detectable clinical correlate. The cyclic muscle artifact is either due to contralateral 'ictal' muscle tone or cyclic arousal with nonspecific increase in muscle tone when more stimulated, with the PLEDs present in the more awake portion of the cycle. Also note the persistent asymmetry with more power on the left (downgoing green relative asymmetry index tracing and blue on the asymmetry spectrogram, maximal in the theta range). Finally, the cyclic pattern can be seen on the suppression ratio (bottom panel).

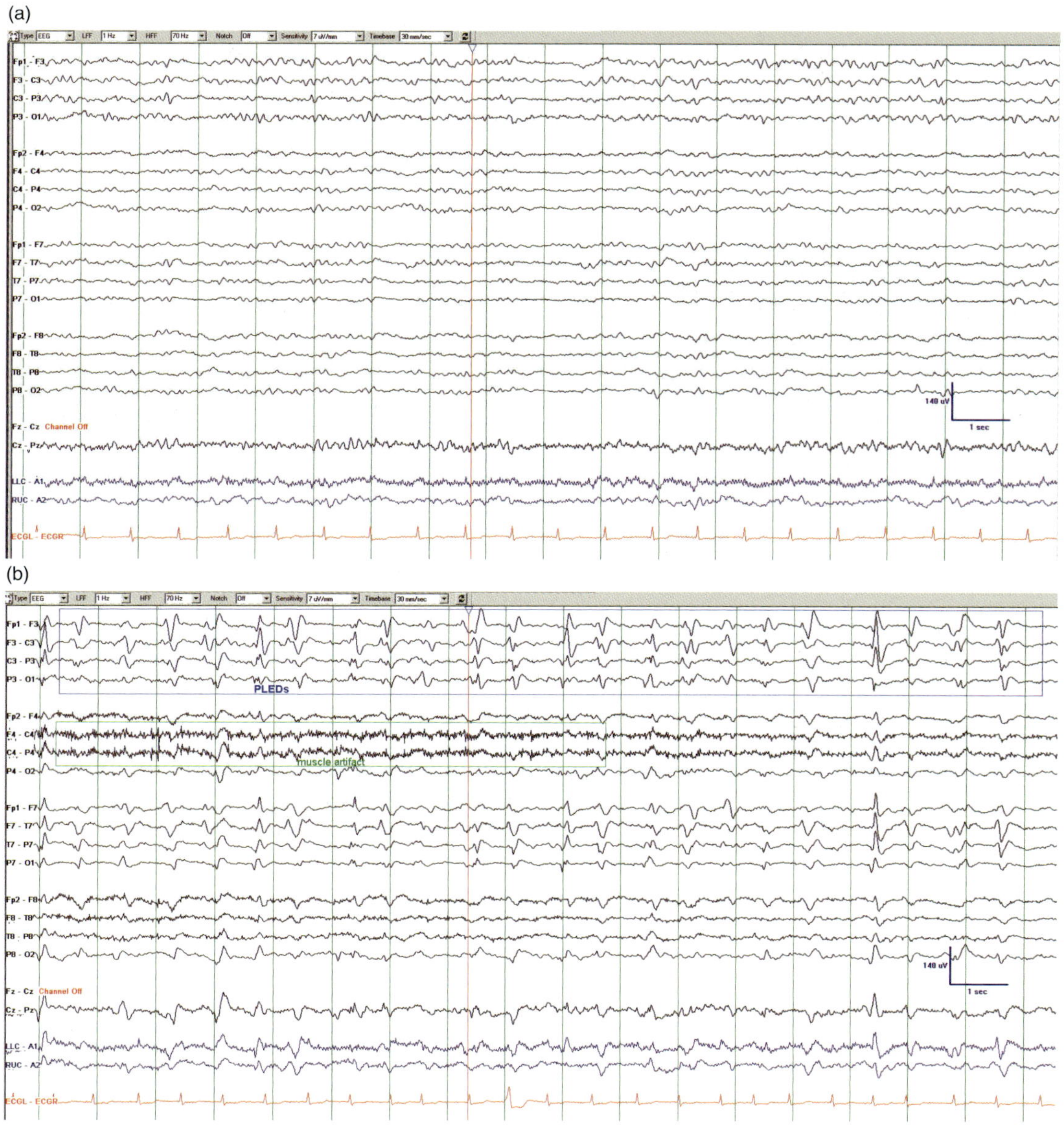

Figure 7.21 (*Continued*) The suppression ratio shows the percent of the record that is suppressed (below a certain amplitude, such as 5 uV), and is mainly used to quantify suppression-burst patterns. The asymmetry can be seen in this tracing as well, with higher suppression ratios on the right (red) than left (blue). **(a)** EEG at A: portion without PLEDs, showing mostly theta range activity, higher amplitude on the left. **(b)** EEG at B: portion with left PLEDs averaging ∼1.5 Hz with some spread to the right, and right-sided muscle artifact.

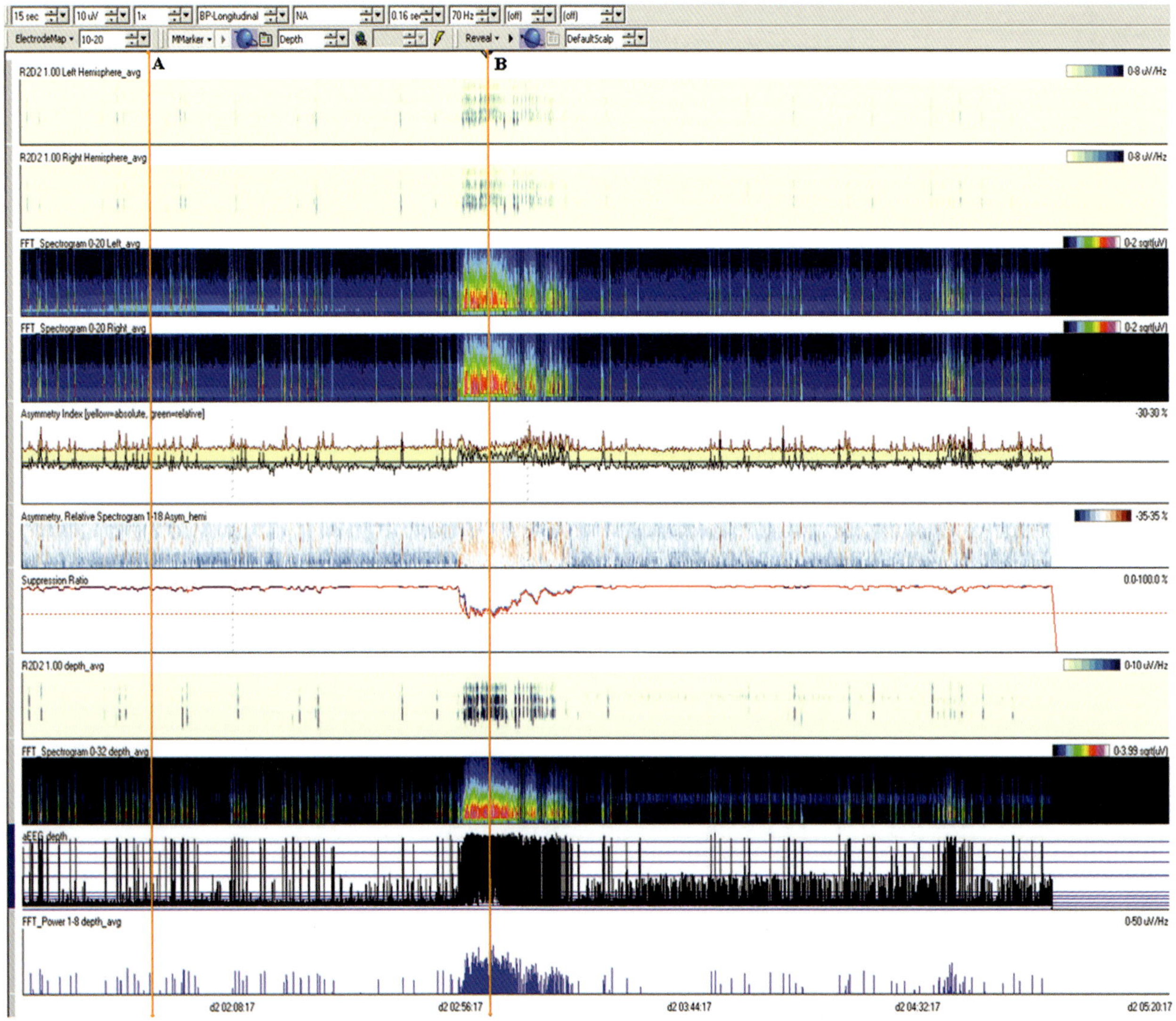

Figure 7.22 Pentobarbital coma, suppression-burst, depth electrode and QEEG alarms. **Main:** Four hours of QEEG in a 27-year-old woman with encephalitis. The patient was being treated with pentobarbital for refractory status epilepticus with a goal of near-complete suppression because frequent seizures continued to arise from any lower degree of suppression. Note the suppression ratio (the percent of the record that is 'flat', or below 5 uV in this setup; seventh panel) was around 100% for most of the record. It then dropped down to just under 50% (B), crossing the alarm threshold set at the bedside (dotted red line on the suppression ratio panel) and resulting in an increase in pentobarbital. Alarms can be set on almost any QEEG parameter and can result in bedside alarming and/or multiple forms of remote notification. The bottom four panels in this case show QEEG calculations on a single miniature eight contact depth electrode traversing the

(a)

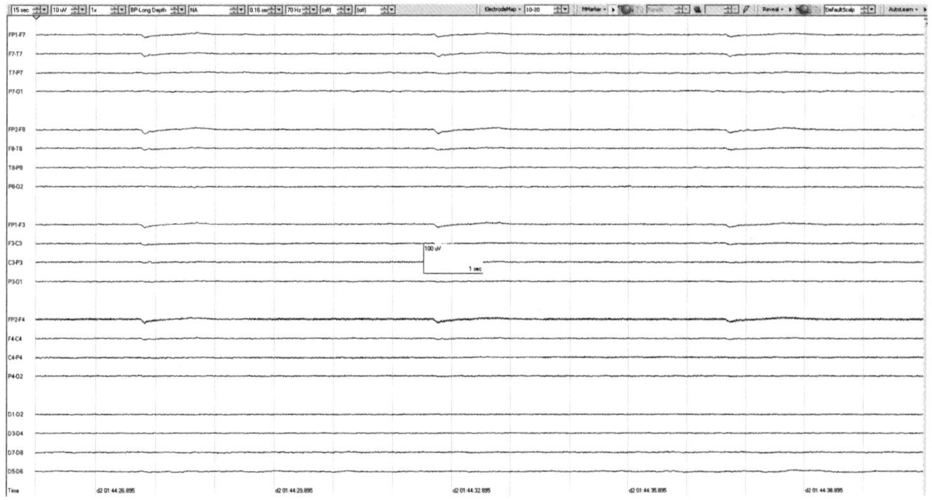

(b)

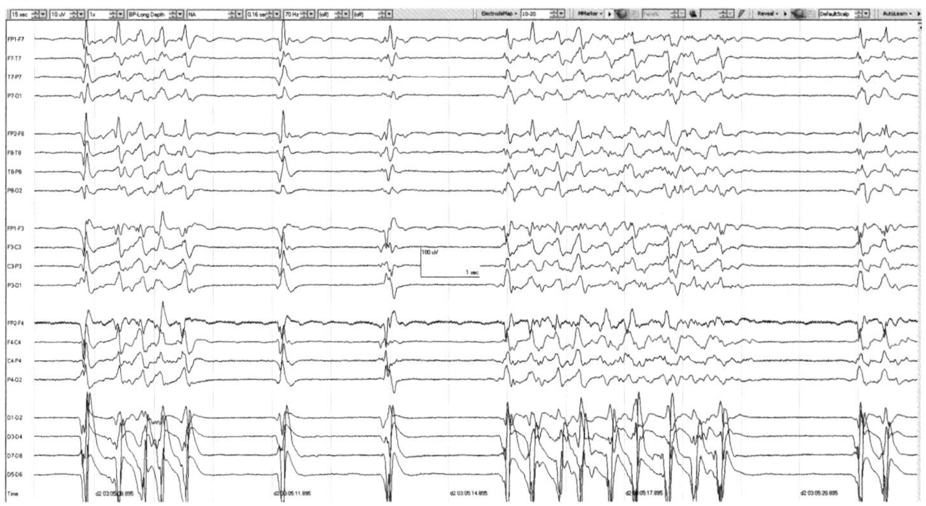

Figure 7.22 (*Continued*) cortex that is placed at the time of placement of other invasive monitoring devices. EEG from these intracranial electrodes has much improved signal-to-noise ratio, allowing much more reliable setting of QEEG alarms for detection of brain events, including seizures and ischemia. **(a)** EEG at A: complete suppression, including on the depth electrode (bottom four channels). **(b)** EEG at B: suppression-burst with about 40% of the record suppressed and the rest containing medium-to-high amplitude epileptiform discharges. This is the pattern that led to alarming of the suppression ratio (became too low), though it could also have been due to increased total power, mean amplitude or rhythmicity on the depth channels (bottom four channels). Alarms on any of these could have been sensitive and specific for this change.

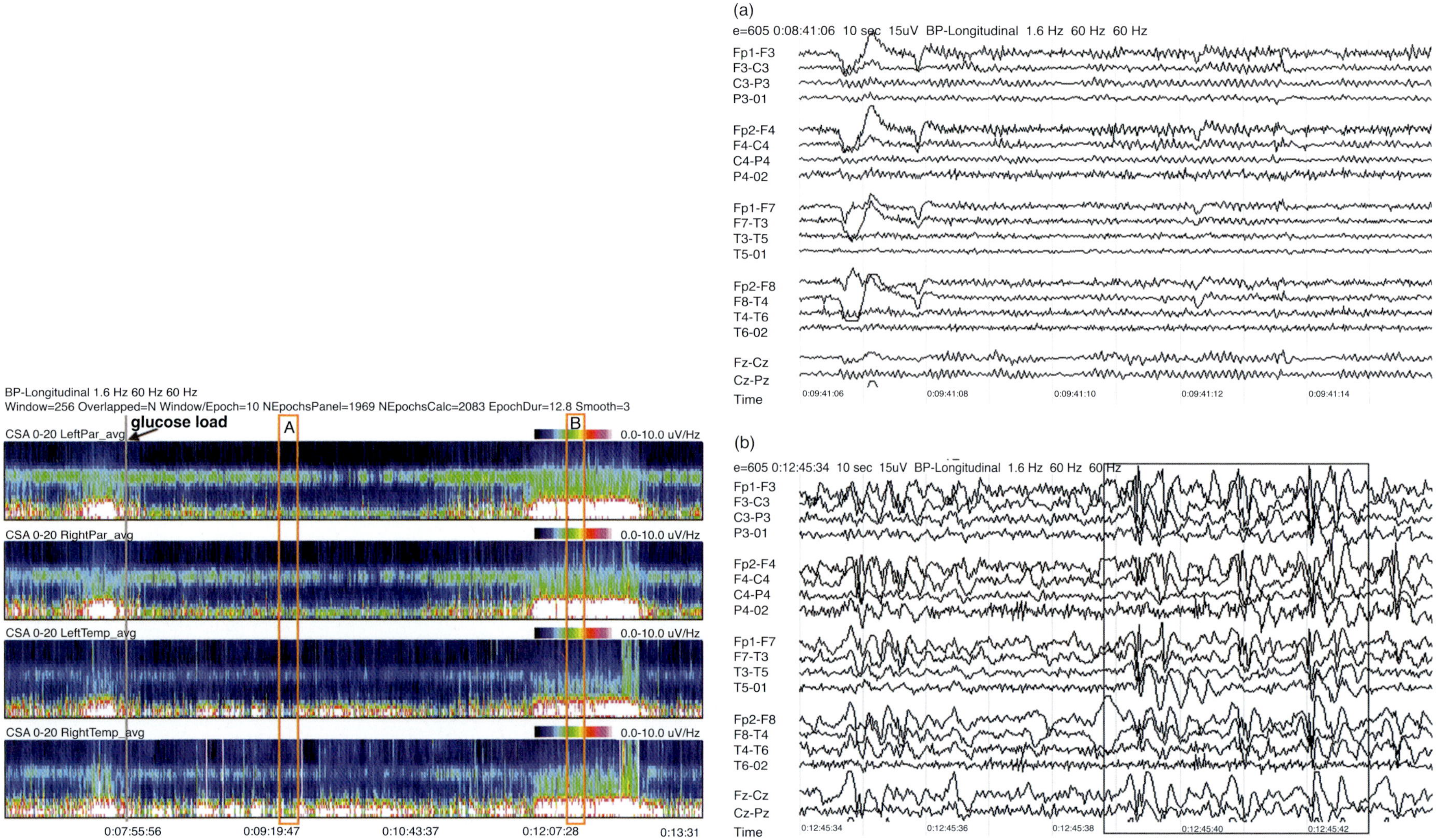

Figure 7.23 Glucose load effect in glucose transporter deficiency. **Main:** Nine hours of QEEG in a child with glut-1 deficiency syndrome, a condition with low CSF glucose due to a defect in the glucose transporter glut-1, which transports glucose into the central nervous system across the blood–brain barrier. Many patients with this syndrome, also known as De Vivo syndrome, have seizures and generalized epileptiform discharges. This example shows periods of high delta power due to frequent generalized spike-wave discharges (before the glucose load and at B) that resolve with a glucose load (gray line and A), then return after fasting for 5–6 h (B). **(a)** EEG at A: no epileptiform discharges. **(b)** EEG at B: frequent irregular generalized spike-wave discharges (box), resulting in marked increase in delta power.

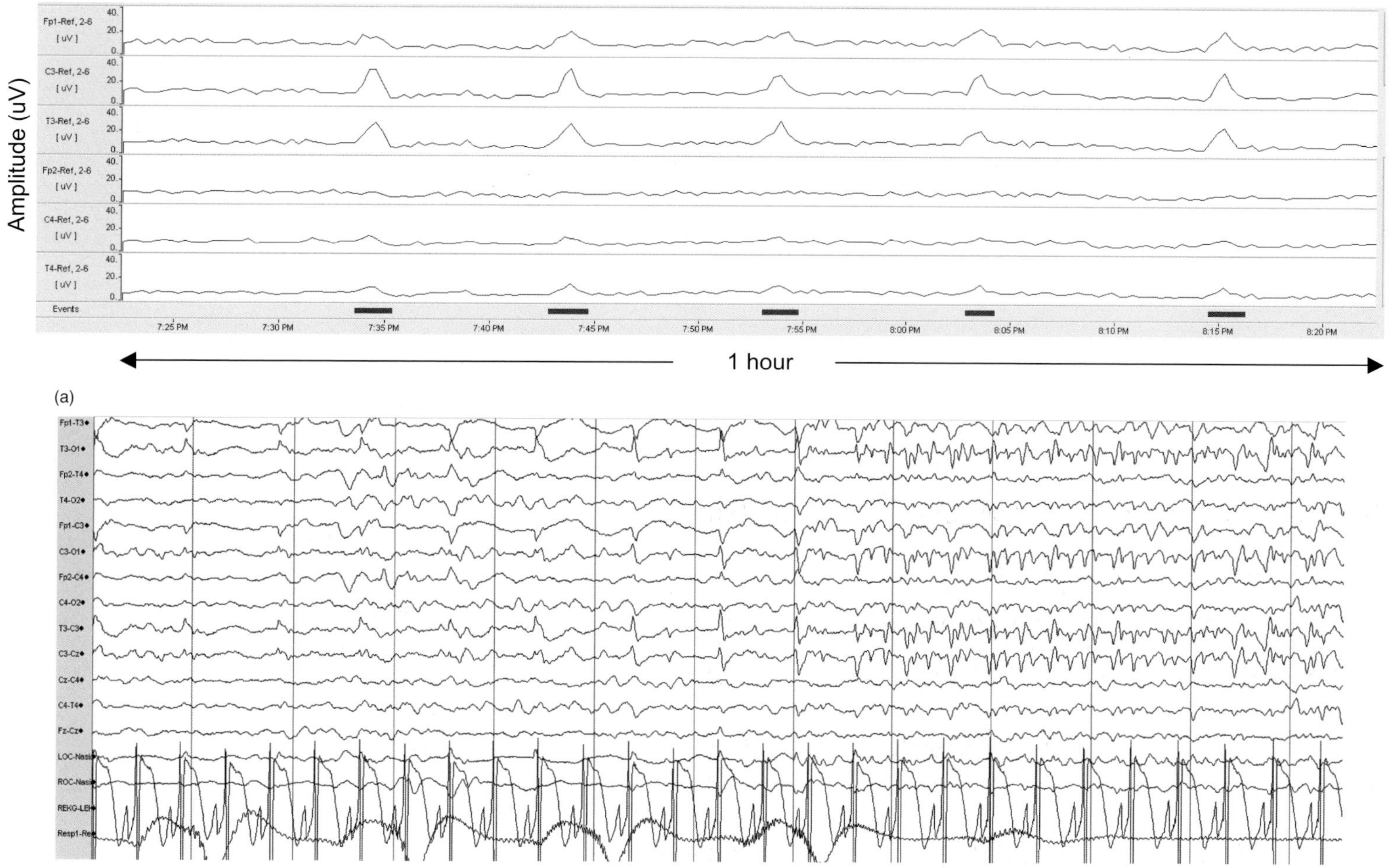

Figure 7.24 Envelope trend analysis for neonatal seizure recognition. **Main:** One-hour envelope-trend tracing in a term neonate with discrete recurrent seizures secondary to hypoxic-ischemic encephalopathy. Envelope trending selects waveforms within a specified frequency range (e.g. 2–6 Hz as in this example) and plots the median amplitude of waveforms within this frequency range over a specified period of time (usually 10–20 s). The vertical axis is in microvolts and the horizontal axis is time. (This is similar to the total power panel shown in Figure 7.16) Display of 2–4 h per screen is usually optimal for seizure detection with envelope trend. In neonates with acute encephalopathy, the background is often slow or discontinuous and suppressed. Seizures contain a rhythmic series of waves, often in the 2–6 Hz range, and thus result in an increase in the median amplitude within that range, which is displayed as an upward deflection. Plotting the median amplitude rather than the mean amplitude reduces false detections from brief artifacts such as movement or electrode artifact. In this example, the flatter periods contain delta activity that is excessively discontinuous. The large upward deflections in the left hemisphere (C3, T3) are seizures, as confirmed on the corresponding raw EEG as always. Seizures identified by standard EEG interpretation are marked by the black bars below the envelope trend. **(a)** EEG showing onset of the first marked seizure using a standard neonatal montage. (Images courtesy of Nicholas Abend, MD and Susan T. Herman, MD, USA).

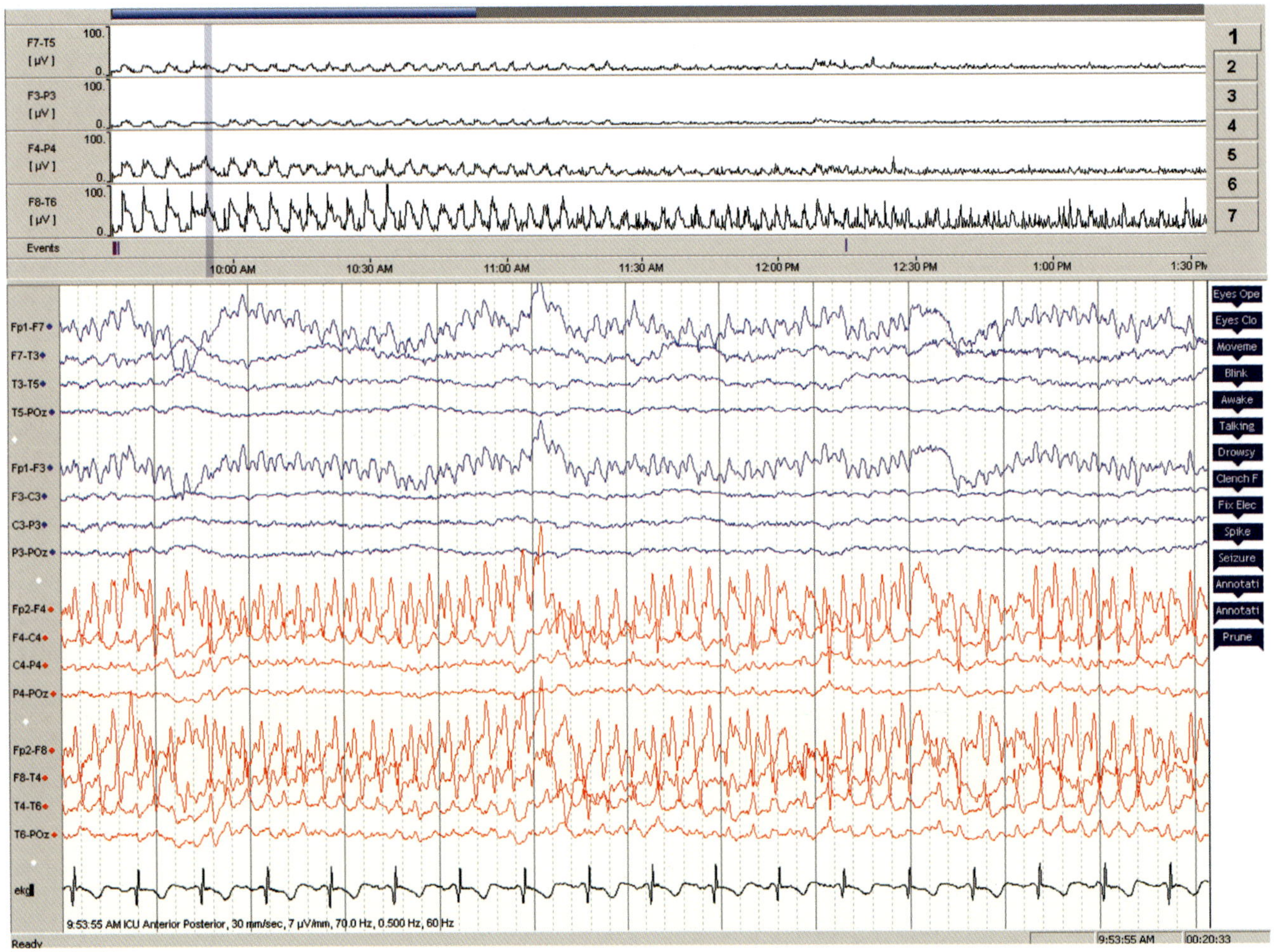

(a)

Figure 7.25 Envelope (amplitude) trending: multiple seizures in an adult. **(a)** 61-year-old woman s/p right frontal meningioma resection and prolonged confusion post-operatively. Envelope (amplitude) trend reveals frequent, periodic amplitude peaks on the right, each corresponding to an electrographic seizure (example at the gray bar shown).

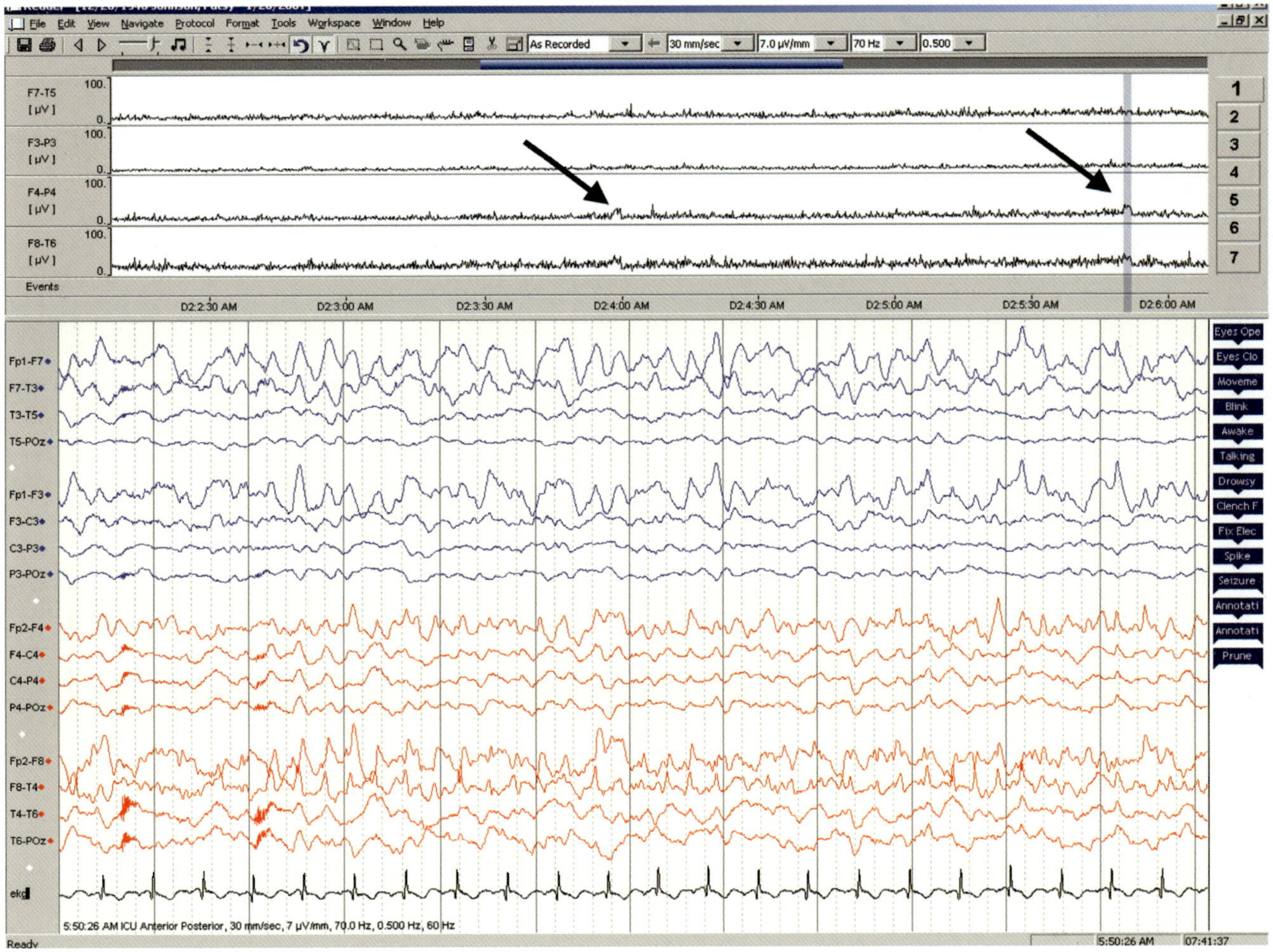

(b)

Figure 7.25 (*Continued*) **(b)** Same patient two days later after treatment for partial, nonconvulsive status. Envelope trend reveals two small peaks in amplitude corresponding to more subtle, isolated electrographic seizures, maximal at F8 (example at the gray bar shown). (Images courtesy of Suzette Laroche, MD, USA).

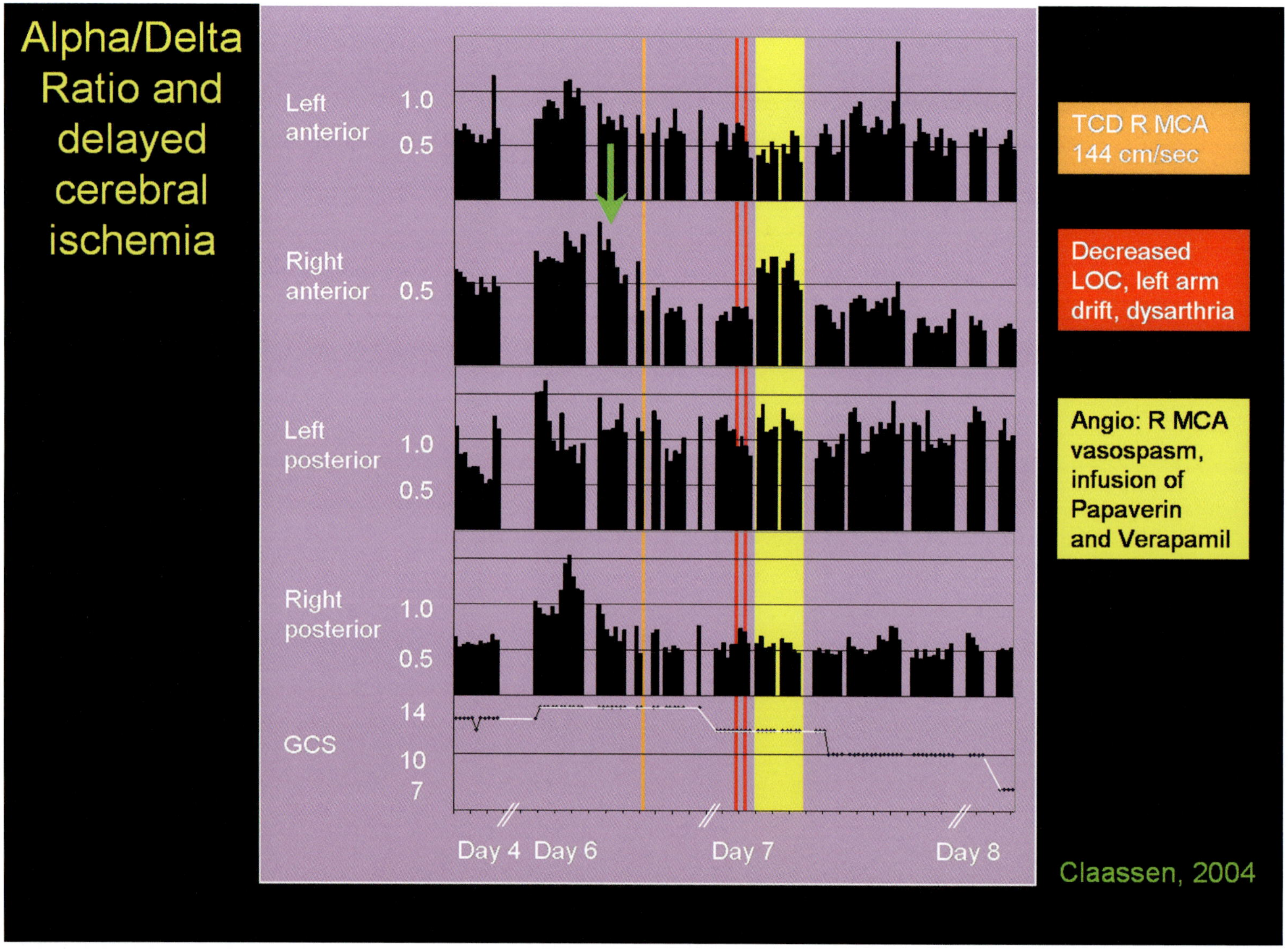

Figure 7.26 Multimodality monitoring for vasospasm after subarachnoid hemorrhage (SAH); alpha-delta ratio. **Main:** Alpha-delta ratio (ADR) calculated every 15 min and Glasgow Coma Score (GCS) shown for days 6–8 of continuous EEG (cEEG) monitoring. A 57-year-old woman admitted for acute subarachnoid hemorrhage (admission Hunt-Hess grade 4) from a right posterior communicating aneurysm. Admission angiography did not show vasospasm. The aneurysm was clipped on SAH day 2. No infarcts were seen on postoperative CT, day 2 (shown on next page). Postoperatively she had a GCS of 14. CEEG monitoring was performed from SAH days 3 to 8. The alpha/delta ratio progressively decreased after day 6, particularly in the right anterior region (green arrow), to settle into a steady trough level later that night, reflecting loss of fast frequencies and slowing over the right hemisphere in the raw EEG (also shown on next page). On SAH day 6, flow velocity in the right middle cerebral artery (MCA) was marginally elevated (144 cm/s), but the patient remained clinically stable with hypertensive-hypervolemic therapy (systolic blood pressure >180 mmHg). On day 7, the GCS dropped from 14 to 12 and a CT scan showed a right internal capsule and hypothalamic infarction (see day 7 CT).

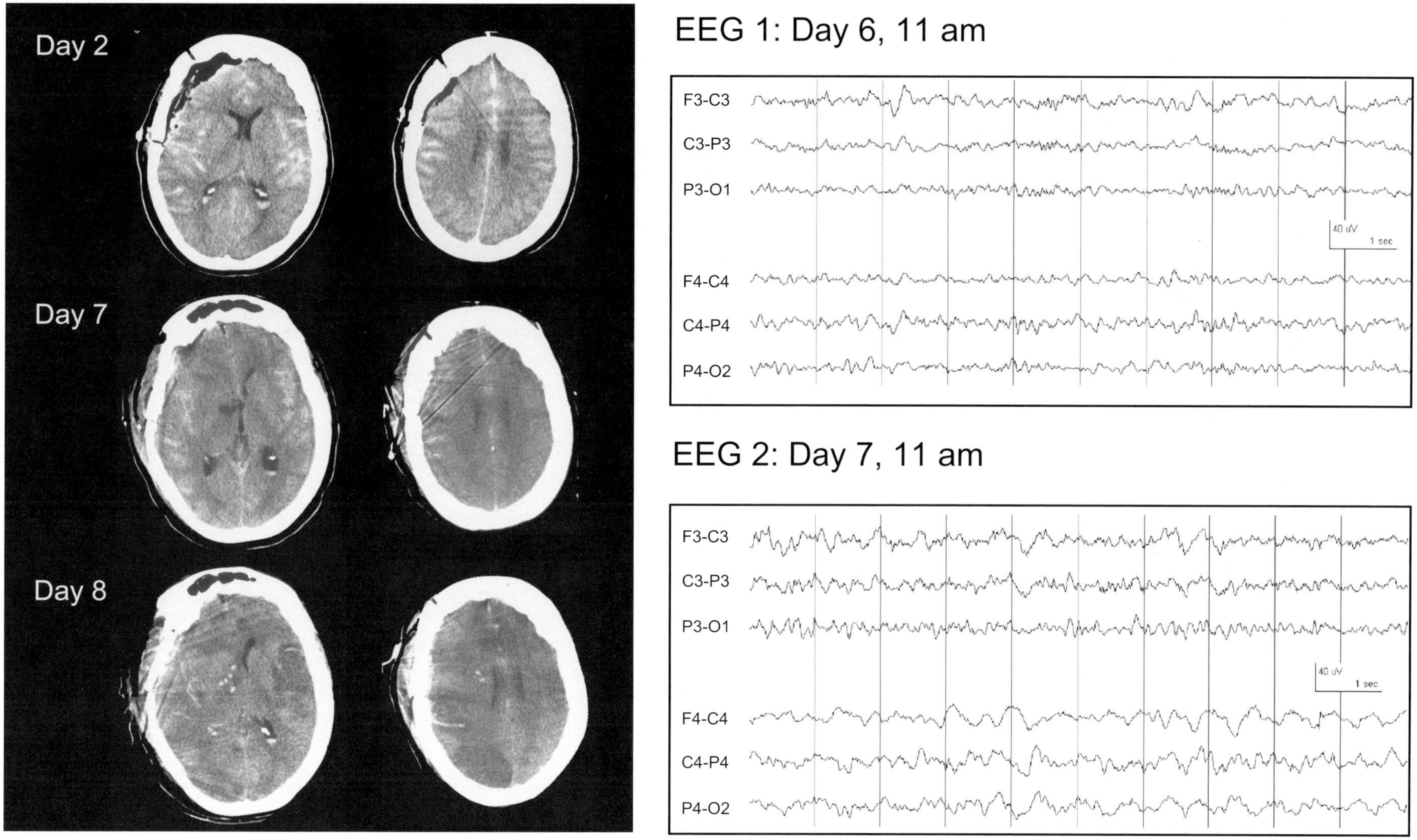

Figure 7.26 (*Continued*) Angiography demonstrated severe distal right MCA and left vertebral artery spasm; however, due to the marked tortuosity of the parent vessels and the location of vasospasm, a decision was made not to perform angioplasty, but to infuse verapamil and papaverine. This resulted in a marked, but transient increase of the right anterior and posterior alpha/delta ratios (yellow shaded area). Later that day the patient further deteriorated clinically to a GCS of 7, with a new onset left hemiparesis, and died on SAH day 9 from widespread infarction due to vasospasm (see day 8 CT). *CT scans*: CT scans obtained on SAH days 2, 7, and 8. *EEGs*: Sample of raw EEG prior (SAH day 6) and during (SAH day 7) change in the alpha/delta ratio. There is an increase in delta and decrease in faster activity, more pronounced on the right (bottom three channels) in EEG 2 compared to EEG 1. (From Claassen *et al.*, 2004, with permission)

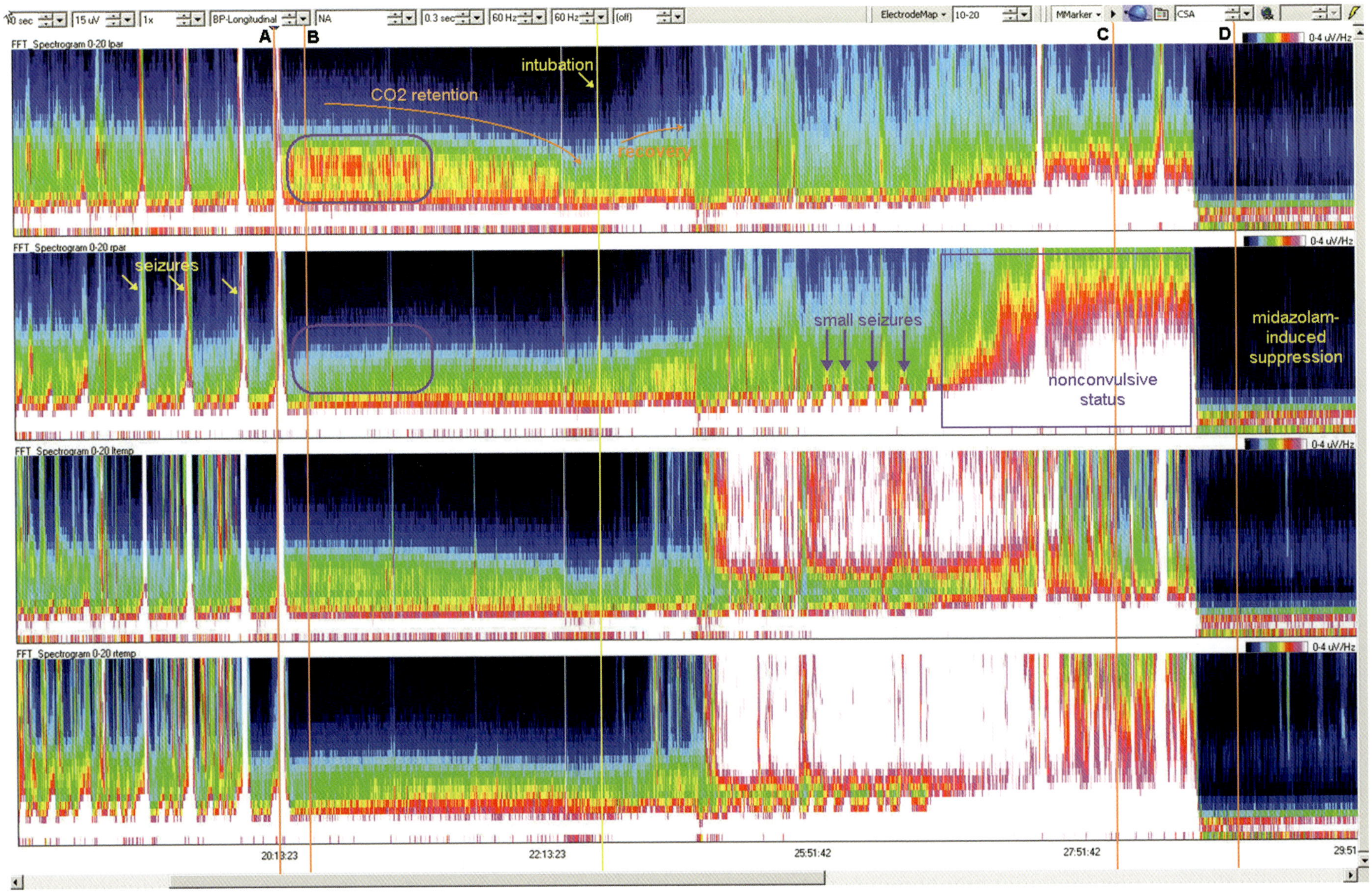

Figure 7.27 CO_2 retention, acidosis and resolution of nonconvulsive seizures. **Main:** Spectrogram showing 12 h of EEG in a man in his 60s with a right-sided subdural hematoma and refractory nonconvulsive seizures. He was still having two or three nonconvulsive seizures per hour (labeled, with example at A) in the first few hours of this sample; intubation was being avoided if possible. The seizures resolved without specific intervention, but the patient then became sleepier. The spectrograms showed an asymmetry with attenuation of theta/alpha in the right parasagittal region

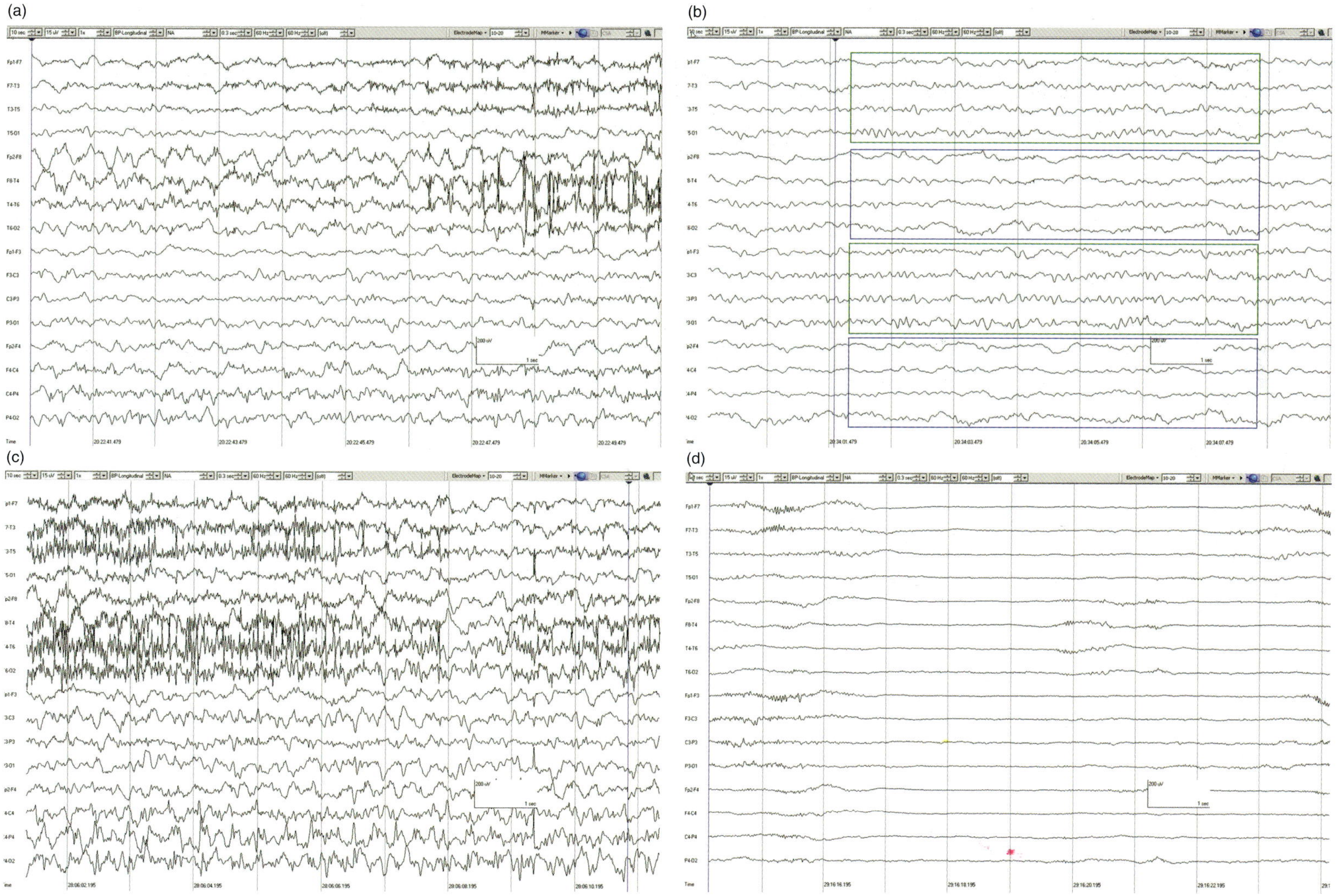

Figure 7.27 (*Continued*) (blue ellipses and B), likely due to the extra-axial collection on the right. After the seizures resolved, the background EEG on the healthier side (the left) began to attenuate gradually (orange-curved arrow labeled 'CO_2 retention'); arterial blood gas revealed CO_2 retention and acidosis with a pH of 7.1. He was then intubated (yellow line) and background began to recover (curved arrow labeled 'recovery') as his CO_2 and pH normalized. However, smaller seizures then appeared (labeled 'small seizures'), followed by nonconvulsive status epilepticus (C) that eventually had a clinical component. Midazolam drip was then started, seizures stopped and background was attenuated (D). The acidosis is probably what stopped the seizures. **(a)** EEG at A: right hemisphere seizure. **(b)** EEG at B: attenuation of faster frequencies on the right (blue boxes [right] compared to green boxes [left]). **(c)** EEG at C: during nonconvulsive status epilepticus, with ictal activity maximal in the right parasagittal region, especially the bottom three channels. **(d)** EEG at D: suppressed due to midazolam.

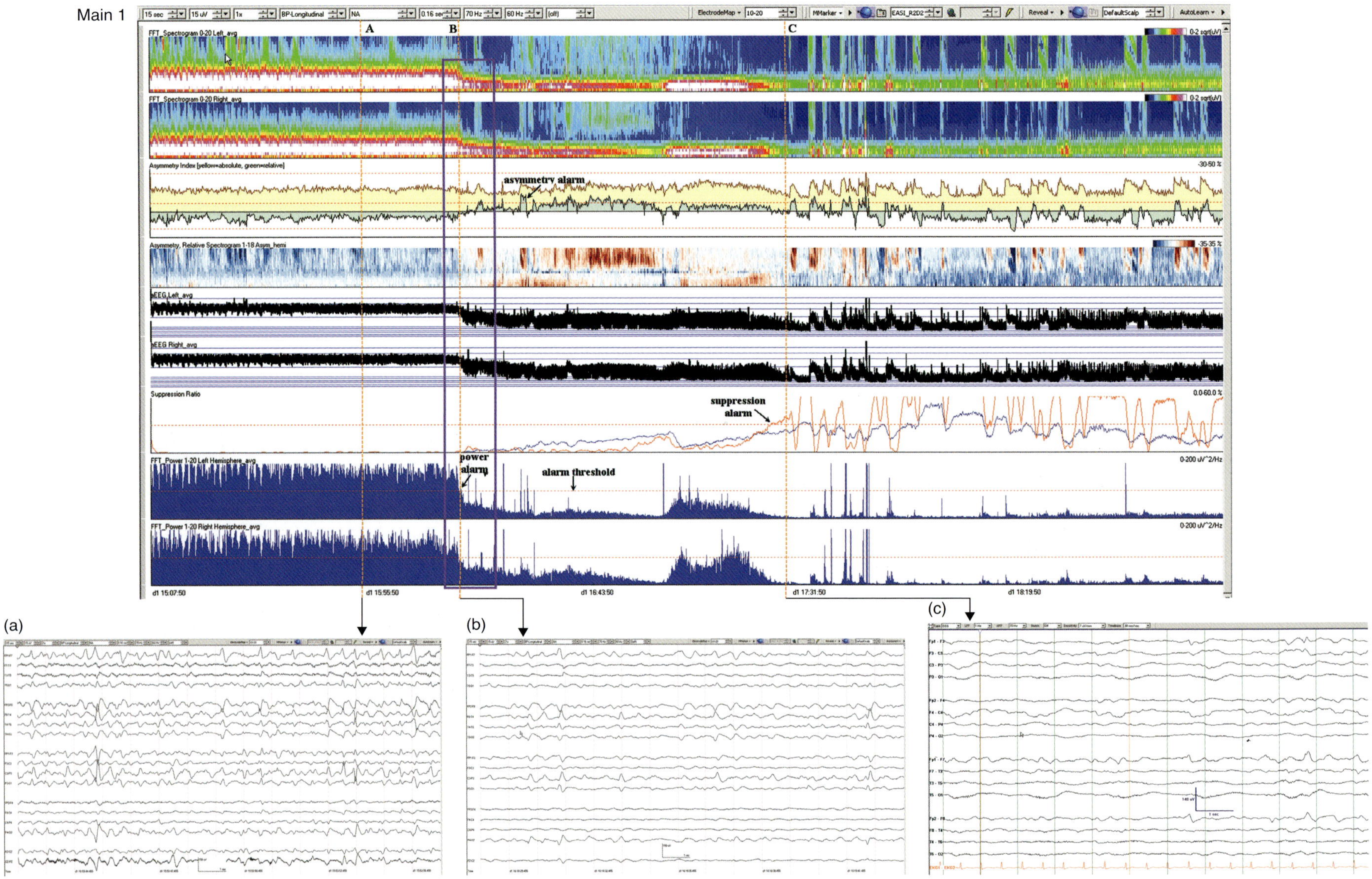

Figure 7.28 Hydrocephalus and multiple QEEG alarms. **Main 1:** Four hours of EEG in a 61-year-old woman with hepatic encephalopathy, cryptococcal meningitis and a lumbar drain to help manage raised intracranial pressure (ICP). The drain stopped functioning and ICP went up (purple box). Total power (bottom two panels) rapidly dropped, and dropped below the alarm threshold (dashed red line) quickly (labeled 'power alarm'). Shortly after, the asymmetry alarm threshold is crossed (labeled), followed by the suppression alarm about an hour later (suppression ratio above 25% in this example).

Main 2

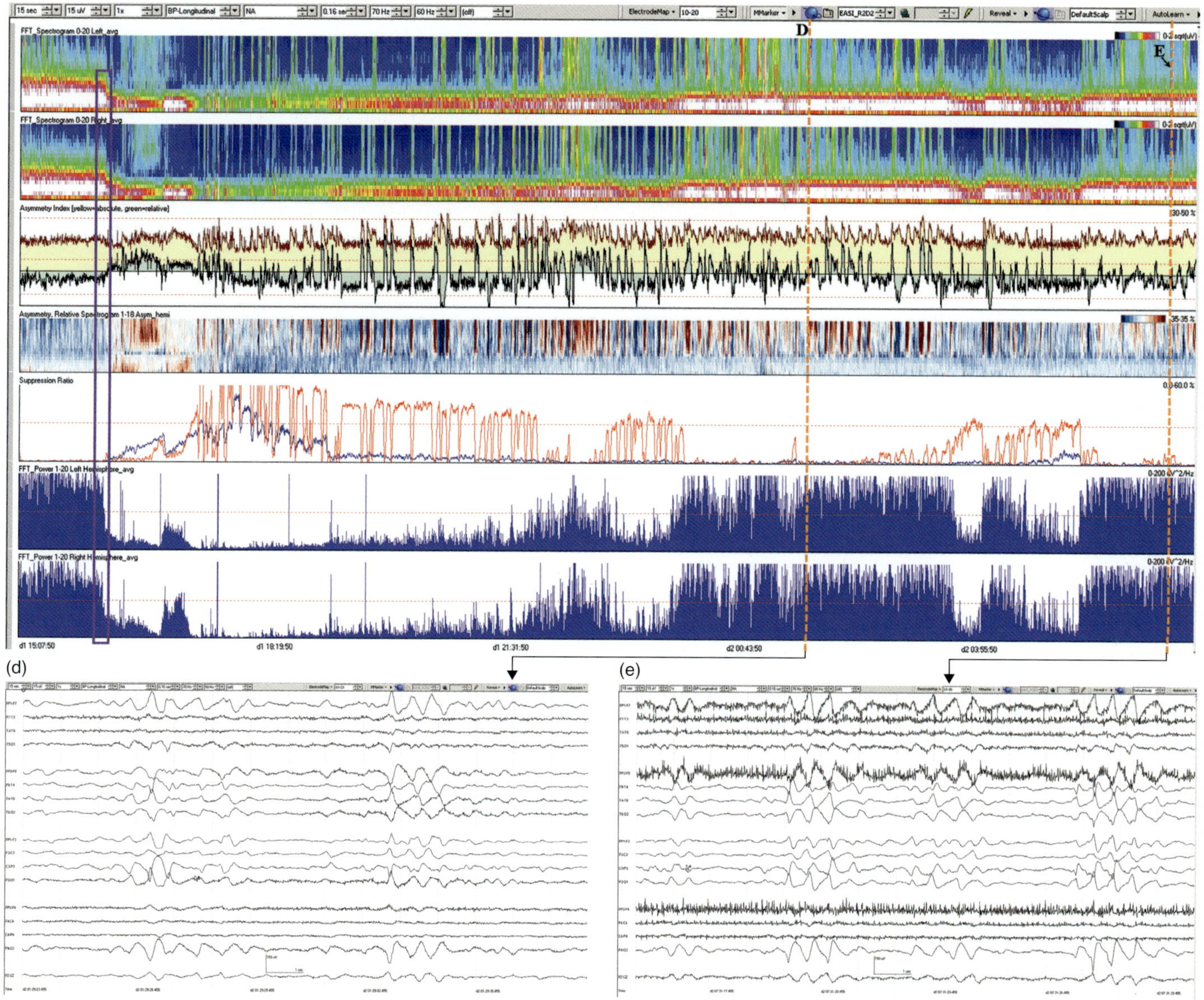

Figure 7.28 (*Continued*) Alarms can also be set on the aEEG tracing using the average amplitude (not shown). **(a)** EEG at A: baseline abnormal EEG. **(b)** EEG at B: diffuse attenuation compared to baseline as ICP rises. **(c)** EEG at C: more attenuated (and now unreactive, not shown). **Main 2:** Sixteen-hour view in the same patient starting at the same time. The acute change can be seen in the first few hours. By the second half of this 16-h period, EEG has begun to recover after the lumbar drain was fixed and ICP came back down. **(d)** EEG at D: early recovery of EEG; now reactive (reactivity not shown). **(e)** EEG at E: further recovery of EEG.

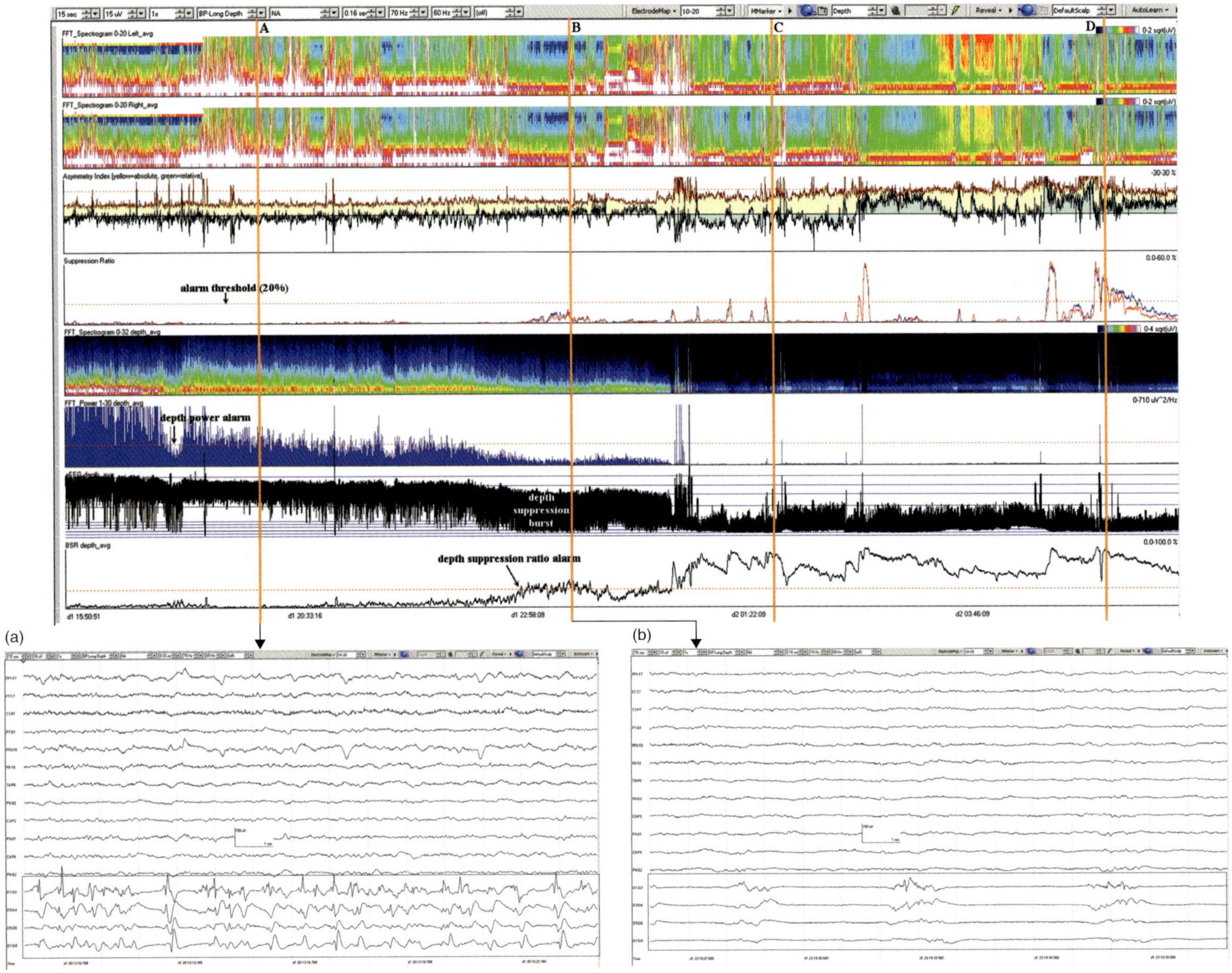

Figure 7.29 Detecting delayed cerebral ischemia after subarachnoid hemorrhage, including setting alarms and use of depth electrode. **Main:** Sixteen hours of QEEG in a 70-year-old woman s/p Hunt and Hess grade 3–4 subarachnoid hemorrhage. The patient developed sepsis, bilateral vasospasm and bilateral infarcts during this time period. The top four panels are based on the standard scalp EEG, whereas the bottom four are based on intracranial EEG recorded from a miniature, eight contact, cortical minidepth electrode placed in the right frontal lobe (see scout X-rays, parts e and f). Alarm thresholds can be seen as dotted red lines, set on the scalp asymmetry index, the scalp suppression ratio, depth total power (1–30 Hz), depth average amplitude (red line not shown) and depth suppression ratio. On the scalp QEEG tracings, it is difficult to appreciate major changes until the second half of this time period, when asymmetry increases and the suppression ratio eventually rises, at least intermittently. On the depth QEEG tracings, the changes can be seen much earlier and more clearly, and a long gradual trend can be seen in the first third of this sample.

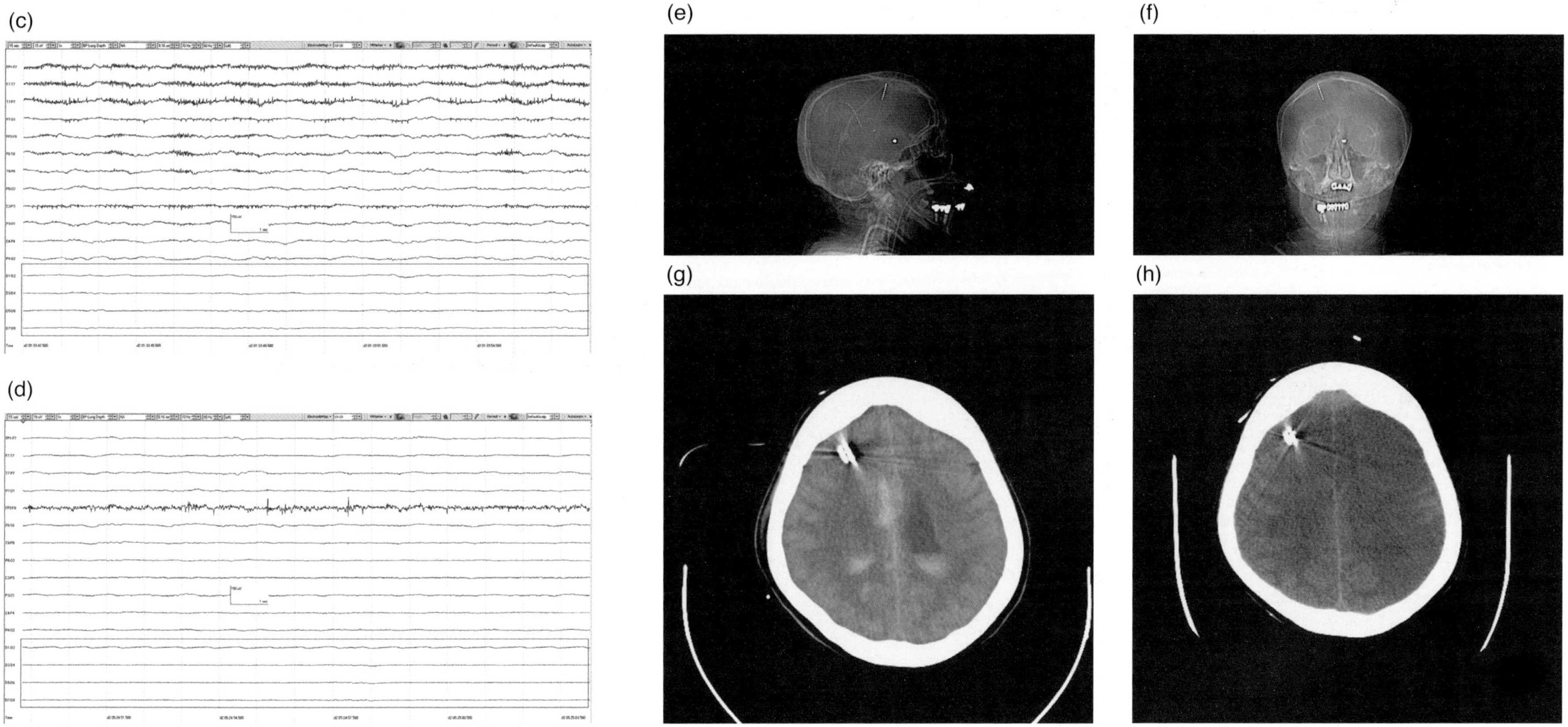

Figure 7.29 (*Continued*) The bottom three panels all triggered alarms, beginning with a drop in total power in the depth (labeled 'depth power alarm'), then a drop in average amplitude (not shown), then a rise in the suppression ratio (labeled 'depth suppression ratio alarm'). Also note the thick band that developed in the depth amplitude-integrated EEG panel (labeled in second panel from bottom) corresponding to intracranial suppression-burst (both high and low amplitudes in each epoch). By the second half of this time period, the depth EEG pattern appears to be nearly flat, with low power in all frequencies, low amplitudes and high-suppression ratios. The patient went on to develop bilateral anterior cerebral artery and left middle cerebral artery (MCA) infarcts with rising intracranial pressure by the end of this time period. She died 2–3 days later. **(a)** EEG at A: diffuse slowing on the scalp EEG, but continuous epileptiform activity in the depth EEG (bottom four channels). This is not an unusual occurrence, with seizure-like activity on the depth recording only. **(b)** EEG at B: diffuse slowing and attenuation on the scalp and suppression-burst in the depth EEG. **(c)** EEG at C: depth EEG recording is now flat, with the scalp EEG showing some muscle artifact and diffuse attenuation. The scalp recording is not quite low enough to qualify as suppressed in the scalp suppression ratio calculation, possibly due to the muscle artifact. **(d)** EEG at D: scalp and depth recordings are now flat. The suppression ratio on the scalp (as well as the depth) is now above 50%. **(e and f)**: Skull X-ray (scout views during the CT scan), showing the eight contact depth electrode in the right frontal lobe; there is a ventricular catheter right next to it (placed via same burrhole). **(g)** CT scan before the vasospasm and infarcts. The artifact in the right frontal lobe is from the ventricular catheter and the depth electrode combined. **(h)** CT scan after the vasospasm and infarcts, showing bilateral infarcts, worse on the left.

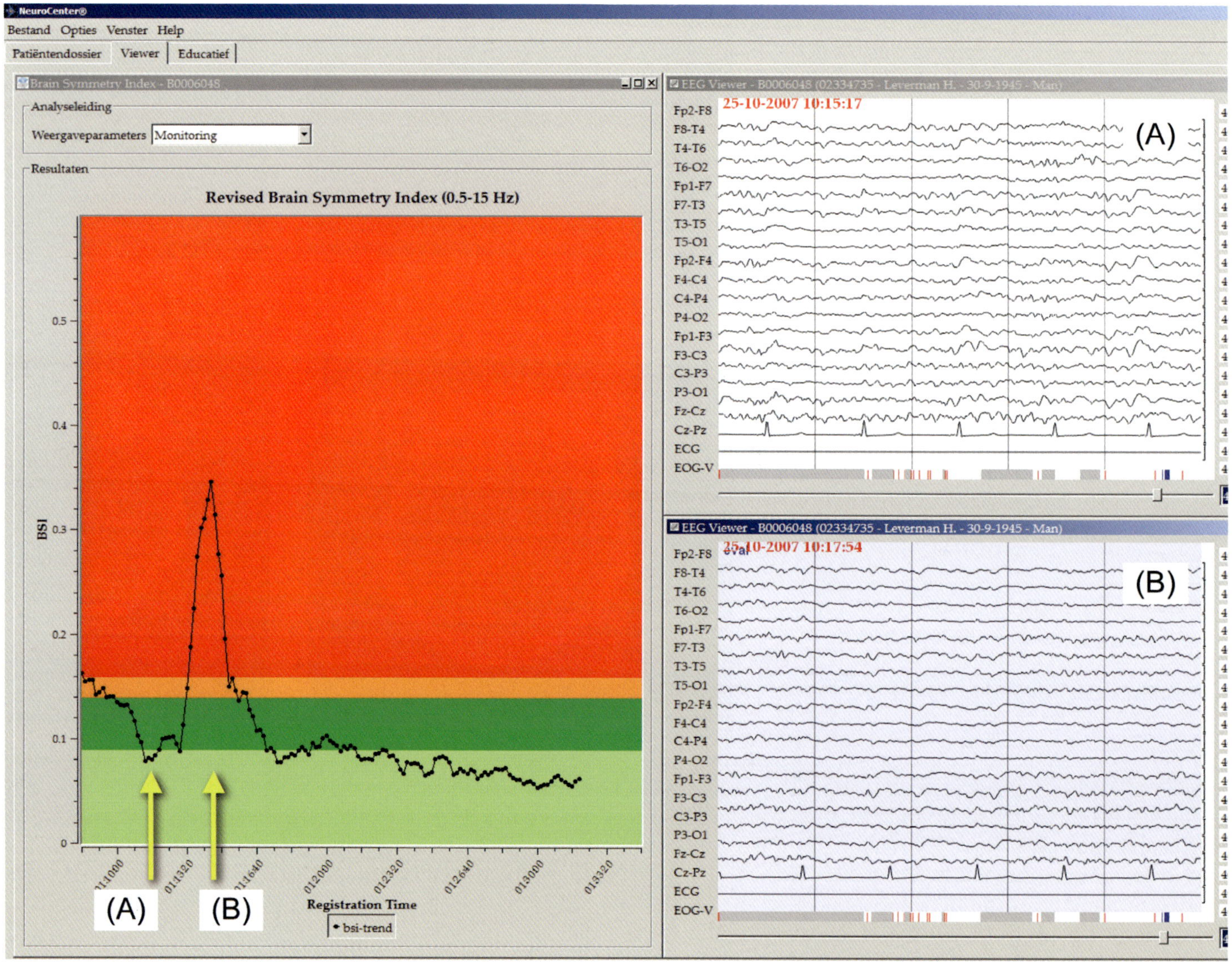

Figure 7.30 Brain Symmetry Index during carotid clamping. The Brain Symmetry Index (BSI) is a single numerical measure of total asymmetry, essentially summing the absolute values of the differences at each homologous electrode pair for all frequencies (similar to the yellow total absolute asymmetry index in prior images; see Figure 7.6 for initial description). This example shows the rise in asymmetry after clamping of the carotid artery during an endarterectomy. Note the right-side attenuation after clamping on the raw EEG (B). The BSI correlates with clinical stroke scales and has been used to follow the evolution of stroke and the effects of tPA administration (see van Putten and Tavy, 2004, 2007; de Vos *et al.*, 2008). (Image courtesy of Michel JAM van Putten, MD, PhD, The Netherlands)

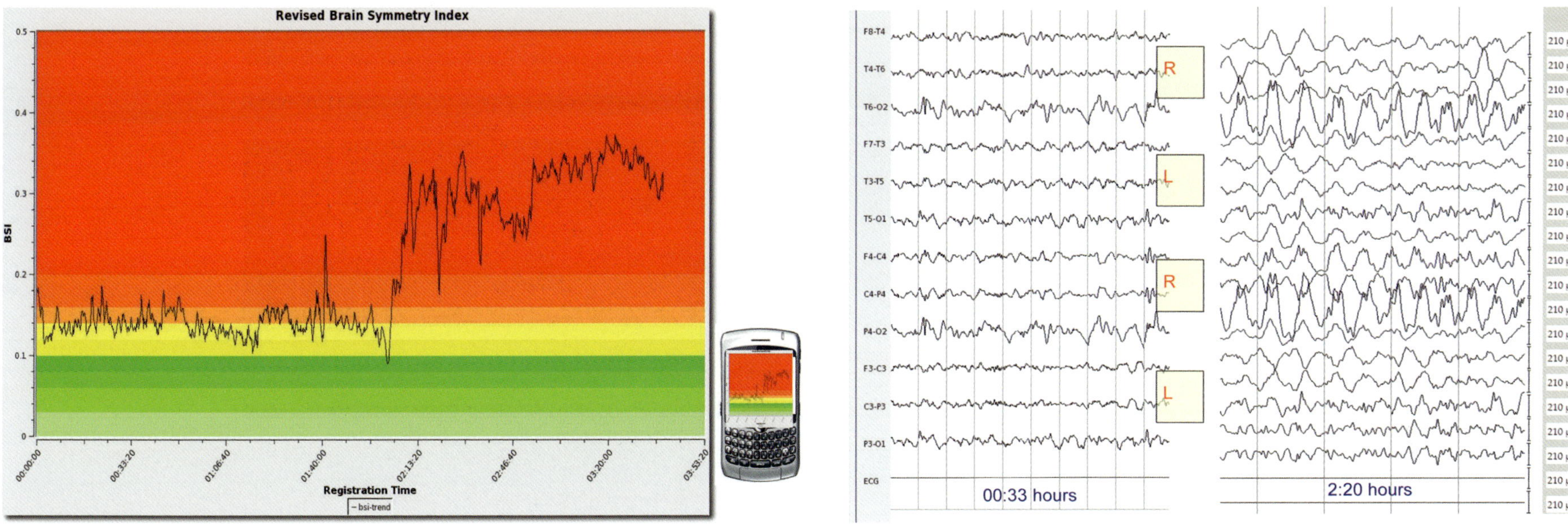

Figure 7.31 Brain Symmetry Index (BSI) and seizures. **Main:** A 4-h tracing of the BSI in a 3-year-old with right hemisphere seizures. The prominent and sustained rise in BSI (increasing asymmetry) was due to seizure activity on the right. The inset shows the ability to have screenshots sent remotely to a handheld device. **(a)** EEG before and after the rise in BSI. The second EEG shows ictal activity in the posterior right hemisphere. (Images courtesy of Michel JAM van Putten, MD, PhD, The Netherlands)

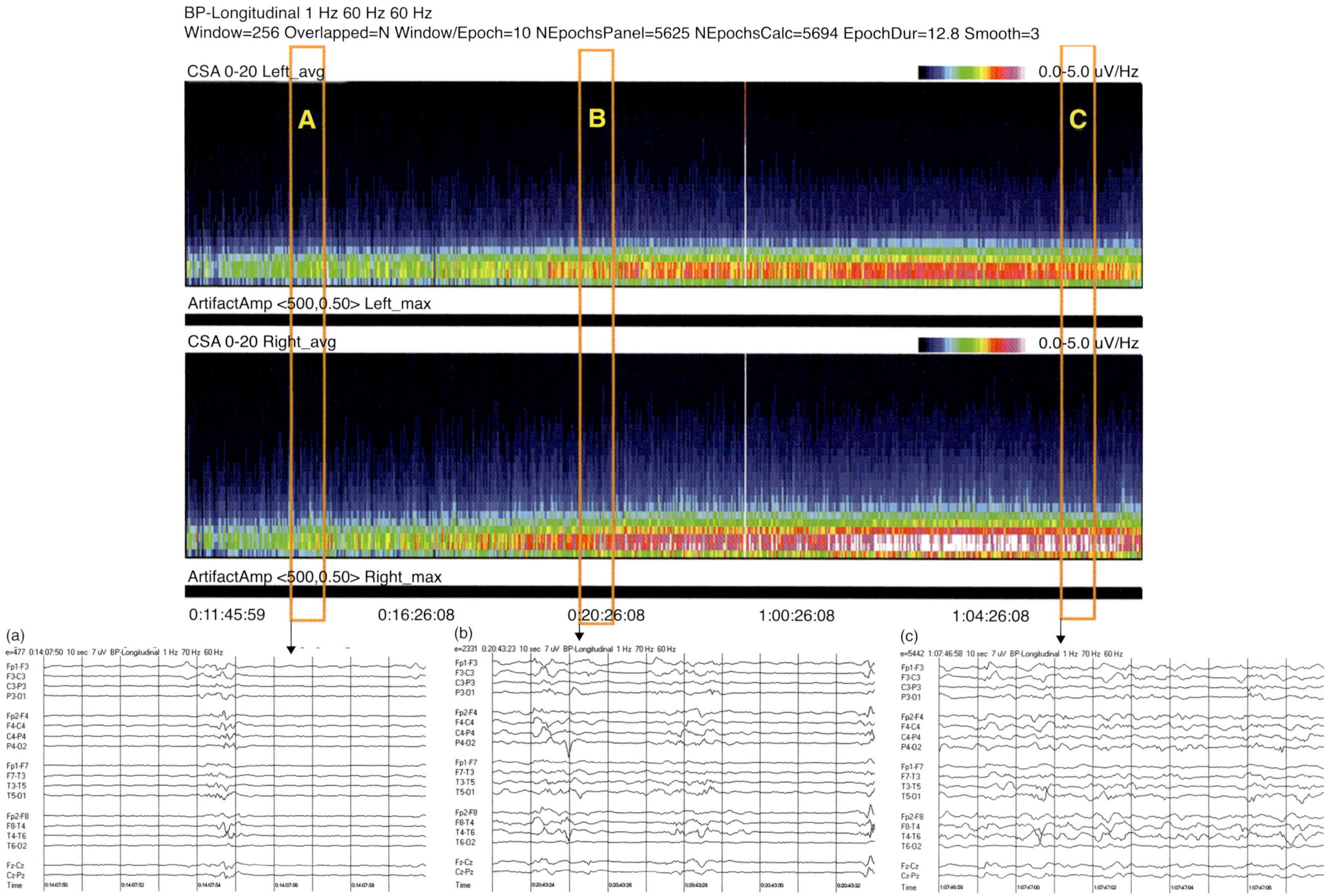

Figure 7.32 Long-term trends: wearing off of pentobarbital. **Main:** Spectrogram showing about 20 h of EEG during pentobarbital-induced coma in a 6-month-old boy with a left frontal hemorrhagic infarct and refractory status epilepticus. By showing this many hours of EEG at once, it is easy to appreciate the long gradual wearing off of the pentobarbital effect. The suppression ratio or amplitude-integrated EEG would be additional good QEEG methods for following this. **(a)** EEG at A: suppression-burst, with just one short burst on this 10-s page. **(b)** EEG at B: suppression-burst, with more frequent bursts. **(c)** EEG at C: emergence out of suppression-burst.

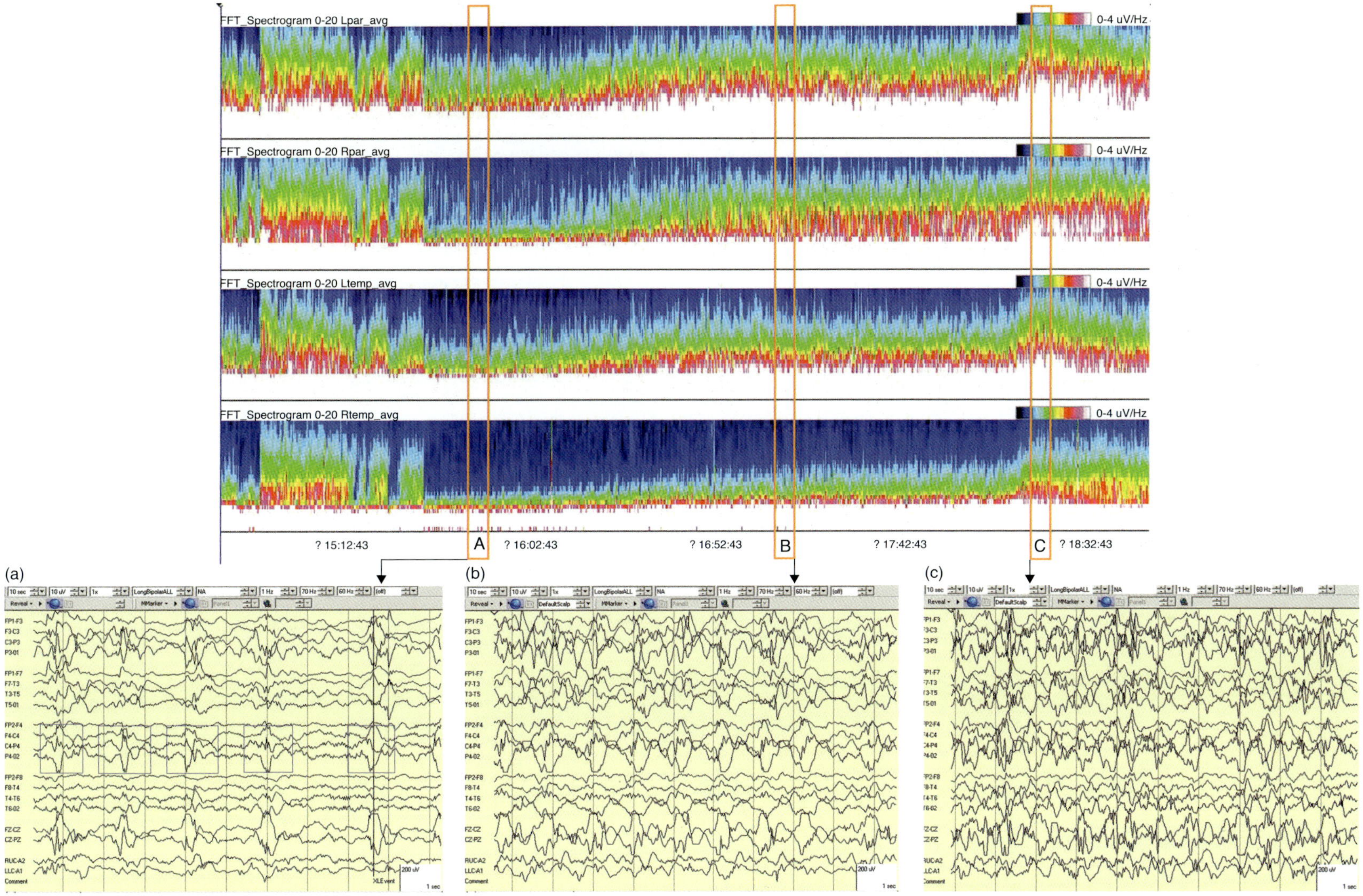

Figure 7.33 Long-term trends: worsening of nonconvulsive status epilepticus (NCSE); ictal-interictal continuum. **Main:** Spectrogram showing 4 h of EEG in a 4-month-old boy with refractory nonconvulsive seizures. Although treatment had stopped NCSE just prior to A, the ictal pattern gradually resumed and worsened over the next several hours. This is also a good example of the interictal-ictal continuum, as there is a gradual, smooth transition from one to the other in this patient. **(a)** EEG at A: periodic complexes every 2 s (boxes), bisynchronous and maximal in the parietal regions. This is most likely not an ictal pattern. **(b)** EEG at B: higher amplitude complexes, more epileptiform and twice as fast, now at 1 Hz and with minimal or no interdischarge interval. This is probably an ictal pattern at this point, though again the exact point at which interictal became ictal is arbitrary. **(c)** EEG at C: even higher amplitude, continuous, unequivocally ictal EEG pattern at this point. There was no clear clinical correlate.

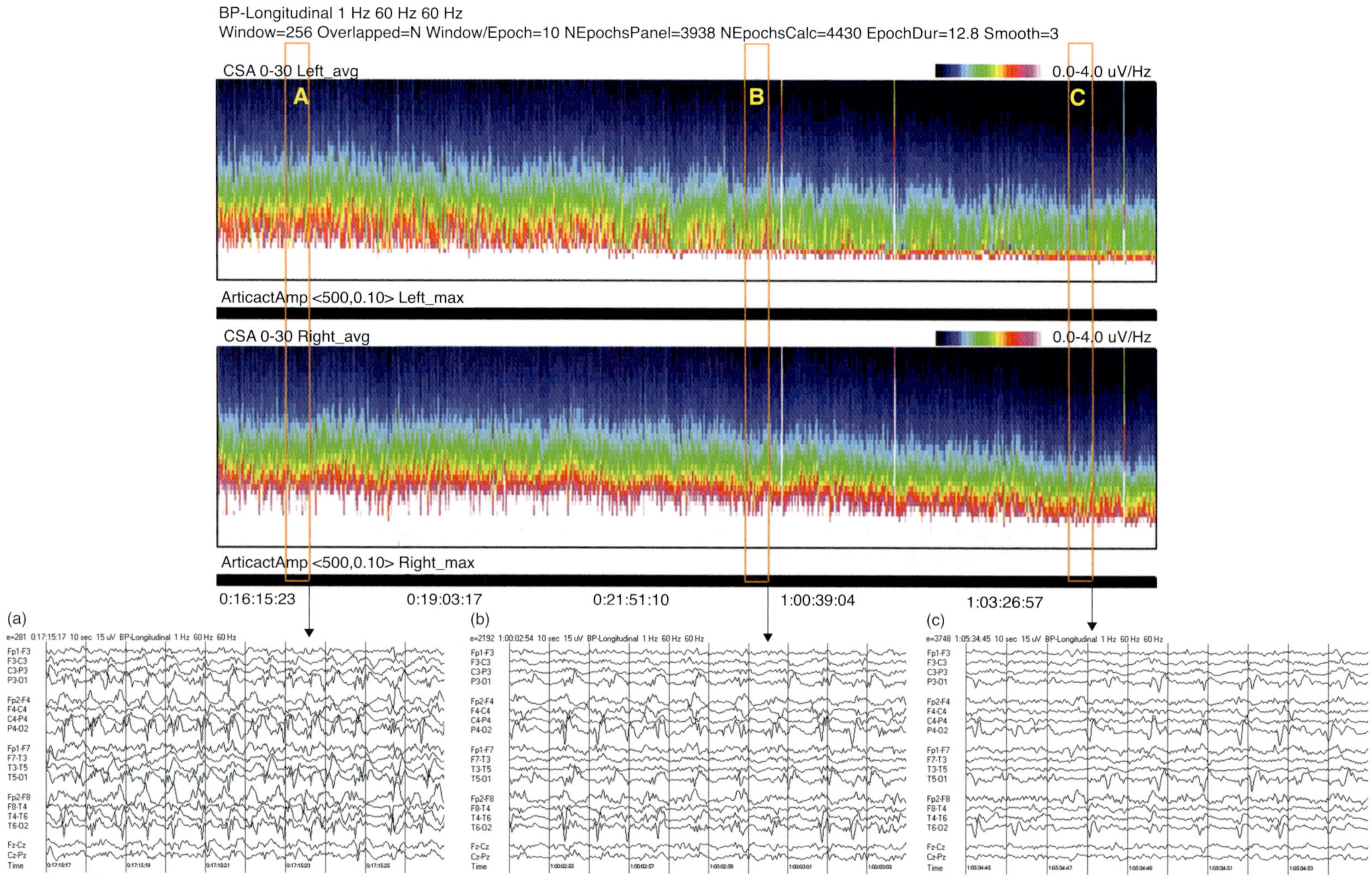

Figure 7.34 Long-term trends: gradual resolution of nonconvulsive status epilepticus (NCSE); ictal-interictal continuum and bilateral independent PLEDs (BIPLEDs). **Main:** Twelve-hour spectrogram in a 3-year-old s/p cardiac surgery showing gradual resolution of NCSE. This example also supports the concept of an ictal–interictal continuum as this patient has gradual transition for ictal to interictal, with a necessarily arbitrary cutoff point if trying to dichotomize. **(a)** EEG at A: posterior-predominant, ~1.5 Hz periodic epileptiform discharges, mostly but not always bisynchronous, often polyspikes, superimposed on a background of rhythmic delta. This pattern is on the ictal–interictal continuum, interpreted as ictal at this point. **(b)** EEG at B: similar pattern, but a bit slower, with brief breaks in the rhythmicity for half a second or so, and with more restricted field and more evidence of a bilateral independent pattern. This is still on the ictal–interictal continuum and was interpreted as BIPLEDs-plus, more prominent on the right (also known as BIPDs-plus in the new nomenclature; see appendix). **(c)** EEG at C: bilateral independent posterior-predominant PLEDs (BIPLEDs, or BIPDs), slower than 1 Hz and probably not ictal at this point.

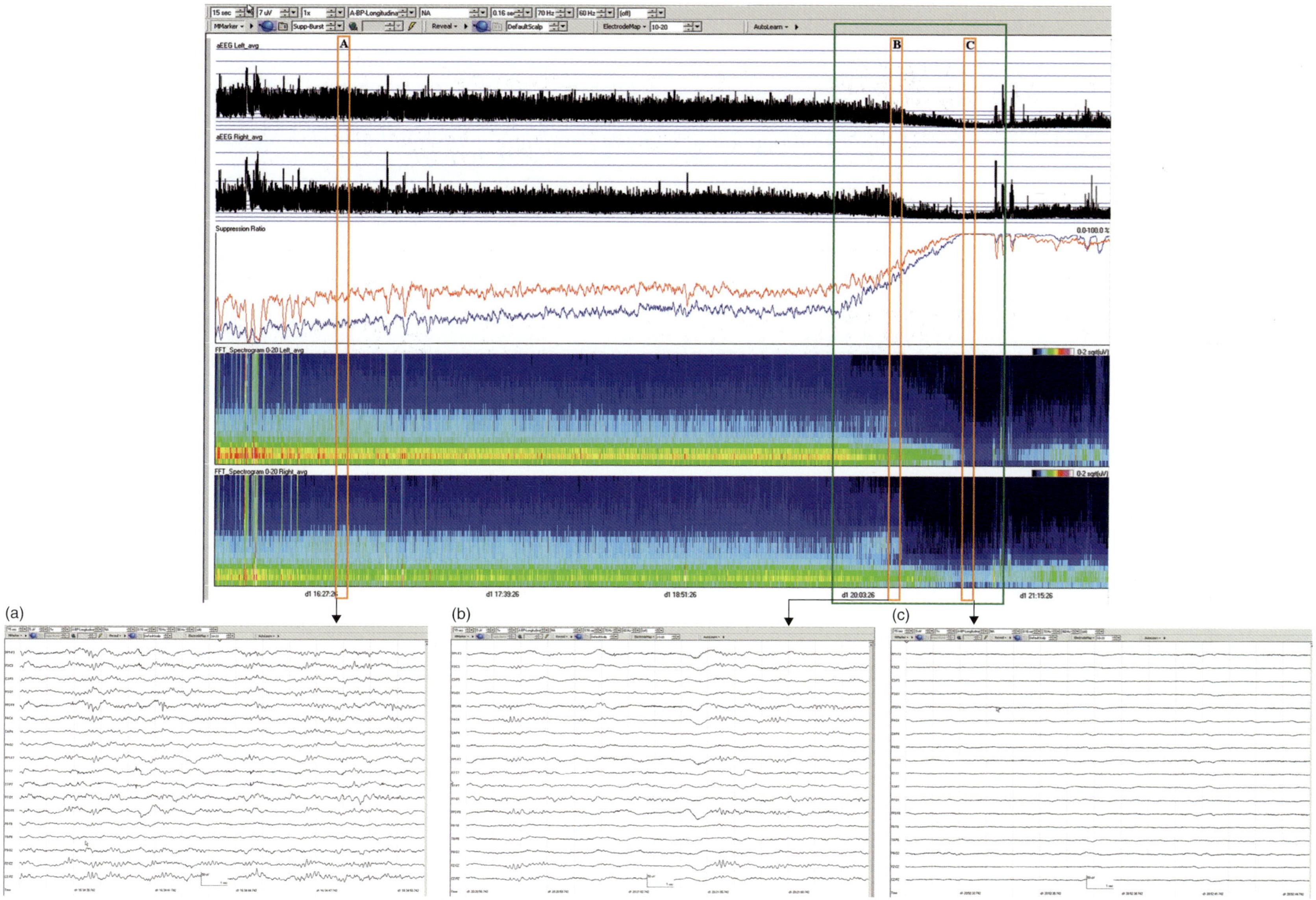

Figure 7.35 Long-term trends: patient death. **Main:** Six hours of QEEG in a middle-aged woman with cancer, septic encephalopathy and do-not-resuscitate status. There is a mild asymmetry, with more attenuation on the right as seen on the amplitude-integrated EEG (first two panels, with the tracing lower on the right), the suppression ratio (higher on the right; red = right), and the spectrogram. Near the end of this time period (green box), there is gradual loss of all power on both sides, with suppression rising to 100% as cerebral blood flow ceased. **(a)** EEG at A: mild right-sided attenuation. **(b)** EEG at B: more attenuation diffusely. **(c)** EEG at C: flat EEG.

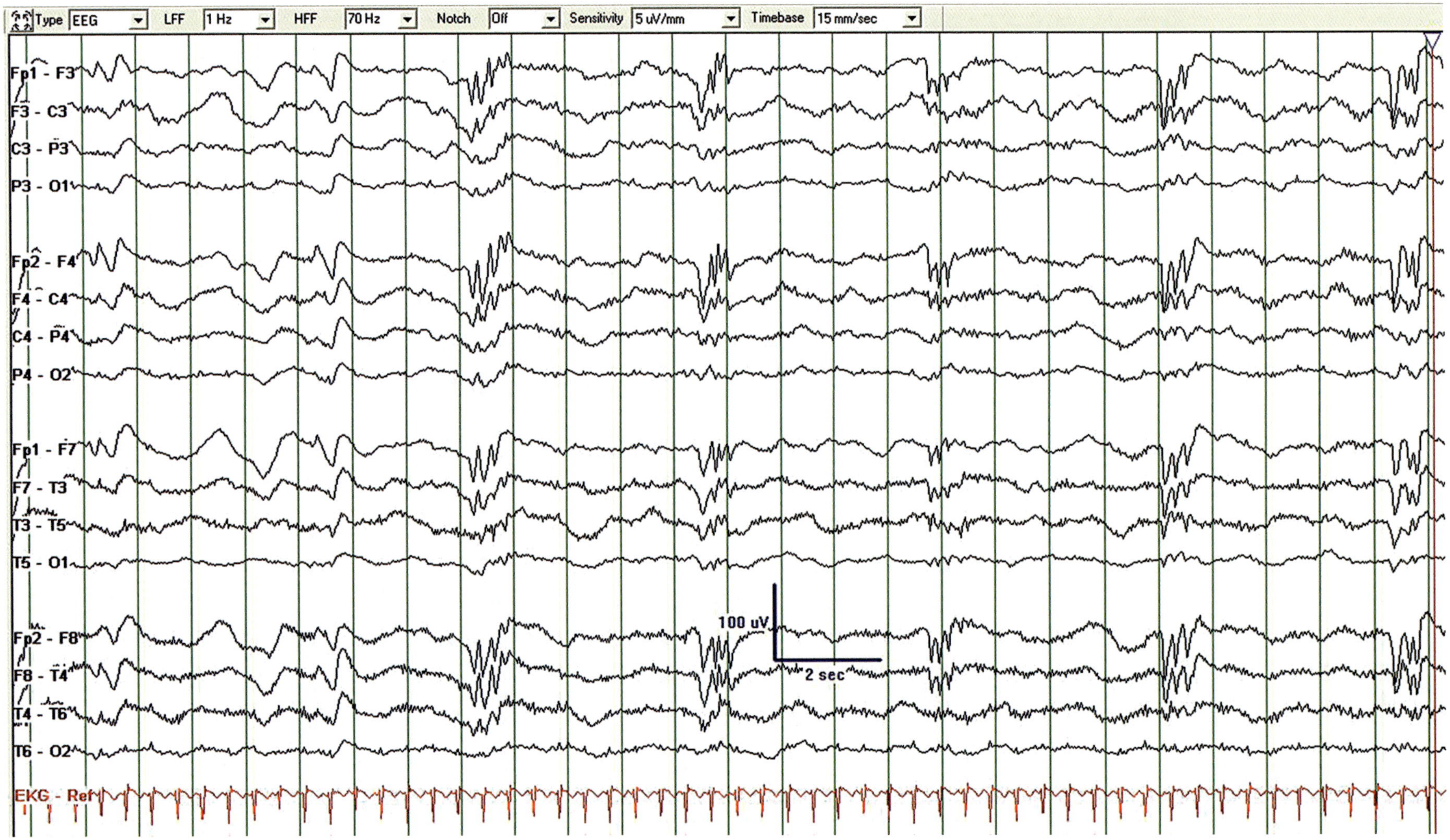

Figure 7.36 Ventilator artifact. EEG in a young HIV-positive woman with a left hemisphere infarct and right hemisphere abscess. EEG (at 15 mm/s rather than the usual 30) shows generalized, frontally predominant, polyspike-like discharges every 4–5 s. Review of video showed that this corresponded with ventilator-delivered breaths and resolved after clearing fluid from the ventilator tubing.

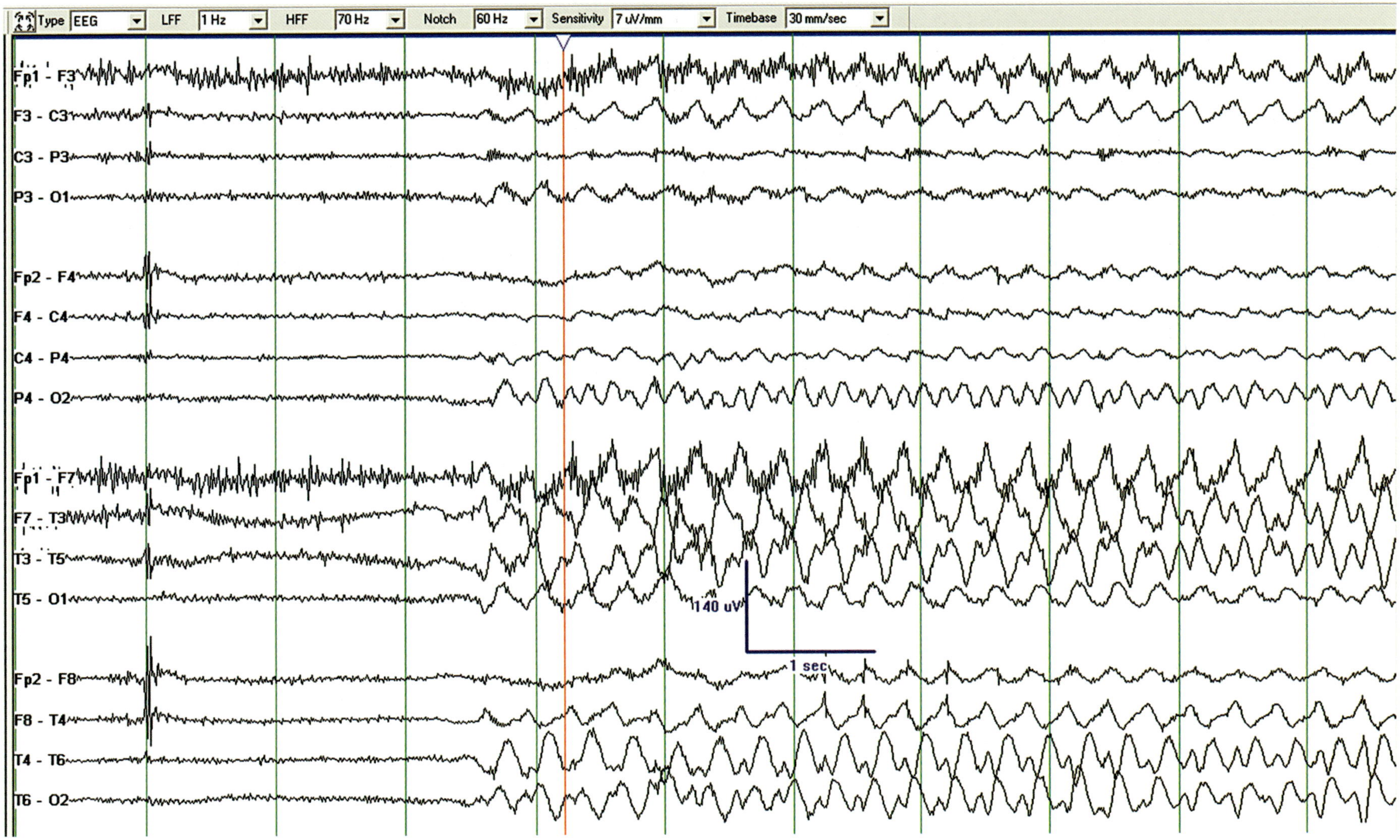

Figure 7.37 Chest percussion artifact. Paroxysmal rhythmic pattern due to chest percussion by a respiratory therapist in a 34-year-old with AIDS, end-stage renal disease and seizures. Recording video allows rapid confirmation of the artifactual nature of this pattern. This is a common rhythmic artifact in the ICU and can mimic seizures quite effectively at times.

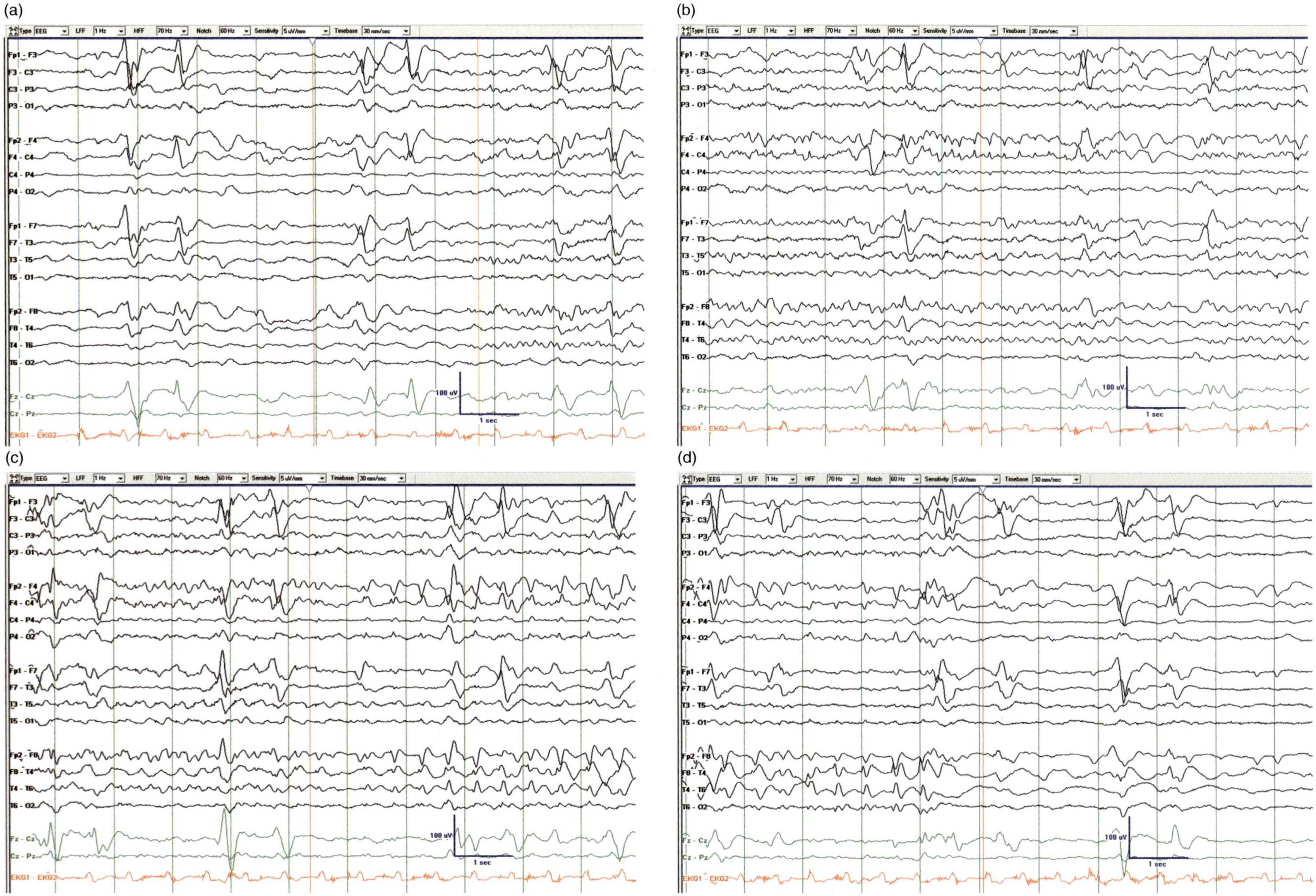

Figure 7.38a–d Chest percussion artifact: four consecutive pages of EEG in an elderly woman s/p meningioma resection with postoperative convulsive seizure and impaired mental status. There is a rhythmic pattern that starts at the end of A, settles into the right fronto-temporal region in B, evolves in morphology and frequency in C with a physiological field, then stops suddenly in D. Review of video showed that this was due to chest percussion and was artifact, not seizure. Without video, this pattern is likely to be misinterpreted as a seizure.

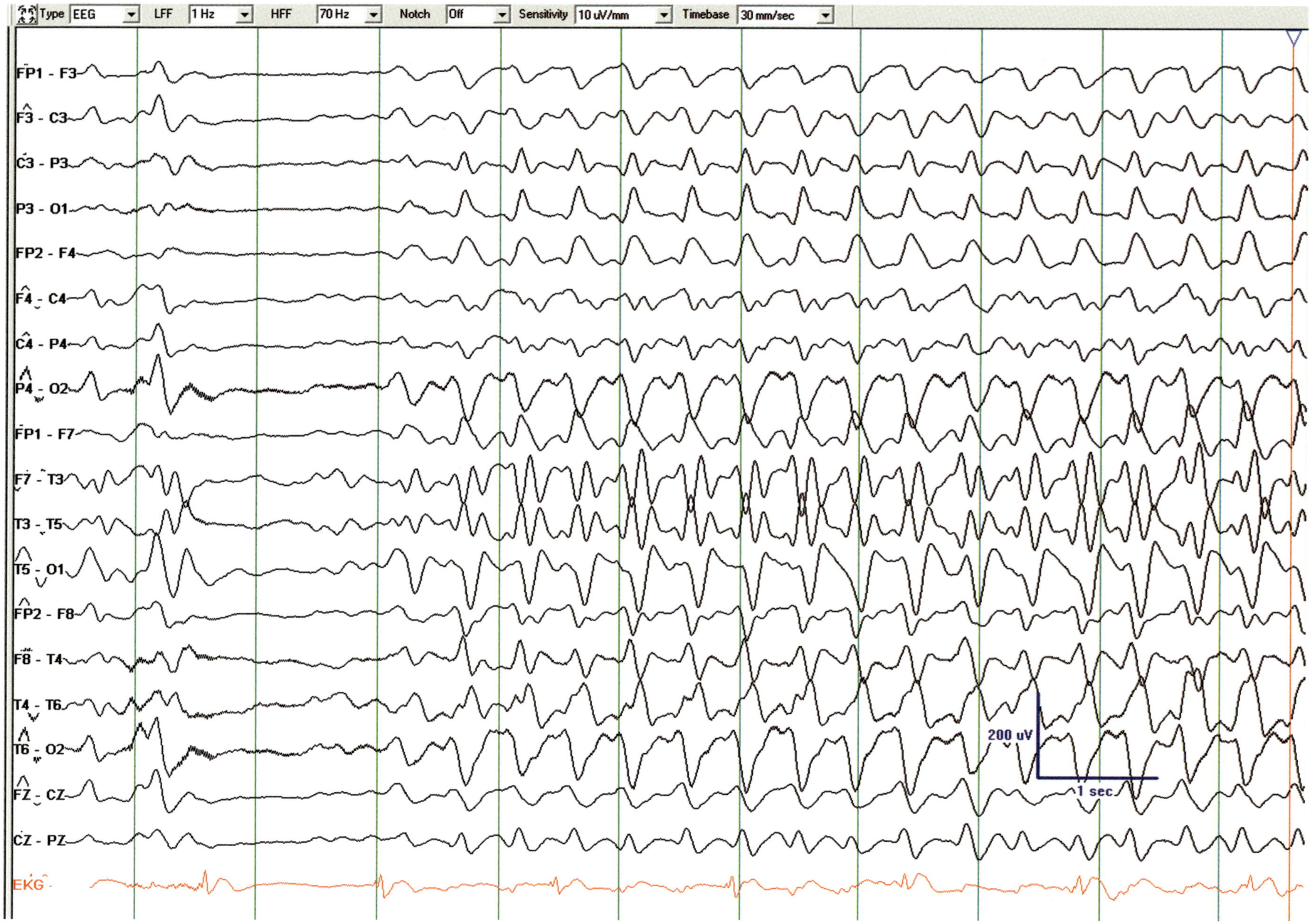

Figure 7.39 Chest percussion artifact. An additional example in a young woman with anoxic encephalopathy.

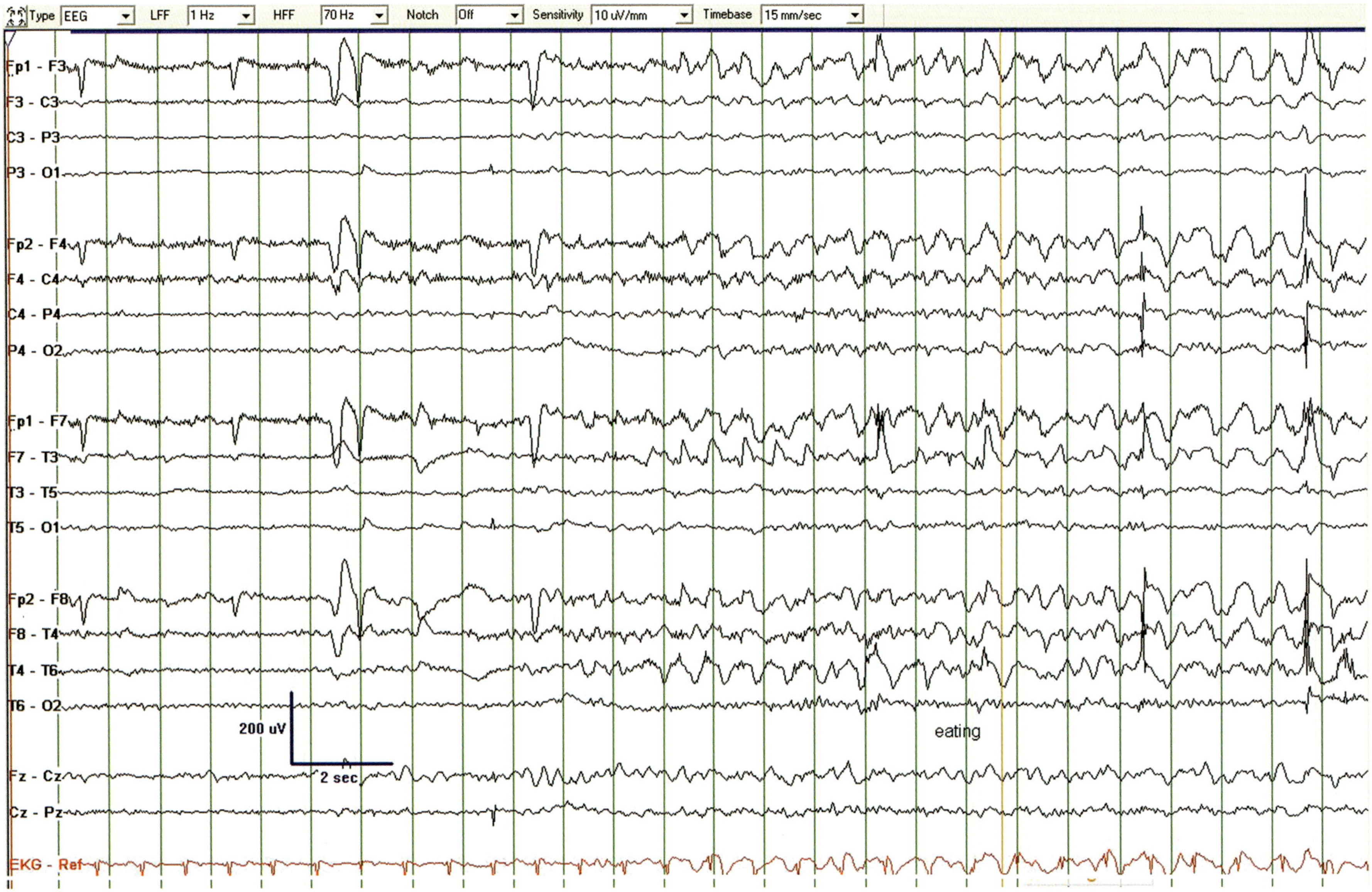

Figure 7.40 Chewing (glossokinetic) artifact: EEG (at 15 mm/s rather than the usual 30) in a man in his 70s with seizures s/p evacuation of a left subdural hematoma, shows a rhythmic pattern, maximal in the right temporal lobe. Video revealed that this was due to chewing and was reproduced after each mouthful of food. This is a more prominent glossokinetic artifact than is typically seen, but again shows the importance of video for avoiding misinterpretation of rhythmic artifacts. Note that the pattern is absent at the vertex (Cz), typical of most artifacts.

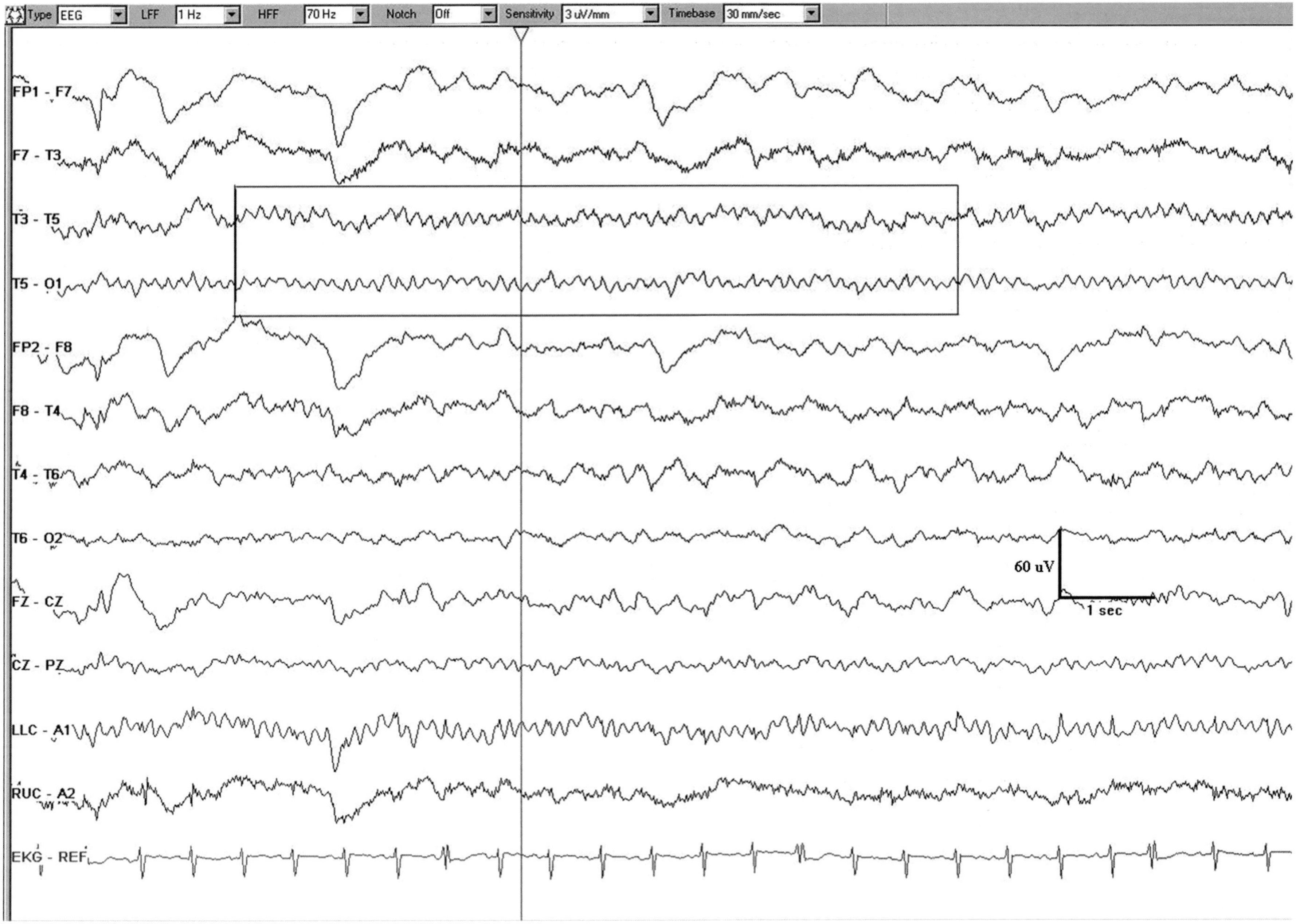

Figure 7.41 'Pseudoalpha' artifact: There appears to be a well-developed posterior dominant 'alpha' rhythm on the left in this comatose patient. This was due to an oscillating bed.

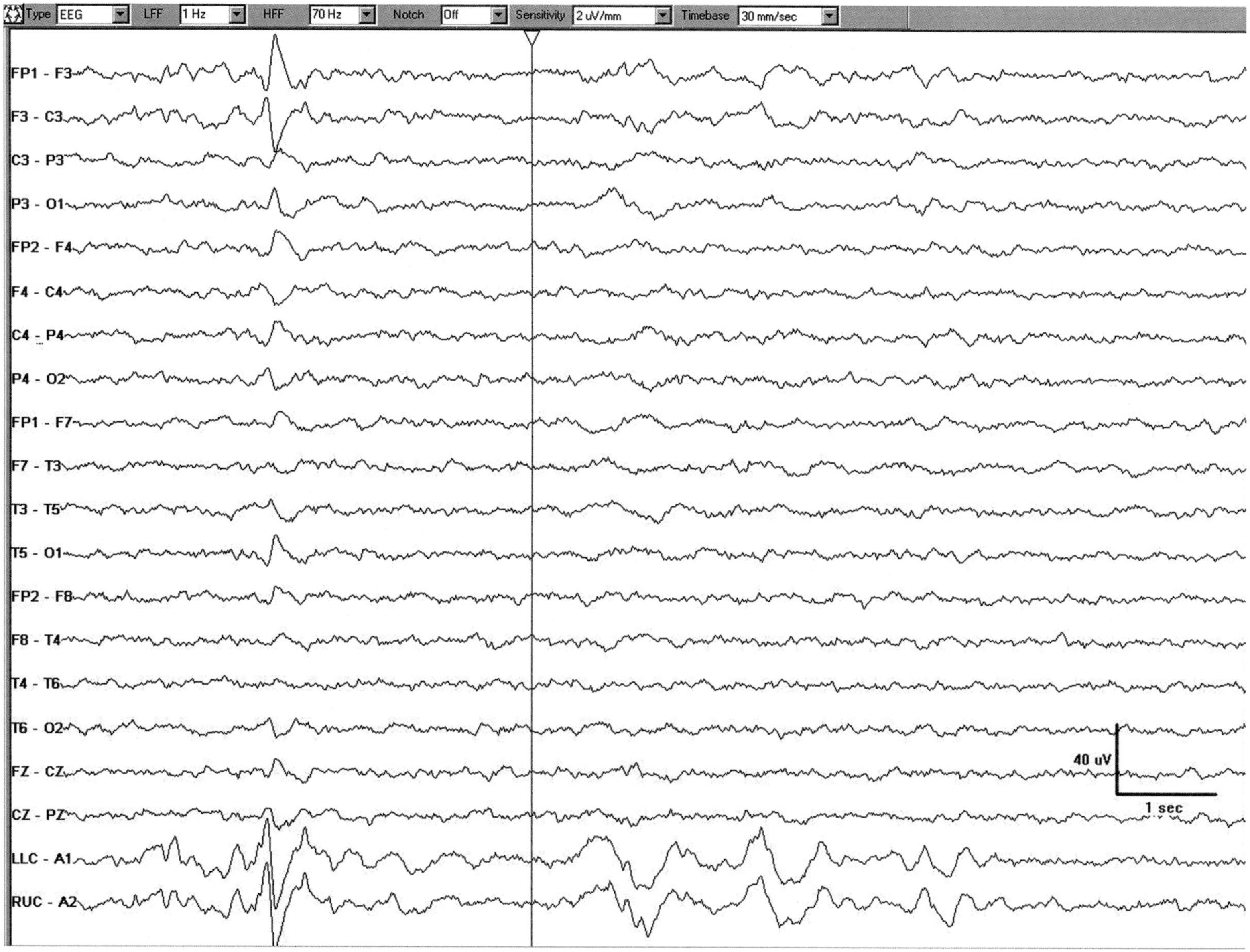

Figure 7.42 'Virtual'or disconnected patient. There appears to be diffuse attenuation and slowing, but there is actually no patient in the room as the patient was rushed to an emergency scan in the middle of the night. This is the pattern seen when no electrodes are plugged into the headbox (jack-box). Note the very high gain of 2 uV/mm (but the 60 Hz, or notch filter, is not on, as electrical noise is not recorded when nothing is connected to the headbox). Video confirmed the lack of a patient in the room.

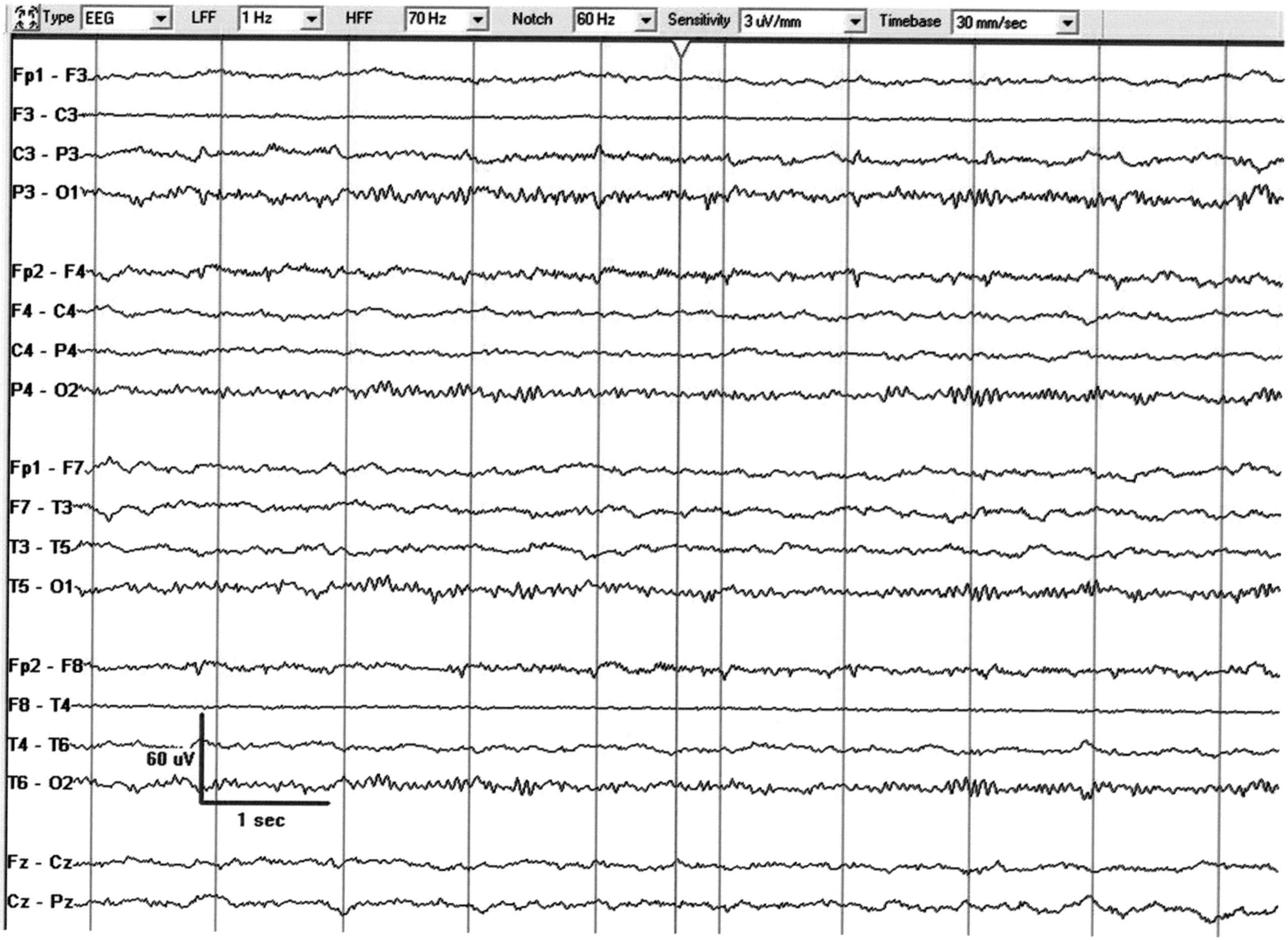

Figure 7.43 'Virtual' or disconnected patient. In this case, the patient is no longer in the room, but the electrodes are still plugged into the headbox. There appears to be diffuse slowing and attenuation. Note the high gain of 3 uV/mm and the use of the 60 Hz (notch filter). Without the 60 Hz filter, this EEG was overwhelmed by 60 Hz artifact (electrical noise; this would be 50 Hz in many countries).

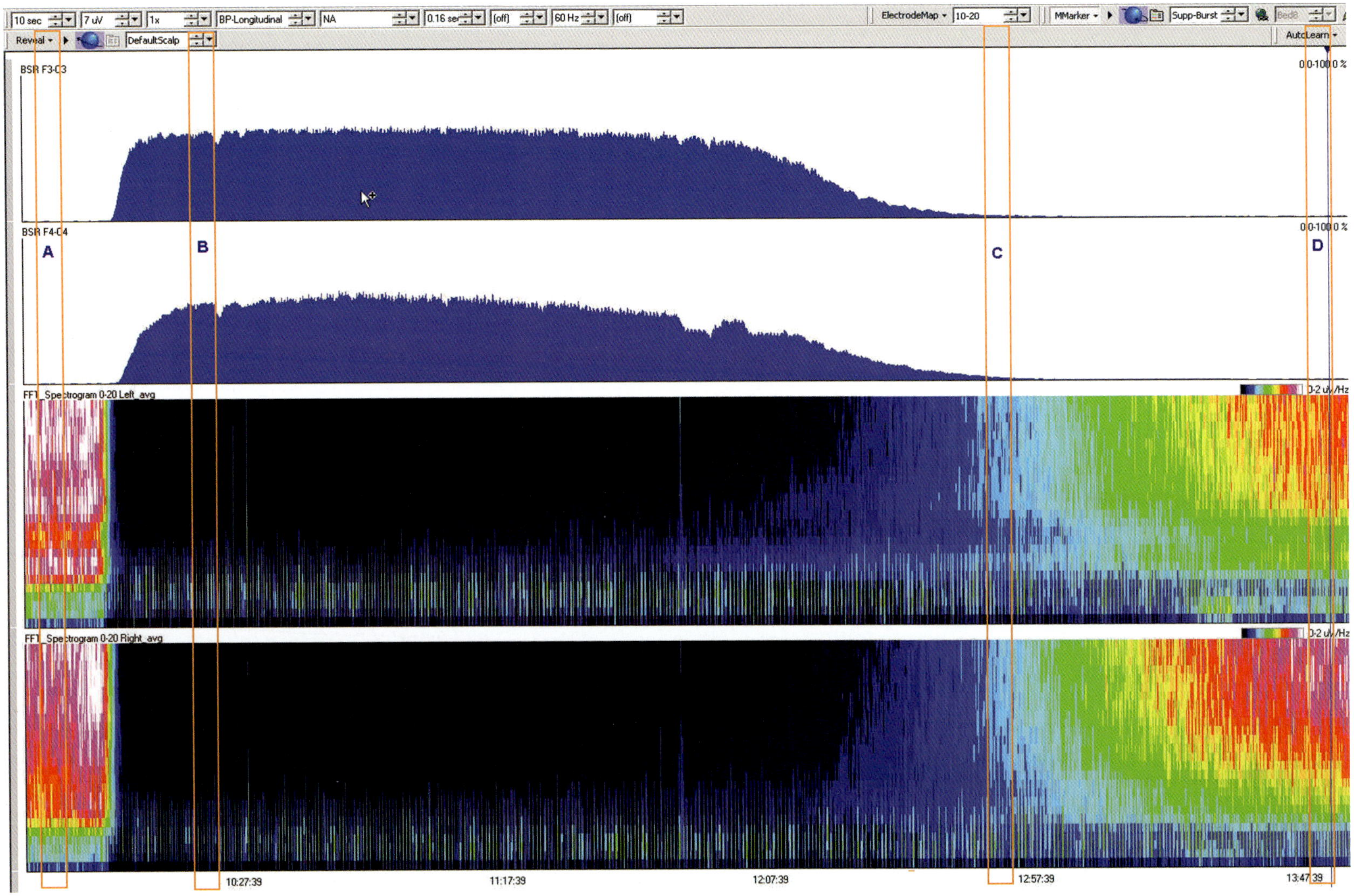

Figure 7.44 Wearing off of paralytic; shivering artifact. **Main:** Four hours of QEEG in a 75-year-old woman s/p cardiac arrest being treated with hypothermia. The initial EEG (A) is obscured by continuous muscle artifact, likely due to shivering related to hypothermia (often 'micro-shivering' that is difficult to notice clinically). A paralytic was administered between A and B, removing all muscle artifact. Underlying EEG shows marked suppression with low-amplitude bursting (B). The suppression ratio (top two panels, labeled 'BSR' in this example) rises rapidly and remains high for a couple of hours before gradually declining before C (causing a humpback whale shape). On the spectrogram, muscle artifact can be seen gradually returning (C) and increasing in power until again prominent (D). **(a)** EEG at A: prominent muscle artifact. **(b)** EEG at B: muscle artifact no longer present after paralytic. **(c)** EEG at C: muscle artifact returning. **(d)** EEG at D: muscle artifact prominent again.

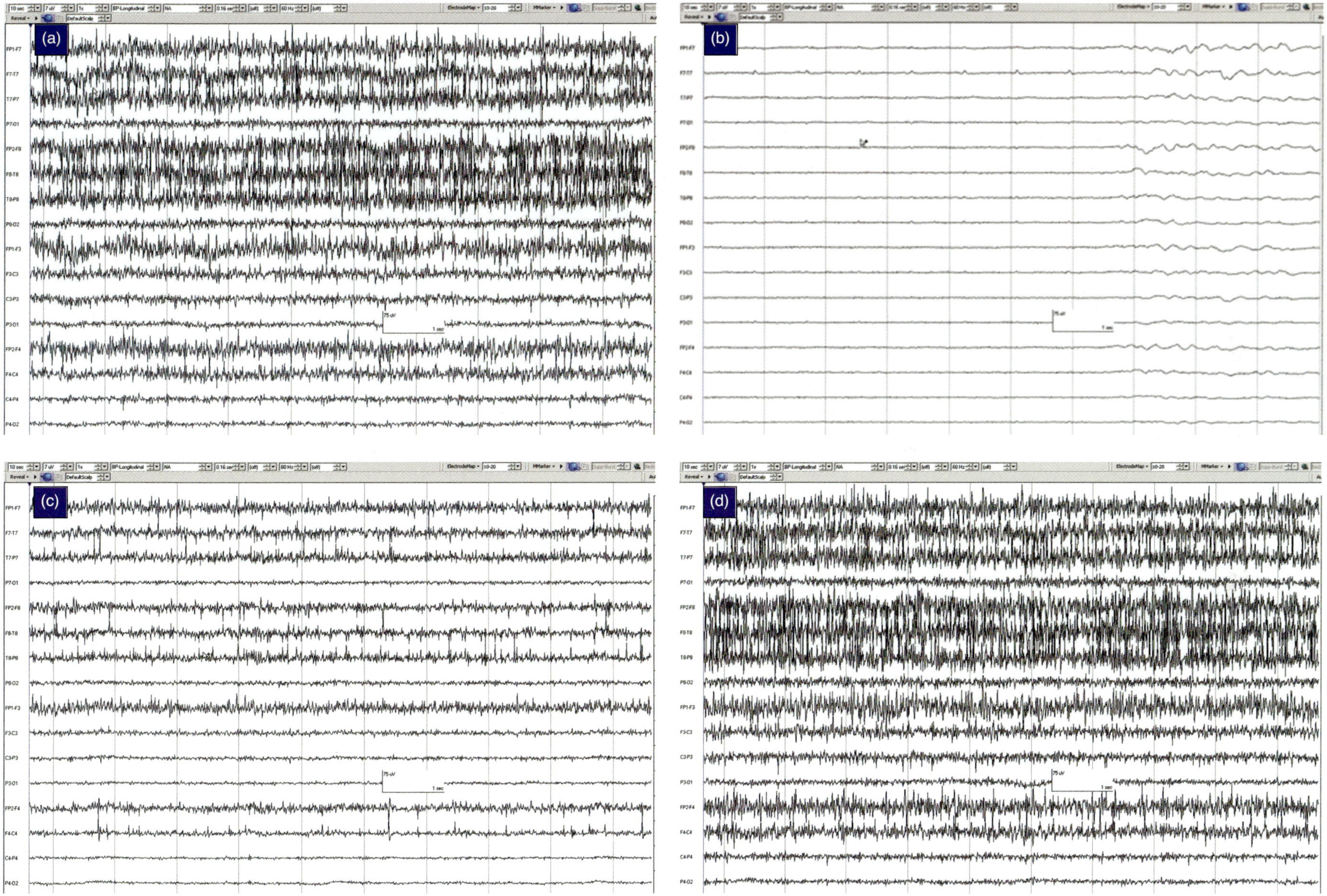
(a)
(b)
(c)
(d)

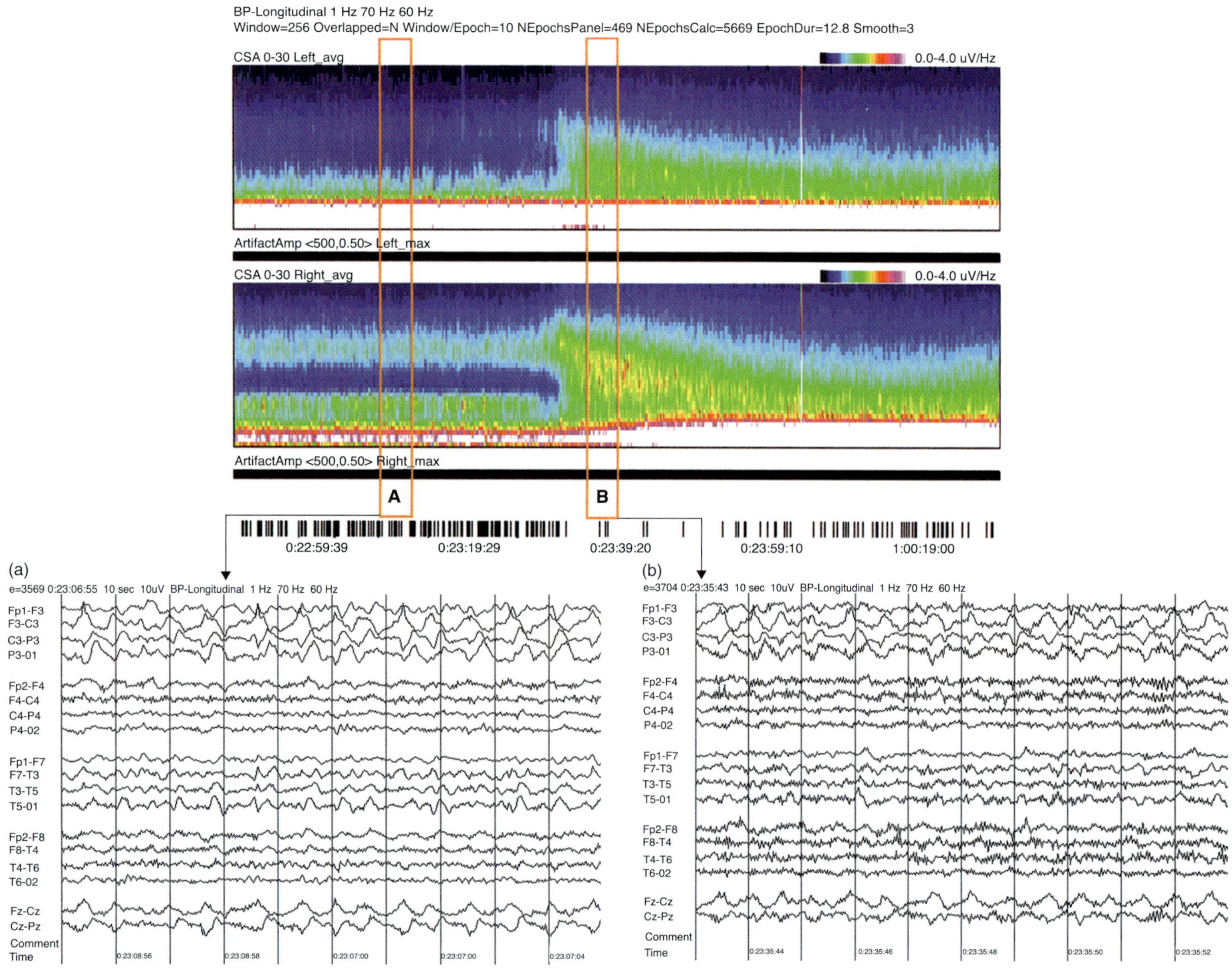

Figure 7.45 Drug-induced beta and asymmetry. **Main:** Spectrogram showing 2 h of EEG from 1 to 30 Hz in a 4-year-old with status epilepticus (with right body twitching at times), treated with midazolam drip. There is an asymmetry with slowing (more delta power) and attenuation (less power in alpha/beta ranges) on the left (A). A benzodiazepine bolus (midazolam) is then administered and a marked increase in fast activity can be seen (B), still greater on the right (the healthier side). **(a)** EEG at A: marked left-sided slowing, maximal parasagittally and consisting of semirhythmic delta. There is attenuation of normal faster activity on the left as well, but fairly prominent on the healthier right side. **(b)** EEG at B: much more fast activity (enhanced beta), a common effect of benzodiazepines and barbiturates; this is increased on both sides, but still asymmetric.

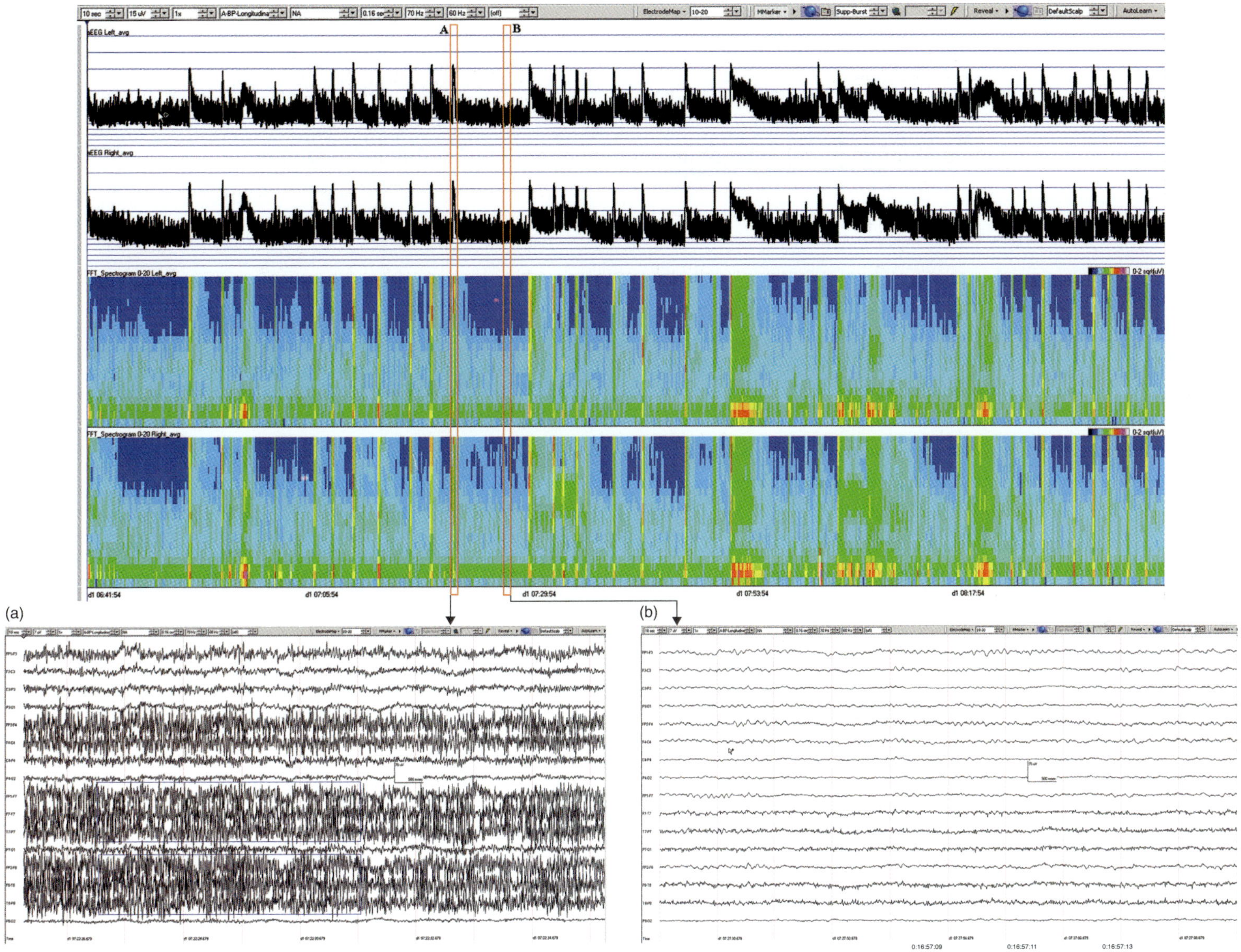

Figure 7.46 Artifact mimicking seizures on amplitude-integrated EEG (aEEG). **Main:** 2 h of QEEG in a 44-year-old woman with AIDS, sepsis, meningitis and prior seizures. Note frequent paroxysmal increases in amplitude (such as A) that look like typical seizures on the aEEG tracing. However, this patient had no seizures, but rather had intermittent muscle artifact. This is a reminder of the dangers of interpreting aEEG traces without expert review of the corresponding raw EEG. **(a)** EEG at A: muscle artifact, which caused the increase in amplitude on aEEG. **(b)** EEG at B: baseline, with less muscle artifact.

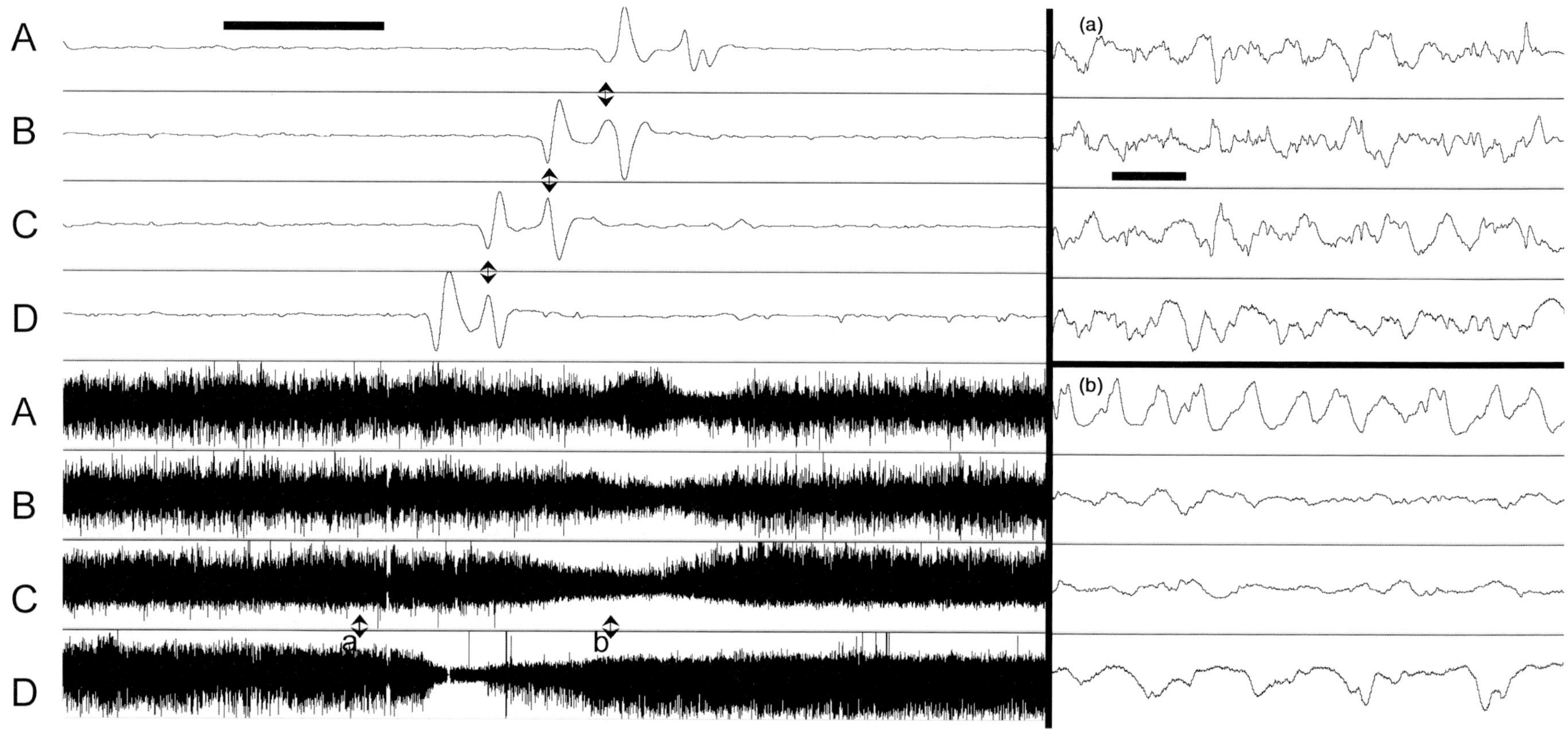

Figure 7.47 Electrocorticogram (ECoG) of cortical spreading depression of Leão (CSD) in the human brain. It has been recognized recently that cortical spreading depression and peri-injury depolarizations are common in patients with acute brain injuries, including trauma, infarct and subarachnoid hemorrhage. Furthermore, there is extensive evidence that they contribute to secondary injury (see Dreier *et al.*, 2006; Fabricius *et al.*, 2006; Strong *et al.*, 2007). This example is from a 65-year-old female, who four days previously suffered a subarachnoid hemorrhage and an intracerebral hematoma due to a ruptured aneurysm of the left middle cerebral artery (MCA). After clipping of the aneurysm on the second day, a subdural strip was placed over the left frontal cortex. Four channels of ECoG were recorded from five platinum electrodes, 1 cm apart, and connected in a bipolar chain (A–D). The initial 40 h of recording showed irregular delta activity and intermittent trains of spikes. Over the subsequent 70 h, 16 episodes of CSD were recorded. The patient died 10 days post ictus due to respiratory failure. *Left panel*: 60 min recording, bar: 10 min. Upper four traces: 0.05 Hz low pass filtered, full scale 4 mV, *lower four traces*: same recording as upper traces, but now 0.5 Hz high pass filtered, full scale 1 mV. *Right panels*: **(a)** and **(b)**: high resolution samples, bar: 1 s, same amplification and filtering as lower left. **(a)** shows background activity a few minutes before onset of CSD commencing in channel D and subsequently spreading to channels C, B and A. **(b)** indicates the time when activity is depressed in channel B and C, but nor yet in channel A, while channel D is recovering after CSD. CSD is caused by a severe, long-lasting depolarization of the cortical tissue as evidenced by the huge change of the DC-potential recorded in the same channels and visualized in the upper four, low pass filtered, curves. A slow potential change (SPC) commences in channel D and spreads from electrode to electrode as evidenced by the phase shift of the SPC between channels D and C, C and B and B and A (double arrows). CSD spread at 3 mm/min in accordance with Leão's observations in the rabbit (Leão, 1944). (Image courtesy of Martin Fabricius, MD, Denmark)

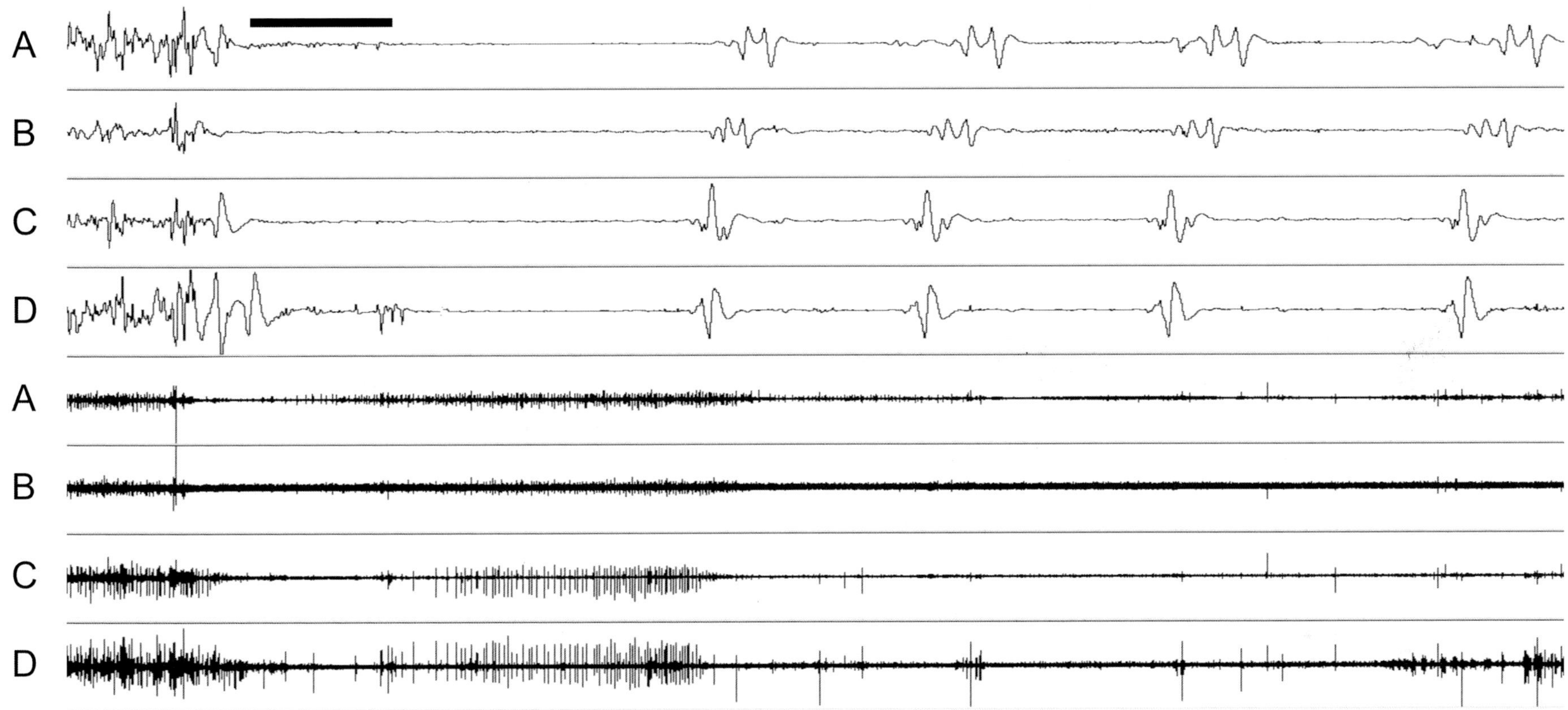

Figure 7.48 Electrocorticogram (ECoG) of periinjury depolarisations (PIDs) in the human brain. This 67-year-old male had a fall, and was admitted with a right frontal lobe contusion and acute subdural hematoma. After evacuation of the hematoma, a subdural strip was placed over the right middle frontal gyrus (see previous figure for details). Baseline ECoG activity showed burst-suppression pattern with long flattened periods. The patient remained comatose and died two days later. Upper four traces: 0.05 Hz low pass, full scale 4 mV. Lower four traces: same recording as upper traces, but now 0.5 Hz high pass, full scale 2 mV. Bar: 20 min. 200 min of the recording is shown commencing 18 h after ictus. Two episodes of cortical spreading depression (CSD) accompanied by stereotyped slow potential changes (SPCs) are seen at the far left (channels A to D) and in the middle (D to A), 1 h apart. Recovery of ECoG background activity after the first CSD was delayed and incomplete, but after the second CSD the ECoG activity remained depressed in all channels. Then another three episodes of very stereotyped SPCs are seen spreading from channel D to A at a velocity of 2–3 mm/min and occurring at approximately 30 min intervals. Arterial oxygen saturation remained $>90\%$ and no extra sedative was administered to the patient in this period to explain the lack of cortical activity. The ECoG remained depressed indicating compromised metabolism. The event was therefore classified as a PID, i.e. a depolarization wave spreading slowly through an area of the cortex where perfusion is too low to maintain nerve cell signaling, but where the cells are still viable. Animal experiments suggest that repeated PIDs expand the final volume of injured cortex by energy depletion and vasospasm (Fabricius *et al.*, 2006). (Images courtesy of Martin Fabricius, Denmark, and Anthony J. Strong, UK)

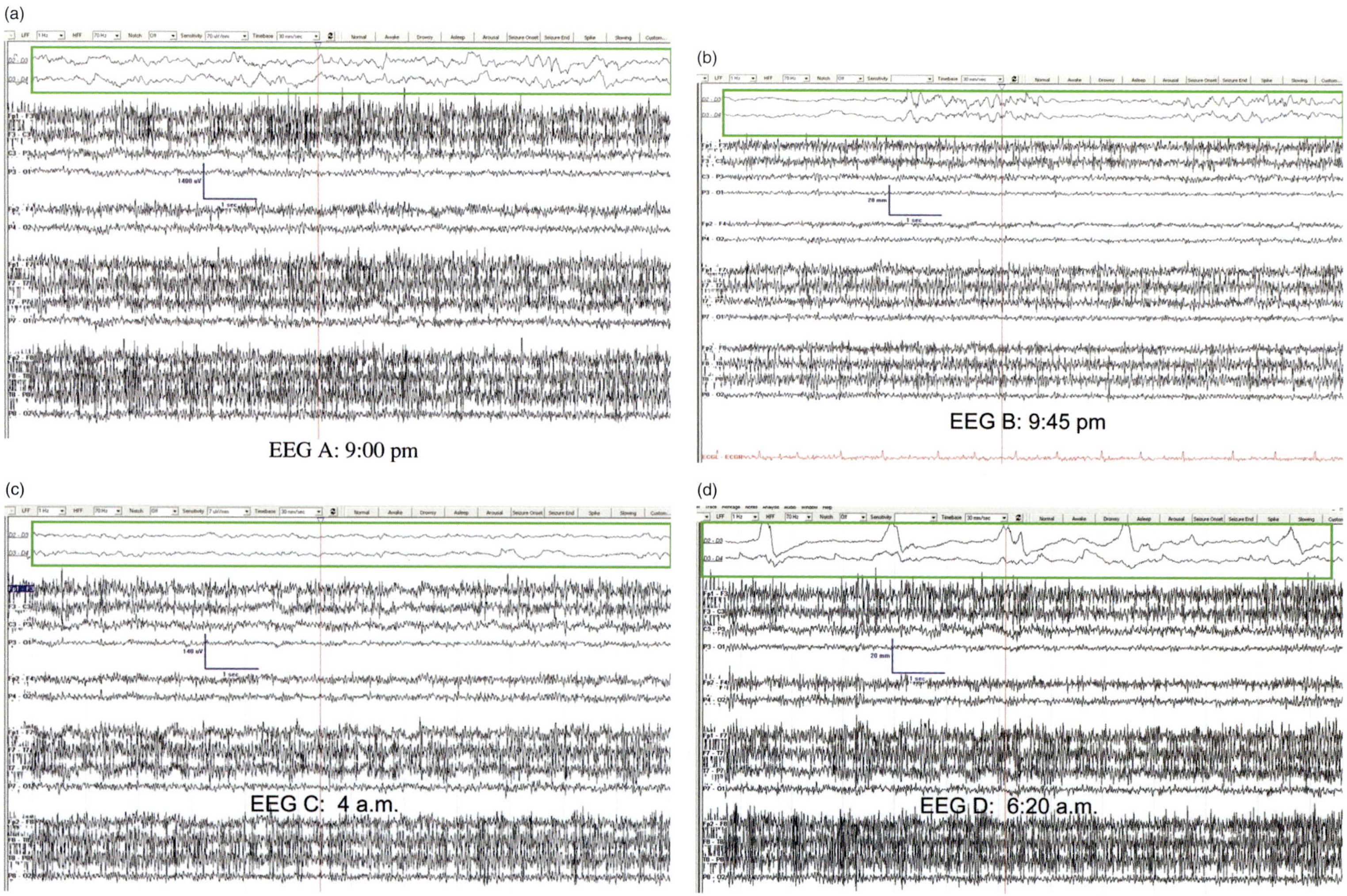

Figure 7.49 Multimodality monitoring of hemorrhagic transformation of a large infarct, including with depth electrode. (This patient was previously presented; see Waziri *et al.*). **(a)–(e)** 73-year-old man with a large right hemisphere infarct (see CT scan, part g) undergoing invasive monitoring for raised intracranial pressure (ICP), and being treated with hypothermia. An eight-contact miniature depth electrode was placed in the right frontal lobe in the ischemic penumbra, along with the ICP monitor, a brain tissue oxygen tension monitor and a cerebral microdialysis catheter. Baseline EEG at 9:00 pm is shown in (a), including continuous mixed frequency in the depth electrode recordings (top two channels, and in green box); scalp recording is obscured by muscle artifact, likely from micro-shivering (see Figure 7.44). The scale legend *y*-axis represents 1400 uV for the depth channels and 140 uV for the scalp channels for all EEGs in this case. At 9:45 pm (b), the depth EEG becomes discontinuous, with suppression-burst suddenly appearing, later found to be due to hemorrhagic transformation of the infarct; the scalp shows no significant change. By 4:00 am (c), the depth EEG is flat, and the scalp EEG remains uninformative. The intracranial EEG begins to recover, with periodic delta waves

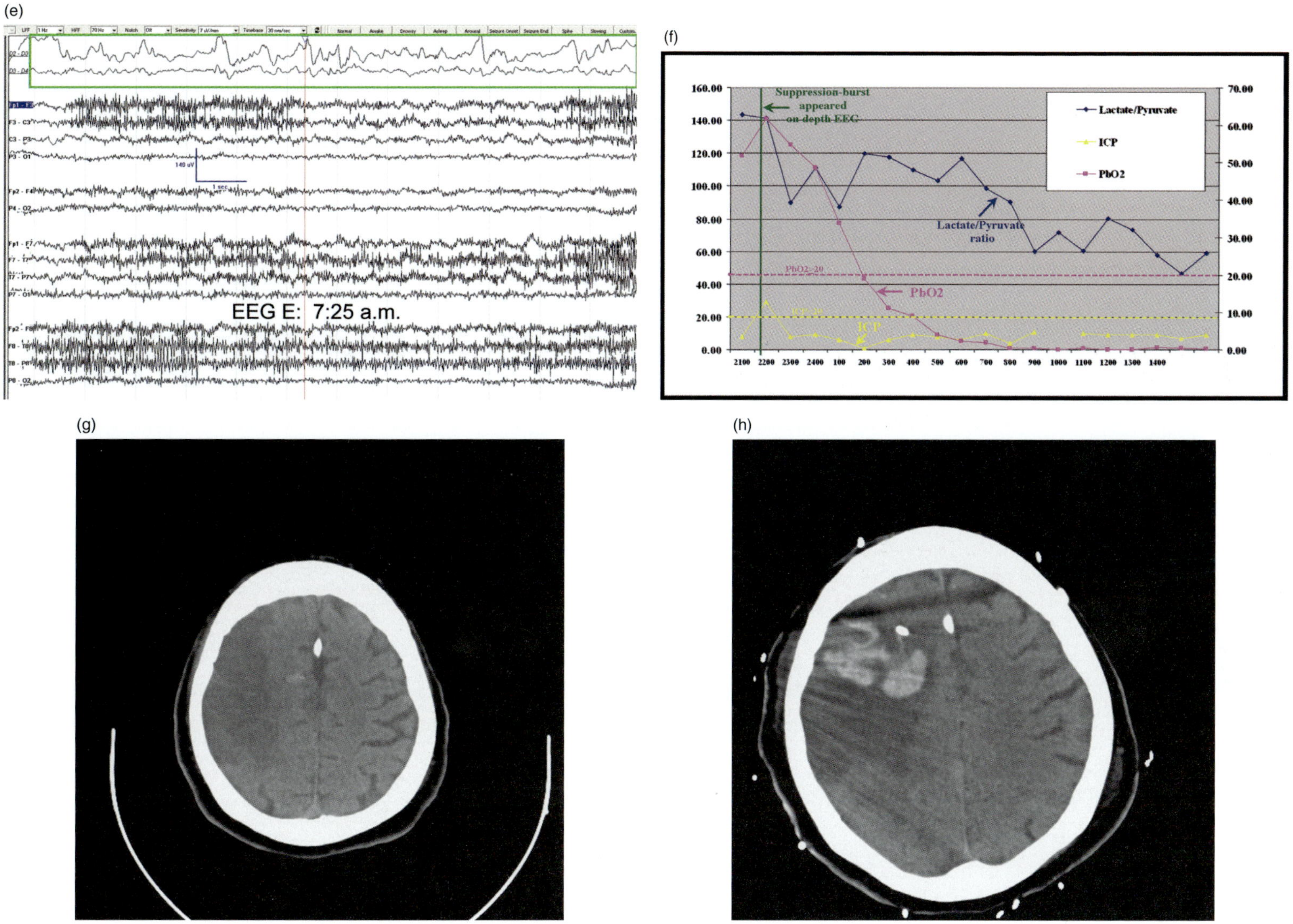

Figure 7.49 (*Continued*) by 6:20 am (d), and resumption of a continuous pattern by 7:25 am (e). **(f)** Multimodal graph: the prominent EEG change (green line) occurred a few hours before brain tissue oxygen tension dropped significantly. ICP bumped slightly above normal at the probable time of the hemorrhagic transformation, but rapidly returned to normal. The parenchymal microdialysate lactate/pyruvate ratio (a standard measure of neuronal stress, with normal <30) was markedly elevated throughout and thus was not helpful (it was actually improving during this time). No clinical change was noted until the next day. Thus, intracranial EEG seemed to be the earliest and best indicator of an acute event in this case. It also allowed monitoring of the EEG without paralyzing the patient, which would have been necessary to monitor using the scalp EEG. **(g)** Head CT scan prior to placement of invasive monitors, showing the large right hemisphere infarction. Falx calcification can also be seen. **(h)** Head CT scan after hemorrhagic transformation. A ventricular catheter can be seen as well; the miniature depth electrode was more superior (and more superficial, as it barely reaches the white matter).

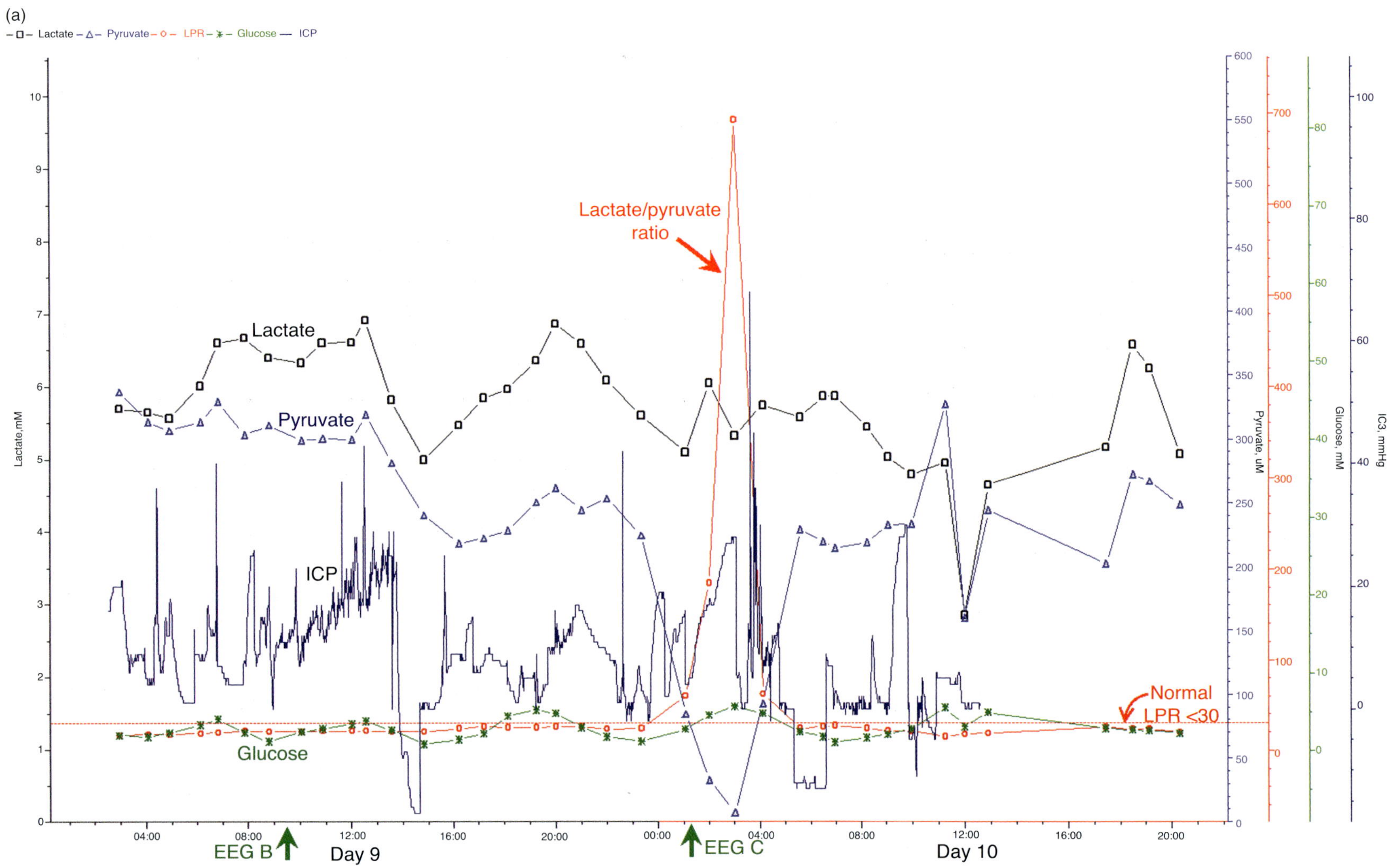

Figure 7.50 Multimodality monitoring of seizures on intracranial EEG after meperidine bolus. **(a)–(c)** 61-year-old woman with a Hunt and Hess grade V subarachnoid hemorrhage, s/p placement of a left frontal eight-contact mini-depth electrode and cerebral microdialysis catheter, and a right frontal ventricular drain. Almost 48 h of multimodal data is shown in the graph (a). There was a dramatic rise in the lactate/pyruvate ratio from 1:00 to 4:00 am, which occurred shortly after administration of meperidine. The increase in this ratio was not due to a rise in lactate as is seen with ischemia, but rather to a drop in pyruvate, as can be seen with increased substrate utilization, such as with seizures. Intracranial pressure (ICP) went up as well, but had been quite variable prior to this. EEG at baseline (b) showed no epileptiform discharges. At the time of the dramatic rise in lactate/pyruvate ratio (c), the depth electrode (top 11 channels, with labels starting with 'D') showed nearly continuous epileptiform discharges, especially with any alerting stimuli (SIRPIDs, or stimulus-induced rhythmic, periodic or ictal discharges). The scalp EEG (bottom 10 channels) did not show

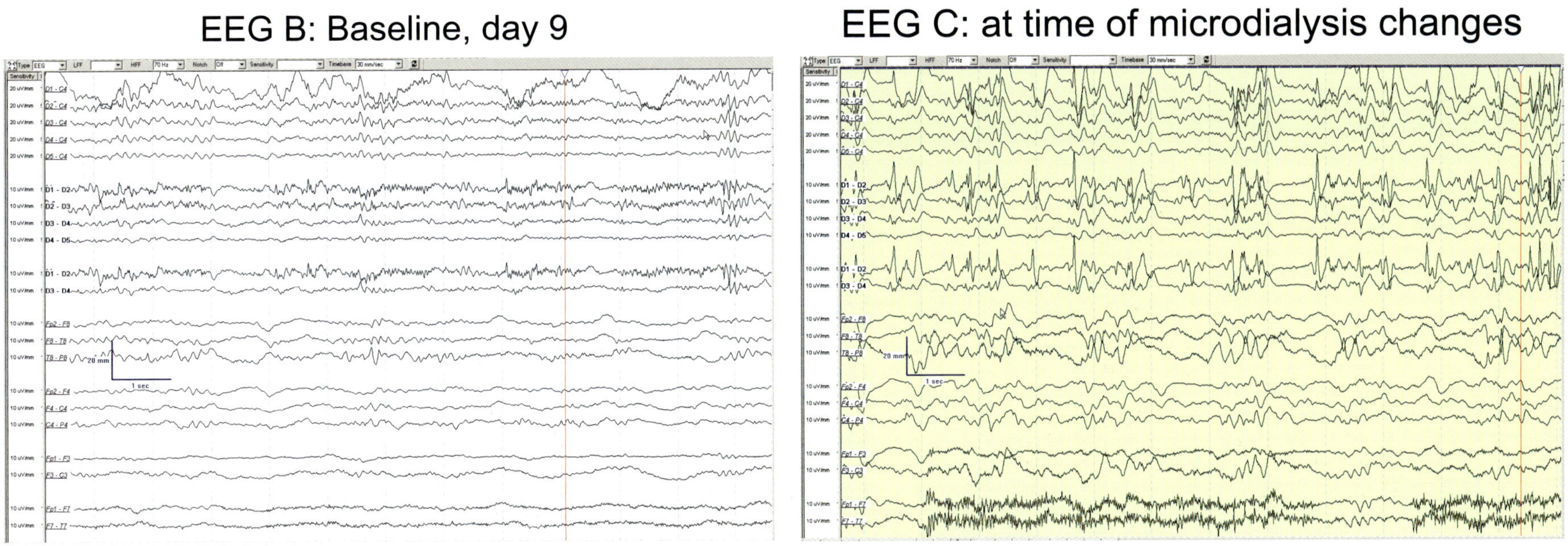

Figure 7.50 (*Continued*) any obvious epileptiform discharges. This example presumably shows the adverse physiological effects (markedly elevated lactate/pyruvate ratio (LPR) with decreasing pyruvate) of these epileptiform discharges. When an epileptiform EEG pattern is associated with this type of physiological effect in a given patient, we are more likely to treat it aggressively than if these changes are not seen. In this case, it resolved after a few hours and meperidine was avoided to prevent recurrence. Without the intracranial recording, we would not have known that seizure activity was the explanation for the rising LPR, though this physiological pattern (rising LPR with dropping pyruvate) raises that possibility even if depth EEG is not being recorded.

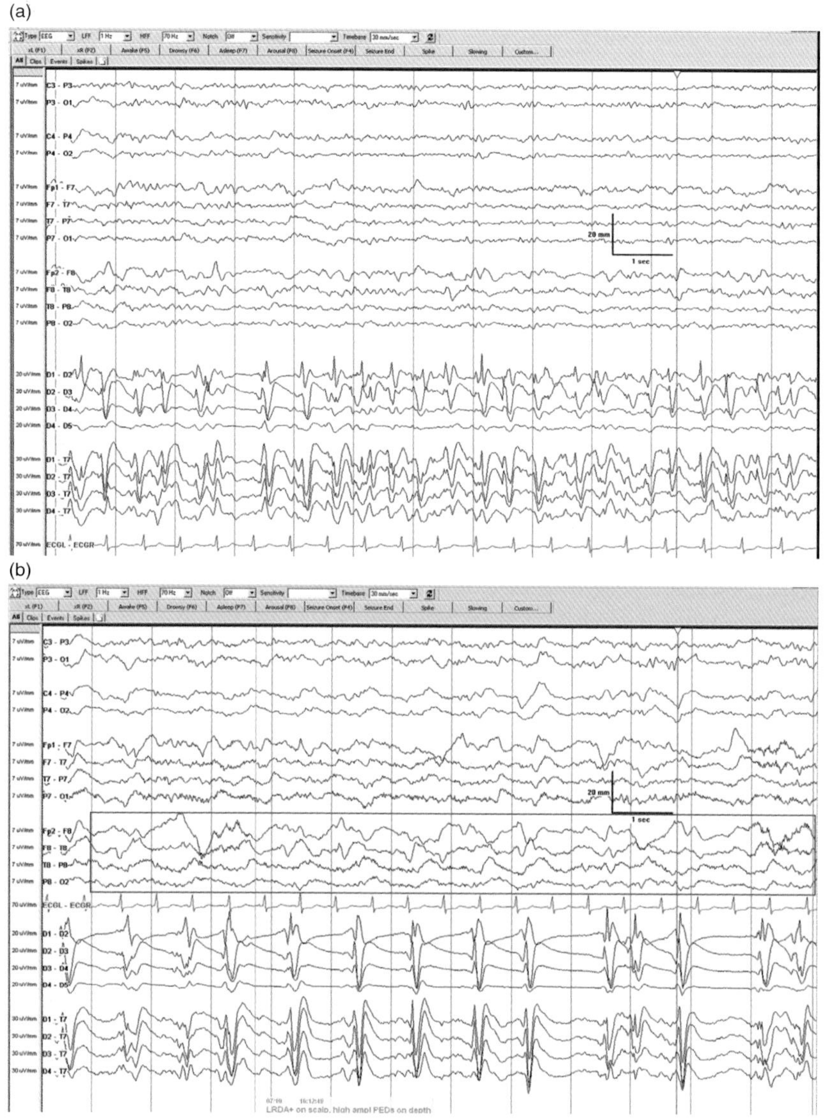

Figure 7.51 Seizures and periodic discharges on intracranial EEG only. **(a)** and **(b)** Two samples of EEG from an older woman with a poor-grade subarachnoid hemorrhage, ventricular extension and right frontal intracerebral hemorrhage. The bottom eight channels are from an eight-contact mini-depth electrode placed in the superficial cortex of the right frontal lobe near the hemorrhage, but in normal-appearing brain. The remaining channels are from standard scalp electrodes. There were frequent times with ictal-appearing intracranial EEG (a) but no hint of a correlate on the scalp. There were other times with prominent periodic epileptiform discharges (b) on the depth channels; this was sometimes accompanied by quasirhythmic delta as in this sample (box in B; also known as lateralized rhythmic delta activity or LRDA). When the ictal-appearing pattern replaced the periodic discharges, the scalp EEG appeared to normalize (quasirhythmic delta resolved; 'pseudonormalization').

(a)

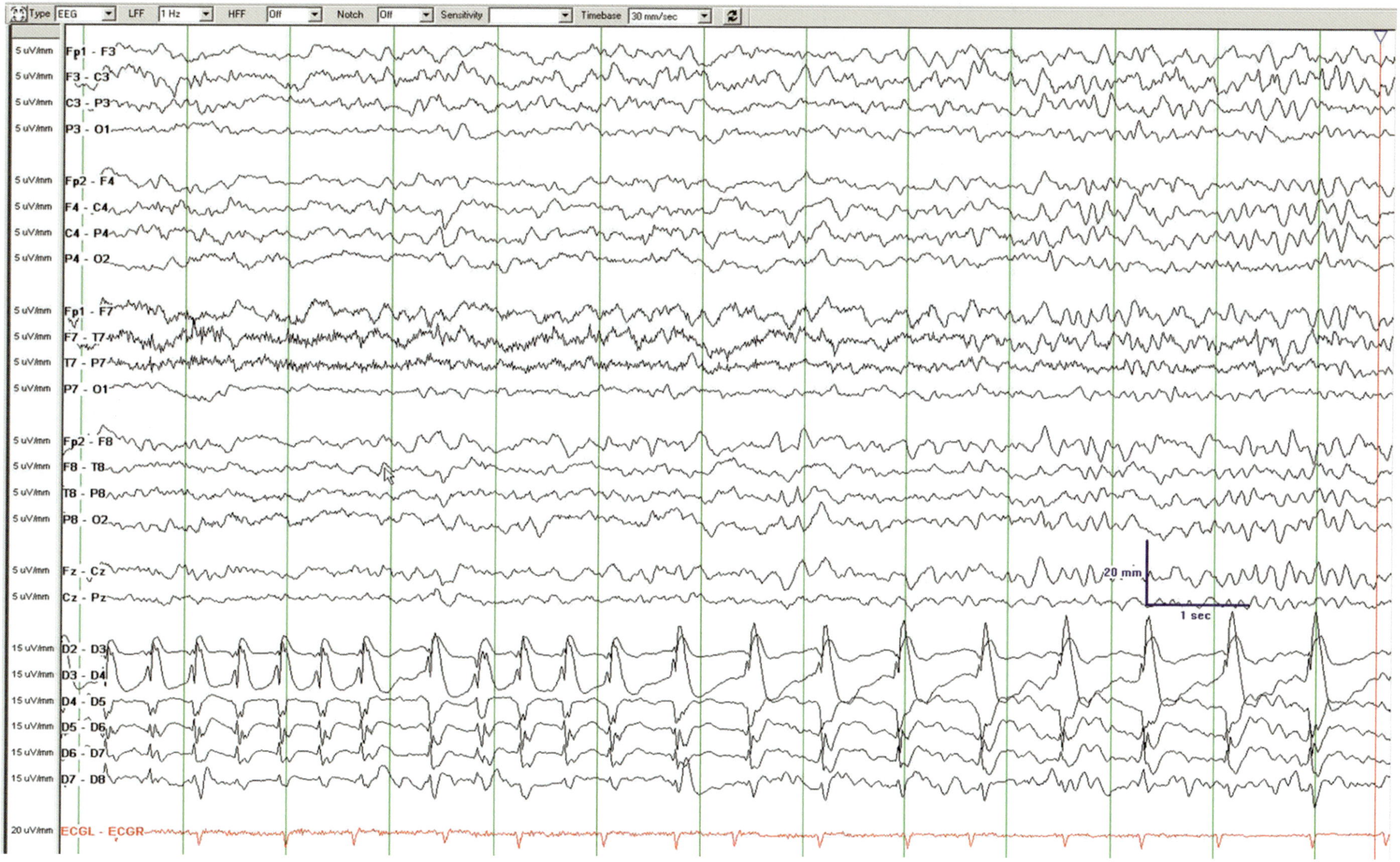

Figure 7.52 Cyclic seizures on intracranial EEG only. **(a)** EEG sample from an older woman with a Hunt and Hess grade III subarachnoid hemorrhage and a left frontal mini-depth electrode. She had no seizures for some time, then had a 5-h period with cyclic seizures in the depth electrode only, each lasting about one minute and recurring every few minutes. A typical seizure is shown here. The bottom six channels show a clearly evolving seizure, with no hint of it seen on the scalp channels despite a high-quality recording with no missing electrodes.

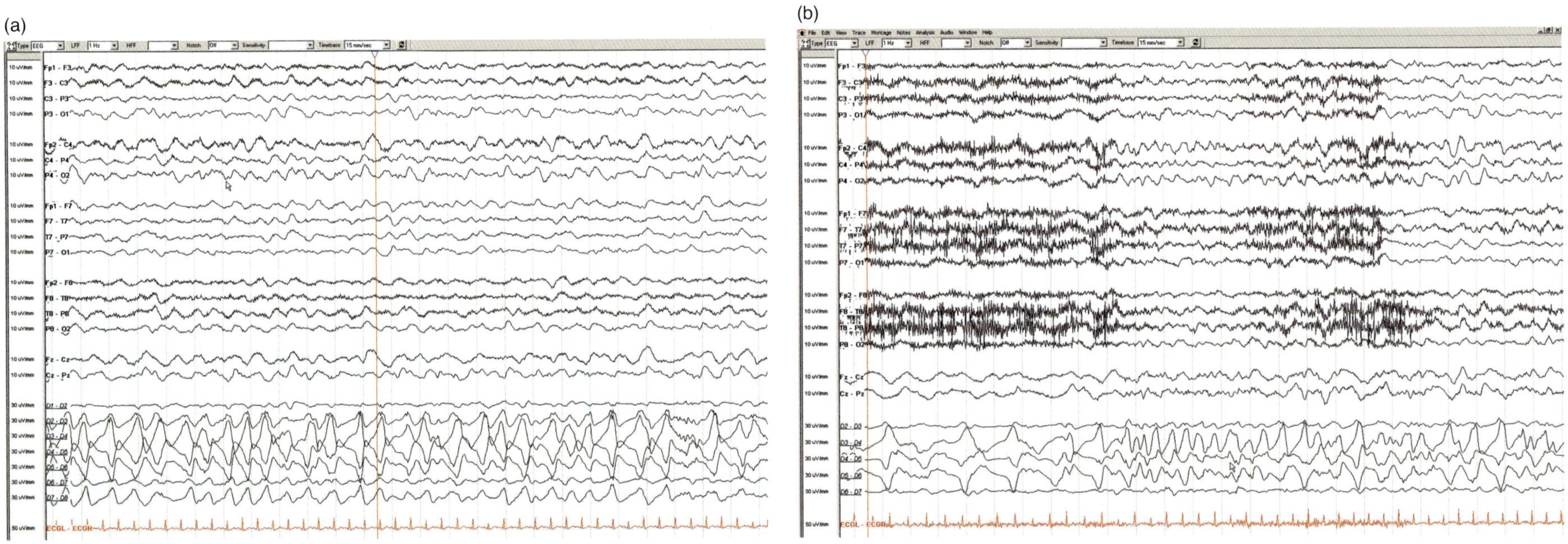

Figure 7.53 Multimodality monitoring after traumatic brain injury (TBI), including depth electrode. **(a)** and **(b)** 20-year-old pedestrian hit by a car, sustaining a small right frontal contusion with subarachnoid hemorrhage, intraventricular hemorrhage and basilar skull fracture. She was arousable to painful stimuli only. No clinical seizures were noted. Invasive monitors were placed in the right frontal lobe, including an eight-contact mini-depth electrode, brain tissue oxygen tension monitor, intracranial pressure (ICP) monitor and cerebral microdialysis catheter. Scalp EEG ((a) and (b), all but the bottom five channels) showed only moderate diffuse slowing, but depth (intracranial) EEG (bottom five channels on (a) and (b), labeled as 'D#') showed new appearance of rhythmic, high amplitude, sharply contoured delta, sometimes evolving (b). This pattern waxed and waned but

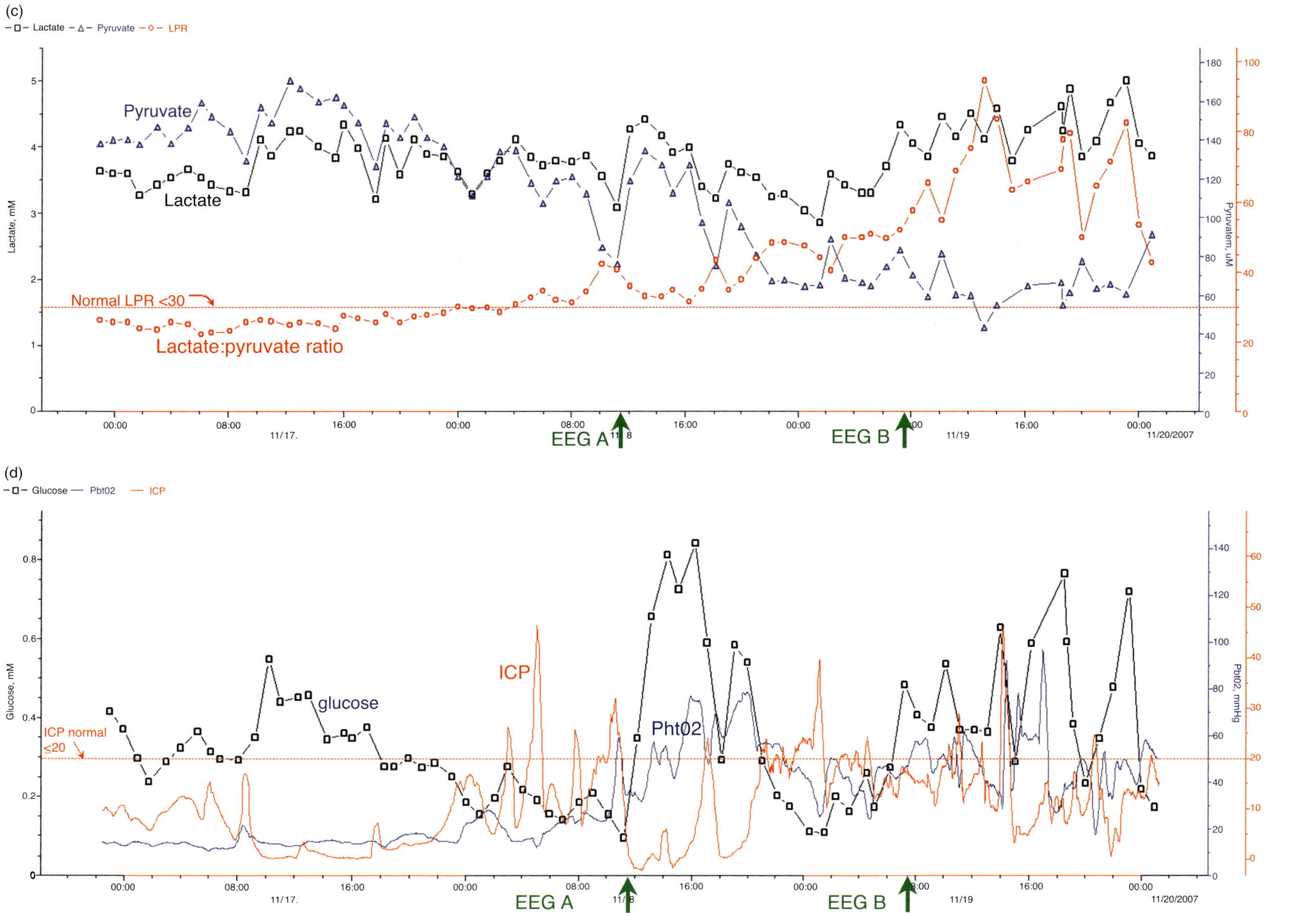

Figure 7.53 (*Continued*) became more prominent and persistent over 1–2 days. **(c)** and **(d)** Multimodal graphs (3–4 days shown) reveal that the lactate/pyruvate ratio was gradually rising on the days of the above findings. This was due to declining pyruvate, not rising lactate, suggesting excessive substrate utilization such as that seen with seizure activity, rather than ischemia. ICP was also intermittently elevated during this time period. Thus, due to this evidence of neuronal stress with potentially permanent secondary neuronal injury, this pattern was treated more aggressively.

(a)

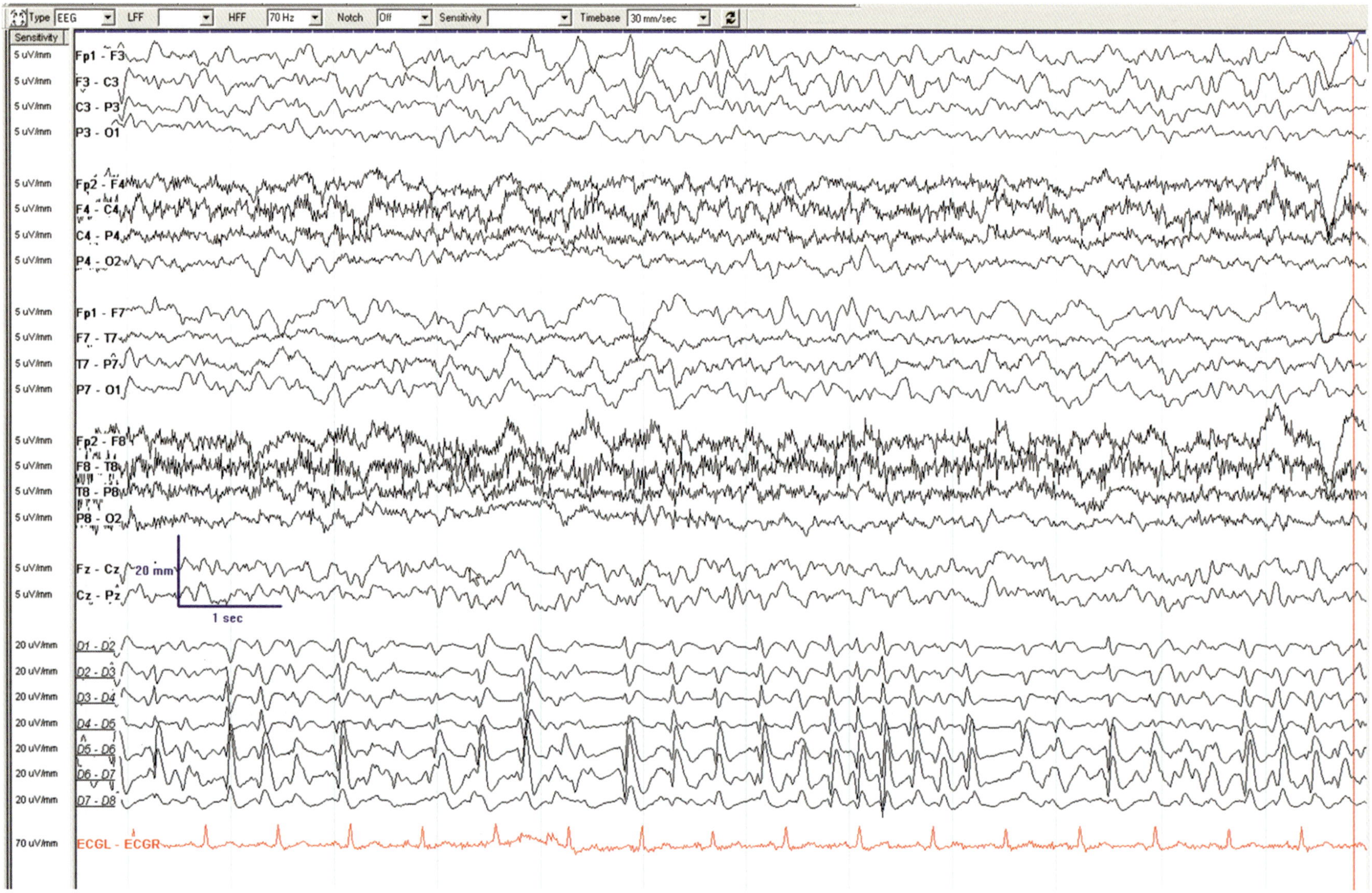

Figure 7.54 Ictal-appearing SIRPIDs on intracranial EEG only. **(a)** EEG sample from another older woman with a subarachnoid hemorrhage and a left frontal eight-contact mini-depth electrode. When stimulated (suctioning, examination, loud noise, pain, etc.), she had ictal-appearing runs in the depth EEG only, as shown here. The bottom seven EEG channels are from the depth. There was left hemisphere slowing, but no hint of seizures on the scalp recording. Thus, these were ictal-appearing SIRPIDs (stimulus-induced rhythmic, periodic or ictal discharges) that were visible on the intracranial EEG but not the scalp.

8 Evoked and event-related potentials in the ICU

David A. Houlden,* Amanda Taylor,* Michael Schwartz,* Corrine Davies-Schinkel† and G. Bryan Young†

**Sunnybrook Health Sciences Centre and the University of Toronto Toronto, Ontario, Canada*
†University Hospital and the University of Western Ontario London, Ontario, Canada

Figure list

Figure 8.1 Effect of number of stimuli on evoked potential tracing.

Figure 8.2 Normal median nerve somatosensory evoked potential (SSEP).

Figure 8.3 Worsening on serial SSEPs after traumatic brain injury.

Figure 8.4 Improvement on serial SSEPs after traumatic brain injury.

Figure 8.5 Algorithm for decision-making after cardiac arrest.

Figure 8.6 SSEPs in acute hepatic encephalopathy.

Figure 8.7 Normal brainstem auditory evoked potentials (BAEPs).

Figure 8.8 Flash visual evoked potentials.

Figure 8.9 Event-related potentials: mismatch negativity.

Evoked potentials (EPs) are signals generated in the central nervous system (CNS) in response to a stimulus. Evoked potentials have low amplitude and hence are buried in other ongoing nervous system activity and a variety of electrical artifacts. In order to visualize the EP, repetitive stimulation and computer averaging are used. Electrographically recording the CNS activity at frequent intervals after the stimulus captures the wanted EP as well as the unwanted surrounding activity. Fortunately, the EP is time-locked to the stimulus but the surrounding activity and electrical artifact is not, hence repeating the test over and over again allows the EP to summate in the computer while the random surrounding activity 'averages out' or approaches a zero value. This is illustrated in Figure 8.1, which shows the gradual buildup of the N20 response from the primary sensory cortex in response to contralateral median nerve stimulation. Evoked potential waveform names are derived from the polarity (N = negative, P = positive) and from the typical latency in milliseconds. Thus, the N20 is a negative peak normally occurring approximately 20 ms after stimulation.

Evoked potentials can be classified according to the sensory modality being tested: usually visual, auditory or somatosensory. Evoked potentials can also be considered by their latencies (early, middle and late), which reflect the degree of CNS processing of the signal. The early EPs are usually those from the primary sensory cortex of the specific sensory modality.

Atlas of EEG in Critical Care Lawrence J. Hirsch and Richard P. Brenner

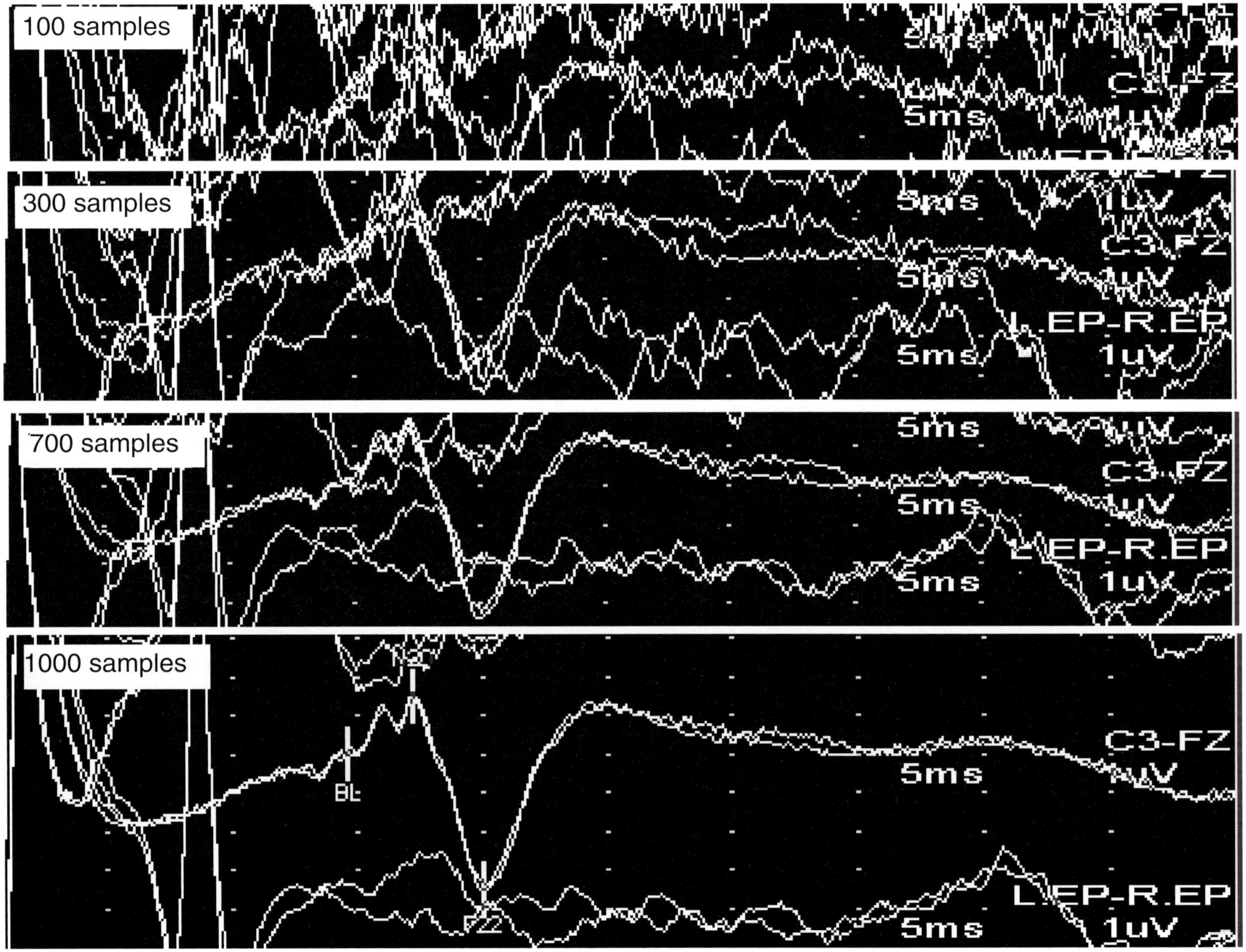

Figure 8.1 Effect of number of stimuli on evoked potential tracing. Repetitive median nerve stimulation with recording and averaging from over the contralateral primary sensory area (C3-Fz). Note the better definition of wave forms and reduction of 'noise' as the number of repetitions increases. The N20-P22 (also referred to as P25) response from the primary sensory cortex is labeled in the bottom row.

8.1 Median nerve somatosensory evoked potentials

Methods

Somatosensory evoked potentials (SSEPs) are obtained using commercially available EP machines. Most machines have at least four channels. The median nerve is alternately stimulated at each wrist with a stimulus intensity 1.5 to 2 times that necessary to evoke a visible thenar muscle twitch. Typical stimulus pulse duration is 0.2 ms with the stimulus rate being 3.1 Hz. Typical locations for three recording electrode pairs are (1) ipsilateral Erb's point-frontal pole electrode (Fpz) to record peripheral nerve activity, (2) the C2 spinous process (Cv2)-Fpz to record mainly spinal cord and distal brainstem activity and (3) the scalp overlying the contralateral somatosensory cortex (C3' or C4')-Fpz to record activity generated above the brainstem. A fourth channel (contralateral somatosensory cortex-contralateral Erb's point) may be used to clarify subcortically generated waveforms. A fifth channel (contralateral somatosensory cortex-ipsilateral somatosensory cortex) may be used to isolate the parietal lobe contribution to the SSEP (since Fpz may contribute unwanted frontal activity). SSEP recordings are obtained from surface electrodes and/or subdermal needle electrodes. Skin/electrode impedance should be below 5000 ohms. The SSEP is the averaged result of about 500 stimulus presentations. The amplifier gain is typically 10–20 μV/division and the recording band pass is 3–2000 Hz. The sweep time should be at least 70 ms. Most machines allow for the display scale (amplitude) to be adjusted for optimum presentation of the SSEP waveforms. To avoid interpretation errors, we do not use a display scale that is less than 1.2 μV/division. At least two SSEPs from each limb should be superimposed for waveform reproducibility.

Interpretation

From our normative data, the response is abnormal when the scalp recorded N20-P25 amplitude is less than 0.9 μV or 2.5 times smaller than the contralateral P25 amplitude (recorded from contralateral somatosensory cortex-Fpz). A response is also considered abnormal if the central conduction time through the brain, measured by P/N13-N20 interpeak latency (Figure 8.2), is greater than 7.2 ms.[1] The response from scalp overlying contralateral somatosensory cortex is absent when N20, P25 and all other subsequent waveforms are lost. If a scalp recording electrode is over an area where a skull bone flap has been removed, the SSEP cortical amplitude cannot be properly interpreted (unless it is absent) since the recording electrode from the scalp is closer to the near-field generated brain response, thereby erroneously increasing its amplitude.

SSEPs in traumatic brain injury

In patients with traumatic brain injury (TBI), SSEPs have been used to determine whether neurological deficits are from an injury to the brain, spinal cord or peripheral nerve.[2] For example, from our recent experience, 7% of comatose patients with TBI had acute nerve injury or peripheral neuropathy, and another 5% had spinal cord injury. Considerations that may confound the interpretation of SSEP are previous stroke, anoxic-ischemic brain injury after cardiac arrest or aspiration, limb amputations and previous dementia or schizophrenia. When traumatic injury to the nervous system is confined to the brain, SSEP testing within the first week after injury is the best single predictor of outcome when compared to clinical examination, CT scan, age, intracranial pressure (ICP) and EEG recordings.[3–5]

Early investigators determined that the median nerve SSEP conduction time through the brain (central conduction time) obtained within 3.5 days after the injury correctly predicted the outcome in 30 of 41 patients with a head injury.[6] Others have shown that a distortion of the early cortically generated SSEP waveform (N20-P25) mainly reflected cortical brain damage, whereas a prolonged central conduction time in combination with a distorted N20-P25 correlated with subcortical lesions.[7] Many studies have shown that absent cortically generated SSEP waveforms in the early stages after a head injury always predicted death or a persistent vegetative state, while normal cortical SSEPs predicted a good outcome in adult patients.[1,8,9] Despite the

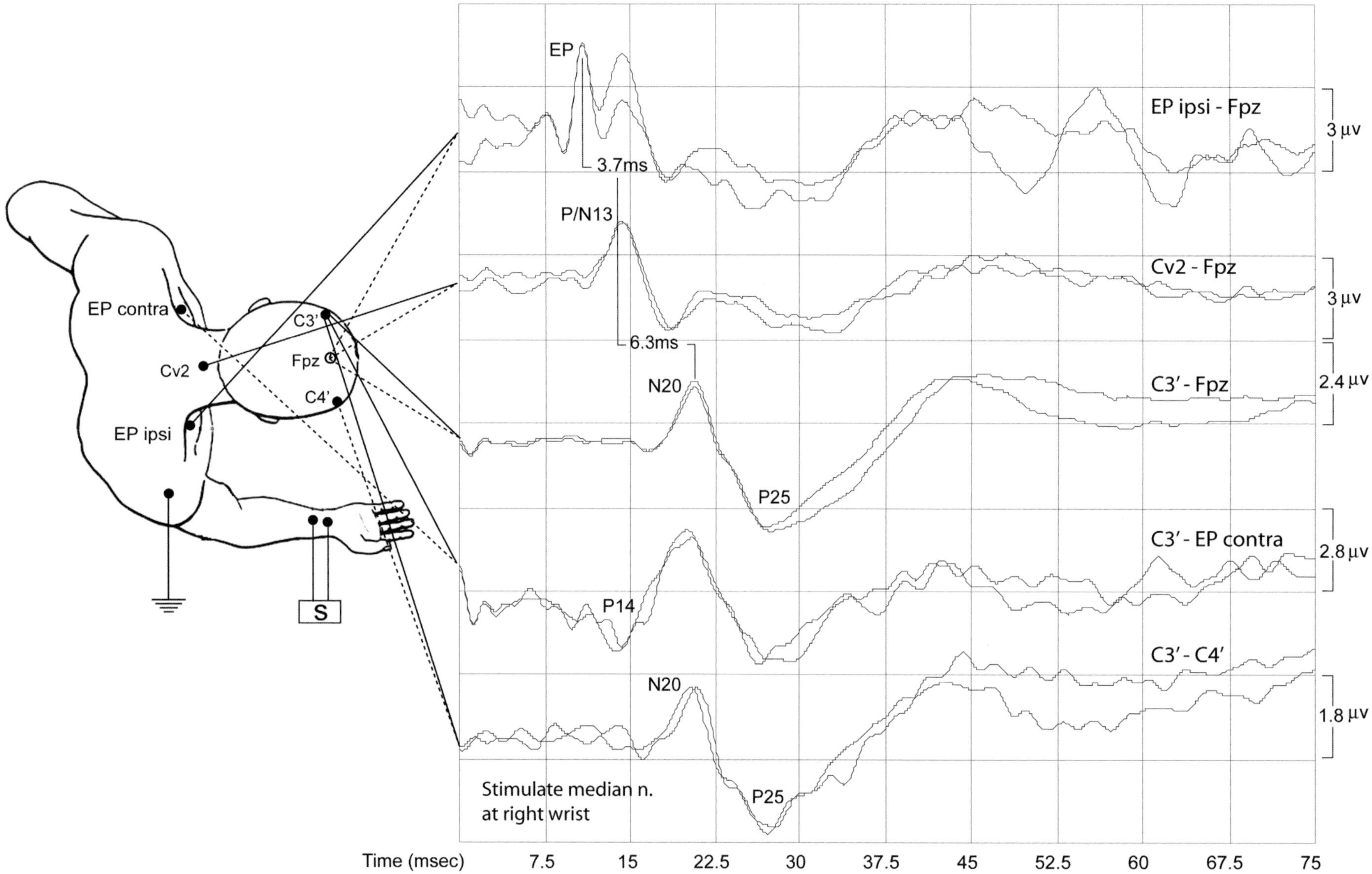

Figure 8.2 Normal nerve SSEP. The right median nerve is stimulated at the wrist and recording electrodes are placed over Erb's point (EP; activity from the ipsilateral brachial plexus), the high cervical region (Cv2; P/N13 activity from high spinal cord/base of medulla) and the scalp overlying the contralateral somatosensory cortex for the hand (C3′; N20/P25 activity from primary somatosensory cortex). The P/N13–N20 interpeak latency and N20–P25 amplitude are used to determine if the SSEP is abnormal.

overall power of SSEP grading for predicting outcome in all comatose patients with TBI,[1,9] intermediate SSEP grades (i.e. SSEPs that are present but bilaterally abnormal) have a weaker association with outcome than low or high grades. For patients with intermediate SSEP grades, SSEP grade changes in the early stage following injury may have a stronger association with outcome than the SSEP grade itself (Figures 8.3 and 8.4).

SSEPs in anoxic-ischemic encephalopathy

In 2006, the American Academy of Neurology (AAN) published a practice parameter for establishing the prognosis for patients who were comatose after resuscitation for cardiac arrest.[10] An algorithm for decision making taken from that paper is presented in Figure 8.5. If patients do not meet the criteria for brain death and if they do not have myoclonic status epilepticus (associated with a uniformly unfavorable outcome, at least prior to the era of therapeutic hypothermia), SSEPs are prognostically useful.

The somatosensory-evoked response is one of the most useful predictors of poor outcome.[10–12] Bilateral absence of the N20 component of the SSEP with median nerve stimulation at the wrist had greater predictive value for poor outcome than EEG, with studies showing false-positive rates (FPRs) of 0%. The AAN has recommended that the test be applied for prognostic purposes after 3 days.[10] It should be noted that this was based on a meta-analysis of the literature antedating the use of hypothermia for comatose survivors of cardiac arrest. The influence of hypothermia and modest doses of sedative drugs are not likely to alter the validity of these findings. Indeed, the N20 response is minimally altered by (or even during) the modest hypothermia utilized in such patients. We have found that if the N20 response is lost, it is not regained. It may take up to three days for the response to be lost after cardiac arrest, so the three-day recommendation by the AAN is reasonable[13].

Most of the patients with post anoxic coma and preserved N20 responses still have poor outcomes. The combination of preserved N20 and absent N70 response is associated with recovery of consciousness in only 15% of patients.[14]

The following are reliable predictors of an outcome no better than severe disability and total dependency after cardiac arrest when hypothermia was not utilized: myoclonic status epilepticus in the comatose state, loss of pupillary light reflex and no better than extensor response by three days (or loss of motor response beyond six days for those treated with hypothermia), bilateral absence of the N20 SSEP to median nerve stimulation at the wrist by day 3 and elevation of serum neuron specific enolase (NSE) to >33 μg/l between 24 and 72 h from the arrest. Further work needs to be done to better define the role of EEG, S-100 protein and predictors of favorable outcomes.

SSEPs in acute hepatic encephalopathy

Acute hepatic failure is commonly associated with cerebral edema. We have found that cerebral edema is accompanied by a decrease in the amplitude and a prolongation of the N20 response latency with median nerve stimulation in patients with acute fulminant hepatic failure (Figure 8.6). More work is needed in this area, but SSEPs hold promise as a means of monitoring such patients for cerebral edema and raised ICP. Direct ICP measurement is difficult due to the associated coagulopathy in such patients.

8.2 Brainstem auditory evoked potentials

Brainstem auditory evoked potentials (BAEPs) are useful to check central auditory pathways in the brainstem, especially when SSEPs cannot be performed because of nerve or spinal cord compromise.

Methods

BAEPs occur within 10 ms after an auditory (usually click) stimulus delivered via earphones or ear inserts. The stimulus duration is 100 μs and the stimulus rate is approximately 10 Hz. Stimulus intensity is usually 60 dB above hearing threshold, or at 90–100 dB if this is not known. The

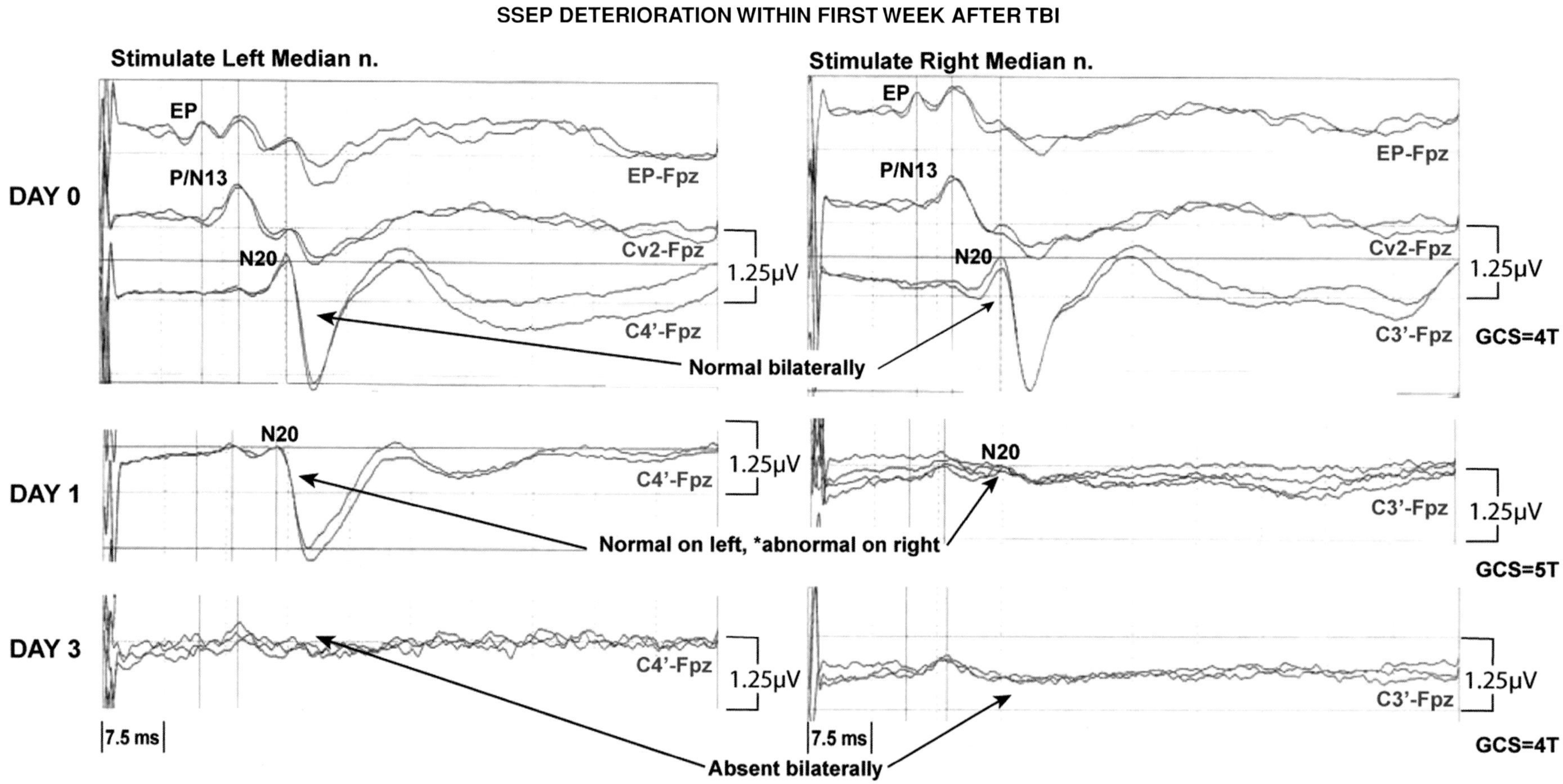

Figure 8.3 SSEP deterioration between days 0 (12–24 hours), 1 and 3 after traumatic brain injury. On day 0 the SSEP was normal bilaterally, but on day 1 the N20-P25 waveform was severely reduced in amplitude after right median nerve stimulation despite a small improvement in GCS. The subcortical waveform (P/N13) was unchanged bilaterally (not shown). By day 3 the N20-P25 waveform was absent bilaterally. This patient had diffuse axonal injury, subarachnoid hemorrhage and brainstem injury. He died before day 7. EP, peripheral nerve action potential recorded from Erbs point; P/N13, subcortical activity recorded from neck-Fpz; N20 and P25, cortically generated activity recorded from the scalp; GCS, Glasgow Coma Score; T, intubated.

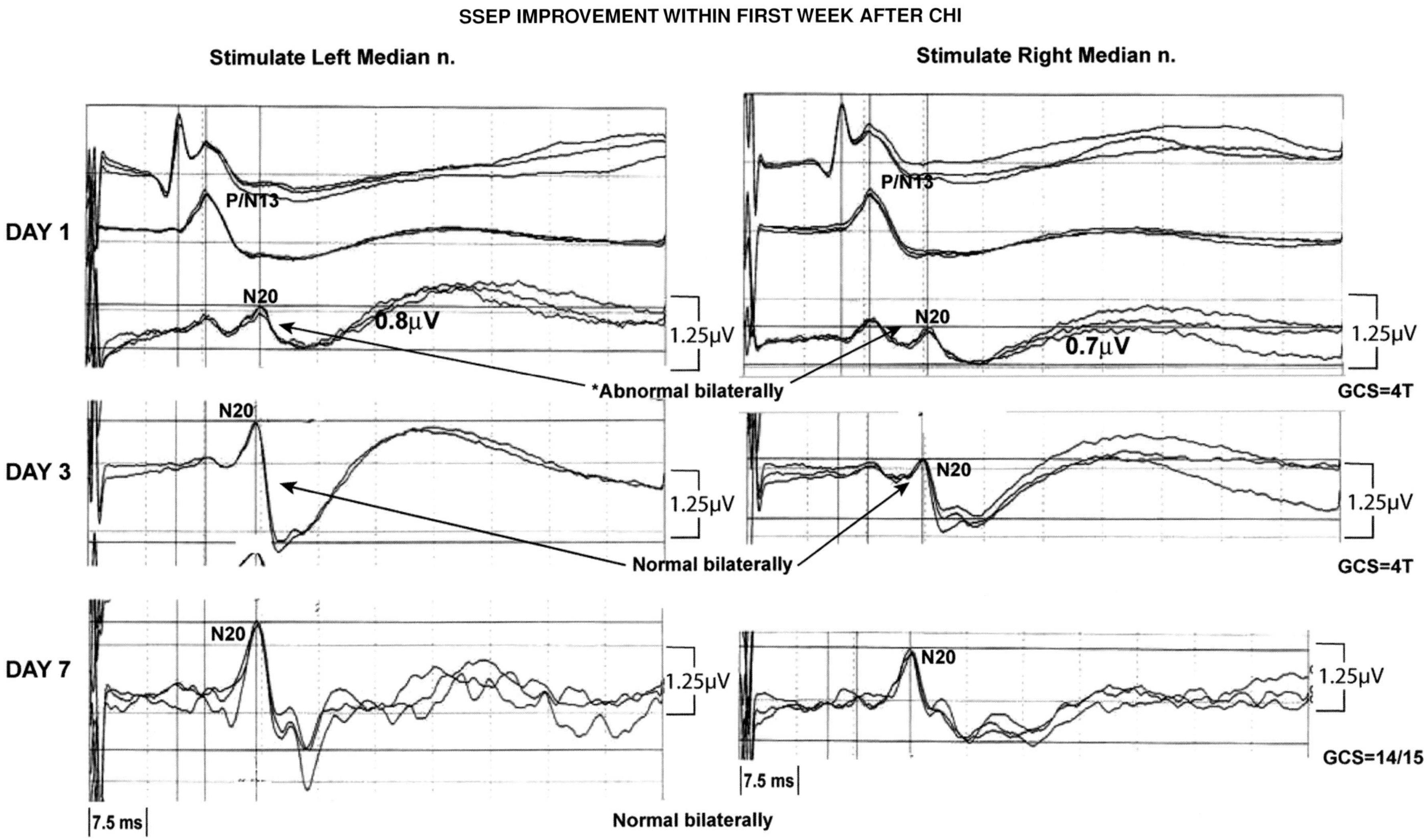

Figure 8.4 SSEP grade improvement between days 1 and 3 after traumatic brain injury. On day 1 the amplitude of the N20-P25 waveform was abnormal bilaterally (<0.9 µV). By day 3 the N20-P25 amplitude increased to within normal range bilaterally despite no change in GCS. This patient had diffuse axonal injury, intraventricular hemorrhage and subarachnoid hemorrhage. He returned to work and part-time studies by one year after injury. EP, peripheral nerve action potential recorded from Erb's point; P/N13, subcortical activity recorded from neck-Fpz; N20 and P25, cortically generated activity recorded from the scalp; GCS, Glasgow Coma Score; T, intubated.

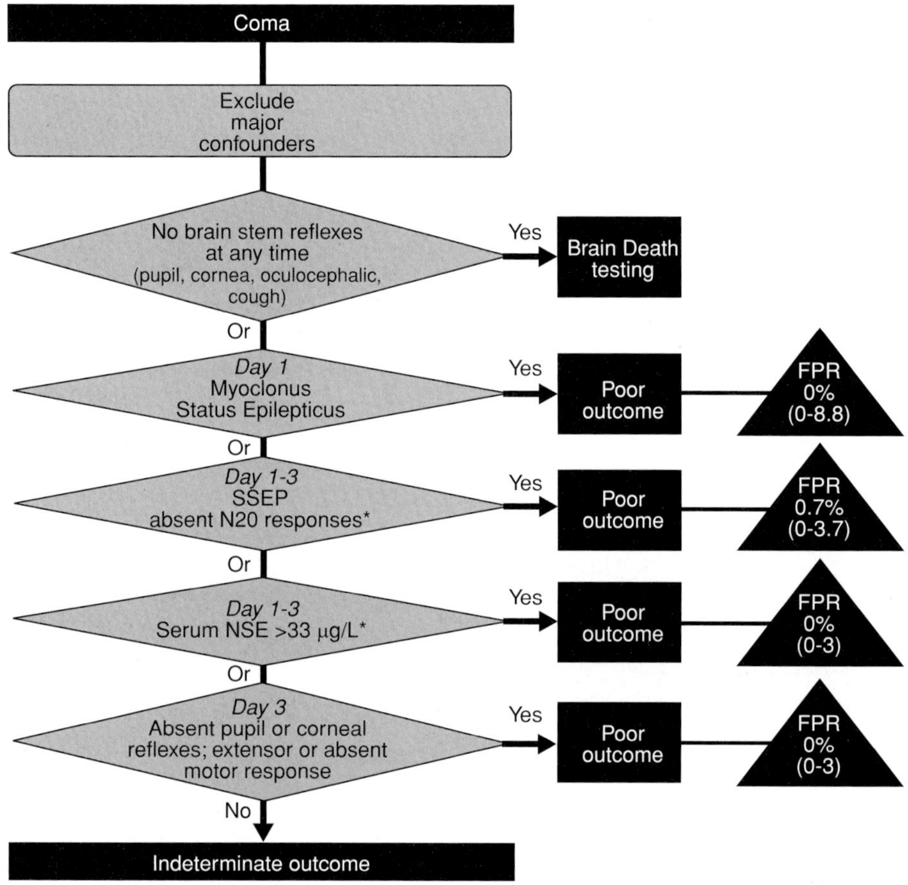

Figure 8.5 Algorithm for decision-making after cardiac arrest.

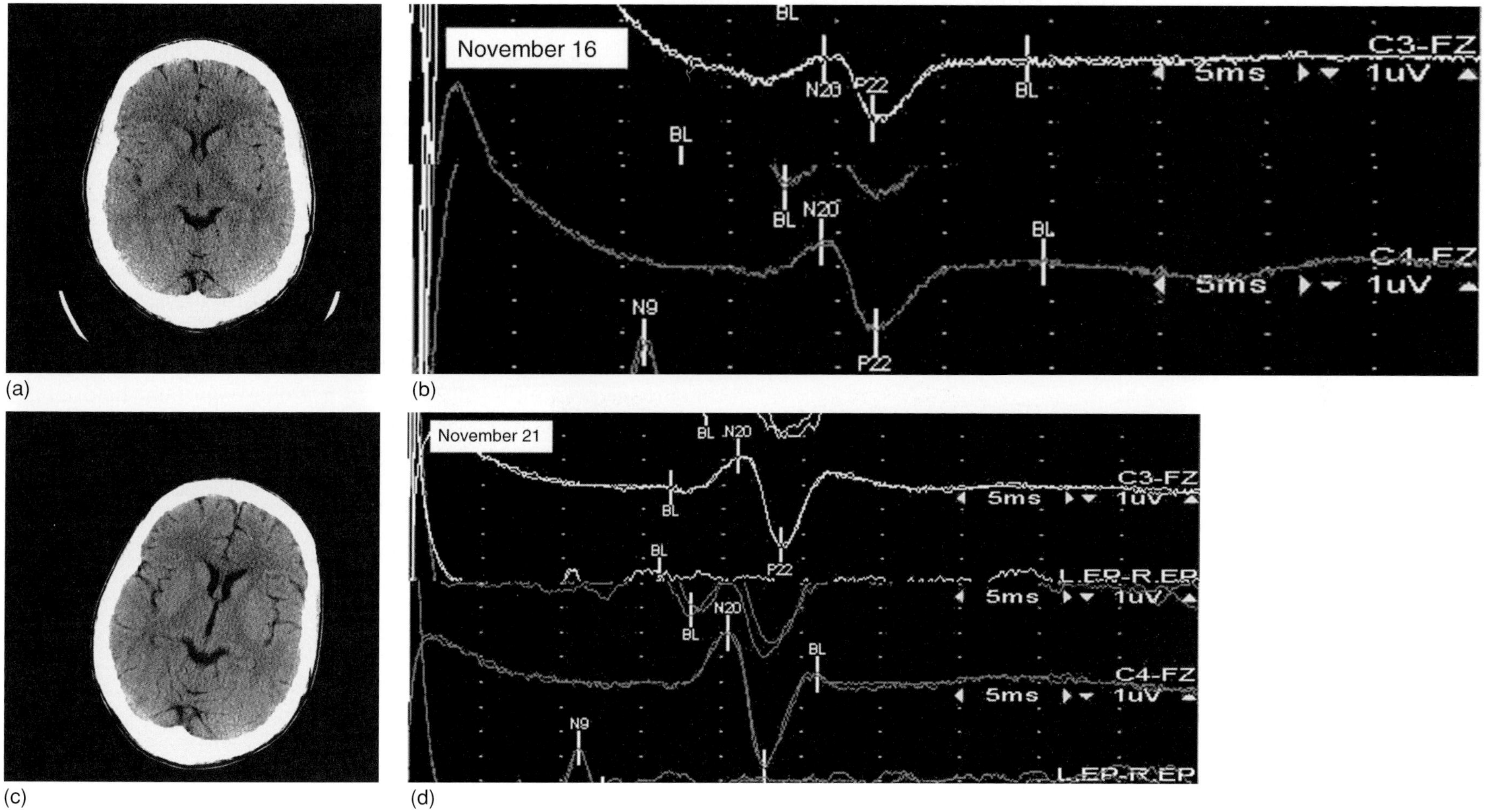

Figure 8.6 The patient developed acute fulminant liver failure secondary to B-cell lymphoma infiltration (there was no involvement of the brain or meninges by the lymphoma). On November 16 the patient was deeply comatose with cerebral edema affecting both cerebral hemispheres (Figure 8.6a; note the narrow ventricles and sulci of the cerebral hemispheres.) His SSEP studies showed N20-P22 (also referred to as P25) amplitudes of 0.03 and 0.54 μV for left and right hemispheres, respectively, on that date (Figure 8.6b). After chemotherapy he improved neurologically and biochemically; this correlated with an improvement in his CT scan (Figure 8.6c; now showing slightly wider ventricles and sulci). N20-P22 improved with amplitudes of 1.34 and 1.68 μV (Figure 8.6d). Latencies did not change significantly. All recordings used the same sensitivities.

ear contralateral to stimulation opposite ear is masked with white noise usually 30–40 dB less than the click intensity. Brainstem auditory evoked potentials are usually recorded from two channels: (1) vertex electrode (Cz)-ipsilateral mastoid process and (2) Cz–contralateral mastoid. The sweep time is 10–15 ms. The amplifier gain is typically 10 μV/division and the recording band pass is 100–3000 Hz. The display scale should be adjusted for optimum presentation of the BAEP waveforms (usually not less than 0.1 μV/division). Two BAEPs from each side should be superimposed for waveform reproducibility. The BAEP is the averaged result of 1000–2000 stimulus presentations (Figure 8.7).

Interpretation

Wave I is thought to be generated by the auditory nerve and wave III by the ipsilateral cochlear nucleus. Wave V is generated in either the upper pons or inferior colliculus of the midbrain.[15] Waves VI and VII are generated in the midbrain and above, probably in the thalamus (medial geniculate body) or thalamocortical projection; since waves VI and VII are not always well-defined, they are less useful clinically. Waves II–V are recordable from the Cz electrode but wave I is recordable by only the ipsilateral mastoid electrode. Accordingly, a second channel, Cz-contralateral mastoid, records waves II–V (from Cz) but not wave I. Simultaneous recording of both channels may help in waveform recognition by corroborating waves II–V. In comatose patients, wave presence or absence is helpful in predicting outcome. As a caveat, wave I should be present, in order to conclude that the problem lies in the brainstem and is not just a peripheral lesion of the eighth cranial nerve or the cochlea. If wave I has poor resolution then its amplitude may be improved by replacing the ipsilateral mastoid electrode with a needle electrode inserted in the external ear canal. When wave I is present and wave V absent, patients have poor outcomes.[16,17] Interpeak latencies (between waves I and V, I–III or III–V) and the amplitude ratios of waves I to V have been used to assess intrinsic brainstem dysfunction. Victims of stroke, trauma and intracranial hemorrhage with prolonged conduction time (wave I–V interpeak latency) do poorly.[17] Brainstem auditory evoked potentials are not very susceptible to the effects of sedative drugs, which make them reliable in the ICU setting. However, BAEPs rarely offer more than is clinically available because, unlike the cerebral cortex, the brainstem can be well examined clinically in the comatose patient.

8.3 Flash visual evoked potentials

Method and interpretation

The FVEP (Figure 8.8) is useful when there is a question about the integrity of the visual pathway from the retina to occipital lobe. It may also be used to assess cortical function when the SSEP cannot be interpreted because of nerve or spinal cord compromise. It is evoked by a luminance (flash) delivered through the eyelids by commercially available goggles containing light emitting diodes, or by a stroboscopic lamp held approximately half a meter from the eyes. The eyes may be stimulated separately or together. The stimulus is usually delivered at 0.5–1 Hz. Recordings are obtained from electrodes placed on the scalp overlying the occipital lobe (Oz) and referred to the vertex (Cz). Usually up to 50 stimulus presentations are contained in the averaged response. The amplifier gain is 50 μV/ division and the band pass is 1–100 Hz. The sweep time should be 500 ms. The display scale may be decreased to 5 μV/division for optimal presentation of waveforms. At least two FVEPs should be superimposed for waveform reproducibility. The interpretation of the FVEP is purely qualitative; either the FVEP waveforms after 100 ms are present (FVEP present), or they are absent.

8.4 Event-related potentials

Event-related potentials (ERPs) are usually considered separately from EPs as they are more temporally remote from the stimulus and require a discriminative function of the brain. Although EPs reflect ‘hard-wired’ responses from the primary and associate sensory cortex, ERPs reflect more widespread, integrated processing. For example, mismatch negativity (MMN) testing relies on the brain’s ability to discriminate an ‘oddball’ tone pip that is different from those presented more regularly. After the randomly presented ‘oddball’ sound, computer averaging reveals a positive wave over the parietal regions in patients whose brains

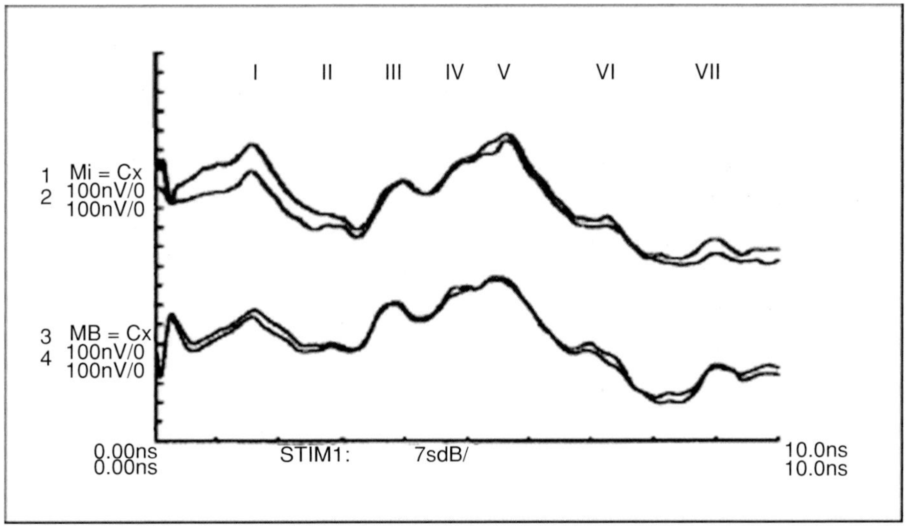

Figure 8.7 Normal BAEPs. Normal BAEP waveforms elicited by monaurally presented click sounds with contralateral sound masking. The sound stimulation was set at 78 dB normal hearing level (NHL), while the sound masking was at 60 dB NHL. The stimulation frequency was set at 10 Hz. Waveforms were recorded at the mastoids (M1, M2) referred to the vertex (Cz). The upper two superimposed lines were the BAEP waveforms evoked by left ear stimulation and ipsilateral recording (M1–Cz) while the bottom two lines by right ear stimulation (M2–Cz). (Adapted from Hu, C.J., Chan, K.Y., Lin, T.J. *et al.* (1997) Traumatic brainstem deafness with normal brainstem auditory evoked potentials. *Neurology* **48**, 1448–1451.75 Reprinted with permission from Williams & Wilkins, Lippincott.)

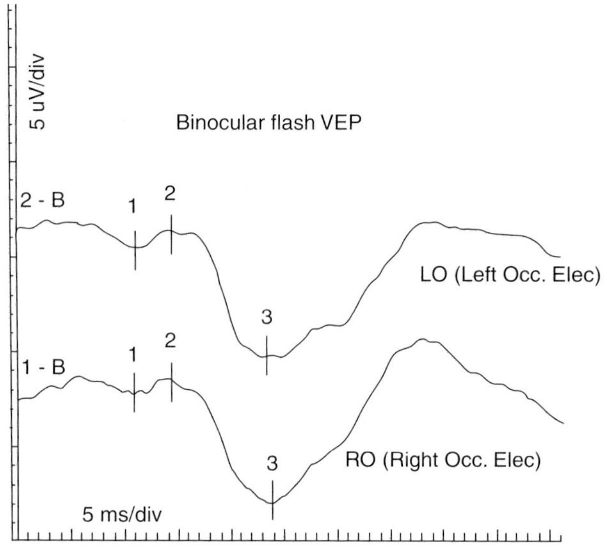

Figure 8.8 Binocular flash visual evoked response, performed to note the symmetry of response (from Brown, M.C., Southern, C.L., Anbarasu, A. *et al.* (2006) Congenital absence of the optic chiasm: demonstration of an uncrossed visual pathway using monocular flash visual evoked responses. *Doc Ophthalmology* **113**, 1–4, with permission.)

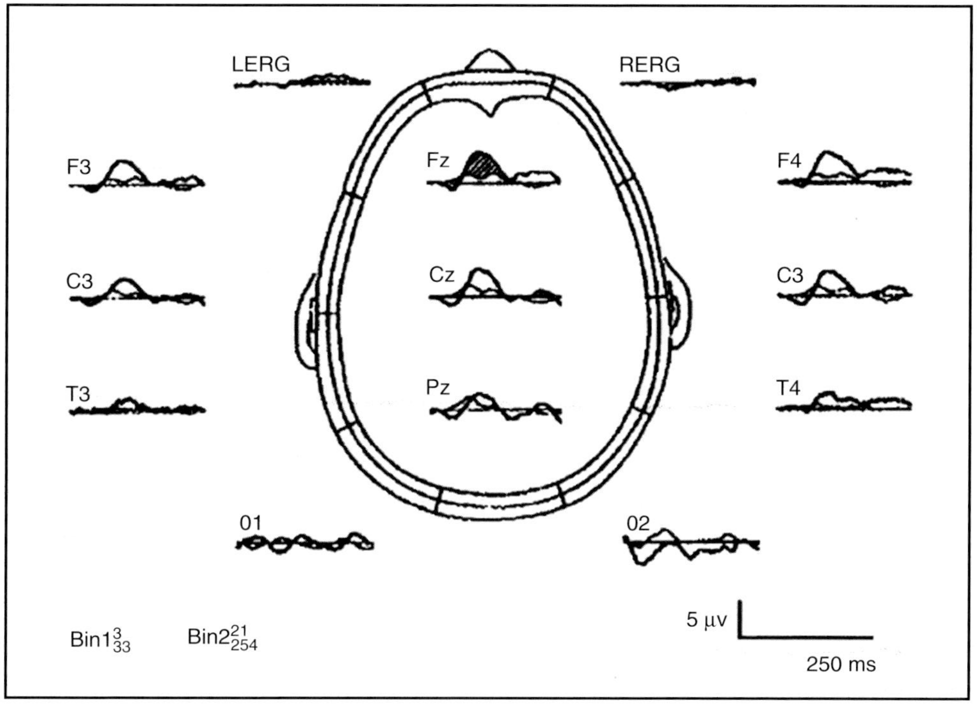

Figure 8.9 Mismatch negativity (MMN). Normal MMN recorded in a passive oddball paradigm. Waveforms were recorded from 11 scalp recording sites, referred to the earlobes. The deviant auditory tone was set at 1600 Hz and presented randomly with a probability of 10% while the standard tone was at 800 Hz. Both stimuli were presented binaurally via earphones using a stimulation intensity of 110 dB sound pressure level (SPL). The deviant tone evoked a negative, upward waveform (bold line) with respect to the waveform elicited by the standard tone (thin line). The MMN was shaded at the Fz electrode. (Adapted from Kane, N.M., Curry, S.H., Rowlands, C.A. *et al.* (1996) Event-related potentials – neurophysiological tools for predicting emergence and early outcome from traumatic coma. *Intensive Care Medicine* **22**, 39–46.143 Reprinted with permission from Springer Verlag ©.)

are able to make the distinction of sounds. Event-related potentials usually depend on wakefulness and vigilance. They include the P300, the N400 and the MMN response.

The following technical description is for auditorially presented items, as these are the only practical ones used in the ICU.[18,19] They require the presence of alertness, except for MMN, in which the response can be present in cases of traumatic coma.[20]

- With MMN (Figure 8.9),[20] the EEG is recorded with filters 0.1–100 Hz with 500 Hz sampling rate, averaging at FZ, F7, F8, CZ, PZ, P3 and P4 referenced to the nose. Recordings start from 50 ms pre-stimulus (baseline prior to the auditory stimulus, i.e. the tone) to 500 ms post-stimulus and amplitude is measured in 50 ms periods from 100–500 ms post-stimulus. Stimuli are presented in 12 blocks of 500 stimuli each. The standard (90%) tone frequency that is presented in 90% of the acquisitions is commonly 500 Hz and 75 ms in duration. The deviant (10%) frequency, which generates the MMN, is of different frequency and is of different (e.g. 25 ms) duration. The probability of a second deviant after the first deviant is 1%; deviant frequencies are presented randomly. The tones are presented with a 600 ms inter-stimulus interval (ISI). Event-related potentials are then averaged to obtain responses to the standard frequency tone (preceded by at least three standards) and then responses to the deviant frequency. The presence of an ERP is a harbinger of consciousness (but not necessarily good outcome) and few comatose patients have an ERP in the acute stage. Furthermore, its absence does not necessarily imply lack of consciousness recovery.[21] This, combined with the fact that ERPs are more sensitive to sedation than short latency BAEPs and SSEPs, limits their clinical utility in the acute stage after traumatic brain injury.

Suggested reading

1. Houlden, D.A., Li, C., Schwartz, M.L. *et al.* (1990) Median nerve somatosensory evoked potentials and the Glasgow Coma Scale as predictors of outcome in comatose patients with head injuries. *Neurosurgery* **27**, 701–707.
2. Houlden, D.A., Schwartz, M.L. and Klettke, K.A. (1992) Neurophysiologic diagnosis in uncooperative trauma patients: confounding factors. *Journal of Neurotrauma* **33**, 244–251.
3. Narayan, R.K., Greenberg, R.P., Miller, J.D. *et al.* (1981): Improved confidence of outcome prediction in severe head injury. *Journal of Neurosurgery* **54**, 751–762.
4. Moulton, R.J., Brown, J.I.M. and Konasiewicz, S.J. (1998) Monitoring severe head injury: a comparison of EEG and somatosensory evoked potentials. *Canadian Journal of Neurological Sciences* **25**, S7–S11.
5. Carter, B.G. and Butt, W. (2005) Are somatosensory evoked potentials the best predictor of outcome after severe brain injury? A systematic review. *Intensive Care Medicine*, **31**, 765–775.
6. Hume, A.L. and Cant B.R. (1981) Central somatosensory conduction after head injury. *Annals of Neurology* **10**, 411–419.
7. Walser, H., Emre, M. and Janzer, R. (1986) Somatosensory evoked potentials in comatose patients: Correlation with outcome and neuropathological findings. *Journal of Neurology*, **233**, 34–40.
8. Chiappa, K.H. and Hill, R.A. (1998) Evaluation and prognostication in coma. *Electroencephalography and Clinical Neurophysiology*, **106**, 149–155.
9. Wang, J.T., Young, G.B. and Connolly, J.F. (2004) Prognostic value of evoked responses and event-related brain potentials in coma. *Canadian Journal of Neurological Sciences* **31**, 438–450.
10. Wijdicks, E.F.M., Hijdra, A., Young, G.B. *et al.* (2006). Practice Parameter: Prediction of outcome of comatose survivors after cardiopulmonary resuscitation (an evidence-based review). *Neurology* **67**, 203–210.
11. Zandbergen, E.G., de Haan, R.J., Stoutenbeek, C.P. *et al.* (1998) Systematic review of early prediction of poor outcome in anoxic-ischaemic coma. *Lancet* **352**, 1808–1812.
12. Sherman, A.L., Tirschwell, D.L., Micklesen, P.J. *et al.* (2000) Somatosensory potentials, CSF creatine kinase BB activity and awakening after cardiac arrest. *Neurology* **54**, 889–894.
13. Young, G.B., Doig, G. and Raggazoni, A. (2005) Anoxic-ischemic encephalopathy: clinical and electrophysiological associations with outcome. *Neurocritical Care* **2**, 159–164.
14. Zandbergen, E.G., Koelman, J.H., de Haan, R.J. *et al.* PROPAC-Study Group. (2006) SSEPs and prognosis in postanoxic coma: only short or also long latency responses? *Neurology* **67**(4), 583–586.

15. Chiappa, K.H. (1997) *Evoked Potentials in Clinical Medicine*, 3rd edn. Lippincott-Raven, New York.

16. Karnaze, D.S., Weiner, J.M. and Marshall, L.F. (1985) Auditory evoked potentials in coma after closed head injury: a clinical-neurophysiologic coma scale for predicting outcome. *Neurology* **35**, 1122–1126.

17. Lindsay, K.W., Pasaoglu, A., Hirst, D. *et al.* (1990) Somatosensory and auditory brainstem conduction after head injury: a comparison with clinical features in prediction of outcome. *Neurosurgery* **26**, 278–285.

18. Alho, K., Sams, M., Paavilainen, P. *et al.* (1989) Event-related potentials reflecting processing of relevant and irrelevant stimuli during selective listening. *Psychophysiology* **26**, 514–528.

19. Connolly, J.F. and D'Arcy, R.C.N. (2000) Innovations in neuropsychological assessment using event-related brain potentials. *International Journal of Psychophysiology* **37**, 31–47.

20. Fischer, C., Morlet, D., Bouchet, P. *et al.* (1999) Mismatch negativity and later auditory evoked potentials in comatose patients. *Clinical Neurophysiology* **110**, 1601–1610.

21. Daltrozzo, J., Wioland, N., Mutschler, V. *et al.* (2007) Predicting coma and other low responsive patients outcome using event-related potentials: a meta-analysis. *Clinical Neurophysiology* **118**, 606–614.

A ACNS Standardized EEG Research Terminology and Categorization for the investigation of rhythmic and periodic patterns encountered in critically ill patients: July 2009 version

Report of the American Clinical Neurophysiology Society Critical Care Monitoring Committee

Chair: Lawrence J. Hirsch, MD

Initial published proposal 1/2005

Revised 12/2005, 10/2006, 11/2006, 6/07, 9/07, 1/08, 10/08, 11/08, 12/7/08, 03/03/09, 5/27/09, 7/02/09

This nomenclature is still undergoing testing and revision

Background

Continuous EEG monitoring is becoming a commonly used tool in assessing brain function in critically ill patients. However, there is no uniformly accepted nomenclature for EEG patterns frequently encountered in these patients such as periodic discharges, fluctuating rhythmic patterns and combinations thereof. Similarly, there is no consensus on which patterns are associated with ongoing neuronal injury, which need to be treated or how aggressively to treat them. The first step in addressing these issues is to standardize terminology to allow multicenter research projects and to facilitate communication. To this end, we gathered a group of electroencephalographers with particular expertise or interest in this area in order to develop standardized terminology to be used primarily in the research setting. One of the main goals was to eliminate terms with clinical connotations, intended or not, such as 'triphasic waves', a term that implies a metabolic encephalopathy with no relationship to seizures to many clinicians. We also avoid the use of as 'ictal', 'interictal' and 'epileptiform' for equivocal patterns that are the primary focus of this report.

Atlas of EEG in Critical Care Lawrence J. Hirsch and Richard P. Brenner

A standardized method of quantifying interictal discharges is also included for the same reasons, with no attempt to alter the existing definition of epileptiform discharges (sharp-waves and spikes (Noachtar *et al.*, 1999). Similarly, we are not necessarily suggesting abandonment of prior terms such as periodic lateralized epileptiform discharges (PLEDs) and triphasic waves for clinical use. Finally, we include suggested categorizations of background EEG activity.

This proposal is the result of several revisions due to solicited feedback of the initial version (Hirsch *et al.*, 2005) and interim versions, with feedback obtained from within and outside this committee and society, and including public presentation and discussion in several venues, including at the 2006 ACNS annual meeting in Chicago, November 2006.

Objective

To standardize terminology of periodic and rhythmic EEG patterns in the critically ill in order to aid in future research involving such patterns.

Secondary objective: To avoid terms with associated clinical connotations.

Not included in this nomenclature

Unequivocal electrographic seizures including the following: generalized spike-wave discharges at 3/s or faster; and clearly evolving discharges of any type that reach a frequency >4/s, whether focal or generalized. These would still be referred to as electrographic seizures. However, their persistence, duration, frequency and relation to stimulation should be stated as described below when being used for research purposes.

Corollary

The following patterns are included in this nomenclature and would not be termed electrographic seizures for this research purpose (regardless of whether or not these patterns are determined to represent seizures clinically in a given patient): generalized spike and wave patterns slower than 3/s and evolving discharges that remain slower than or equal to 4/s. This does not imply that these patterns are not ictal, simply that they may or may not be.

Note: This terminology can be applied at all ages, but was not intended for use in neonates.

Proposed nomenclature

A. Rhythmic or periodic patterns

All terms consist of main term #1 followed by #2, with modifiers added as appropriate.

Main terms

(1) **Generalized** (**G**; for this purpose, the term 'generalized' refers to any bilateral, relatively symmetric and bisynchronous pattern, even if it has a restricted field (e.g. bifrontal)) OR **Lateralized** (**L**; includes unilateral focal/regional and bilateral synchronous but asymmetric; specify side) OR **Bilateral Independent** (**BI**) OR **Multifocal** (**Mf**, rarely encountered).
  - (a) Additional localizing information (specify in all cases for databasing):
    - (i) For **L, BI** or **Mf**: Specify lobe(s) involved (F, P, T, O) and bilateral asymmetric vs. unilateral. If bilateral asymmetric, specify involved lobes in both hemispheres.
    - (ii) For **G:** Specify frontally predominant (defined as having an amplitude in anterior derivations that is at least 50% greater than that in posterior derivations on an ipsilateral ear, average or noncephalic referential recording), occipitally-predominant or 'truly' generalized

(2) **Periodic Discharges (PDs) OR Rhythmic Delta Activity (RDA) OR Spike-Wave (SW**; includes sharp-wave**)**

Rhythmic: Repetition of a waveform with relatively uniform morphology and duration and no interval between consecutive waveforms. The duration of one cycle (i.e. the period) of the rhythmic pattern should vary by <50% from the duration of the subsequent cycle for the majority (>50%) of cycle pairs to qualify as rhythmic.

Periodic: Repetition of a waveform with relatively uniform morphology and duration with a definable and quantifiable inter-discharge interval between consecutive waveforms and recurrence of the waveform at nearly regular intervals. This applies only to *single discharges* (defined as a discharge with no more than three phases (i.e. crosses the baseline no more than twice) or any discharge lasting 0.5 s or less, regardless of number of phases) and not to *bursts* (defined as discharges lasting more than 0.5 s and possessing at least four phases (i.e. crosses the baseline at least three times)). 'Nearly regular intervals' is defined as having a cycle length (i.e. period) varying by <50% from one cycle to the next in the majority (>50%) of cycle pairs.

Spike-wave: Spike or sharp wave consistently followed by a slow wave in a regularly repeating and alternating pattern (spike-wave-spike-wave-spike-wave), with a consistent relationship between the spike (or sharp wave) component and the slow wave.

Notes:

(1) A pattern can qualify as rhythmic or periodic as long as it continues for at least 3 cycles (e.g. 1/sec for 3 seconds, or 3/sec for 1 second).

(2) If a pattern is alternating between two or more main terms (e.g. between rhythmic and periodic or between generalized and lateralized), all patterns lasting >10 continuous seconds should be coded. If multiple patterns are observed to last >10 consecutive seconds, all of these should be recorded as present in the database even if only one of these multiple patterns is predominant. If a single pattern appears from a background with no other rhythmic/periodic pattern and lasts <10 s but for at least 3 cycles, it should still be coded as present (with duration 'very brief' as described below).

(3) If a pattern qualifies as both GPDs and RDA simultaneously, it should be coded as GPDs+ rather than RDA+ (see modifier 8 below for description of '+').

Most of the following sections can be applied to research on any EEG phenomenon. Although many of the categorizations are arbitrary, our hope is that standardization will allow systematic, scientific and collaborative investigation of these EEG features.

Modifiers:

(1) **Persistence:** *Specify* percentage of record or epoch (see section B below). When categorizing, use the following. Suggested equivalent clinical terms are given as well. If 2 or more patterns are equally or almost equally prominant (e.g. ~30% GRDA, 30% GPDs, and 40% BIPDs) record the presence and persistence of each one.
(a) >90% of record/epoch ('continuous')
(b) 50–89% of record/epoch ('abundant')
(c) 10–49% of record/epoch ('frequent')
(d) 1–9% of record/epoch ('occasional')
(e) <1% of record/epoch ('rare')

(2) **Duration**: *Specify* typical duration of pattern if not continuous. When categorizing, use the following. Also record total duration over the entire record/epoch or 24-h period ('burden') and longest continuous duration.
(a) >1 hour ('protracted')
(b) 5–59 min ('prolonged')
(c) 1–4.9 min ('intermediate duration')
(d) 10–59 s ('brief')
(e) <10 s ('very brief')

(3) **Frequency**: Rate per second: *specify* typical rate and range for all patterns, e.g. 1/s and 0.5–2/s;
When categorizing, use the following (record typical, minimum and maximum frequency).
<0.5/s, 0.5/s, 1/s, 1.5/s, 2/s, 2.5/s, 3/s, 3.5/s and ≥4/s

(4) **Sharpness**: Specify for both the predominant phase (phase with greatest amplitude) and the sharpest phase if different. For both

phases, describe the *typical* discharge. Applies only to PDs and SW, not RDA. If SW, specify for the spike/sharp wave only. Categorize as one of the following:
(a) spiky (qualifies as a spike, i.e. duration of that component [measured at the EEG baseline] is <70 ms)
(b) sharp (qualifies as a sharp wave, i.e. duration of that component is 70–200 ms)
(c) sharply contoured (but does not qualify as sharp or spiky)
(d) blunt.

(5) **Amplitude:**
(a) Absolute: Typical amplitude measured in standard longitudinal bipolar 10–20 recording in the channel in which the pattern is most readily appreciated. For PDs, this refers to the highest amplitude component. For SW, this refers to the spike/sharp wave. Amplitude should be measured from peak to trough (not peak to baseline). Specify for RDA as well.
Categorize amplitude as:
(i) <20 uV ('very low')
(ii) 20–49 uV ('low')
(iii) 50–199 uV ('medium')
(iv) ≥200 uV ('high')
(b) Relative: For PDs *Only* (PDs require two amplitudes, absolute and relative). Typical ratio of amplitude of the highest amplitude component to the amplitude of the background between discharges measured in the same channel and montage as absolute amplitude. Categorize as ≤2 or >2.

(6) **Stimulus-Induced (SI)**: Repetitively and reproducibly brought about by an alerting stimulus, with or without clinical alerting; may also be seen spontaneously. If never clearly induced by stimulation, report as 'spontaneous'. If unknown, unclear or untested, report as 'unknown'.

(7) **Evolving** or **Fluctuating**: Both terms refer to changes in frequency, location or morphology. If neither term applies, report as 'static'. *Evolving* is defined as follows: unequivocal sequential change in frequency, morphology or location lasting for at least 10 discharges or cycles; evolution in *frequency* is defined as a change in the same direction for two consecutive time periods by at least 0.5/s, e.g. from 2 to 2.5 to 3/s, or from 3 to 2 to 1.5/s); evolution in *morphology* is defined as at least two consecutive changes to a novel morphology; and evolution in *location* is defined as sequentially spreading into or sequentially out of at least two standard 10–20 electrode locations. The criteria for evolution must be reached without the pattern remaining unchanged in frequency, morphology and location for 5 or more minutes. *Fluctuating* is defined as follows: at least three changes, not more than one minute apart, in frequency (by at least 0.5/s), at least three changes in morphology or location (by at least one standard inter-electrode distance), but *not qualifying as evolving*. This includes patterns fluctuating from 1 to 1.5 to 1 to 1.5 Hz; spreading in and out of a single electrode repeatedly; or alternating between two morphologies repeatedly. Change in amplitude or sharpness alone would not qualify as evolving or fluctuating.
(a) For databasing, if evolving or fluctuating, a minimum and maximum frequency should be specified under 'frequency' above. For non-generalized patterns, specify degree of spread (none, unilateral or bilateral).

(8) **Plus (+)**: Additional feature which renders the pattern more ictal-appearing than the usual term without the plus. For periodic discharges (PDs), this includes superimposed fast activity with each discharge, or superimposed rhythmic or quasi-rhythmic activity of any frequency. For rhythmic delta activity (RDA), this includes frequent intermixed sharp waves or spikes (where "frequent" is defined as one to five sharp waves or spikes every 10 seconds, i.e. 10 to 49% of the seconds for that epoch) or RDA that is sharply contoured. This does not apply to SW. If absent, database as 'no +'.
(a) Subtyping of '+': all cases with '+' should be subtyped as follows into +F, +R, +FS or +FR:
(i) '+F': superimposed *fast* activity – can be used with PDs or RDA.

(ii) '+R': superimposed *rhythmic* or quasi-rhythmic activity – applies to PDs only.
(iii) '+S': superimposed *sharp* waves or *spikes*, or *sharply contoured* – applies to RDA only.
(iv) It is possible to have '+FR' for PDs, or '+FS' for RDA if both subtypes apply.

NOTE 1: Re: Bilateral "+" vs. unilateral: If a pattern is bilateral and qualifies as plus on one side, but not on the other, the overall main term should include the plus (even though one side does not warrant a plus).
NOTE 2: Re: +F: If a pattern qualifying as RDA or PDs has superimposed continuous fast frequencies, this can and should be coded as +F if the fast activity is not present in the background activity when the RDA or PDs is not present. In other words, if the superimposed fast activity is part of the RDA or PD pattern and not simply part of the background activity.

Minor modifiers

(All except "quasi-" are required for database studies; record presence or absence of each)

(1) *Quasi-*: This term is to be applied only when using computer-assisted analysis. Used to modify rhythmic or periodic, as in *quasi-periodic* or *quasi-rhythmic*. (quasi preferred over pseudo- or semi-). Quasi is defined as having a cycle length (i.e. period) varying by 25–50% from one cycle to the next in the majority (>50%) of cycle pairs. If >50% variation in the majority of cycles, the pattern would not qualify as rhythmic or periodic and would not be included in this nomenclature. If the variation is <25%, the modifier quasi- would not be appropriate. When not using computer analysis, quasiperiodic is coded as periodic, and quasirhythmic as rhythmic.
(a) *Sudden onset* or *gradual onset* (sudden onset preferred over paroxysmal): Sudden onset is defined as progressing from absent to well-developed within 3 s.
(b) *Triphasic morphology*: Three phases, negative-positive-negative, with each phase longer than the previous and the second phase of highest amplitude.
(c) *Anterior-posterior lag* or *reverse lag*: Applies if a consistent measurable delay of ≥100 ms appears to be present from anterior derivations to posterior derivations; specify typical delay in msec from anterior to posterior (negative = posterior to anterior lag) in both longitudinal bipolar and in a referential montage, preferably with an ipsilateral ear reference.

B. Minimal time epochs to be reported/databased separately

(1) First ~30 min (equivalent to a 'routine' EEG).

(2) Each 24-h period.

If significant changes occur in the record during this time period, report additional epochs separately as needed.

C. Quantification and categorization of sporadic (non-rhythmic and non-periodic) epileptiform discharges (includes sharp waves and spikes as previously defined (Noachtar et al., 1999)).

- ≥1/(10 s), i.e. averaging at least one per typical EEG page, but not periodic ('abundant')
- ≥1/min but less than 1/(10 s) ('frequent')
- ≥1/h but less than 1/min ('occasional')
- <1/h ('rare')

D. Background EEG

Symmetry: (1) Symmetric; (2) mild asymmetry (consistent asymmetry in amplitude on referential recording of <50% or consistent asymmetry in frequency of 0.5–1 Hz); (3) marked asymmetry (≥50% amplitude or >1 Hz frequency asymmetry).

- Breach effect (note presence, absence, or unclear)
- When any of the following features are asymmetric, they should be described separately for each hemisphere.

Posterior dominant 'alpha' rhythm: Specify frequency (to the nearest 0.5 Hz) or absence.

Predominant background EEG frequency: Delta, theta and/or ≥alpha. If two or three frequency bands are equally prominent, record each one.

Variability: Yes, no or unknown/unclear/not applicable. The last choice might apply, for example, in a 30-min awake record.

Reactivity: Change in cerebral EEG activity to stimulation: Yes, no or unclear/unknown/not applicable. Appearance of muscle activity does not qualify as reactive.

Voltage: (1) Normal, (2) low (most or all activity <20 uV in longitudinal bipolar with standard 10–20 electrodes [measured from peak to trough]) or (3) suppressed (all activity <10 uV). If discontinuous, this refers to the higher amplitude portion.

Stage II sleep transients (K-complexes and spindles): (1) Normal (K-complexes and spindles both present and normal), (2) present (at least one) but abnormal or (3) absent (both absent).

Continuity: (1) Continuous, (2) brief periods of attenuation (describe duration and persistence as above), but periods of attenuation occupying <10% of the record; if >10%, would qualify as discontinuous or suppression-burst; (3) discontinuous (but with interburst interval voltage ≥10 uV; specify typical duration of bursts and interburst intervals, and sharpest component of a typical burst using the sharpness categories defined above under modifier 4) or (4) suppression-burst (discontinuous with interburst interval voltage remaining <10 uV; specify typical duration of bursts and interburst intervals, and sharpest component of a typical burst). Bursts must average more than 0.5 s; if shorter, they should be considered single discharges (as defined above under main term 2). A 'flat' or continuously suppressed record would be categorized as continuous.

Examples of appropriate terms:

Continuous 1–2/s fluctuating GPDs

Occasional 30–0 s bursts of 1.5/s SI-LRDA

Abundant 1–3-min periods of 0.5–1.5/s LPDs-plus

Occasional 10-s periods of 1/s BIPDs

Other examples of corresponding new terms for older terms (some could have alternative new terms depending on exact pattern):

OLD term	NEW term
triphasic waves, most of record	continuous 2/s GPDs (with triphasic morphology)
PLEDs	LPDs
BIPLEDs	BIPDs
GPEDs/PEDs	GPDs
FIRDA	Occasional frontally predominant brief 2/s GRDA (if 1–10% of record)
PLEDS+	LPDs+
SIRPIDs* w/ focal evolving RDA	SI-Evolving LRDA
Lateralized seizure, delta frequency	Evolving LRDA
Semirhythmic delta	Quasi-RDA

Suggested reading

Hirsch, L.J., Brenner, R.P., Drislane, F.W. *et al.* (2005) The ACNS Subcommittee on Research Terminology for Continuous EEG Monitoring: Proposed standardized terminology for rhythmic and periodic EEG patterns encountered in critically ill patients. *Journal of Clinical Neurophysiology* **22**, 128–135.

Noachtar, S., Binnie, C., Ebersole, J. *et al.* (1999) A glossary of terms most commonly used by clinical electroencephalographers and proposal for the report form for the EEG findings. *EEG Clinical Neurophysiology* (Suppl 52), 21–41.

Abbreviation list

BI = bilateral independent

EDs = epileptiform discharges

G = generalized

L = lateralized

Mf = multifocal

PDs = periodic discharges

RDA = rhythmic delta activity

SI = stimulus-induced.

SW = spike-wave or sharp-wave

+ = Plus = additional feature which renders the pattern more ictal-appearing than the usual term without the plus:

+F = superimposed fast activity
+R = superimposed rhythmic activity
+S = superimposed sharp waves or spikes, or sharply contoured

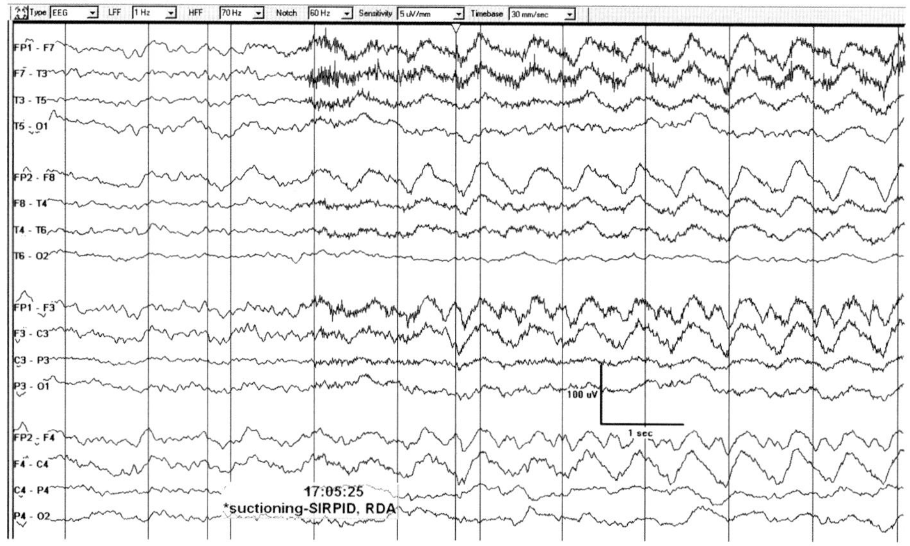

Figure A.1 SI-GRDA. Stimulus-induced generalized rhythmic delta activity (RDA). In this case, the pattern was elicited by suctioning the patient.

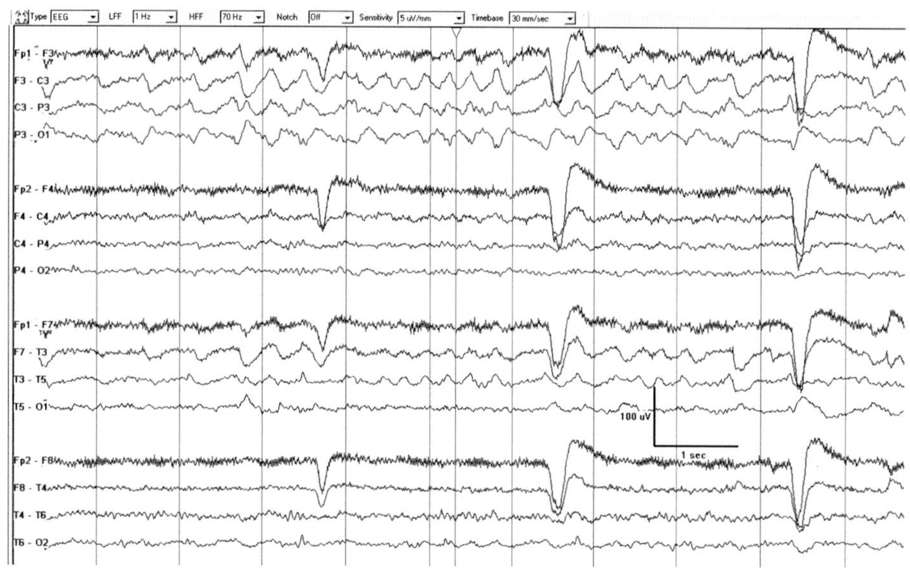

Figure A.2 Evolving LRDA. Lateralized rhythmic delta activity that evolves in morphology and frequency. It begins as low voltage sharply contoured 1.5 Hz delta in the left parasagittal region, evolves to 3 Hz rhythmic delta, then again slows.

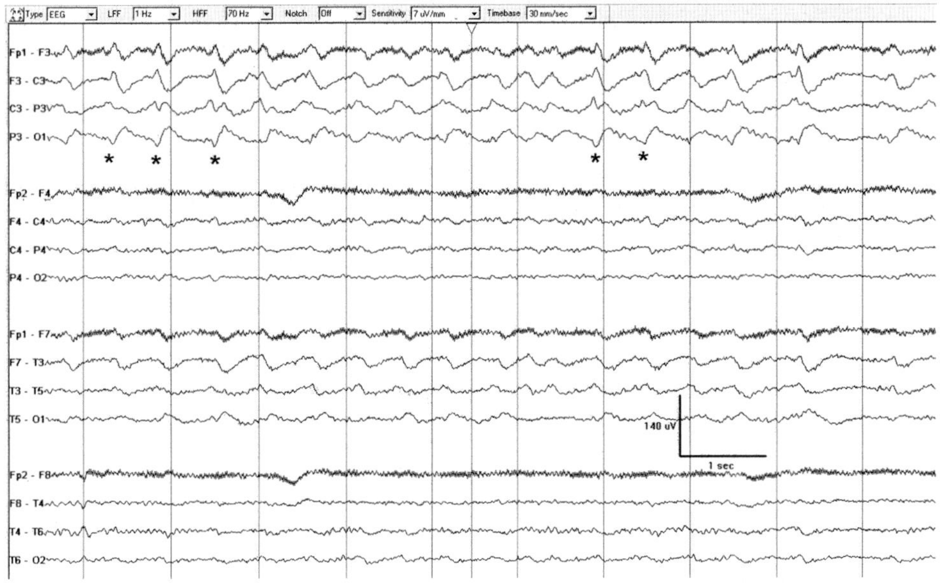

Figure A.3 LRDA + S. LRDA with superimposed repetitive sharp waves (several marked with asterisks).

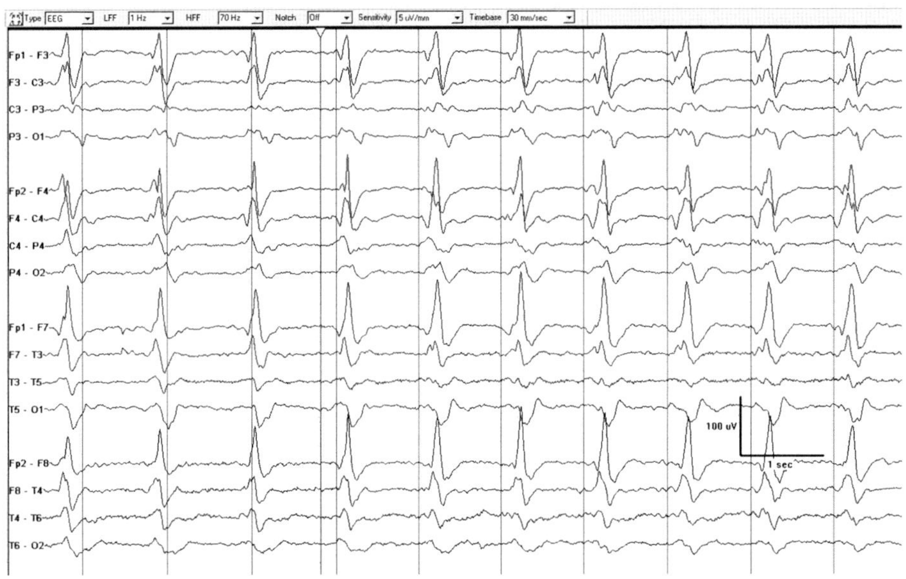

Figure A.4 GPDs. One per second generalized periodic discharges.

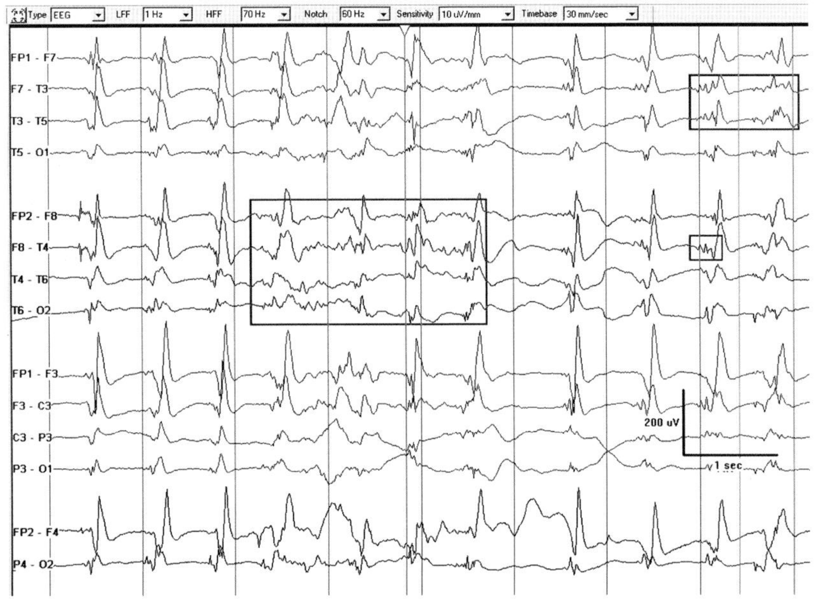

Figure A.5 GPDs + FR. 1–1.25 per second GPDs with superimposed low-amplitude quasi-rhythmic sharp fast activity (highlighted in boxes).

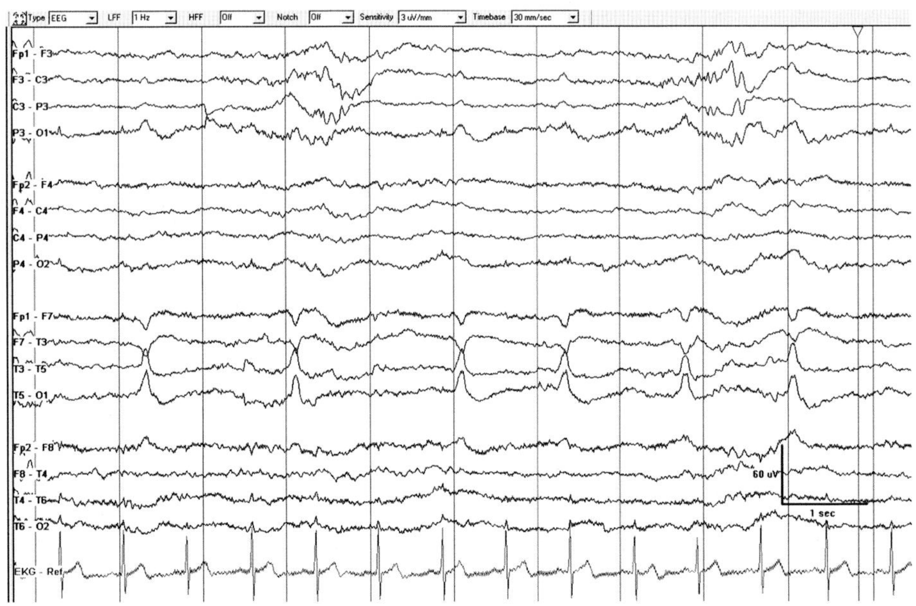

Figure A.6 LPDs. 0.5–0.75 per second lateralized periodic discharges in the left temporal region.

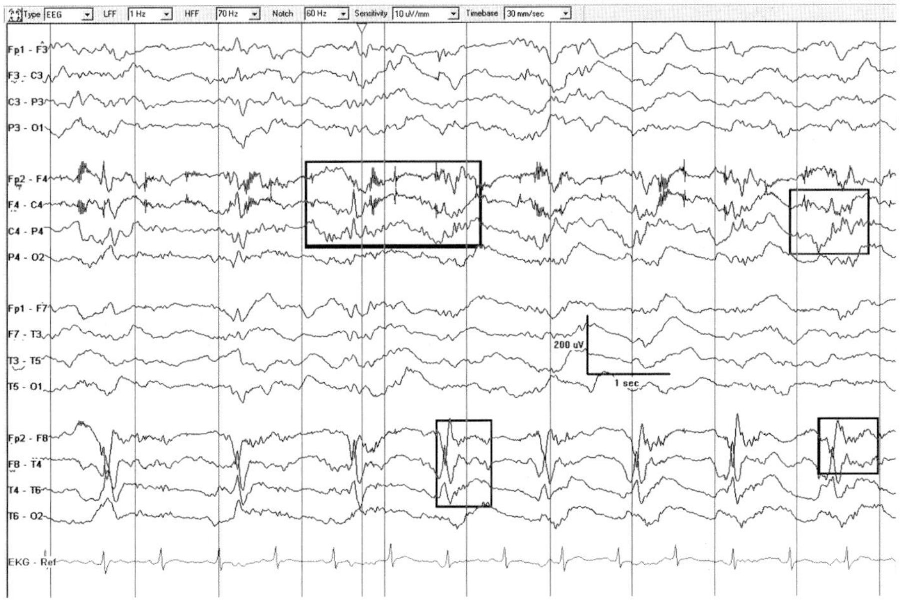

Figure A.7 LPDs + F. 0.5–1 per second LPDs with superimposed bursts of low amplitude fast activity with each periodic discharge (highlighted in boxes).

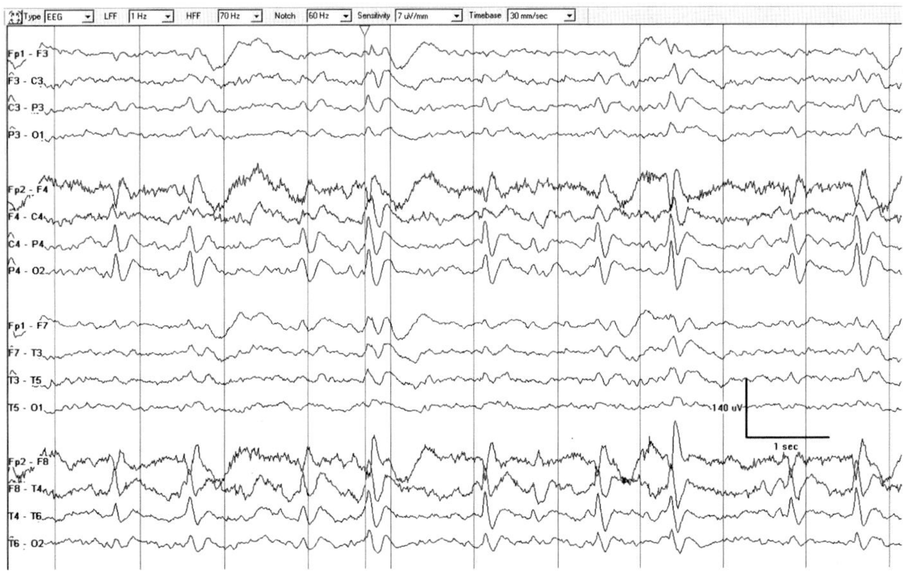

Figure A.8 LPDs + R. Irregular (in morphology and repetition rate) 0.5–1 per second quasi-periodic discharges with superimposed quasi-rhythmic delta activity in the right hemisphere with occasional spread to the left. Less 'stable' pattern and more ictal-appearing than LPDs alone; compare with Figure A.6.

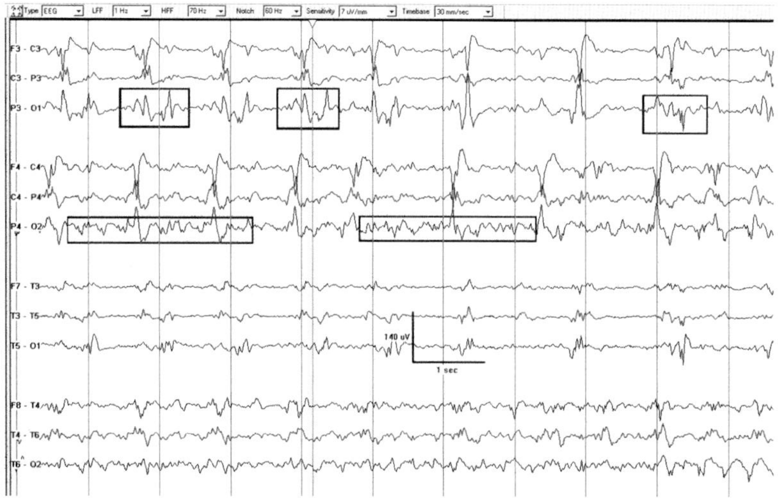

Figure A.9 BIPDs + FR. Bilateral independent periodic discharges at 0.5–1 per second, most prominent centroparietally on both sides. The periodic discharges are associated with low-amplitude sharply contoured quasi-rhythmic fast activity (see boxes), especially posteriorly, and more prominent on the right where the fast activity is nearly continuous (see longer boxes).

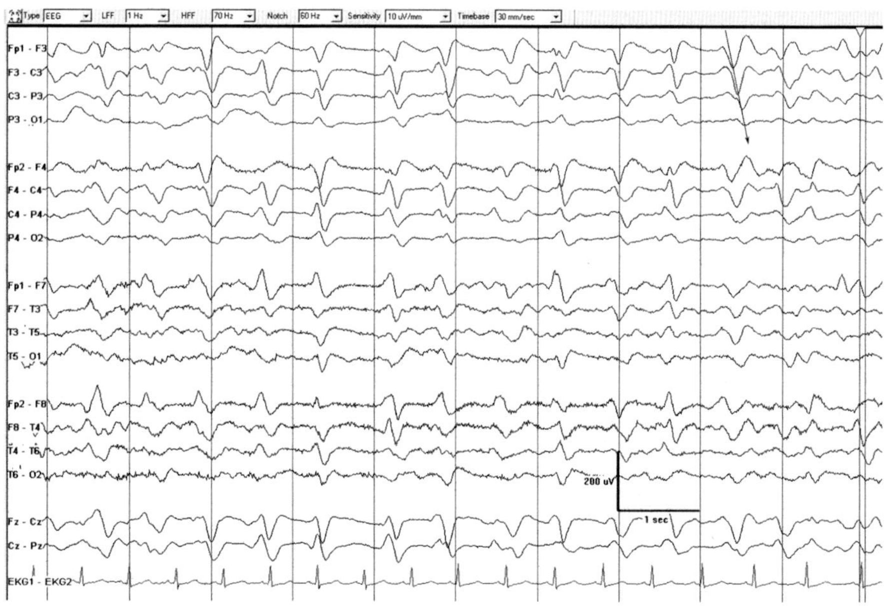

Figure A.10 GPDs with triphasic morphology and A-P lag. Generalized periodic discharges at just under 1.5 per second. In this case there is also a triphasic morphology and an anterior-posterior lag, highlighted with the diagonal line in the upper right of the figure.

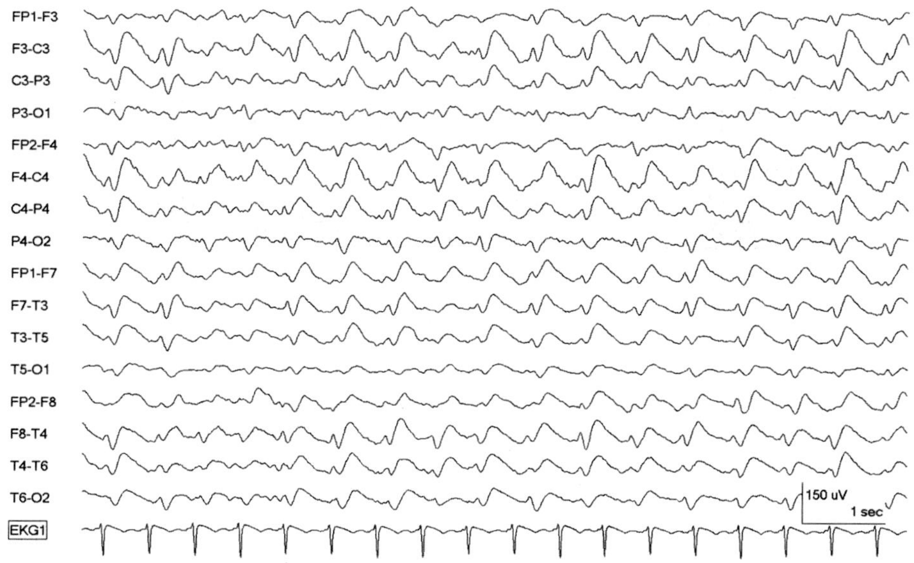

Figure A.11 GSW with triphasic morphology. Blunt generalized sharp and wave at two per second with a triphasic morphology.

Index

Numbers in *italics* refer to Figures

14 and 6 Hz positive spikes, *65–6*

acetaminophen *77*
acidosis *264–5*
active reference 3, *14–16, 28–32*
alarms *257, 266–9*
alerting and arousal 39, *43, 45–6*, 130, *146*, 318
  see also stimulus-induced rhythmic, periodic or ictal discharges
alpha rhythm 4–5, *8–10, 13, 281*, 320
alpha-delta ratio (ADR) *229–31, 262–3*
Alzheimer disease 129
ammonia *43*
amplitude *268–9, 273*
  trending *258–61*
amplitude-integrated EEG (aEEG) *229, 232–5, 238, 249, 267–9, 272, 275, 281, 287*
  artifacts *280, 287*
  long-term trends *272–5*
aneurysms *59, 185–6, 262–3, 288*
angiography *262–3*
anoxia *132, 279, 284*
  see also postanoxic coma
anoxic-ischemic encephalopathy 301, 303
anterior-posterior lag *243*
aphasia *170*
arousal *see* alerting and arousal
artifacts 3, 4, 5, 187–90, *201–3, 205, 209, 216*, 219, *259, 280*
60Hz *282–3*
cardioballistic 187, 189, *214*
chest percussion *277–9*
chewing 187, *200, 280*
dialysis *210*
EKG *67, 68, 111*, 187–9, *208, 211, 214*
electrical 299
electrodes *107*, 189, *202–4, 212, 257*
eye movements *11–12, 18, 33*, 187–8, *199, 210, 213, 215*
externally sourced 189,
glossokinetic *48–9, 280*
humpback whale *284*
mechanical 189, *227, 236, 252–3*
mimicking seizures 187–92, *206–7, 287*
muscle artifacts 3, *8–9, 13, 17–18, 284, 287*
  cyclic PLEDs *254–5*
  mimicking seizures 187–9, *191–8, 206–7*
  QEEG *225, 227, 234–5, 238–40, 246–8*
  seizures *119–21*
  shivering *284, 289–90*
  SIRPIDs *148*
myogenic 5
pacemaker 187, 189
pseudoalpha *282*
pulse *111*, 187, 189, *212*
QEEG *245, 268–9, 284–6*
rejection *228–31*
respiration 187, *208, 216*
ventilator *216, 276*
shivering 188, *197, 284*
  snoring *208*
  sweat 187, 188, *199*
  twitching *191–2*
  ventilator *216, 276*
asymmetry *55, 56, 268–9, 275*
  breach rhythm *201, 209*
  BSI *270–71*
  ischemia *228–31*
  QEEG *228–31, 234–5, 238–9*
  seizures *248–9*
  spectrograms *234–6, 238–9, 248–9, 252, 254–5*
  stroke *164–8, 170–2*
attenuation 5, *10, 55, 67–8*, 161, *228–9*
  diffuse *157, 225, 266–7*
    encephalopathy *43, 52–3, 67–8*
  focal *95, 285*
  hydrocephalus *266–7*
  postictal *114, 250, 251*
  regional *91–5*
  stroke *163, 164–5, 166, 168–1*
  unilateral *55, 163–6*

baclofen 39, 40, *88*, 129
barbiturates 4, 39, 40, *83–4, 86–7, 241, 286*
bed oscillation or vibration *227, 236, 252–53, 281*
Bell's phenomenon *9*
benzodiazepines 4, *14–16*, 39–40, 130, *286*
beta rhythms 4–5, *14–16, 95, 245*
  artifacts 188, *196, 201, 206*
  excessive *14–16*, 40, *84, 297*
  ischemia 161

Atlas of EEG in Critical Care Lawrence J. Hirsch and Richard P. Brenner

beta rhythms (*cont.*)
  SIRPIDs *145, 157*
  stroke *164*
bilateral independent periodic discharges (BIPDs) *142–3, 274*, 320, *326*
bilateral independent PLEDs (BIPLEDs) 129, *142–3, 274*, 320, *326*
bipolar montages 1–4, *11, 17, 96*
blinks *8–9, 11–12, 13, 183, 202–4, 238–9*
blunt spike and wave 129
body movements *see* muscle artifacts
brain death 40, *69*, 188–9, *275*, 301
brain injury 89, 129, 217, *287–8*
  see also traumatic brain injury
Brain Symmetry Index *270–71*
brain tissue oxygen *290–91, 296–7*
brainstem 39–40, *213*
  SSEPs 299, 301, 303, *307, 309, 311*
brainstem auditory evoked potentials (BAEPs) 303, 308, 312–13
breach effect and rhythm 5, *201, 205, 209, 234–5, 246–7*, 319
burr hole 5, *59, 269*
burst-suppression and suppression-burst *289*, 320
  long-term trends *272, 275*
  QEEG *232–3, 236, 241, 254–5, 256, 268–9*

cancer *275*
  tumors *57, 238–9, 246–7*
carbon dioxide (CO_2) retention *264–5*
cardiac arrest *143, 145–6, 193–4, 251, 284*
  postanoxic encephalopathy 40, *67, 70–6*
  SSEPs 300–301, *306*
cardiac surgery *274*
cardioballistic artifact 187, 189, *214*
carotid clamping *270*
carotid endarterectomy *83–4*
cefepime 39, *79–80*, 129, *151–2*
cerebellar hemorrhage 161, *173*
cerebral blood flow *275*
cerebral death 40, *69*, 188–9, *275*, 301
cerebral edema 301, *307*
cerebral function monitor *232–3*
cerebral silence *see* electrocerebral inactivity
cerebrovascular disease 161–2, *163–86*
chest percussion artifacts *277–9*
Cheyne-Stokes breathing *254–5*
chromosomal abnormalities *142*
clonic jerking *119–20*
cognitive potentials *313*
coma 39–40, *43–4, 50, 53, 61–2, 65–6, 81–4, 86–7*, 89
  alpha coma *76*
  BAEPs 302
  BIPLEDs 129, *143*
  ERPs 301
  GPEDs *134, 144, 151–2*
  hemorrhage *173, 183*
  pentobarbital *272*
  QEEG *236, 241, 256*
  SIRPIDs *14, 145–6, 151–2, 157–60*
  Spindle coma *78, 173*
  SSEPs 300–301, *306–7*
  see also postanoxic coma
compressed spectral array (CSA) *222–33, 236*
  artifacts *285–6*
  long-term trends *272–5*
continuous video recordings 130
convulsive status epilepticus 129
CO_2 retention *264–5*
cornea *9, 11–12, 19–20*, 187, *215*
cortical spreading depression (CSD) *288–9*
craniectomy *176–7, 184*, 189, *205*
cranioplasty *115–24*
craniotomy 5, *201, 206*
Creutzfeldt-Jacob disease 39, 129
cyclic PLEDs *254–5*
cyclic seizures *250–4, 295*
  nonconvulsive *250–53*
Cz-reference *24, 32, 36, 185–6*, 189

De Vivo syndrome *258*
death 188–9, *275, 288*
  SSEPs 300, *307*
delayed cerebral ischemia *262–3, 268–9*
delta activity 4–6, 161, *222–3, 259, 288, 294*
  artifacts 188–9, *199*
  bursts *47–9*
  focal slowing *35, 37*
  hemorrhage *176, 262–3*
  intracranial EEG *293, 296–7*
  ischemia 161, *228–31*
  multimodality monitoring *290, 292, 296–7*
  neonates *259*
  nomenclature 319–20, *321, 324*
  seizures *104, 113, 115, 240, 246–9, 258*
  SIRPIDs *147–8, 151*
  stroke *172*
  see also frontal intermittent rhythmic delta (FIRDA); rhythmic delta
dementia 39, 301
density spectral array (DSA) *222*
  artifacts *285–6*
  long-term trends *272–5*
depth electrodes *256–7, 268–9, 290–8*
  multimodality monitoring *262, 290, 292, 296*
dialysis artifact *210*
diffuse axonal injury *304–5*
diffuse slowing *101–5*, 161, *177, 242, 244, 269*
  encephalopathy 40, *50–3, 61–2, 77, 85, 87*
dipoles 1, 3, *9*, 187
discontinuity *54*
drowsiness 4–5, *19–20, 65–6, 199, 232–3*
drug effects *see* medication effects
drug-induced beta *286*

edema, cerebral 303–07
EEG nomenclature 317–18
electrical noise *282*
electrocardiogram (EKG) 3, 187–9, *236*
  artifacts *67, 68, 111*, 187–9, *208, 211, 214*
electrocerebral inactivity 4, 39–40, *67–9, 86–7*
  artifacts 188
electrocorticogram *288*
electrode artifacts *107*, 189, *202–4, 212, 259*
electrode nomenclature 1–4
electroretinogram (ERG) 187–8
encephalitis *252, 256*
encephalopathy 39–42, *43–9, 51–5, 57–62, 64–5, 67–8, 70, 72–7, 79–84, 86–8*, 89, 129–30
  hepatic *52*, 129, *266*, 301, *307*
  neonatal *259*

renal failure 40, *51, 79–80*
septic *275*
endarterectomy *83–4, 228, 270*
envelope-trend analysis *259–61*
epidural hemorrhage 161
epilepsy *169, 242*
epileptiform discharges (EDs) *116–24*, 161, *258*, 315–18
vs. artifacts *196, 209*
on intracranial EEG *293*
multimodality monitoring *291–2*
see also GPEDs; PEDs; PLEDs; BIPLEDs
event-related potentials (ERPs) 308, *311*, 312
evoked potentials (EPs) 299–302, *310*
see also BAEPs; SSEPs; VEPs; cognitive EPs
evolution *179, 270*, 318, *321*
in cyclic seizures *250–53*
in seizures 89, *93, 106–14, 116–24, 235, 245, 248–9*
in SIRPIDs *156–60*
extra-axial fluid 161, *163–5*
extraocular muscle spikes *17–18, 33–4, 114, 215*
eye closure *8–9, 10*, 187
eye movement artifacts *33*, 187–8, *210, 213, 215*
horizontal *11–12, 18, 199*
vertical 187–8, *213, 215*
eye opening 5, *10, 45*, 188
eyelid flutter 187–8, *202–4*

facial twitching *135*
far-field *305*
fast-Fourier transformation (FFT) *222–3*
fasting *258*
filters 188, *195–6*
flash visual evoked potentials (FVEPs) 302, *312*
'flat' tracings 39–40, *69*
focal attenuation *95, 286*
focal motor seizures *110, 115–24*, 130, 189
focal seizures *91–5, 100–14, 178–80*
nonconvulsive *246–7*
PLEDs 129, *137–8*
SIRPIDs *157–60*
focal slowing 5, *35–7, 95, 201, 234–5, 285*
hemorrhage 161, *176–7, 185–6*
stroke *170–1*
focal status epilepticus *91–5*
frontal intermittent rhythmic delta (FIRDA) 39, *47–50, 188*, 318
hemorrhage 161, *175*
frontal slowing 188

generalized periodic discharges (GPDs) *132–4, 147–52, 181*
encephalopathy 39–40,*70–1, 79–80, 88*
nomenclature 317, 319, *322–23, 325*
generalized periodic epileptiform discharges (GPEDs) 129, *132–4, 144, 147–8, 151–2*
encephalopathy 39–40, *70–1, 79–80*
hemorrhage *181*
mimicked by artifacts 187–90, *191–216, 234–5, 278–81, 287*
multimodality monitoring *262, 290, 292, 296*
neonatal *259*
nomenclature 320
QEEG *258*
generalized polyspikes *72*
generalized spike waves *82, 127, 211, 258*, 316, *326*
glossokinetic artifacts *48–9*, 187–8, *280*
glossokinetic potential (GKP) *48–9*, 187–8, *280*
glucose transport deficiency *258*
glut-1 deficiency *258*
GPEDs *see* generalized periodic epileptiform discharges (GPEDs)

harmonics *236*
Hashimoto encephalopathy 40, 129
head trauma *91–5, 127, 209*
headbox *282*
hemicraniectomy *176–7*
hemiparesis *167–8, 170, 228, 263*
hemorrhage 161, *173–4, 178–81*, 217
asymmetry *182–84*
FIRDA 161, *175*
focal slowing 161, *176–7, 185–6*
hemorrhage *177, 182–4*
hemorrhagic transformation *290–91*
hepatic encephalopathy *52*, 129, *266–7*, 303, *307*
hepatic failure *43, 65–6, 77, 100*, 303, *307*
herpes simplex encephalitis (HSE) 39, 129, *135, 137–8*
high frequency filter (HFF) 188, *195–6*
HIV/AIDS *276, 287*
horizontal eye movement 5, *11–12, 17–18, 114*, 188, *199*
REM sleep *33–4*
Slow, roving *19–20*
humpback whale pattern *284*
hydrocephalus 217, *266–7*
hyponatremia 40
hypothermia treatment 40, 188, *284, 290–1*, 303
hypoxic-ischemic encephalopathy *259*

ictal-interictal continuum *150, 152, 273–74*
ifosfamide 39, 129
infant seizures *250, 272–73*
infarcts *58, 157–60, 161, 268–9*
hemorrhagic *183, 185–6, 272*
long-term trends *272*
inferior orbital electrodes *49*, 188
instrumentation artifacts 189
intensive care unit (ICU) 89, 129–30, 217, 303, 308
artifacts 187, *259, 280*
intracranial EEG *290–97*
intermittent rhythmic delta activity (IRDA) *47–9*
see also FIRDA
international 10–20 system 2, 7
intracerebral hematoma *288*
intracerebral hemorrhage 89, 161, *174, 176, 215*
cyclic seizures *254–5*
intracranial EEG *257, 268, 288–98*
multimodality monitoring *262, 290, 292, 296*
intracranial hemorrhage 161, 308
intracranial pressure (ICP)
multimodality monitoring *262, 290, 292, 296*
raised 39, 161, *266, 290*
intraventricular hemorrhage 161, *175*
intubation *264–5*
invasive monitoring *290–92*
ischemia 161, 217, *228–31, 245, 257, 262–3, 268–70*

K-complexes 4–5, *29–32*, 39, *173, 233*, 319

lactate/pyruvate ratio (LPR) *291–3, 297*
lambda waves *17–18*, 189
laminar necrosis *228–31*
lateral eye movements *see* horizontal eye movements
lateral rectus (muscle) spikes *18, 33–4*

lateralized periodic discharges (LPDs) *321–22*; see also periodic lateralized epileptiform discharges
lateralized rhythmic delta activity (LRDA) *294, 321–22*
leukodystrophy *222–3*
Licox monitor *see* multimodality monitoring
lithium 39, 40, 129
liver transplant *50, 63–4*
locked-in syndrome 39
long-term trends *243, 272–75*
lorazepam *94–5, 99, 125–6*
low-pass filter 188, *195–6*
lumbar drain *266–7*
lung and heart transplant *110–14*
lupus *139*

mechanical artifacts 189, *227, 236, 252–3*
median nerve 299–302, *304–5*
medication effects 4, *14–16*, 40, *81–2*
meningioma *260, 278*
meningitis *147–8, 243, 266–7, 287*
  cryptococcal *266–7*
meningoencephalitis *243*
mental retardation *96–7, 142*
meperidine *291–2*
metabolic encephalopathy 39–40, *79–80*, 129–30, *244*, 315
  FIRDA *175*
  GPEDs *133, 151–2*
  SIRPIDs *150, 151–2*
metastatic carcinoma *199*
microdialysis *290–93, 296–7*
micro-shivering *290*
midazolam *265, 286*
midline derivations *193, 197–8, 200, 206*
mini-depth electrodes *293–8*
minimally conscious state 40
mismatch negativity (MMN) 308, 311–12
motor vehicle accidents *53, 61–2, 132, 183*
mu rhythm 4–5, *11–12, 13*
multimodality monitoring 217, *262, 289–97*
muscle spikes 188
myoclonic status epilepticus *72, 74–5*, 303, *306*
myoclonus 39
myogenic artifact 5

N20 response 299, *300, 302–7*, 313
neonates 4, *259*, 316
neoplasm *see* tumors
neuroleptic malignant syndrome 40
neurosurgery 40, *60*, 161, 217
neurotelemetry 217
nomenclature 130, *137*, 314–20, *321–6*
nonconvulsive seizures 39, 89, *91–5*, 130
  CO_2 retention *264–5*
  cyclic *250–3*
  focal *246–7*
  intracranial EEG *294–5*
  QEEG 217, *222, 238, 246, 248–9, 259–61*
nonconvulsive status epilepticus (NCSE) *91–9, 125–7*, 130, *211*
  generalized *96–7, 127*
  long-term trends *273–74*
  multimodality monitoring *296–7*
  QEEG *240, 241, 244, 246, 268*
nonphysiological artifacts 187, 189–90
non-REM sleep 5, *21, 25, 29*
normal QEEG *232–3*
notch filter *282–3*
nystagmus 187–8, *215*

obtundation 129
ocular bobbing *213*
oddball paradigm *311*
optic pathways *310*
overdose *77*
oxygen *289–90, 296*

pacemaker artifact 187, 189
papaverine *263*
paralysis and paralytics *74–5*, 188, *284*
Parkinson disease 189
partial seizures *91–5*
partial status epilepticus *91–5*
pediatric *241, 258, 271, 285*
  cyclic seizures *250, 252–3*
  long-term trends *272–4*
pentobarbital *83–4, 86–7, 236, 241, 256, 272*

peri-injury depolarizations (PIDs) 217, *288–9*
periodic discharges (PDs) 129–31, *132–60, 294*
  long-term trends *273–4*
  nomenclature 315–18
  see also GPEDs, PLEDs, BIPLEDs, triphasic waves
periodic epileptiform discharges (PEDs) *292, 294*, 320
  see also GPEDs, PLEDs, BIPLEDs, triphasic waves
periodic lateralized epileptiform discharges – plus *135*
periodic lateralized epileptiform discharges (PLEDs) *58*, 129, *135–41, 191*
  cyclic *254–5*
  encephalopathy 39, *58*
  hemorrhage 161, *174*
  mimicked by artifacts *191–2*
  nomenclature 314, 318
  seizures *101–5, 106–9*
  stroke *164–5, 167–9*
persistent vegetative state (PVS) 40, *67–8*, 301
phase reversal 2–3, *11, 25, 27, 57–8*
phenytoin *85*
ping-pong seizures *252–53*
PLEDs *see* periodic lateralized epileptiform discharges (PLEDs)
polarity 1–4, *11–12, 19–20*, 188, 299
  POSTS *21–4*
  V-waves *25–8*
polyspikes *72, 82, 191–2*
positive discharges *17–18*
positive occipital sharp transients of sleep (POSTS) 4–5, *21–4, 29–32*
positive spikes, 14 and 6 Hz *65–6*
postanoxic coma *76*, 129, *143, 145–6*
  SSEPs 303, *306*
posterior dominant rhythm 5, *8–9, 10, 281*
postictal state *169*
POSTS *see* positive occipital sharp transients of sleep (POSTS)
propofol 39, 40, *45, 54, 81–2, 133*
pseudoalpha artifact *281*
pseudonormalization *294*
psychogenic process 39
pulse artifacts *111*, 187, 189, *212*
pyruvate *297*

quantitative EEG techniques (QEEG) 217, *222–39, 258, 266–8*
artifacts *245, 269, 284*
CO_2 retention *264–5*
cyclic seizures *250*
hydrocephalus *266–7*
long-term trends *272–5*
seizure detection *240–49*

raised intracranial pressure (ICP) *see* intracranial pressure (ICP), raised
reactivity 39, *43, 44, 45, 46, 144*
referential montages 1–4, *9, 12, 15–16, 18, 20*
artifacts 189, *204*
focal slowing *35*
POSTS *22, 24, 30*
REM sleep *34*
seizures *97, 114*
stroke *168, 171*
V-waves *26, 28*
REM (rapid eye movement) sleep 5, *33–4*
renal failure *167–8, 210*
encephalopathy 40, *51, 79–80*
end-stage *151–2, 277*
seizures *101–5, 125–6*
respiration artifacts 187, *208, 216*
respirator *see* ventilator
respiratory failure *288*
respiratory therapy *see* chest percussion
retina *9*, 187–8, 308
rhythmic delta activity (RDA) *113, 176, 214, 294,* 316–18, *321*
SIRPIDs 130, *145–6, 153–6*
rhythmic or periodic patterns 316–19
rhythmic run detector *235, 238, 248, 257, 274*
rhythmic slowing *212*
rhythmicity *234–5, 238–9, 248–9, 257*
Rolandic region 5, *100*
roving eye movements *20*

schizophrenia 300
secondary injury *288, 296–7*
sedation and sedatives 4, *14–16*, 39–40, *289,* 303, 308, 312
seizures 89–90, *91–2, 94–5, 99, 104, 112, 114, 119–23, 125–6*, 161, 217, *240, 252–3*, 316, 320
basics of detection *240–49*
bilateral independent *240–41*
BIPLEDs 129, *142*
BSI *270*
cyclic *250–55, 295*
focal seizures *91–5, 100, 101–5, 106–9, 110–14, 178–80*
nonconvulsive *246–7*
PLEDs 129, *137–8*
SIRPIDs *157–60*
mimicking stroke *169*
nomenclature 315, 316
PLEDs 129, *135, 138, 192*
QEEG *242, 247*
SIRPIDs *see* stimulus-induced rhythmic, periodic and ictal discharges
sepsis *268–9, 287*
serotonin syndrome 40
sharp waves *57, 125–6*, 129, *137, 202*, 316–19, *322*
generalized *326*
shivering artifacts 188, *197, 284*
short distance bipolar recording 2–3
SIRPIDs *see* stimulus-induced rhythmic, periodic or ictal discharges
skull defects 5, *115–24*
artifacts 187, 189, *201, 205, 209*
hemorrhage 161, *177, 182, 184*
QEEG *234–5, 246*
skull fracture *59, 296–7*
sleep 3, 4–6, 39, *78, 224, 226, 232–3*
artifacts 188
non-REM 5, *21, 25, 29*
POSTS 4–5, *21–4, 29–32*
REM (rapid eye movement) sleep 5, *33–4*
stage II *25, 29–32, 232–3*, 319
sleep spindles 4–6, *25–8, 30*, 161, *226, 232*, 319
encephalopathy 39, *78*
hemorrhage *173, 182*
stroke *163, 164–5, 172*
slow continuous ultra filtration (SCUF) *210*
slow lateral eye movements *19–20*
slow potential change (SPC) *288–9*
slow wave sleep 5, *232–3*
slow waves *172*
slowing 39–40, *225, 286*
artifacts 188, *199, 209*
diffuse slowing *101–5*, 161, *177, 242, 244, 269*
encephalopathy 40, *50–3, 61–2, 77, 85, 87*
encephalopathy 39–40, *50–3, 56–7, 61–2, 77, 85, 87*
focal slowing 5, *35–7, 95, 201, 234*
hemorrhage 161, *176, 177, 185–6*
stroke *170–1*
frontal 188
ischemia 161, *228–9*
regional *91–5*
seizures *110, 113, 246–9*
stroke *170–1, 172*
temporal *35–7, 57, 186*
unilateral *56*
virtual patient *282–83*
snore artifact *208*
somatosensory evoked potentials (SSEPs) 299–308, 312–13
spectrograms *222, 228, 234, 236*
asymmetry *234–5, 238–9, 248–9*
cyclic seizures *250–54*
hydrocephalus *266–7*
ICU artifacts *284–86*
ischemia *228–29, 268–9*
long-term trends *272–5*
mechanical artifacts *227, 236*
pentobarbital coma *272*
seizures *240–45, 256–7, 264–5*
spike waves 189, *191–2*, 316–19
generalized (GSW) *82, 127, 211, 258*, 316, *326*
spindle coma *78, 173*
spindles *see* sleep spindles
spreading depression 217, *288*
stage II sleep *25, 29–32, 232–3*, 317
state changes *224, 226, 232–3*
status epilepticus 39, 89–90, *91–126, 236, 286*
convulsive, 129
cyclic seizures *252–3*
focal *91–5*
GPEDs *133*
refractory *81–2, 241, 256, 272*
status epilepticus terminans *133*

stimulus-induced generalized rhythmic delta activity (SI-GRDA) *321*
stimulus-induced rhythmic, periodic or ictal discharges (SIRPIDs) 130, *144–60*, 320
  focal *165*
  hemorrhage *181*
  intracranial EEG *298*
  multimodality monitoring *292–3*
  stroke *164–5*
stroke *91–5*, 161, *163–70, 172, 213*
  BAEPs 302
  cyclic PLEDs *254–5*
  ischemia 161, *228–31, 268*
  multimodality monitoring *262–63*
  PLEDs *129, 136, 167–9*
  QEEG *246, 268–9*
  SSEPs 300
  unilateral attenuation *163–6*
strokectomy *106, 115–24, 163–5*
subarachnoid hemorrhage (SAH) 89, 161, *181, 185–6, 268–9, 288*
  intracranial EEG *294–5*
  multimodality monitoring *292–3, 296–7*
  QEEG *246, 248*
  SSEPs *304–5*
  vasospasm *262–63*
subcortical waveform *307*
subdural EEG *287–8*
subdural hematoma *106, 110*, 161, *177, 178–80, 182–4, 234–5, 264–5, 289*
  artifacts *205, 209, 280*
subtle status epilepticus *133*
superior orbital electrodes 188
superior rectus spikes *215*
suppression 161, *164–5, 166*
  encephalopathy *54, 55, 67–8*
  intermittent *54*
  unilateral *55*
suppression ratio *254–5, 266–9, 284*
  long-term trends *272, 275*
suppression-burst *see* burst-suppression
swallowing *47–9*
sweat (perspiration) artifact 187–8, *199*

temporal slowing *35–7, 57, 186*
terminal EEG 274
theta rhythm 4–5, 161, *227*, 319
  artifacts mimicking seizures *194*
  CO_2 retention *264–65*
  cyclic seizures *254–5*
  encephalopathy 39, *77, 81–2, 85*
  excess *85*, 161
  seizures *103–4, 240*
  SIRPIDs *145, 19, 151*
  stroke *172*
thresholds *266–9*
tissue plasminogen activator (tPA) 161, *270*
Todd's paresis *169*
tongue movements *48–9*, 187–8
tonic seizures *198*
tonic-clonic seizures *58, 140, 242*
total power *247, 257, 266–9*
toxic encephalopathy 39, 129, *175*
traumatic brain injury *44*, 89, *183*, *296–7, 312*
  SSEPs *301*, 303–5, *307*
tremors 187, 189
trends and trending *243, 272–5*
triphasic waves *125–6, 243*
  encephalopathy 39–40, *63–4, 70–1, 79–80, 88*
  GPEDs 129–30, *133, 147–8*
  nomenclature 315–16, 320, *324–5*
  SIRPIDs *147–8, 149–50, 153–6*
  stroke *167–8*
tumors *57, 238–9, 246–7*
twitching artifact *191–2*

unilateral attenuation *163*
unplugged recording *282–83*
uremia *151–2*

vasospasm *244, 262–3, 268–9, 289*
vecuronium *74–5, 192, 194, 207*
vegetative state *see* persistent vegetative state
ventilator artifacts *216, 276*
verapamil *263*
vertex waves 4–6, *25–8*
vertical eye movements 4, *33–4, 48–9*
  artifacts 187–8, *213, 215*
virtual patients *282–83*
visual evoked potentials (VEPs), flash, 308, *310*
visual evoked responses (VERs) 308, *310*
visual scanning *17*
V-waves 4–6, *25–8*
V-waves and spindles *25, 27*

wakefulness 4–6, 39, *51*, 89, 312